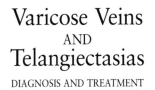

Varicose Veins
AND
Telangiectasias
DIAGNOSIS AND TREATMENT

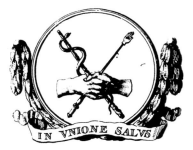

Emblem of Hunczovsky*

This graphic symbol with its caption, "In Union Health," depicts the age-old emblems of medicine: the Aesculapian rod with a serpent and another rod showing a hand with an eye in its palm. Bringing these two emblems together in this way represents a unification of the disciplines of medicine and surgery to form a combined medical practice. In 1787 such a unification was hoped to be successful in improving total patient care and offering an advantage to all who were sick.

The occasion for the development of this symbol was the second anniversary of the opening of the 2000-bed Vienna General Hospital and its merger with the 1200-bed Academia Medico-Chirurgica "Iosephina." These two institutions were combined to provide the best possible care with the best equipment available. The new institution was founded by Emperor Joseph II, who had traveled throughout Europe and learned of the improvements in education of military surgeons in France and the elevation of surgeons to academic rank by King Louis XV.

The great Vienna General Hospital eventually became the site of a massive collection of precious medical books, surgical instruments, and the historical anatomic wax museum. It was also the location of the military medical school known as the Josephinum. In the twentieth century the symbol of the Vienna General Hospital became the signet of the Austrian Society of Surgeons as a reminder of the original attempt to create modern surgery approximately 200 years earlier.

In its original form, this emblem was chosen by the Working Group for Phlebology of the Austrian Society of Dermatology. This choice was appropriate because the rod of Aesculapius represents academic theoretical traditions of medicine and conservative nonsurgical care. The seeing hand, which "sees" what the hand does, is the symbol for both experience in medicine and the manual dexterity associated with surgical skill.

To physicians dedicated to the care of patients with varicose veins and telangiectasias, the symbol is a reminder of the union of surgery and sclerotherapy, an alliance that is necessary for optimum care of the venous insufficiency produced by microphlebectasias and macrophlebectasias. Chosen to be the logo for the Fifth European-American Venous Symposium in Vienna, this symbol is an appropriate frontispiece for this book.

---

*Modified from Holubar H. "In Unione Salus": A short historical perspective on the development of surgical education in Austria in the 18th century. Vasa 20:10-11, 1991.

Varicose Veins
AND
Telangiectasias

DIAGNOSIS AND TREATMENT

SECOND EDITION

EDITED BY

Mitchel P. Goldman, M.D.

Associate Clinical Professor of Medicine
(Dermatology), University of California,
Los Angeles, California

Robert A. Weiss, M.D.

Assistant Professor, Department of Dermatology,
Johns Hopkins University School of Medicine,
Baltimore, Maryland

John J. Bergan, M.D., Hon. F.R.C.S. (Engl.)

Professor of Surgery, Loma Linda University, Loma Linda, California;
Clinical Professor of Surgery, University of California, San Diego, California;
Clinical Professor of Surgery, Uniformed Services University of
Health Sciences, Bethesda, Maryland; Professor Emeritus,
Northwestern University Medical School,
Chicago, Illinois

Quality Medical Publishing, Inc.

ST. LOUIS, MISSOURI
1999

PUBLISHER   Karen Berger
EDITOR   Beth Campbell
PROJECT MANAGER   Carlotta Seely
BOOK DESIGN   Susan Trail
COVER DESIGN   Diane M. Beasley

Quality Medical Publishing, Inc.
11970 Borman Drive, Suite 222
St. Louis, Missouri 63146
Telephone: 1-800-348-7808
Web site: http://www.qmp.com

LIBRARY OF CONGRESS CATALOGING-IN-PUBLICATION DATA

Varicose veins and telangiectasias: diagnosis and treatment / edited
   by Mitchel P. Goldman, Robert A. Weiss, John J. Bergan. — 2nd ed.
         p.   cm.
      Includes bibliographical references and index.
      ISBN 1-57626-097-6
      1. Varicose veins. 2. Telangiectasia. I. Goldman, Mitchel P.
   II. Weiss, Robert A. III. Bergan, John J., 1927-
      [DNLM: 1. Varicose Veins—therapy. 2. Varicose Veins—diagnosis.
   3. Telangiectasis—therapy. 4. Telangiectasis—diagnosis.   WG 620
   V299 1999]
   RC695.V35   1999
   616.1′43—dc21
   DNLM/DLC
   for Library of Congress   98-32317
                                                                  CIP

VT/WW/WW
5   4   3   2   1

Contributors

John J. Bergan, M.D., Hon. F.R.C.S. (Engl.)
Professor of Surgery, Loma Linda University, Loma Linda, California; Clinical Professor of Surgery, University of California, San Diego, California; Clinical Professor of Surgery, Uniformed Services University of Health Sciences, Bethesda, Maryland; Professor Emeritus, Northwestern University Medical School, Chicago, Illinois

Pierre Boivin, M.D.
Co-director of Phlebology Courses, University of Paris VI; Vascular Surgery Service, Salpetrière Hospital; Vascular Medicine Service, Broussais Hospital, Paris, France

Philip D. Coleridge Smith, M.A., F.R.C.S.
Reader in Surgery and Consultant Surgeon, Department of Surgery, University of Middlesex School of Medicine, London, England

André Cornu-Thénard, M.D.
Co-director of Phlebology Training, Cardiology and Surgery Services, St. Antoine Hospital, University Hospital Center, Paris, France

Ralph G. DePalma, M.D.
Associate Dean and Vice-Chairman of Surgery, University of Nevada, Reno, Nevada

David M. Duffy, M.D.
Assistant Clinical Professor of Medicine (Dermatology), University of California, Los Angeles, California; Associate Professor of Medicine (Dermatology), University of Southern California, Torrence, California

Sandra Eifert, M.D.
Research Instructor in Surgery, Department of Surgery, Uniformed Services University of Health Sciences, Bethesda, Maryland

Mitchel P. Goldman, M.D.
Associate Clinical Professor of Medicine (Dermatology), University of California, Los Angeles, California

Abraham Lechter, M.D.
Professor of Surgery and Chief, Department of Surgery, Escuela Militar de Medicina y Hospital Militar Central, Bogota, Colombia, South America

Gregory L. Moneta, M.D.
Associate Professor of Surgery, Department of Surgery, Division of Vascular Surgery, Oregon Health Sciences University, Portland, Oregon

Peter Neglén, M.D., Ph.D.
Vascular Surgeon, River Oaks Hospital, Jackson, Mississippi

H.A. Martino Neumann, M.D.
Professor of Dermatology, Department of Dermatology, University Hospital Maastricht, Maastricht, The Netherlands

John M. Porter, M.D.
Professor of Surgery and Head, Department of Surgery, Oregon Health Sciences University, Portland, Oregon

Pauline Raymond-Martimbeau, M.D.
Director, Dallas Noninvasive Vascular Laboratory, Dallas, Texas

John D.S. Reid, M.D., F.R.C.S.(C), F.A.C.S.
Clinical Assistant Professor, Department of Surgery, Division of Vascular Surgery, University of British Columbia, Vancouver, British Columbia, Canada

Sidney S. Rose, F.R.C.S. (Engl.)
Consultant Vascular Surgeon, Department of Surgery, University Hospital of South Manchester, Manchester, England

Ulrich Schultz-Ehrenburg, M.D.
Professor of Dermatology, Department of Dermatology, St. Josef Hospital, Ruhr-University of Bochum, Bochum, Germany

John H. Scurr, B.Sc., M.B.B.S., F.R.C.S.
Consultant Surgeon and Senior Lecturer, Department of Surgery, Middlesex and University College Hospitals, University of London, London, England

Joseph G. Sladen, M.D., F.R.C.S.(C)
Clinical Professor of Surgery, Department of Vascular Surgery, St. Paul's Hospital, University of British Columbia, Vancouver, British Columbia, Canada

David S. Sumner, M.D.
Professor, Department of Surgery, and Chief, Section of Peripheral Vascular Surgery, Department of Surgery, Southern Illinois University School of Medicine, Springfield, Illinois

Dig J. Tazelaar, M.D.
Department of Dermatology, De Tjongerschans, Algemeen, Ziekenhuis Heerenveen, Heerenveen, The Netherlands

Paul K. Thibault, M.D.
Director, Newcastle Laser Center, Newcastle, New South Wales, Australia

Olav Thulesius, M.D., Ph.D.
Professor, Department of Clinical Physiology, Faculty of Health Sciences, University of Linkoping, Linkoping, Sweden

Paul S. van Bemmelen, M.D., Ph.D.
Assistant Professor of Surgery, Department of Surgery, State University of New York, Stony Brook, New York

J. Leonel Villavicencio, M.D.
Professor of Surgery and Director, Venous and Lymphatic Teaching Clinics, Walter Reed Army and National Naval Medical Centers, Bethesda, Maryland

Margaret A. Weiss, M.D.
Assistant Professor, Department of Dermatology, Johns Hopkins University School of Medicine, Baltimore, Maryland

Robert A. Weiss, M.D.
Assistant Professor, Department of Dermatology, Johns Hopkins University School of Medicine, Baltimore, Maryland

To my loving wife

Dianne

M.P.G.

To my loving family

Marge, Michael, David, and **Jonny**

R.A.W.

To my lovely wife

Elisabeth

J.J.B.

Preface to the Second Edition

In the 6 years that have passed since the first edition of this volume was published, great strides have been made in the diagnosis and management of venous insufficiency. Perhaps the most significant of these changes has been an increased interest in venous disorders in general and venous insufficiency in particular. Commenting on this development, Georges Jantet noted, "Until recently in Great Britain, the practice of phlebology was almost exclusively in the hands of surgeons. Now, however, this discipline is enriched by the input from dermatologists, physicians/angiologists, radiologists, specialists in the field of the new investigative techniques which have developed, as well as from surgeons and gynecologists."* Currently, duplex ultrasonography is generally accepted in the diagnostic testing of patients with varicose veins and telangiectasias. Gradually, sclerotherapy has become directed toward selective treatment of telangiectasias, with varicose vein clusters being dealt with through ambulatory phlebectomy techniques. A better understanding of the causes of cutaneous changes associated with severe chronic venous insufficiency has emerged, and new methods of photoablation of telangiectasias and endovenous restoration of valve competence offer promise. These changes and others are elaborated on in this new edition of *Varicose Veins and Telangiectasias: Diagnosis and Treatment*.

The present volume holds the same purpose as the first edition—to bring together observations, facts, and theories to guide physicians in the care of patients with varicose veins and telangiectasias.

In the fundamental considerations of this book, the physiologic observations by Olav Thulesius remain basic and virtually unchanged, except for a greater appreciation of the origin of hydraulic forces that cause elongation, dilation, and valvular incompetence within varicosities and telangiectasias. Fundamental anatomy changes little, and this subject is described by Mr. Rose of Manchester. However, the interpretation of anatomic patterns does change; for example, an increased appreciation of the origin of varicose clusters in relation to perforator vein outward flow has developed.

*From Jantet G. Foreword. In Tibbs DJ, Sabiston DC, Davies MG, Mortimer PS, Scurr JH, eds. Varicose Veins, Venous Disorders, and Lymphatic Problems in the Lower Limbs. Oxford: Oxford University Press, 1997.

With the latest information integrated, the molecular biology of the pathogenesis of varicose veins and chronic venous insufficiency is summarized by Drs. Coleridge Smith and Scurr in a chapter on fundamental considerations.

The objective evaluation of varicose veins has been updated by Drs. van Bemmelen and Sumner, and the question of appropriate diagnostic testing is discussed by Dr. Schultz-Ehrenburg. This subject leads to the classification of venous disease, which has been drawn up by an ad hoc committee of the American Venous Forum. Although there are flaws in this classification, its overall precepts have been well and universally accepted.

Among the treatment options available, conservative therapy is considered fundamental. Such therapy and the historical development of varicose vein surgery remain largely as they were described in the last edition of this book. However, the prescient observations of Dr. Neglén on comparative studies in interventional treatment of varicose veins have been borne out by the passage of time; that is, ligation of the saphenofemoral junction in combination with any other techniques has proven to be inferior to segmental proximal stripping of the saphenous vein in combination with ablation of varicose clusters. This subject is described in a fascinating dialogue between Drs. DePalma, Rose, and Bergan.

Endovenous interventions are promising and have not been addressed in earlier textbooks. In this volume the newest endovenous technique to emerge is described in a full chapter on the subject by Dr. Weiss.

Sclerotherapy continues to be applied in various ways, and the different approaches are the subject of individual chapters. The contentious problem of greater saphenous vein sclerotherapy is fully described by Dr. Raymond-Martimbeau. The difficulties associated with the use of compression sclerotherapy for large veins and perforating veins is addressed by Drs. Sladen and Reid. Drs. Cornu-Thénard and Boivin present an overview of sclerotherapy, and Dr. Goldman describes the complications and adverse sequelae that may supervene and discusses various methods for minimizing their occurrence.

A revolutionary change has occurred in the treatment of severe chronic venous insufficiency. This change has been engendered by the advent of endoscopic techniques for perforator ablation, which are described in the chapters on complex problems involving varicose veins. Hemangiomatous malformations can be handled through surgical intervention, as described by Drs. Villavicencio and Eifert. Although a role for conservative treatment of severe chronic venous insufficiency certainly exists, this approach has come under criticism recently, and a special chapter has been devoted to this subject. Likewise, the pelvic congestion syndrome currently does not call for surgical intervention but interventional radiology instead, and the latter approach is described in this volume. Treatment of telangiectatic leg veins assumed a new importance when relief of the pain associated with this condition was described by Drs. Weiss and Weiss, who have expanded on this subject in this volume. The new method of treating telangiectasias with lasers and high-intensity pulsed light is addressed in detail in another chapter by Drs. Goldman and Weiss.

Gathering diverse viewpoints on the subject of the diagnosis and treatment of varicose veins and telangiectasias has been a pleasurable employment for us, the editors of this volume. We believe that this information can be used to improve the care of patients with venous disorders. If this goal is achieved, we will consider ourselves amply rewarded.

Mitchel P. Goldman
Robert A. Weiss
John J. Bergan

Preface to the First Edition

The purpose of this volume is to bring together observations, facts, and theories that can guide physicians in the care of patients with varicose veins and telangiectasias. In the past, medical literature on this subject focused on elements of the problem without providing unifying explanations of etiology and pathogenesis to guide specific treatments. Furthermore, an emphasis on the etiology of venous stasis in general and a focus on the causes of venous stasis ulcerations in particular have produced confusion in the treatment of simple varicosities and telangiectasias.

Treatment has been further obscured by the rise and fall of alternative techniques in care. In addition, a decreasing interest in the treatment of venous problems by cardiovascular surgeons has hampered the teaching of diagnosis and care of varicose veins and telangiectasias in academic environments. It is paradoxical that those individuals who should have the greatest interest in treating venous stasis in its various manifestations have a vested interest in preservation of the saphenous vein as a conduit in coronary revascularization and peripheral bypass. For these reasons we thought that it was time to bring this volume through the arduous process of publication.

The thoughtful reader of this book will quickly note the differing methods of diagnosis, disagreements in explanation of phenomena, alternative indications for intervention, and even completely different techniques that appear in the chapters that follow. Students of this field will recognize that rapid developments in knowledge of venous phenomena and their treatment reach disparate medical centers in a nonsimultaneous fashion. Further, in a field of endeavor characterized by few absolutes, there is room for alternative views and explanations.

Not long ago, an editorial in *Lancet* stated: "Varicose veins is probably the commonest as well as the worst treated disorder presenting to general surgeons" (Lancet 2:311, 1975). In response, the respected vascular surgeon Adrian Marston wrote: "To call a condition which is found in 50% of the adult European population a disorder is scarcely logical." Mr. Marston said further that "a sizable minority, perhaps a third of people attending varicose vein clinics, require no treatment at all." He correctly indicated that "most come simply because they do not like the appearance of their legs" (Marston A. Lancet 2:453, 1975). It is precisely those individuals with cosmetic complaints who see advertisements in newspapers and then attend the clinics that advertise sclerotherapy for varicose veins. Neither the patients nor the physicians realize that optimum care is achieved through precise diagnosis and utilization of all, not just one, of the various modalities available for care.

This issue was summarized in a wise editorial in the *British Journal of Surgery* by a well-known general/vascular surgeon and phlebologist, Bo Eklöf. In citing the Latin phrase *ad utrumque paratus,* from the seal of the University of Lund in Sweden, he pointed out that this phrase, which means "to be prepared for both the sword as well as the book," could be "transcribed for the modern treatment of varicose veins: use the knife as well as the syringe." Eklof noted that simple physical examination supplemented by nondirectional Doppler ultrasound could be used routinely. With this approach, evaluation for obstruction, patency, or reflux in both the superficial and the deep venous systems could be accomplished. Further, Eklof stated that the vascular laboratory and phlebography would be necessary in the few cases in which symptoms and clinical findings correlate poorly, when a problem of deep venous insufficiency is involved, or for patients with congenital angiodysplasia.

In this volume an analogy is drawn between the anatomic aspects of telangiectasias and varicose veins. Both are collections of elongated, dilated, tortuous venous vessels with incompetent valves. The thoughtful reader will see that treatment of the gross anatomic abnormality is best achieved by surgical removal and that treatment of the almost microscopic pathologic vessels is best achieved by obliteration through sclerotherapy. Since patients will present to the interested physician with both forms of phlebectasia, a treatment plan guided by accurate diagnosis will be recognized as essential.

Attention must be given to socioeconomic considerations in the diagnosis and treatment of varicose veins and telangiectasias. Since both conditions are very common, it is incumbent on the medical profession to decrease the costs of care for society without compromising the quality of care to the individual. This balance can be achieved by eliminating the hospital stay and employing ambulatory surgery. Correct selection of compression sclerotherapy will further reduce cost. In fact, it has been calculated that 20% of patients can be treated with compression sclerotherapy as an alternative to surgery. This approach could reduce the total cost of treatment of varicose veins by at least one third in comparison with the sole use of inpatient surgery (Eklof B. Br J Surg 75:297, 1988).

The chapters that follow will attempt to shed light on the obscure problems that comprise the diagnosis and treatment of varicose veins and telangiectasias. Some of the confusion in current practice is related to the history of diagnosis and treatment of the condition. Without returning to the fascinating investigations of the ancients, one can learn much from events that occurred after 1900. In 1916 Homans described the postphlebitic limb and discussed the effects of deep vein thrombosis. Although the clarification of these effects and Homans's notation that incompetence of perforating veins of the calf and ankle occurred in "venous disease" were important advances, his use of the terms "varicose ulcers" and "venous ulcers" did not help to explain the situation. Now, in looking back on the observations of Homans, we can say that cure of advanced manifestations of venous stasis can be achieved through complete elimination of superficial reflux. On the other hand, palliation is the only thing that can be achieved in the treatment of patients with severe deep venous insufficiency. Homans's emphasis on the importance of valve incompetence has been reinforced by subsequent investigations (Homans J. Surg Gynecol Obstet 22:143, 1916).

It was not until 1953 that Cockett described the three constant perforating veins in the medial aspect of the lower third of the leg. The importance of this observation has been obscured by recent investigations. However, the truth of Cockett's thesis remains: Perforating vein incompetence results in high pressure transmitted from the calf pump during exercise directly to the unsupported veins superficial to the membranous fascia and the intradermal vessels of the skin. The result of this high-pressure "leak" is elongation, tortuosity, dilation, and valve incompetence in the affected vessels (Cockett FB, Jones DEE. Lancet 1:17, 1953).

Another important observation that seems to have gone unrecognized by subsequent physicians is that perforator incompetence can exist without complete incompetence of the deep veins of the leg (Dodd H, Cockett FB. The Pathology and Surgery of the Veins of the Lower Limb. Edinburgh: Churchill Livingstone, 1976). This fact supports the hypothesis that treatment of superficial incompetence can cure a patient whereas treatment of incompetence associated with deep venous insufficiency is merely palliative.

Another confusing factor in treating varicose veins is that some workers believe that no venous ulcer can exist without perforator incompetence (Burnand KG, et al. Surgery 82:9, 1977). Others have pointed out that cutaneous ulceration has been demonstrated in patients with only saphenous insufficiency (Wright DDI, et al. Br J Surg 75:395, 1988). Even the marvelously executed studies of Bjordal in the early 1970s led to some confusion. It has been understood by many that Bjordal demonstrated that incompetent perforating veins contributed little to increased pressure in the superficial system. In fact, Bjordal's studies clearly show that flow through perforating veins in the patients he studied was bidirectional, both inward and outward (Bjordal RI. Acta Chir Scand 138:251, 1972). The fact that Bjordal concluded that most of the flow was directed inward does not detract from the other part of his observation, that outward flow was, indeed, present. Such outward-directed flow conforms to the observations of Cockett that high exercising pressure is transmitted directly to the most poorly supported venules of the skin and subcutaneous veins.

Another concept related to the etiology of varicosities has added to the confusion. This matter is the observation of arteriovenous anastomoses in association with varicose veins and the increased oxygen content of such veins (Haimovici H, et al. Ann Surg 164:990, 1966; Schalin L. In Eklof B, et al., eds. Controversies in the Management of Venous Disorders. London: Butterworth, 1989, p 182). Although many have criticized the interpretation of those observations, not many have questioned the observations themselves. Because of respect for the wisdom of Browse, the criticism leveled by him in a commentary on the work of Schalin has been cited. Browse argued that demonstrating a fistula requires physiologic techniques, and he pointed out that radiologic results are also open to subjective interpretation. Nevertheless, there is direct evidence of pathologic fistula development in limbs with venous disease. This evidence comes from the work of Gius, who described the existence of arteriovenous anastomoses at operation through the use of a dissecting microscope. Gius noted that the histology of these vessels showed a uniformly hypertrophied muscle coat (Haimovici H, et al. Radiology 87:696, 1966). Further work has shown that these anastomoses are of capillary caliber and are thought to open in response to alterations in temperature or pressure (Ryan TJ, Copeman PWM. Br J Dermatol 81:563, 1969). This last observation lends credence to the importance of arteriovenous anastomoses in the development of varicose veins and telangiectasias. A unifying hypothesis of increased hydrostatic and hydrodynamic pressure being transmitted to the veins and venules of the lower extremity could very well lead to a breakdown in the capillary barrier and to the development of direct arteriovenous connections.

In the preparation of this volume, it became clear that a review of the vast literature on the subject of venous disease suggests that many old theories are founded on signs whereas others are based on conjecture. As will be shown in this book, a great degree of understanding about venous stasis and venous ulceration was achieved even in ancient times. On the other hand, throughout the ages there have been many misconceptions about venous disease, some of which have been transmitted directly to us today. Like Eklof, we can only hope that increased international awareness of the problem of venous disease, venous stasis, and telangiectasias will produce an increased level of scientific inquiry and activity. Ultimately, if this book contributes to improved management of the common, if not lethal, disorder of venous stasis, then we will feel rewarded indeed.

John J. Bergan
Mitchel P. Goldman

Contents

Part One ▪ **FUNDAMENTAL CONSIDERATIONS**

1   Physiologic Observations on Causes of Varicose Veins   3
    Olav Thulesius

2   Anatomic Observations on Causes of Varicose Veins   12
    Sidney S. Rose

3   Pathogenesis of Varicose Veins and Chronic Venous Insufficiency
    Syndrome   42
    Philip D. Coleridge Smith and John H. Scurr

4   Common Anatomic Patterns of Varicose Veins   70
    John J. Bergan

Part Two ▪ **DIAGNOSTIC EVALUATION**

5   Classification of Venous Insufficiency   87
    John J. Bergan

6   Laboratory Evaluation of Varicose Veins   94
    Paul S. van Bemmelen and David S. Sumner

7   Pretreatment Testing of Patients With Varicose Veins and Telangiectatic
    Blemishes   110
    Ulrich Schultz-Ehrenburg

Part Three ▪ **TREATMENT OPTIONS**

8   Compression Therapy   127
    H.A. Martino Neumann and Dig J. Tazelaar

9   Historical Development of Varicose Vein Surgery   150
    Sidney S. Rose

10 Treatment of Varicosities of Saphenous Origin: Comparison of Ligation, Selective Excision, and Sclerotherapy   175
Peter Neglén

11 Treatment of Varicosities of Saphenous Origin: A Dialogue   193
Ralph G. DePalma, Sidney S. Rose, and John J. Bergan

12 Controlled Radiofrequency–Mediated Endovenous Shrinkage and Occlusion   217
Robert A. Weiss and Mitchel P. Goldman

13 Treatment of Varicose Veins by Sclerotherapy: An Overview   225
André Cornu-Thénard and Pierre Boivin

14 Compression Sclerotherapy for Large Varicose Veins and Perforator Veins: Details of an Empty Vein Technique   247
Joseph G. Sladen and John D.S. Reid

15 Role of Sclerotherapy in Greater Saphenous Vein Incompetence   265
Pauline Raymond-Martimbeau

16 Complications and Adverse Sequelae of Sclerotherapy   300
Mitchel P. Goldman

Part Four ▪ COMPLEX PROBLEMS INVOLVING VARICOSE VEINS

17 Chronic Venous Insufficiency and Its Surgical Care   383
John J. Bergan

18 Treatment of Varicose Veins Associated With Congenital Vascular Malformations   397
J. Leonel Villavicencio and Sandra Eifert

19 Varicose Veins and Venous Ulceration: Rationale for Conservative Treatment   414
Gregory L. Moneta and John M. Porter

20 Pelvic and Vulvar Varices: Pelvic Congestion Syndrome   425
Abraham Lechter

Part Five ▪ TELANGIECTATIC LEG VEINS

21 Treatment of Telangiectasias   451
Paul K. Thibault

22 Treatment of Leg Telangiectasias With Laser and High-Intensity Pulsed Light   470
Mitchel P. Goldman and Robert A. Weiss

23 Painful Telangiectasias: Diagnosis and Treatment   498
Robert A. Weiss and Margaret A. Weiss

24 Techniques of Small Vessel Sclerotherapy   518
David M. Duffy

Index   549

PART ONE

Fundamental Considerations

Chapter 1

Physiologic Observations on Causes of Varicose Veins

Olav Thulesius

VARICOSE VEINS AND VENOUS INSUFFICIENCY

Venous insufficiency is defined as any abnormality of the peripheral venous system that reduces or impedes venous return. It includes not only the veins themselves and their patency, wall properties, and valves but also the important extravascular factors that largely determine venous return from the extremities, such as the muscle pumps of the foot, calf, and thigh, which, in turn, are dependent on proper neuromuscular function and the mobility of joints (especially the ankle) and connective tissue support by fascia.

Varicose veins per se may or may not be an integral part of the full-blown picture of venous insufficiency, characterized by venous hypertension, edema, and leg ulcers. The spectrum of varicose veins is great: they can be an early sign of venous insufficiency, which should be treated to prevent disease progression, or they may be a late sign, appearing as dilated collaterals.

Varicose veins are dilated, tortuous veins exhibiting reflux because of valvular insufficiency. Dilatation of the veins may be primary, initiated by an unknown process, or it may be the result of postthrombotic changes, arteriovenous fistula, or diverted flow (collateral flow) resulting from blockage of deep veins. The question, however, arises about the site and mechanism of the initial fault in primary varicose veins, which initiated the disease process. The most likely candidates are defective venous valves that are unable to close properly or weakness of the venous wall that leads to distention and reflux.

Venous Valves

A functional evaluation of venous valves can be made by determining the pressure at which leakage occurs after retrograde filling of isolated veins. A study of saphenous veins of the thigh from 20 healthy controls and 20 patients with distal varicose veins revealed a significantly lower leak pressure in long saphenous varicose veins (79 mm Hg) as compared to that of normal veins (197 mm Hg).[1] Surprisingly, however, there were five cases without immediate leakage in controls and three cases with normal leak pressure (200 to 300 mm Hg) in patients with varicose veins. These results are not consistent with the concept of a generalized tendency toward leaky valves in cases of primary venous insufficiency; moreover, even individuals without venous disease can have incompetent valves.

Venous Wall

Most evidence about varicose veins suggests that they are caused by a primary abnormality of the venous wall that results in increased distention. The wall elements responsible for distensibility characteristics are connective tissue and smooth muscle. These elements, which reside in the media, may be affected by the disease process. Since alterations of venous wall viscoelastic properties are important in regard to the development of varicose veins, the fundamental principles are discussed here.

The venous viscoelastic properties can be viewed as a three-component mechanical model (Figure 1-1). The model is composed of smooth muscle (internal elastic element and a viscous dashpot) and connective tissue (parallel elastic element). The latter can be recruited in the relaxed state or at maximal distention. When stretch is applied to this model, elongation (length) and stress (tension) can be measured. This action is best depicted in a length-tension diagram (Figure 1-2). The slope of the length-tension relationship is an expression of the elastance (stiffness) of the stretched wall elements. When smooth muscle is contracted, stretch elongates the internal elastic elements and the dashpot. This change is reflected in a slight slope of the length-tension curve, which indicates low elastance. In a dilated vein, with relaxed smooth muscle, the length-tension curve initially has a flat

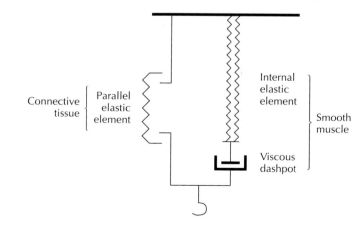

FIGURE 1-1. Three-component mechanical model characterizing the viscoelastic properties of a normal vein with two parallel elastic elements, one inside the contractile portion of smooth muscle and the other in the connective tissue. The latter is recruited only in fully dilated veins. The viscous dashpot element is also part of the smooth muscle.

slope because of filling from the partially collapsed state to the filled round transection. Thereafter the wall elements become stretched, demonstrating a steeper slope than that of the contracted state. In this stretched state, the parallel elastic elements of connective tissue become weight-bearing and are responsible for measured elastance. Therefore stiffness is higher in relaxed veins.

Connective tissue and lysosomal enzymes. In primary varicose veins, the initial interest was focused largely on the weakness of connective tissue elements and the possibility of a destructive process initiated by the local release of lysosomal enzymes. Niebes[2] demonstrated elevated serum levels of beta-glucoronidase and N-acetyl-beta-glucaminidase in cases involving primary varicose veins. We were able to confirm these findings, but we later found that this abnormality was not confined to patients with primary varicose veins but also could be demonstrated in postthrombotic states.[3] Therefore it is likely that lysosomal enzymes and tissue damage may be involved in the fully developed disease process of venous insufficiency but not in the initial state. A loosening of connective tissue, however, may be considered a result of hormonal changes associated with varicosis of pregnancy.

The concept of lysosomal enzymes and cytokines has recently received renewed attention in patients with leg ulcers. Coleridge Smith et al.[4] presented evidence that trapped white blood cells release enzymes that damage wall elements, induce increased capillary permeability, and promote thrombus formation.

Smooth muscle. Evidence is accumulating to implicate a deficient contractile function as a cause of varicose veins. In lower extremity veins, the amount of smooth muscle increases from proximal to distal, with a thicker muscle coat in foot veins compared to thigh veins. This increase can be viewed as an adaptive process that enables distal veins to withstand hydrostatic pressure better than proximal veins do. Therefore smooth muscle must play an important role in the physiologic function of lower extremity veins. This role involves serving as a local control mechanism rather than maintaining centrally governed vasomotor control through the sympathetic nervous system.

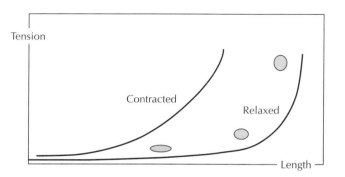

FIGURE 1-2. Length-tension diagram showing the action of a vein when contracted and relaxed during the process of filling and stretching. Steepness of the slope indicates the elastance (stiffness of wall). Characteristics of the wall are evident only in filled veins. Low initial slope of the relaxed (dilated) vein is only an indication of the expansion of the partially collapsed vein.

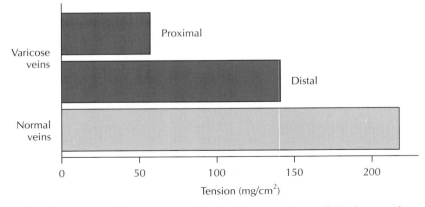

FIGURE 1-3. In vitro contractile responses of isolated preparations of the long saphenous vein in patients with varicose veins and in controls.

The in vitro measured maximal contractile force of varicose saphenous vein preparations to norepinephrine was shown to be lower than that of controls[5] (Figure 1-3). Also, it has been shown that alpha-adrenergic responsiveness of superficial hand veins in patients with varicose veins was lower than that of healthy controls.[6]

Another important parameter of smooth muscle function not related to shortening or generation of tension is associated with viscoelastic wall properties. Contrary to what one would expect, resistance to deformation is lower in contracted (vs. relaxed) vascular preparations.[7] We have been able to show that foot veins in patients with venous insufficiency display a reduced compliance (increased stiffness) and a higher elasticity modulus, a finding that is in agreement with the assumption of damaged smooth muscle in varicose veins.[8] Another indication of smooth muscle derangement is the loss of or reduction in stress relaxation and stress-release contraction in varicosis[9] (Figure 1-4). Stress relaxation in leg veins implies that the increase in venous volume that takes place with distal translocation of blood volume in a change from the supine to the upright position or with temporary outflow impediment is balanced and retarded. Alternatively, emptying of a normal vein is followed by venous contraction, as happens after venous emptying during exercise; that is, the reduction in volume is retarded because of smooth muscle hysteresis.

Superficial veins are involved in thermoregulation since venous blood flow favors dissipation of heat. Therefore a rise in local and overall body temperature results in venodilatation. Venoconstriction favors preservation of body heat since it diverts surface blood flow to deep veins surrounding arteries and promotes countercurrent heat exchange with precooling of arterial blood directed to acral regions. Normal superficial veins are sensitive to cooling, with vasoconstriction elicited by a very effective mechanism that is independent of sympathetic vasoconstrictor nerves but based on the blockade of the NA^+,K^+-ATPase (sodium pump).[10] This mechanism is not operative in varicose veins (Figure 1-5).

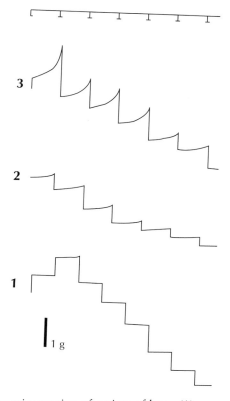

FIGURE 1-4. Recording of passive tension of a piece of latex *(1)*, a venous preparation from a varicose vein *(2)*, and a normal vein *(3)*. Stress relaxation (slow decrease of tension) is clearly seen in the normal vein. Curves were obtained by stepwise stretch of 0.2 mm of a preparation measuring 10×4 mm. Time marking: 1 minute at top (*Note:* Record should be read from right to left). (From Thulesius O, Gjöres JE. Reactions of venous smooth muscle in normal men and patients with varicose veins. Angiology 25:145-154, 1974. Reproduced with permission of the copyright owner: Westminster Publications, Inc., Roslyn, N.Y. All rights reserved.)

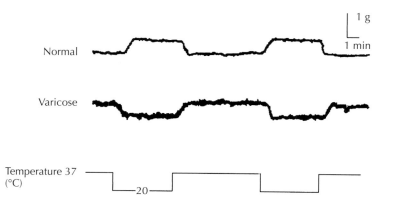

FIGURE 1-5. Effect of cooling on the tension of the human great saphenous vein. Note that cooling from 37° to 20° C in the normal vein induces contraction and dilatation in the varicose vein. (Recordings indicate tension of strips from isolated human great saphenous veins in a thermostated organ bath. *Top:* Normal preparation; *middle:* varicose vein; *bottom:* record of temperature.)

Raju et al.[11] presented evidence to show that the degree of deep venous insufficiency is related to changes in venous wall compliance.

Endothelium

The role of endothelium in controlling local vasomotor function has been clearly established. The existence of an endothelium-derived relaxing factor has been consistently demonstrated in arteries. The situation on the venous side is the opposite of that of the arterial side: saphenous vein endothelium has a contraction-facilitating effect in response to stimulation with norepinephrine. In varicose veins, however, endothelium-mediated enhancement of vasoconstriction induced by norepinephrine is reduced as a result of endothelial damage. This effect also has been documented by ultrastructural studies.[12] Therefore local dilatation of veins with the development of varicose veins can be initiated by endothelial damage.

DEVELOPMENT OF VARICOSE VEINS

The pathophysiologic process of the development of varicose veins is presented in Figure 1-6. This concept takes into account the development of both primary and secondary (postthrombotic) varicose veins. In the primary category, knowledge is accumulating to show that the initial abnormality resides in the smooth muscle coat of the media of veins and is caused by hereditary weakness, hormonal influences during pregnancy, or endothelial damage. (In the case of hormonal influences during pregnancy, a loosening of connective tissue elements also may occur.) The primary abnormality induces venous distention with secondary valvular insufficiency, reflux, and venous hypertension.

In secondary, or postthrombotic, varicose veins, the scenario is different. The condition begins with the inflammatory process of recanalization (phlebitis), which can damage the delicate valve leaflets and lead to valvular insufficiency and reflux. Other aspects of the postthrombotic state are characterized by incomplete recanalization and phlebofibrosis (Figure 1-7).

Perforator Veins

The superficial and deep veins of the lower extremity are connected by short perforator veins that transverse the deep fascia, usually at an oblique angle. The function of perforator veins is to drain blood from the superficial to the deep venous system, except in the foot, where drainage is from inside to outside. The normal direction of blood flow in perforator veins is guided by two factors: the presence of valves and the moving fascia, both of which direct blood flow from outside to inside on the thigh and the calf. Since there are approximately 30 perforator veins on the thigh and 40 on the calf and the foot, when the surface area of the various parts is considered, it can be seen that the density of perforators increases distally.

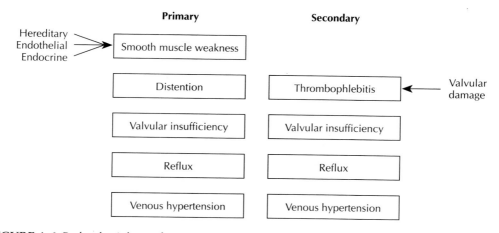

FIGURE 1-6. Pathophysiology of varicose veins in primary and secondary (postthrombotic) varicose veins.

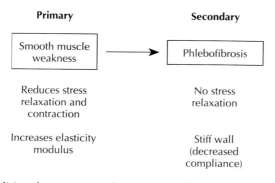

FIGURE 1-7. Abnormalities characterizing the venous wall in primary and secondary (postthrombotic) varicose veins.

As a consequence of thrombotic injury to valves or flow-induced dilatation and valvular incompetence, the direction of venous blood flow may become inverted, with a "blowout" flow occurring during exercise. (The flow-induced dilatation of perforator veins usually takes place after long-standing superficial venous insufficiency in the long, or greater, saphenous vein.) Blowout flow in a single insufficient ankle perforator vein during dorsiflexion of the foot can be in excess of 100 ml/min and may be greater with weight-bearing exercise such as walking.[13]

Some clinically important perforators that drain the long saphenous vein are found on the medial aspect of the calf, 5 to 25 cm above the sole of the foot ("Cockett's perforators"), on the dorsal aspect of the calf, and (a few) on the thigh. The pathophysiologic importance of perforator insufficiency is related to recurrence of varicose veins and local venous hypertension.

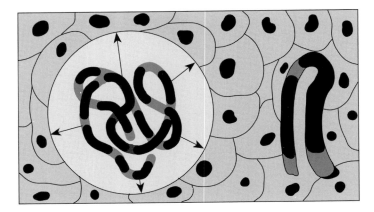

FIGURE 1-8. Schematic representation of a microvarix surrounded by a halo of edema. (From Bollinger A, Fagrell B. Clinical Capillaroscopy. Toronto: Hofgrefe & Huber, 1990, p 32.)

Microvarices

With superficial varicose veins, coiled and distended skin capillaries occur in a patchy distribution. With advanced deep venous insufficiency and venous hypertension, capillary distention leads to the development of microvarices, or glomerulus-like tortuous capillaries surrounded by a halo formation caused by local edema[14] (Figure 1-8).

Reticular varices are small ectatic cutaneous veins, probably dilated venules in the upper corium. Also called hyphen webs, they can be present together with large truncal varices of the saphena system or can occur in isolation. These varices usually have no functional consequences in themselves if they are not associated with other abnormalities.

REFERENCES

1. Thulesius O, Ekman L, Gjöres JE. Functional study of isolated venous valves, with special comments on the etiology of varicose veins. In American European Symposium on Venous Diseases. Montreux, 1974, pp 74-76.
2. Niebes P. Determination of enzymes and degradation products of glucosaminoglycan metabolism in the serums of healthy and varicose subjects. Clin Chim Acta 42:399-403, 1972.
3. Thulesius O, Gjöres JE, Eriksson O, Berlin E. Mechanical and biochemical factors in chronic venous insufficiency. Vasa 13:195-200, 1984.
4. Coleridge Smith PD, Thomas P, Scurr JH, Dormandy JA. Causes of venous ulceration: A new hypothesis. BMJ 296:1726-1727, 1988.
5. Thulesius O, Ugaily-Thulesius L, Gjöres JE, Neglén P. The varicose saphenous vein, functional and ultrastructural studies, with special reference to smooth muscle. Phlebology 3:89-95, 1988.
6. Blöchl-Daum B, Schuller-Petrovic S, Woltz M, Korn A, Böhler K, Eichler H-G. Primary defect in alpha-adrenergic responsiveness in patients with varicose veins. Clin Pharmacol Ther 49:49-52, 1991.
7. Gow BS. The influence of vascular smooth muscle on the viscoelastic properties of blood vessels. In Bergel DH, ed. Cardiovascular Fluid Dynamics, vol 2. London: Academic Press, 1972, pp 65-110.

8. Norgren L, Thulesius O. Pressure-volume characteristics of foot veins in normal cases and patients with venous insufficiency. Blood Vessels 12:1-12, 1975.
9. Thulesius O, Gjöres JE. Reactions of venous smooth muscle in normal men and patients with varicose veins. Angiology 25:145-154, 1974.
10. Thulesius O, Yousif MH. Na+, K+-ATPase inhibition. A new mechanism for cold-induced vasoconstriction in cutaneous veins. Acta Physiol Scand 141:127-128, 1990.
11. Raju S, et al. Observations on the calf venous pump mechanism: Determinants of post-exercise pressure. American Venous Forum, Third Annual Meeting. Fort Lauderdale, Fla., Feb. 1991.
12. Thulesius O, Said S, Shuhaiber H, Neglén P, Gjöres JE. Endothelial mediated enhancement of noradrenaline induced vasoconstriction in normal and varicose veins. Clin Physiol 11:153-159, 1991.
13. Thulesius O, Gjöres JE, Berlin E, Grip A, Kristoffersen K. Blood flow in perforator veins of the calf. In May R, Partsch H, Stabesand J, eds. Perforating Veins. Munich: Urban & Schwarzenberg, 1981.
14. Bollinger A, Fagrell B. Clinical Capillaroscopy. Toronto: Hofgrefe & Huber, 1990.

Editor's Note

The concept of the development of varicose veins as explained by Thulesius includes both primary varicose veins and those that follow an episode of severe deep venous thrombosis. Although Thulesius characterizes primary varicosities as having a vein wall weakness and emphasizes that secondary varicosities are linked to valvular damage produced by the thrombosis, it may be that both vein wall and valve deficits are occurring simultaneously in primary varicose vein development and that perforator vein incompetence is linked to the development of secondary varicose veins. This possibility is suggested by the comments made by Thulesius in describing perforator vein malfunction. He describes blowout flow as being in excess of 100 ml/min. Others have expressed muscular contraction pressure within compartments as ranging from 150 to 300 mm Hg. Such pressure transmitted through failed perforator vein valves can explain the development of both primary and secondary varicosities.

Chapter 2

Anatomic Observations on Causes of Varicose Veins*

Sidney S. Rose

The idea of valvular venous incompetence that allows reversal of blood flow and resultant dilatation was first conceived by William Harvey in 1628.[1] It was the natural corollary to his theory of circulation of the blood. Before Harvey's studies the humoral theory had held sway for centuries. Blood in the veins was thought to be thickened by "gross and evil humours" that distended the veins by viscosity. Bandaging the limb was contraindicated because it would drive these humors back into the body.

Harvey's theory was developed after he became interested in studying venous valves while in Padua at the Anatomy School of Fabricius.[2] Harvey made two fundamental observations: (1) the direction of the valve is such that blood can only flow toward the heart, and (2) the heart is a pump, not merely a receptacle (as was formerly thought). It is ironic that the final and third link in the circulatory chain—the capillaries—was described by Malpighi[3] only 8 years after Harvey's death.

The theory of valvular incompetence proposed by Harvey was the subject of heated debate for the next 20 years. It was finally accepted, along with the theory of primary valvular incompetence, as the cause of varicose veins. This mechanical theory, as it has become known, has been propagated in most surgical texts since the time of Harvey, and surgical treatment of varicose veins has been governed by this theory. This approach has stimulated various forms of proximal ligation of incompetent veins to replace incompetent valves.

Since the results of such surgery have not been universally successful, many generations of surgeons have been motivated to vary their techniques. As a result,

*Modified from Hobbs J, Nicolaides AN, Yao JST, eds. Investigation of Chronic Venous Insufficiency. London: Med-Orion Publishing, 1993.

THEORETICAL CAUSES OF VARICOSE VEINS

Heredity
Race
Gender
Posture
Gravitational back pressure
Pregnancy
Hormonal influence
Weight
Primary valvular incompetence
  Decreased number of valves
  Aging

Incompetent perforating veins
Arteriovenous communications
Vein wall weakness
Vein wall abnormality
Secondary valvular incompetence
  Phlebitis
  Deep vein thrombosis

various additions and modifications to the operative treatment have been developed. Ultimately, even Harvey's theory was called into question. Additional theories have included vein wall weakness and perforating vein incompetence. Other less popular theories have been advanced, and they are discussed here (see accompanying box).

GENERAL FACTORS AFFECTING VEIN WALL

The common element in the cause of varicose veins is a basic genetic defect. Gender, pregnancy, hormones, enzymes, and other humoral factors all are superimposed on this genetic element. Gravitational back pressure also plays a role. Whether such pressure is primary or secondary is debatable. The debate involves consideration of the contribution of each of these factors individually and as a whole. It is important to remember that the total effect may be greater than the sum of its parts.

Heredity

No doubt exists that an inherited genetic defect is present in patients with varicose veins. There is also a familial tendency. Whole families may be affected, and it is common for a mother and a daughter to have the same pattern of varicosities. Sometimes a generation is skipped. Occasionally the link is established only through maternal or paternal aunts. Congenital anatomic abnormalities of veins have been suggested as a cause of varicosities, but this theory has never been verified. The congenital view is contested by Nicholson,[4] who reported that 68% of cases do not develop until an individual reaches the age of 18 years, with the main incidence occurring between the ages of 18 and 35 years.

Race

Inbred racial differences have been observed that support the theory of genetic influence. Varicosity is common in the Western world. However, surgery for varicose veins in East Africa is an extremely rare event. In the Caribbean, where there are people of mixed race who tend to have many pregnancies, varicose veins are present in a high proportion of women. The mass deportations to the Caribbean Islands that occurred during Oliver Cromwell's occupation of Ireland in the seventeenth century led to the introduction of Irish blood, which probably has had a considerable effect on the prevalence of varicose veins.

Gender

Varicose veins occur predominantly in females, with the female:male ratio ranging from 4:1 to 8:1 in North America and Europe. The incidence of varicose veins in these areas is reported to be 2% of the adult population.

Posture

Upright posture has a detrimental effect on varicose veins. Although such posture causes the symptoms, it probably is not the primary cause of varicosity. However, once the vein has become incompetent, it will be affected by gravitational back pressure.

In comparing the habits of races in which varicose veins are rare, one striking postural difference is a natural adoption of the squatting position during defecation and parturition by Africans. In this position strain is transmitted into the pelvis rather than the groin, as occurs with these acts in Western nations. In the groin pressure is transmitted to the femoral and saphenous veins. It is interesting to note that the incidence of varicose veins increases among blacks who have moved from Africa to a Western environment, as has been shown in studies in cities in the United States.

Gravitational Back Pressure

Gravitational back pressure is not entirely responsible for vein dilatation; if this were the case, the vein wall would respond uniformly. Such pressure would not explain the localized development of lateral, saccular, and irregular blowouts, as described earlier.

Gravitational back pressure is the main cause of symptoms, however, and therefore it has been held responsible for causation of varicose veins. The patient's complaint of chronic aching pain is the result of stasis that develops gradually over time. Symptoms may be absent or minimal; however, as dilatation continues to extend the affected vein, incompetence of a protecting valve that is located either proximally or in a perforating vein can develop gradually or suddenly. When this occurrence is sudden, such valve incompetence causes rapid development or exacerbation of a varicosity. This action produces localized discomfort in a vein that was previously asymptomatic or not apparent. Pain is caused by reflux and may be quite sharp initially. The pain soon decreases to an ache as the affected vein wall adjusts.

The physiologic response to increased pressure in a normal vein is hypertrophy, not dilatation. This fact is demonstrated in the reversed normal saphenous vein when used as an arterial bypass. In this situation the vein is able to cope with arterial blood pressure. Similarly when an in situ vein graft is performed, the vein, with all its valves destroyed, responds to the raised internal pressure by hypertrophy, not dilatation.

Finally, if hydrostatic pressure is the major cause of varicosities, they should develop at the point of greatest dependency and become larger from below in an upward direction. However, this is not the case. The largest varicose clusters are often found just below the knee. Increased hydrostatic pressure resulting from occupational strain, exemplified in operatic tenors and weight lifters, has been invoked as the cause of varicosity, but it is doubtful whether this change occurs in the absence of a genetic factor. On the other hand, if competent valves are present proximal to a venous blowout, they will become distended by the accumulation of venous blood arriving from the periphery until there is sufficient pressure to empty them. The symptoms therefore are caused by stasis rather than back pressure. Both these factors may coexist.

Pregnancy

Further etiologic clues are found from the study of varicose veins that develop during pregnancy. In this physiologic model varicose veins not only develop but also subsequently disappear. The development of varicose veins during pregnancy sheds some light on vein wall and vein valve theories. Varicose veins of pregnancy appear early and gradually increase during pregnancy; many veins disappear shortly after delivery. This phenomenon demonstrates that the formation of varicose veins is reversible under special circumstances. It also means that any valves that became incompetent were able to regain competence. These valves must not have undergone any basic structural change during pregnancy. Every valid etiologic theory of varicose veins must explain how this happens because varicosities of pregnancy are macroscopically and microscopically indistinguishable from varicose veins that develop independently of pregnancy. For further discussion of the effects of pregnancy and the menstrual cycle, see Chapter 3.

Hormonal Influence

In the past it was thought that uterine pressure was the cause of varicose veins of pregnancy. Actually these varicosities begin to appear long before the uterus is large enough to cause increased back pressure. Now it is accepted that

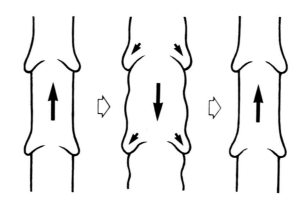

FIGURE 2-1. Diagrammatic representation of development and removal of varicose veins of pregnancy.

venous dilatation is the result of hormonal influences rather than pressure alone. As the hormonal changes begin with the onset of pregnancy, the varicose process begins immediately. Nevertheless, the veins do not become visible until the dilatation has had time to develop, at about the sixth week. Sometimes they appear earlier.

It has been suggested that estrogens and/or progesterones are responsible for venous dilatation of pregnancy. These hormones cause loss of vein wall tone through an effect on genetically susceptible smooth muscle cells and supporting tissues. When the vein becomes dilated, the valve ring expands until the commissure separates and the cusps are unable to meet. Dilatation of the vein wall and valve ring therefore produces secondary valvular incompetence (Figure 2-1).

After pregnancy ends, the circulating hormones return to normal and the situation is reversed. Muscle cells that were marginally affected are able to recover, and veins that were minimally affected regain much of their tone. The valve ring contracts and valves are able to close. Thus valvular competence is restored. In a first pregnancy some veins may not be sufficiently dilated to become clinically obvious, and they appear only with the second pregnancy. Only those veins that have been dilated beyond repair become permanently varicose. This fact explains the aggravation of symptoms that normally occurs during the first day or two of menstruation.

When combined with an underlying genetic defect, pregnancy may cause a female:male predominance of varicosity of 8:1. However, even in the nullipara, the ratio of varicosities is still 5:1. Although genetic background must be the same in both sexes, the added influence of female sex hormones explains why varicose veins occur more frequently in women, even in the absence of pregnancy. On the other hand, varicose veins in men are often much larger, though less symptomatic, than those in women.

Weight

No specific relationship has been established between obesity and truncal varicosities. However, in susceptible individuals there appears to be an increase in the number and irregularity of visible reticular veins in limbs with excessive subcutaneous fat. This condition often is associated with a profusion of intradermal telangiectasias.

Primary Valvular Incompetence

The theory of primary valvular incompetence is based on Harvey's mechanical theory. It has been postulated that an individual with varicose tendency is either born with fewer than normal valves or suffers from atrophy of the valves with advancing age. A combination of the two factors also has been suggested. To this genetic concept of primary valve failure is added the theory of sequential descending valvular incompetence.[5] It has been postulated that the first valve to become incompetent is the uppermost. This valve may be the one at the saphenofemoral junction or the valve in the middle third of the thigh at the adductor canal. It has been suggested that incompetence proceeds peripherally as each successive valve succumbs to increasing back pressure from above. The entire vein and valve complex then responds by venous dilatation.

Although this theory is conceptually attractive, it is not in accord with clinical findings. Furthermore, pathologic changes that occur in the valve have been described only incompletely. The most detailed description of valve pathology comes from Gottlob and May,[6] who investigated changes in valves resulting from phlebitis. In such cases the valve is damaged acutely by blood clot and chronically by fibrosis and atrophy. These facts are not relevant to development of valve failure in primary varicose veins. In primary venous insufficiency it is rare to find any inflammatory reaction unless phlebitis or local trauma has occurred.

The question that arises is whether the valve can lose its tension or can atrophy spontaneously. If so, why and how? Functionally the normal valve is extremely strong. Attempts to rupture it experimentally by increasing intraluminal pressure have shown that valves withstand pressures well over 300 mm Hg.[7,8] The valve ring is the strongest and least distensible part of the vein wall. The ring is seen as a beaded shadow on venograms.

Informative descriptions of normal venous valves are few. Long ago the best description was given by Franklin[9] in his historical monograph.

VENOUS VALVE

The anatomy of the normal venous valve reveals several interesting structural features (Figure 2-2). The facts presented here are from a study of valves obtained during vein surgery and from cadavers.[10,11] In the past the valve was thought to be an inert flap of connective tissue covered on each aspect by a layer of endothe-

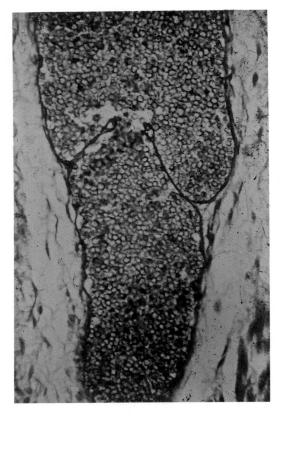

FIGURE 2-2. Macroscopic view of venous valve.

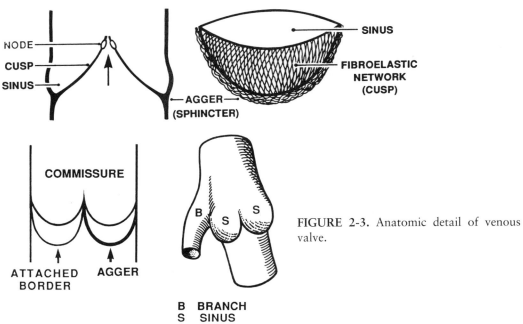

FIGURE 2-3. Anatomic detail of venous valve.

lium. Actually the structure is much more complex. The constituent parts are agger, sinus, cusps, cornua, and commissure (Figure 2-3). In some larger valves a central nodule is found on the free border of the cusp. The valves, other than those at major junctions, often are not easy to identify or isolate. This situation frequently has made it difficult to obtain a meaningful section through the correct plane.

Histology: Light Microscopy

The normal valve leaflet is connected to the venous wall by a complex fibromuscular structure forming a humplike mass originating from the media and extending into the base of the cusp. This mass contains well-identified groups of muscle fibers supported by a collagen matrix (Figure 2-4). According to most authorities, the muscle extends into the base of the cusp and no farther. Franklin,[9] however, described the presence of muscle cells in the cusp, stating that: "They [muscle cells] are said to lie transverse to the long axis of the vein, especially near

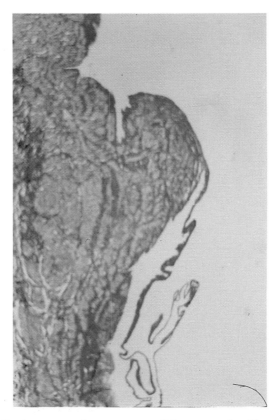

FIGURE 2-4. Valve leaflet is connected to venous wall by a complex fibromuscular structure. This structure forms a humplike mass that originates from the media and extends into the base of the cusp (elastic van Gieson's stain: collagen, red; muscle, pale; elastic tissue, blue/black).

the free border, to occur in some valves, but not in others, and more often in the larger valves." My colleagues and I have not confirmed this, but we have identified a number of scattered fibromyoblasts that may have been the cells to which Franklin referred. The aggregation of circular muscle fibers at the base of the valve that Franklin describes has every appearance of being a localized sphincter. Franklin also agreed with Sappey,[12] who was unable to find any nerve supply. Absence of a nerve supply subsequently has been confirmed by electron microscopy and immunohistochemical techniques not available to Franklin or Sappey.

The internal elastic lamina of the vein wall continues from the subendothelium of the vein in a linear fashion under the luminal surface of the cusp throughout its length. The lamina divides the cusp into two portions, one facing the sinus and the other facing the lumen. The endothelium on the sinus side runs transversely and presents a pitted appearance. The endothelium on the luminal aspect runs longitudinally in common with the rest of the luminal endothelium (Figure

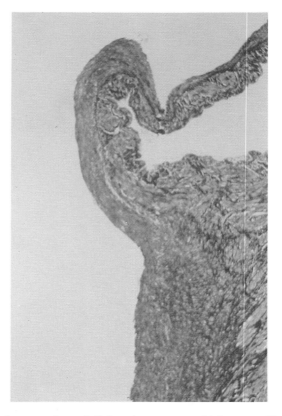

FIGURE 2-5. Venous valve seen through light microscopy on high power. Van Gieson's stain: collagen, red; muscle, pale; elastic tissue, dark. Luminal surface of valve cusp is smooth and continuous with luminal endothelium seen in upper part of section. Endothelium that lines sinus is folded and produces an irregular surface. Elastic tissue is continued into valve cusp, where it divides into two portions longitudinally.

2-5). The result is a much smoother surface. Elastic tissue in the cusp generally extends to the free border, where it fans out, but in some specimens it ends in a nodule consisting of a concentration of elastic fibers lying in whorls of collagen (Figure 2-6). In the cusps of the valve, scattered pale-staining cells that appear to be fibromyoblasts are seen.

The complexity of the whole valve structure—the muscle hump, the arrangement of muscle cells, and the peculiarity of the terminal nodule—suggests that the valve may be more than a passive structure. The valve may be able to open and close actively in response to circulatory demands. Transmission electron microscopy reveals that the total length of the cusps is greater than the diameter of the vein (Figure 2-7, A). This situation is thought to allow expansion of the valve ring during dilatation. The peculiar construction of the cusp suggests that it possesses the ability to "ruche up" when the vein contracts. It is possible that movement begins in the muscle hump and runs out through the leaflet, which elongates and contracts according to intraluminal pressure and flow. This process produces an elongation and contraction of the opposing leaflets to ensure contact and competence in all phases of venous activity. The specialized nodules at the free edge may signal when the leaflets come into contact with each other. Distribution of elastic tissue suggests that this action can be activated from the basal muscle aggregation. Because of the valve length, it is conceivable that some degree of prolapse may oc-

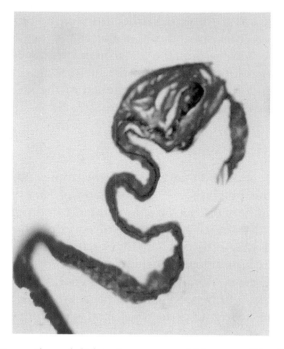

FIGURE 2-6. "Nodule" seen through light microscopy on high power. Van Gieson's stain: collagen, red; elastic tissue, dark (traced through cusp and terminating in nodule).

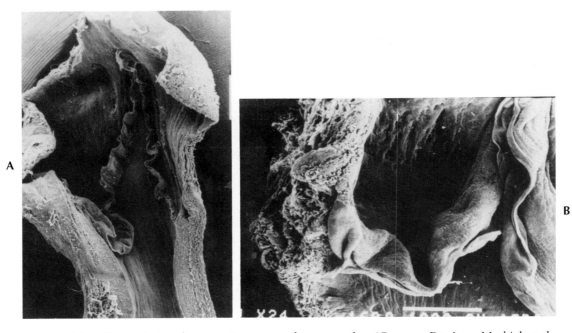

FIGURE 2-7. Transmission electron microscopy of venous valve. (Courtesy Dr. Aron Mashiah and Kaplan Hospital, Rehovot, Israel.)

cur under normal conditions and may be regarded as physiologic. Further, it may be that the floppy valve syndrome of Kistner[13] is a pathologic version of the same phenomenon. However, this possibility is a matter for further research.

Finally, it is noteworthy that the electron microscope scan shows that the endothelium is disposed longitudinally on the luminal aspect of the valve cusp in continuity with the endothelium lining the lumen of the vein while it runs transversely on the sinus aspect of the valve (Figure 2-7, B).

Venous Valve in Varicose Veins

In general, the venous valve in varicose veins shows no pathologic change in the absence of previous phlebitis.[14,15] Examination of varicose and normal valves shows no histologic difference between functionally competent and incompetent valves. In contrast, valves that have been involved in phlebitis show fibrosis, cystic degeneration, and adhesions. Such changes render them incompetent, but this type of lesion is not seen in uncomplicated varicose veins.

In long-standing cases of valvular incompetence, disuse atrophy may occur. This condition is as likely to be secondary as primary. Senile valvular atrophy also has been described in anatomic dissections, but it was not associated with varicose veins.[16]

On balance, evidence supporting the theory of primary valvular insufficiency as a cause of varicose veins is presumptive rather than proven. There is a good deal of argument against it. For example, if valve incompetence were a precipitating factor in causing varicose veins, the involved valve should be the first to show changes; however, what might be described as an early change has never been reported. Instead, Eger and Casper[17] presented anatomic evidence that the valvular defect in primary varicose veins was not the result of damage to the cusps but was caused by dilatation of the valve ring. Also, Leu[14] found that there was no reduction in number of valves with increasing age. The theory of sequential descending incompetence also is questionable. Further, it is difficult to explain the absence of varicosities in reported cases of senile atrophy of saphenous valves.[16] In addition, varicosity may develop in a circumscribed group of veins that communicate with veins of normal caliber, as described by King,[18] who showed that varicose veins could develop equally in an upward or downward direction.

Ludbrook[19] and others have demonstrated that some valves that are competent with the patient in a supine position become incompetent when the subject is erect. This finding focuses attention on the valve ring. Perhaps a weakened valve ring dilates when the patient is in the upright position. This dilatation occurs despite the reflex vasoconstriction that occurs in the erect position. Ludbrook attempted to verify the theory of sequential descending valvular incompetence but was unable to do so. Finally, if the absence of competent valves is the cause of varicose veins, a reversed or in situ saphenous arterial bypass should become varicose because all the valves are inactivated or destroyed. In fact, the opposite occurs. The vein wall follows established physiologic principles and hypertrophies in response to the extra pressure.

INCOMPETENT PERFORATING VEINS

The presence of incompetent valves in perforating veins is believed by many to be a primary cause of varicosity. Early anatomists were aware of the communicating veins between the deep and the superficial venous systems. In particular, surgeons of the French anatomic-pathologic school of the early nineteenth century first described these communicating veins with particular reference to varicose veins. Studies of Bordeu[20] in 1775 and Briquet[21] in 1824 were confirmed by their British counterparts later in the nineteenth century, including Colles (1844),[22] Brodie (1846),[23] and Gay (1868).[24] Further descriptions were offered in the twentieth century with anatomic reports of Kosinski (1926)[25] and Franklin (1927).[9] It was Turner-Warwick[26] and Linton[27] who again drew attention to the perforating veins from a clinical point of view.

In 1947 Myers[28] reintroduced stripping of the internal saphenous vein with a new and improved stripper that he thought would deal with incompetent tributaries including perforators. However, early optimism evaporated as it became apparent that Myers's results were still imperfect.

In 1956 Dodd and Cockett[29] attempted to explain the occurrence of varicosities below a competent valve. They emphasized that failures associated with stripping were caused by uncorrected valvular incompetence in perforating veins. They believed that incompetent perforating veins also played an important part in the causation of varicose veins and that this fact justified a major change in operative technique. This concept was well received, and subsequent surgical treatment was based on this theory. Perforator ligation, alone or in conjunction with stripping, was performed enthusiastically with some improvement in results. The degree of improvement, however, was not commensurate with the increased technical difficulties of the procedure. The operation became increasingly time-consuming. These procedures are still widely practiced, but experience has raised doubts about the importance of the incompetent perforator.

Varicosities often appear in localized clusters that seem isolated; when dissected, they show no obvious connection to incompetent truncal or perforating veins. After numerous dissections Linton showed that normal perforating veins are <2 mm in diameter, and he regarded only those >4.4 mm as pathologic. Linton was surprised to find that in cases of varicose veins 79% of those examined were <2.4 mm. In a more recent report by Schalin,[30] only 21% of perforators were ≥2.5 mm in diameter. Only 8 of 74 perforators were >4 mm. Schalin summarized: "The absence of perforating veins in 47 per cent of varicose veins operated on and no more than eight subfascial branches being equal to or larger than 4 mm out of a total of 131 branches examined, in the 53 per cent of varicose veins in which perforators were found, constitutes a very impressive discrepancy between expectation and observation."

Difficulty in localizing perforating veins in relation to the varicosities has been emphasized by Haeger.[31] By thermography, he counted "hot spots" that were thought to overlie incompetent perforators. When these spots were checked by phlebography, perforators were completely absent in 74 (47%) of 157. Actually, those that were found (83 of 157) were smaller than expected and did not correlate well with thermographic hot spots.

Pflug and Daintree Johnson[32] used perioperative microscopy to reveal that most suspect incompetent perforating veins divide subfascially into two or more normal-looking branches that diverge into the muscle. Instead of increasing in size when dissected inward, they become narrower. In this situation the subcutaneous part of connecting veins shows a greater dilatation that gradually decreases in a centrifugal direction, the opposite of what would be expected. Single dilated incompetent perforators were recorded in both of these reports, but the number is disproportionately small compared with the number of varicosities described.

The direction of flow in perforating veins has been thought to be from superficial to deep, but this flow was reversed when perforators became incompetent. Bjordal[33] used a square-wave flowmeter to show that the net flow in incompetent perforating veins was mainly directed inward. He noted that there was an outward flow, but this flow was more than compensated for by the inward flow. This finding conflicts with current acceptance of the venous refill time after emptying as a standard measure of incompetence. Such testing assumes that reflux occurs entirely through incompetent perforators. In fact, there are at least two perforating veins in the foot that are valveless and that allow open communication between the superficial and the deep venous systems. Incompetent perforators also

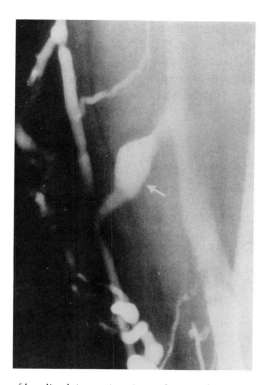

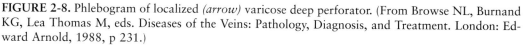

FIGURE 2-8. Phlebogram of localized *(arrow)* varicose deep perforator. (From Browse NL, Burnand KG, Lea Thomas M, eds. Diseases of the Veins: Pathology, Diagnosis, and Treatment. London: Edward Arnold, 1988, p 231.)

may be present as a secondary rather than a primary phenomenon, for example, perforators involved in the varicose process (Figure 2-8). The theory of primary varicosity of deep perforators as the cause of varicose veins therefore has lost many of its advocates.

ARTERIOVENOUS COMMUNICATIONS

Observations by some workers while treating varicose veins have led them to give support to arteriovenous (AV) communications as a theory of causation. These observations may be summarized as follows: blood in varicose veins is often as red as arterial blood. Pigeaux[34] noted this fact as long ago as 1843. He attributed the finding to widening of the capillary bed with increased arterial flow.

Some varicosities may occasionally pulsate,[35] and Blalock[36] found oxygen tension to be increased in blood taken from the internal saphenous vein in a patient with varicose veins. Also, varices are found in association with known AV fistulas. When the fistulas are closed, the varicosities disappear.

The main proponents of the AV fistula causation theory, Wolf,[35] Haimovici,[37] and Schalin,[30] have shown what they believe to be small AV communications exposed at operation. Because these investigators are experienced observers, it is necessary to evaluate the arguments that they have advanced. Blalock's report[36] of raised oxygen levels in blood taken from the saphenous vein has been the source of considerable controversy. His observations have been confirmed by some workers, but they have not been consistently reproduced. The AV connection theory was strongly disputed by de Takats et al.[38]

Venous pulsation in a varicosity is usually transmitted from an adjacent artery. Such pulsation is significant only if it is associated with a known AV fistula or if it occurs in a dilated venous capillary. Varicose veins are associated with peripheral vasodilatation, and venous capillaries are often dilated as part of the process. If the capillary bed is opened in this way, a functional AV short circuit may develop and act as a shunt. This occurrence would explain the "arterialization" of varicose vein blood and the pulsatile flow transmitted from the dilated arterial capillary into the dilated venous capillary. It may be that this action is what has been called an AV communication.

Detection of the capillary changes that are necessary to explain the presence of AV communications is difficult. Such changes that occur in the vascular bed vary in accordance with circulatory demands. This fact may explain why such connections are not found more frequently and why the theory has not gained much support. Haeger[39] claimed that if arterialization of venous blood occurs, it is probably the result of, and not the cause of, varicosity.

It is interesting to note that in the seventeenth century it was thought that the prime cause of varicose veins was an excessive volume of blood being propelled through venous capillaries. This action was said to have a dilating effect on the vein wall. This theory leads us to consideration of the weak vein wall theory, which has gained support in recent years.

VEIN WALL WEAKNESS

The most obvious clinical abnormality in varicose veins is the dilated vein and therefore the vein wall. Traditionally, a weak vein wall has been the main alternative theory to primary valvular incompetence. Although the latter generally has been preferred, the weak vein wall theory has had many followers.[15] The mechanical theory of varicose dilatation states that a weak vein wall is a secondary manifestation of valvular incompetence caused by exposure of the vein wall to pressures it cannot withstand. Examination of this pronouncement, however, raises many questions. For example, what is the reaction of a normal vein to an increase in pressure? The average standing hydrostatic head of pressure from the right atrium to the ankle in the upright position is 85 mm Hg. This pressure may be raised by coughing, breathing against resistance (Valsalva), or straining. Adjustments of the degree of venous wall tone are responsible for maintaining this pressure within normal limits. The degree of tonicity present in a normal saphenous vein is most apparent to vascular surgeons at operation. The vein contracts markedly on handling in preparation for a vein bypass. Even a varicose vein con-

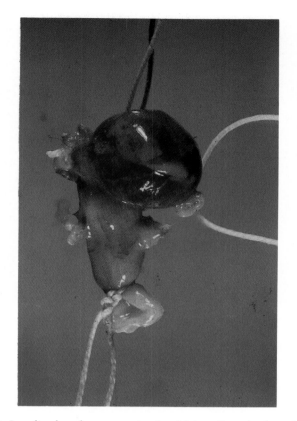

FIGURE 2-9. Localized saphenous varicosity. Main tributaries have been ligated.

tracts on handling—however, to a limited degree in which the response is not uniform. The surgeon can determine the strength of the venous wall by the pressure required to distend the vein to enlarge its lumen. Ackroyd et al.[7] demonstrated that a normal vein wall is capable of withstanding pressures in excess of anything it may be called on to endure.

Several frequently encountered circumstances are not explained by valve incompetence but are explained by weakness of the vein wall. For example, a saphena varicosity is often a saccular dilatation occurring laterally as a blowout (Figure 2-9). The vein wall is involved locally only at the base of the blowout. Furthermore, a varicose vein often consists of a string of dilatations interspersed throughout areas of comparative normality. If dilatation were a result of back pressure alone, the whole venous wall should be affected evenly. Lateral and fusiform blowouts are caused by localized areas of weakness in the vein wall, resulting in an irregular pattern of dilatation of the vein.

Nylander[40] has described this phenomenon as the meandering syndrome (Figure 2-10). He compared the tortuous appearance of a varicose vein to a meandering river and attributed this effect to the same mechanism that produces tor-

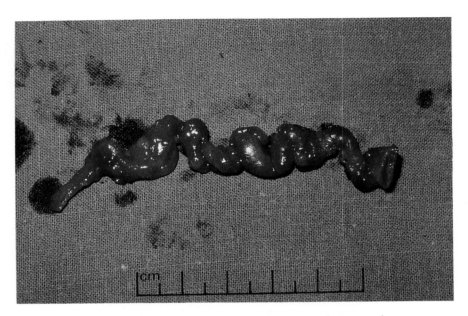

FIGURE 2-10. Tortuous varicosity known as meandering syndrome.

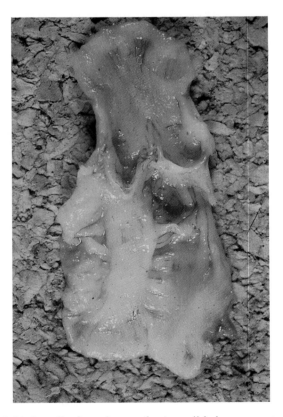

FIGURE 2-11. Localized weakness of vein wall below competent valves.

tuosity in a hose when the water is turned on. However, this picturesque analogy is misleading because tortuosity occurs only when the water is at jet pressure, not at flow levels comparable to those encountered in venous flow.

Tortuosity of a varicose vein is caused by a combination of factors. First is the irregular distribution of involved areas. Second, the varicosity assumes a tortuous course when the vein elongates between two fixed points. Elongation is caused by involvement of longitudinal muscle. Third, vein valve cusps are arranged so that each successive pair is at right angles to the last. This situation tends to produce a degree of torsion in the long axis of the vein that will act in combination with the other changes. Varicosities also can develop below and in between competent valves (Figure 2-11). This occurrence is commonly seen and was fully described by Cotton[41] in 1961. It can be argued that the reason for dilatation below a competent valve is incompetence of an associated perforator, which produces back pressure in the superficial vein. However, pressure in the superficial vein can rise only briefly in response to a rise in deep venous pressure if there is no obstruction to the flow of blood above and below the involved perforator. If there is deep venous obstruction, venous hypertension will develop that should be evenly distributed between the superficial and the deep venous systems.

The response of a normal vein wall to a rise of internal pressure will be a contraction to expel the excess blood. On the other hand, if an inherent weakness of the vein wall is present, pooling of blood in the superficial vein will occur because it cannot contract properly in response to the pressure change. If the valve ring above dilates as a consequence of a weakened vein wall and incompetence develops, gravitational back pressure will cause an exacerbation of symptoms.

VEIN WALL ABNORMALITY

Veins have been regarded purely as valved conduits through which blood is returned to the heart, with little attention paid to vein wall function. However, changes in the venous reservoir can occur during shock and hemorrhage. The reservoir changes are caused by a balance of vasoconstriction and vasodilatation that affects veins as well as arteries. Indeed, changes in venous caliber are much greater than those in arteries and involve extremes of tonal adjustment. It has been suggested that minor variations in tone assist venous return by an effect on the vis a tergo at night when the other mechanisms of venous return are at a low ebb.[15]

The main constituents of the vein wall are muscle layers, collagenous matrix, and elastic tissue, which all interact to maintain tone. Collagen provides strength and prevents overdistention. Muscle provides contractility, and the interaction of elastic tissue with muscle and collagen provides compliance. The degree of venous tone mainly depends on the state of reactivity of the muscle layer. Loss of tone therefore must be in this layer. However, the matrix in which the muscle functions is inseparable from it. The whole structure, together with the venous valve, must act in concert. All vein wall constituents require close scrutiny.

LIGHT MICROSCOPY
Normal Vein

Examination of the normal vein wall reveals the medial coat as the most prominent feature (Figure 2-12). The medial coat consists of a well-developed circular muscle layer arranged in regular whorls that are supported on the scaffold of a tightly packed collagenous matrix. Immediately internal to the medial coat is a thin inner layer of longitudinal cells lying in a matrix of loose subendothelial connective tissue. This layer is separated from the endothelium by a distinct elastic lamina. Other elastic fibers are scattered sparsely throughout the vein wall. Surrounding the medial coat there is an outer longitudinal muscle layer arranged loosely in bundles that merge into the adventitia. The adventitia forms the outer coat in which connective tissue again becomes predominant. It contains numerous vasa vasorum, nerve filaments, and occasional nerve endplates. However, the structure of veins taken from different sites demonstrates a wide variation in wall thickness, muscle content, and number of valves. Changes are related to the site of the vein and the function it serves.

Varicose Vein

In the varicose vein the most striking change is a marked increase of collagenous tissue that appears to invade muscle layers and causes a breakup of the regular cellular pattern, with separation and interruption of muscle cells (Figure 2-13). The intima is intact in early cases, but in long-standing varicosities there is a tendency for some loss of endothelial cover. Desquamation of surface cells ex-

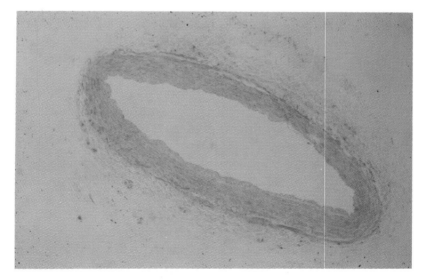

FIGURE 2-12. Normal vein seen through light microscopy on low power. Hematoxylin and eosin stain used. Regularity of muscle pattern is noted in media.

ceeds the rate of replacement. There is no evidence of an inflammatory reaction. In addition to an increase in interstitial collagen, in advanced cases subintimal deposits of collagenous tissue are present that superficially resemble arteriosclerotic plaques (Figure 2-14).

Typically the muscle cell pattern is grossly distorted in affected areas. These

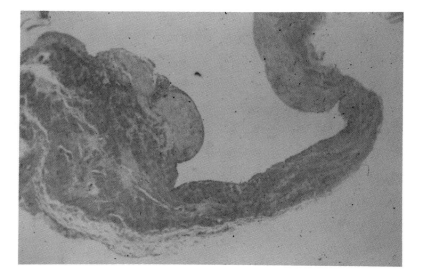

FIGURE 2-13. Varicose vein seen through light microscopy. Hematoxylin and eosin stain used. Shows breakup of muscle pattern and development of callenous infiltration with subendothelial plaque formation.

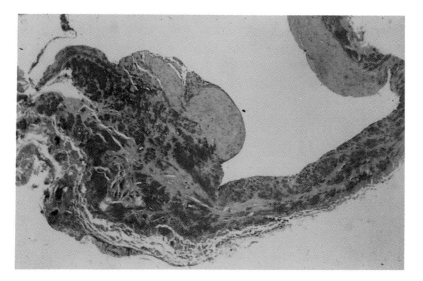

FIGURE 2-14. Same specimen as Figure 2-13 shown with Masson's stain. Collagen, blue; muscle, red.

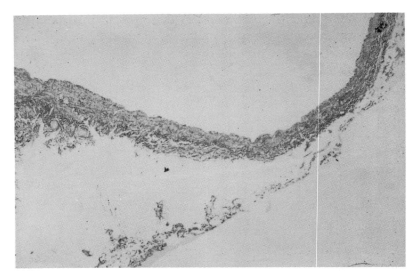

FIGURE 2-15. Varicose blowout seen through light microscopy. Van Gieson's stain: collagen, red; muscle, pale; elastic tissue, dark.

areas are scattered in a patchy distribution, with parts of the wall still retaining a normal pattern. This situation has led to differences in histologic description of varicose veins. In localized blowouts the muscle layer disappears completely and the thinned wall consists mainly of collagen and elastic tissue (Figure 2-15).

TRANSMISSION ELECTRON MICROSCOPY
Normal Vein

In the normal vein muscle cells show well-marked nuclei with a clearly defined chromatin network (Figure 2-16). Cells lie in close proximity to one another and are surrounded by a fine layer of amorphous fibrous tissue. Muscle cells are supported by regularly arranged collagen fiber bundles in vertical and horizontal disposition. The cell cytoplasm contains occasional vacuoles, some of which contain granular material, which suggests secretory activity.

Varicose Vein

In the varicose vein a completely different picture is seen. Muscle cells become separated because of a marked increase in collagenous matrix (Figure 2-17). In areas that are most affected, collagen fibers become packed in an irregular manner between muscle cells. Many elastic fibers are scattered throughout these areas. The fibers are not part of the internal elastic lamina, which is often fragmented.

The increasing infiltration of collagen continues as the condition deterio-

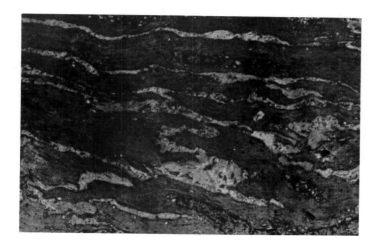

FIGURE 2-16. Transmission electron microscopy of normal vein shows regular pattern of muscle cells lying in close relationship to one another.

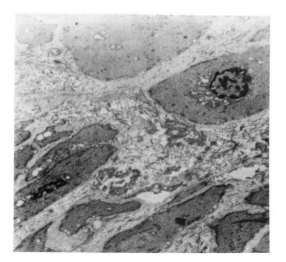

FIGURE 2-17. Transmission electron microscopy of varicose vein. Muscle cells are separated by collagen fibrils and show evidence of vacuolar activity.

rates. Muscle cells become further separated. Eventually, in blowout areas the wall consists entirely of collagen bundles lined by endothelium, with the muscle fibers having completely disappeared (Figure 2-18).

At higher magnifications a marked difference in the cell nucleus is noted. Both normal and varicose cells have a well-differentiated chromatin skein, but the varicose cell shows numerous apparent erosions along its length. In the cytoplasm an increase in "vacuole" formation is present. Some of the vacuoles contain gran-

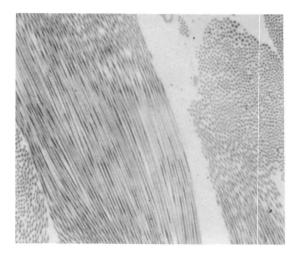

FIGURE 2-18. Transmission electron microscopy of venous blowout. Muscle cells are completely replaced by collagen fibrils, which appear to be normal.

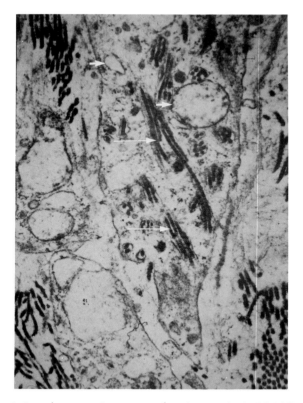

FIGURE 2-19. Transmission electron microscopy of varicose vein (×30,000). Muscle cell contains many vacuoles *(short arrows)* and shows evidence of phagocytosis of collagen fibrils *(long arrows)*.

ules, and others appear to be empty. A pericellular halo of amorphous fibrous tissue is present that seems to have been secreted by the muscle cell itself, probably as a result of increased secretory activity. The cytoplasm of the abnormal cell presents a more disordered appearance than that of its normal counterpart. Both cells possess hemidesmosomes that appear as small intermittent dark areas situated at the margin of the cell membrane. Figure 2-19 shows a varicose muscle cell; at a magnification of $\times 30,000$ it is interesting to find that the muscle cell is capable of phagocytosis. Some collagen fibers appear to have been ingested by the muscle cell. The characteristic banding is still distinguishable.

PROCESS OF VARICOSITY

The main pathologic feature of the process of varicosity is separation of muscle cells by collagen. This characteristic has been described by many authors.[42-46] Since collagen fibers appear to have a normal structure and muscle cells are markedly deranged, it is logical to assume that the latter are responsible for the changes of varicosity. Biologic assay and tissue culture may produce a more definitive answer.

Separation of the muscle cells results in widening of the functional gap between them. This gap needs to be bridged if the contractile state of one muscle cell is to be transmitted to another. When adjustments in venous tone occur, the muscle layer of the vein wall must act as a coordinated whole; this action must occur during the more active process of constriction, as well as during the less active process of dilatation. Communication between muscle cells must be instantaneous. Hemidesmosomes are thought to be involved in this process. These structures are seen as darker areas in cell membranes situated at intervals along their length. It is through these bodies that coordination of muscle cell contraction occurs. This action takes place through a combination of physical, chemical, and electrical stimuli. Hemidesmosomes may be involved in two ways. Small lacunae in the cell membrane in relation to hemidesmosomes may allow protoplasmic fibrils to pass between muscle cells to connect cytoplasms. Glycoproteins such as fibronectin and laminin help to bind muscle cells to the matrix through a network of fibrils attached to a cell wall endplate. The precise area of attachment has not been identified, but it is thought to be related to the hemidesmosome. Both mechanisms enable cells to function as a unified unit. Therefore if the cells become separated, collective action becomes impossible. There is probably an optimum gap between muscle cells that allows their unified function. This gap has been estimated at 0.04 mmu.

Finally, contact between muscle cells and matrix also may occur by chemical or electrical means to enable continuing function during the early stage of separation. As the varicose condition develops, muscle cells undergo changes in form. The cells become larger, irregular, and hypersecretory. They are paler, with many cells appearing shadowy in outline and substance. In short, they show evidence of a severe metabolic disturbance.

FUNCTION OF MUSCLE CELL

The following account of normal cell function is from the work of Vanhoutte and Shepherd.[47] Muscle cells have the basic structure and functional characteristics of vascular smooth muscle cells in general. They contain contractile tissue controlled by contractile proteins that are triggered by an increase in the level of cytoplasmic calcium. The contraction of muscle cells depends on cell length at the moment of stimulation. Longer cells have a more complete contraction. When venous smooth muscle is activated, the constrictor response is determined mainly by local conditions. Intraluminal pressure is the main stimulus brought about by variations in the blood content. It causes mobilization or pooling of blood that adjusts the degree and direction of muscle response. In limb veins contraction of smooth muscle is stimulated by local liberation of cellular neurohumoral mediators. Among these mediators, norepinephrine causes contraction of venous smooth muscle by activation of adrenoceptors on the cell membrane. It is by this means that venous tone is maintained.

In abnormal muscle cells an abnormal metabolic process that interferes with the normal mechanism of contraction is probably taking place. Therefore involved muscle cells may lose their power to contract, at first individually and then collectively as they separate, or even before separating. Weakened muscle cells separate and lose contact, and the muscular grid sags. Simultaneously there is invasion of the intercellular space by collagen together with some elastic tissue. The primary lesion that develops in the muscle cell must be considered to be due to a genetic defect that orchestrates the interplay of factors involved in producing a "varicose" cell.

PHYSICOCHEMICAL FACTORS AFFECTING VEIN WALL

Increased venous wall distensibility found in varicose veins is attributable to a lesion in the muscle layer. Yet since muscle cells, collagen, and elastic fibers must all act in concert, how are other tissues affected? It could be argued that the basic lesion is present in collagen tissue, which, by its overgrowth, engulfs muscle cells and impedes their function. Alternatively, the muscle cell appears to be deranged, whereas collagen and elastic fibers appear to be normal.

Many enzymes have been considered to play a primary role in venous distention, but none has been clearly implicated. Collagenase, increased lysosomal activity,[48] elastase and alteration in collagen, and elastin and adenosine triphosphate content in the vein wall all have been reported as possible causative factors. Plasminogen activator and fibrinolysin levels are reduced, with possible effects on the blood clotting mechanism. The hexosamine content is consistently raised.[44] The effect of estrogens on enzyme activity also is under examination.[49] In addition, circulating noradrenaline has aroused interest as a cause of local vasodilatation.[47,50] The effect of noradrenaline on the vein wall is somewhat paradoxical. It acts as a vasodilator intraluminally and therefore may contribute to turbulence, but it also serves as a contractile stimulant to the muscle fibers in the vein wall. Therefore a distinction must be made between the last two factors. Noradrenaline may be advanced as a primary factor because it is considered to have its vasodilator effect on a normal vein wall, whereas turbulence, even without the mediation of noradrenaline, would presumably be effective on a vein wall that has already undergone pathologic change. The total noradrenaline effect provides a composite stimulus that produces a response in accordance with local needs. Kline and Byrne[51] have suggested turbulence as a physical cause of varicosity because of the relationship of early dilatation to a valve either immediately proximal to or distal to dilatation where turbulence is most pronounced. Turbulence may act physically or through local production of noradrenaline. These factors must be considered, but their relevance to the development of varicose veins has not yet been accurately identified.

Evidence suggests that the basic lesion is located in the muscle cell in the vein wall, but further investigation is necessary, particularly into the activity of various types of collagen, collagenase, elastin, elastase, and the relationship of these substances to the sex hormones.

SUMMARY

The common point of physical, hormonal, and enzyme changes described here is loss of vein wall tone followed by increased distensibility.[8] The vein then begins to dilate locally. The dilatation may remain as a local blowout, but if it extends to valve sphincter level, the vein commissure separates. When this change takes place, secondary valvular incompetence develops. When the valve allows reflux to occur, the already weakened vein distends further and the varicose vein either enlarges or appears clinically for the first time. Eventually, a functionless valve may undergo disuse atrophy, but it is capable of persisting for a long time.

The valve–vein wall argument is summarized by a diagram produced by Edwards and Edwards[52] in 1940. This diagram often has been reproduced without the full caption and used incorrectly to illustrate primary valvular failure as the cause of varicose veins. In fact, the full caption shows it was intended to convey the opposite. Dilatation of the valve ring, not valvular atrophy, is clearly identified as the cause of valvular incompetence (Figure 2-20).

It seems that the solution to this basic problem lies in a study of normal and abnormal metabolic activity of the enzyme-hormone complex in the muscle cell of the vein wall. If this activity is understood, it may be possible to control the tendency to varicosities in susceptible individuals and either limit the extension of the condition or minimize postoperative recurrence. The widespread occurrence of varicose veins and their potential to cause disability justify investigations or modifications of treatment that may contribute to their prevention.

■　■　■

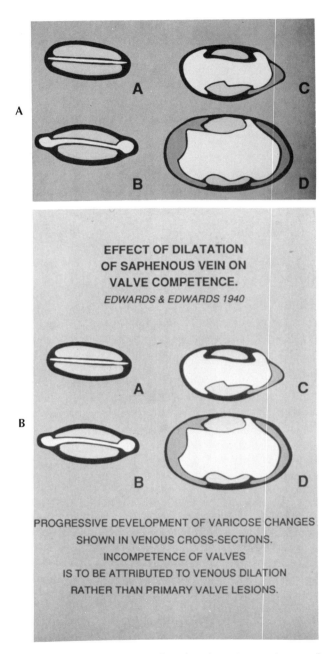

FIGURE 2-20. A, This diagram is often reproduced without its caption, as shown here. Without its caption, the diagram suggests support of the primary valve failure theory. **B,** Full caption shows that the diagram was intended to convey the opposite—that dilatation of the valve ring, *not* valve atrophy, should be identified as the cause of valvular incompetence.

Secondary varicose veins are those that follow an attack of phlebitis. In an attack of moderate severity the affected portion of vein wall and any contained valve are involved in a process of occlusion by thrombosis, fibrosis with organization of the clot, and recanalization, resulting in venous dilatation in all but the smallest veins. If the affected vein is superficial, it is clinically obvious, but if it is deep, the degree of superficial varicosity that follows depends on the degree of deep venous reflux or persisting obstruction. When the wall of a deep perforating vein is involved in the process and its protecting valve is destroyed, a superficial varicosity may result. The majority of varicose veins, however, occur in the absence of a history of deep phlebitis, and less than half the cases of deep phlebitis develop superficial varicosities. Possibly this is because the presence of genetic factors also is required. Therefore it is possible that primary and secondary varicose veins have something in common if it is postulated that varicose veins that develop after deep phlebitis do so only in the presence of genetic factors.

REFERENCES

1. Harvey W. De Motu Cordis, 1628.
2. Fabricius H. De Venarum Ostiolis, 1603.
3. Malpighi M. Opera Omnia [1687]. Bethesda, Md.: National Library of Medicine.
4. Nicholson BB. Varicose veins: Etiology and treatment. Arch Surg 15:351-376, 1927.
5. Zancani A. Über die Varicen der unteren Extremitäten: Experimentelle und klinische Untersuchungen. Arch Klin Chir 96:91, 1911.
6. Gottlob R, May R. The Venous Valve. Berlin: Springer Verlag, 1988.
7. Ackroyd JS, Pattison M, Browse NL. A study of the mechanical properties of fresh and preserved human femoral vein wall and valve cusps. Br J Surg 72:117-119, 1985.
8. Thulesius O, Gjöres JE. Valvular function and venous distensibility. In Negus D, Jantet G, eds. Phlebology 85. London: John Libbey, 1986, pp 26-28.
9. Franklin KJ. The valves in veins. An historical survey. Proc R Soc Med 21:1-33, 1927.
10. Butterworth DM, Rose SS, Clark P, et al. Light microscopy, immunohistochemistry, and electron microscopy of the valves of lower-limb veins and jugular veins. Phlebology 7:27-30, 1992.
11. Rose SS, Mashiah A. The scanning electron microscope in the pathology of varicose veins. Isr J Med Sci 27:202-205, 1991.
12. Sappey R. Traite d'Anatomie, 1869.
13. Kistner RL. Primary venous valve incompetence in the leg. Am J Surg 140:218-224, 1980.
14. Leu HJ. Morphological alteration of non-varicose and varicose veins. A morphological contribution to the discussion on the pathogenesis of varicose vein. Basic Res Cardiol 4:435-444, 1979.
15. Rose SS, Ahmed A. Some new thoughts on the aetiology of varicose veins. Int J Cardiovasc Surg 27:584-593, 1985.
16. Klotz K. Destruction of valves in senile patient without development of varicosities. Arch Anat Physiol Leipzig 1:159, 1888.
17. Eger SA, Casper SL. Aetiology of varicose veins from an anatomic aspect based on dissections of 38 adult cadavers. JAMA 123:148, 1943.
18. King ESJ. Genesis of varicose veins. Aust N Z J Surg 20:126, 1950.
19. Ludbrook J. Valvular defect in primary varicose veins—Cause or effect. Lancet 2:1289, 1963.
20. Bordeu M. Recherches sur les Maladies Chronique. Paris: Presse Médicale, 1775.
21. Briquet P. Trunk, tributaries, tertiaries and telangiectases. Paris: These de Paris, 1824.
22. Colles A. Lectures on the Theory and Practice of Surgery, Bristol, 1844.
23. Brodie B. Lectures on Pathology and Surgery. London, 1846.

24. Gay J. On Varicose Disease of the Lower Extremities. The Lettsomian Lectures of 1867. London: Churchill, 1868.
25. Kosinski CJ. Observations on the superficial venous system of the lower extremity. J Anat 60: 131, 1926.
26. Turner-Warwick W. The Rational Treatment of Varicose Veins and Varicocoele. London: Faber & Faber, 1931.
27. Linton RR. The communicating veins of the lower leg and the operative technique for their ligation. Ann Surg 107:582, 1938.
28. Myers TT, Cooley JC. Varicose vein surgery in the management of the postthrombotic limb. Surg Gynecol Obstet 99:733, 1954.
29. Dodd HJ, Cockett FB. The Pathology and Surgery of the Veins of the Lower Limb, 2nd ed. Edinburgh: Churchill Livingstone, 1976.
30. Schalin L. Arteriovenous communications to varicose veins in the lower extremities studied by dynamic radiography. Acta Chir Scand 146:397-406, 1980.
31. Haeger K. Practical anatomy. In Haeger K, ed. Venous and Lymphatic Disorders of the Leg. Lund: Scandinavian University Books, 1966.
32. Pflug J, Daintree Johnson H. In Proceedings of American-European Symposium on Venous Diseases, pp 56-57. Foundation for International Cooperation in Medical Sciences, 1974.
33. Bjordal R. Circulation patterns in incompetent perforating veins in the calf and in the saphenous system in primary varicose veins. Acta Chir Scand 138:251, 1972.
34. Pigeaux. Maladies des Vaisseaux. A Treatise. Paris, 1843.
35. Wolf G. Praxis 36:41, 1941.
36. Blalock A. Oxygen content of blood in patients with varicose veins. Arch Surg 19:898-905, 1929.
37. Haimovici H. Arteriovenous shunting in varicose veins. J Vasc Surg 2:684, 1985.
38. de Takats G, Quint H, Tillotson BI, Crittenden PJ. Carbon dioxide and oxygen levels in varicose veins. Arch Surg 18:671, 1929.
39. Haeger K. Hot spots, perforating veins and thermography. Triangle 8:18, 1967.
40. Nylander G. Meanders of the great saphenous vein. Angiology 20:587-592, 1969.
41. Cotton LT. Gross anatomy and development of varicose veins. Br J Surg 48:589, 1961.
42. Zwillenberg LO, Lanzt L, Zwillenberg H. Possible influence of smooth muscle on collagen. Angiologia 8:318-346, 1971.
43. Svejcar J, Prerovsky I, Linhart J, Kruml J. Content of collagen, elastin and water in walls of the internal saphenous vein. Clin Res 1:296, 1962.
44. Svejcar J, Prerovsky I, Linhart J, Kruml J. Collagen, elastin and hexosamine in primary varicose veins. Clin Sci 24:325, 1963.
45. Jurukova Z, Milenkov C. Ultrastructural evidence for collagen degradation in the walls of varicose veins. Exp Mol Pathol 37:37-47, 1982.
46. Staubesand J. Intracellular collagen in smooth muscle. Beitr Pathol 1:187-193, 1977.
47. Vanhoutte PM, Shepherd JT. Adrenergic pharmacology of human and canine peripheral veins. Fed Proc 44:37, 1985.
48. Niebes P, Berson I. Determination of Enzymes and Degradation. London: Churchill Livingstone, 1976, p 35.
49. Woolley DE. On the sequential changes in the level of estradiol and progesterone during pregnancy and parturition and collagenolytic activity. In Piez KA, Reddi AH, eds. Extracellular Matrix Biochemistry. New York: Elsevier Science Publishing, 1984, p 138.
50. Crotty TP. Noradrenalin as an inducer of varicosities in the dog vein. J Med Sci 157:166, 1988.
51. Kline AL, Byrne P. Turbulence as a factor in the aetiology of varicose veins. Br J Surg 59:915, 1972.
52. Edwards JE, Edwards EA. The saphenous valves in varicose veins. Am Heart J 19:338, 1940.

Editor's Note

This chapter, which summarizes existing knowledge on the development of varicose veins, is valuable for its completeness. It discusses two conflicting hypotheses about the cause of varicose veins. The first is that valve failure precedes the varicosis, and the second is that a defect in vein wall strength allows venous dilatation. Thulesius[1] summarized these hypotheses, saying that "endothelial damage and dysfunction, weakness of the venous wall leading to distention and reflux" lead to varicosities. Although these two supposedly conflicting theories have dominated past thinking, presently it is possible to link them under observations made directly. One uniform observation in the study of varicose veins has been a decrease in number of functioning valves in the saphenous vein in individuals who have venous varicosities.[2] Cotton[3] recognized this fact nearly 40 years ago, saying, "There are clearly fewer valves in varicose veins than in normal valves but the reduction in the number of valves is unrelated to any of the effects of aging." Others have confirmed Cotton's work more recently.[4] Sales et al.[5] believe that the deficiency in number of valves is the cause of varicosities.

As documentation of the decreased number of valves in refluxing saphenous veins has been accompanied by actual valvular damage,[6] we have taken a different point of view,[7] linking valve destruction to leukocyte infiltration. These observations of infiltration by monocytes into venous valves and venous wall would unify the concept of developing varicose veins into simultaneous destruction of valves and production of vein wall weakness.

REFERENCES

1. Thulesius O. The venous wall and valvular function in chronic venous insufficiency. Int Angiol 15:119-123, 1996.
2. Gradman WS, Segalowitz J, Grundfest W. Venoscopy in varicose vein surgery: Initial experience. Phlebology 8:145-150, 1993.
3. Cotton LT. Varicose veins: Gross anatomy and development. Br J Surg 48:589-598, 1961.
4. Ortega F, Mompeo B, Sarmiento L, et al. Comparison of saphenous veins removed for primary venous insufficiency with cadaver saphenous veins. Vasc Surg 31:663-670, 1997.
5. Sales CM, Rosenthal D, Petrillo KA, et al. The valvular apparatus in venous insufficiency: A problem of quantity? Ann Vasc Surg 12:153-155, 1998.
6. Hoshino S, Satokawa H, Ono T, Igari T. Surgical treatment for varicose veins of the legs using intraoperative angioscopy. In Raymond-Martimbeau P, Prescott R, Zummo M, eds. Phlebologie 92. Paris: John Libbey Eurotext, 1992, pp 1083-1085.
7. Ono T, Bergan JJ, Schmid-Schönbein GW, Takase S. Monocyte infiltration into venous valves. J Vasc Surg 27:158-166, 1998.

Chapter 3

Pathogenesis of Varicose Veins and Chronic Venous Insufficiency Syndrome

Philip D. Coleridge Smith and John H. Scurr

Venous disease has been recognized since the time of the Papyrus of Ebers (c. 3500 BC), and yet the pathogenesis of its most common manifestation, varicose veins, and its most tiresome one, venous ulceration, are incompletely understood. A number of hypotheses have been advanced to explain the mechanism by which varicose veins develop. These theories have been based largely on anatomic and pathologic studies of excised varicose veins or on investigation of anatomic structures in cadavers. Relatively few studies have tried to investigate the development of varicose veins by using functional methods of investigation, largely because until recently this approach necessitated phlebography. Phlebography is a highly invasive method to use for investigation of a benign condition. More recently histologic and immunohistologic methods have been used to investigate changes in the wall structure in varicose veins and some of the metabolic processes involved in the development of varices. Little research has been done with the newer methods of investigation that have become available in recent years to establish why varices develop. We have found few published electron microscopy studies of the valve cusps or the vein wall in venous disease. It seems that much of interest could be discovered in these areas, and yet venous disease is so mundane that it has become unattractive as a subject for research.

DEVELOPMENT OF VARICOSE VEINS

It has been suggested that varicose veins may develop from valve failure caused by increased venous pressure resulting from the lack of valves above the saphenofemoral junction.[1] The upright posture of humans has been suggested as the principal cause of increased pressure, which results in valve failure.[2] Some authors have concluded that the primary problem is a failure of more proximal valves, which is succeeded in turn by incompetence of more distal valves. Others have suggested that the reverse process takes place, with valvular incompetence developing distally and moving proximally.[3]

Trendelenburg[4] was the first to suggest that the failure of proximal valves results in incompetence more distally. He suggested that ligation of the proximal part of the saphenous vein would protect the distal segments. Unfortunately, the results of surgery based on this assumption (proximal ligation of the long saphenous vein) alone reveal that there is a high rate of varicose vein recurrence.

Anatomic studies of the distribution of venous valves in the proximal, femoral, and iliac veins showed that in a proportion of subjects the valves are absent in the common and external iliac veins.[5,6] It was suggested that this situation may predispose the individual to the subsequent development of varicose veins because the hydrostatic pressure of blood resting on the valves below the iliac segment would be increased. Basmajian,[7] in his series of 100 cadaveric dissections, demonstrated that in one limb with long saphenous varicosities and two limbs with short saphenous varicosities competent valves were noted above the entry of these veins into the deep veins. In addition, no varices were found in 40 limbs where there was no valve above the saphenofemoral junction. Clearly the presence or absence of valves in the proximal venous system does not influence the subsequent formation of distal varices.

One possibility in establishing whether or not the sequence of destruction of valves is from proximal to distal is to compare patients with severe and mild varicose veins to determine whether or not long saphenous incompetence precedes incompetence and varicosity of the side branches. Such a comparison has been done by Ludbrook,[8] who used foot vein pressures to judge the severity of the venous incompetence. He was able to show no difference between the severity of valvular incompetence in the groups with mild and severe varicosity, and he concluded that long saphenous vein incompetence might well precede worsening varices in the side branches. There are other possible interpretations of Ludbrook's data, and the matter has been investigated by other authors.

Folse[9] investigated a series of patients with varicose veins by using Doppler ultrasound. He demonstrated venous reflux in the common femoral vein in many of these patients and concluded that varices were likely to be a consequence of descending valve failure. In a few patients Folse found competent proximal saphenous veins with varices arising from a midthigh perforating vein. He concluded that the theories of Fegan and Kline[3] on distal-to-proximal progression of varicosities were incorrect. Folse's reliance on continuous-wave Doppler ultrasound means that he could not be certain that he was insonating the femoral vein; therefore his conclusions must be regarded with caution. In contrast, Rose and Ahmed[10] investigated a series of 300 cases with Doppler ultrasound and preoperative examination and found that 63% of varicosities of the long saphenous vein occurred below a competent saphenofemoral junction. This finding tends to suggest that proximal competence is irrelevant in the development of varices.

The suggestion by Fegan and Kline[3] that valvular incompetence may arise distally and progress proximally is based on the investigation of patients undergoing sclerotherapy for varicose veins. These authors suggested that varicosities appeared first in the branches of the distal long saphenous vein (e.g., in the calf) and then incompetence progressed more proximally. Fegan and Kline used both clinical and Doppler ultrasound examination. They also suggested that appropriate management of distal varices, such as the use of injection sclerotherapy, might restore the competence of proximal valves, as determined by measurements from a tourniquet test. Chant et al.[11] have reported that treatment of distal varices through injection sclerotherapy results in a radiologically demonstrated reduction in diameter of the proximal long saphenous vein. They concluded that saphenofemoral incompetence is a consequence of distal varicosities rather than the cause.

The study of Basmajian[7] suggests that it is unlikely that varicose veins are a consequence of an absence of proximal valves in the iliac or femoral veins. The observations of Rose and Ahmed,[10] Chant et al.,[11] and Fegan and Kline,[3] who used different methods of investigation, imply that distal disease may well determine the severity of proximal venous incompetence. This particular point has not been addressed in any recent study. It should now be possible, through duplex ultrasound imaging, to obtain substantially greater information about the competence or incompetence of distal veins and associated varices.

Calf Perforating Veins: Cause or Effect?

Cockett and Elgan Jones[12] described large perforating veins of the medial calf and their association with overlying varicosities and ulceration. These authors placed considerable emphasis on the treatment of venous ulcers by ligation of these vessels. They complained that these perforating veins were not described in anatomy texts of the time. Our experience with duplex ultrasound imaging suggests that perforating veins tend to be of small diameter (1 to 2 mm) in normal limbs but to increase in size in patients with venous disease. To us the causal association deduced by Cockett is not so obvious; in addition, since the efficacy of perforator ligation in healing ulcers was not rigorously tested by him in a clinical trial, Cockett's assertions must be viewed with care. Subsequent investigation of this problem has resulted in mixed findings, with some authors reporting efficacy[13] but objective studies showing no substantial benefit.[14,15] The authors of a recent study involving functional methods of assessment found it necessary to include both local deep vein incompetence in the calf and calf perforator incompetence in their model of pathogenesis.[16] The precise role of calf perforating veins in the pathogenesis of varicose veins and venous ulceration remains to be fully elucidated. Our own work[17] suggests that the direction of blood flow in these vessels is highly dependent on disease in other veins, with inward or outward flow observed depending on the perturbation of blood flow in other vessels.

Varicose Veins: Vein Wall or Valve Problem?

An alternative explanation for the development of varicose veins is defective structure of the vein wall. King,[18] in an article published in 1950, pointed out that in varicose veins the early swelling of the vein is distal, not proximal, to the valve so that hydrostatic pressure from above the valve is unlikely to be the explanation. He also noted that histologic examination of the vein wall in the early stages of varicosis shows a thickening hypertrophy of the muscle coat and increased vascularity of the adventitia. King suggested that these observations might be attributed to local abnormality of blood flow induced by a chemical stimulus, possibly of hormonal nature. It is apparent that King's observations implied a disease affecting the vein wall that eventually results in loss of mechanical integrity of the wall and dilatation of the vessel with incompetence of its valves.

The question of whether or not vein wall distention is the first stage of the varicosity or occurs as a consequence of valve failure is critical to the pathogenesis. This issue has been studied by Cotton,[19] who also investigated the relationship of varicosities and dilatations of the vein wall to the valves contained within the veins. He investigated veins that were removed at operation and venograms of patients with varicosities. Cotton demonstrated that varicosities usually occurred more distally to the valve, which, in keeping with King's observations, suggests that a failure in the valve wall may precede disruption of a valve itself.

The nature of the failure of the vein wall may be related to a problem with the regulation of the connective tissues. Unfortunately, the biochemistry of the regulation of connective tissues is incompletely understood even today. However, the collagen, elastin, and hexosamine content of the vein wall was investigated in 1962 by Svejcar et al.[20] The principal findings were that the collagen content was significantly lower in varicose veins and potential varicose veins than in normal veins and that varicose veins contain relatively more muscle than normal veins do. Also, the hexosamine content was significantly higher in actual and potential varicose veins than in normal veins, and there was a much greater variation of water and hexosamine content in different segments of varicose veins when compared with the content of different segments of normal veins. Svejcar et al. suggested that the results of their investigation might indicate an inherited anomaly of collagen metabolism. The reliability of these data is open to question because the date of this investigation precedes that of modern monoclonal antibodies; the analyses of Svejcar et al. were made by using biochemical assays. In addition, many different types of collagen that are now recognized were not assessed separately in this study. However, further investigations were carried out by Andreotti et al.,[21] which suggested that there were reduced amounts of collagen and elastin in varicose veins compared with controls.

Subsequently, Haardt[22] investigated the metabolism of the vein wall through monoclonal staining for enzymes. He investigated localization of lactate dehydrogenase, alkaline phosphatase, adenosine, triphosphatase, lysosomal enzymes, beta-glucuronidase, nonspecific esterase, and acid phosphatase. Haardt was able to show an increase in the amount of lysosomal enzyme activity in the varicose veins compared with that of normal veins, with the increase being greater in the media than in the intima. In general, he showed a decline in the activity of the enzymes responsible for energy metabolism in varicose veins, and he suggested that this decrease might be accompanied by a decline in the contractility of the vein wall. Haardt thought that the increase in lysosomal enzymes would reflect the change in collagen with thickening and fibrillation of the individual fibers. It is unclear whether these changes are a cause or a consequence of the varicose process.

More recently Obitsu et al.[23] examined normal and varicose veins with light and transmission electron microscopy. They concluded that valve failure started with depression of the commissure of the valve and involved subsequent expansion of the space between the valve cusps. In this study elongation of the cusps with bulbous thickening of the free-edge cusp was noted. Hyperplasia of the collagen fibers of the valve cusps was also found, but the authors suggested that this finding was a secondary change in response to increased venous pressure.

Histologic Examination

The most prominent change noted on histologic examination is an increase in fibrous tissue, which invades the media and divides the smooth muscle layers into a number of separate bundles. Collagen and fibrous tissue also accumulate in the subintima, and elastic fibers spread throughout the layers of the vein wall, instead of being restricted to the internal and external elastic laminae. All these changes have a patchy distribution. Electron microscopy of smooth muscle cells (SMCs) shows that they contain collagen fibers, which suggests that the SMC has taken on phagocytic properties. The muscle cells are separated from one another by a considerable increase in fibrous tissue, which suggests that the muscle cells are being replaced by fibrous tissue.

Immunohistochemical Study of Vein Wall Components

A detailed immunohistologic study of eight varicose saphenous vein samples and four normal controls was carried out in 1987,[24] when a search for the infiltrating "immune competent" cells in the vessel wall was made. Few infiltrating cells were found, but those present were tissue macrophages carrying the FCR1 receptor. More modern monoclonal antibodies may have revealed a greater influx of inflammatory cells. The most surprising finding was the appearance of class II major histocompatibility antigens on the endothelium, macrophages, and SMCs of the thickened tunica media. Up-regulation of human lymphocyte antigen, HLA-D/DR, was present in all three cell types, but there was preferential up-regulation of HLA-D/DQ in the SMCs. The function of the class II locus is to present processed antigens to T cells that are induced by interferon gamma (IFN-gamma) and tumor necrosis factor alpha (TNFα). At this site D/DQ is probably involved in the maintenance of a chronic inflammatory process. This involvement is almost certainly secondary to the disease process, but the site of D/DQ expression within the thickened media of the vessel suggests a possible active role in the pathology of the disorder.

Chemical Changes in Vein Wall

Plasminogen activator is reduced in varicose veins in comparison with control subjects.[25,26] The reason for this reduction is unclear, although it may be simply associated with the inflammatory process of the varicose veins or it may be related to the development of varicosities. It has been shown that the fibrinolytic processes are down-regulated in varicose veins excised from limbs with lipodermatosclerotic skin.

The research carried out so far suggests that abnormalities are present in both the vein wall and the valve cusps, but the order in which these abnormalities occur is unclear from these investigations. Our findings in color flow–mapped duplex ultrasound suggest that early valve failure is characterized by a small-diameter, high-velocity jet of blood flowing through valve orifices. This activity has been observed in undilated veins, but more rigorous study is necessary to establish the complete pathogenesis of venous valvular failure. One possibility is that turbulent blood flow, which has a substantial effect on the endothelial cells, may result in changes in the metabolism of the endothelial cells, which then produce tissue growth factors. Certainly varicose veins may develop downstream from an arteriovenous fistula.[27] High-velocity retrograde flow through a valve results in turbulent flow, with the overlying vein being subjected to severe turbulence. This force may result in distention of the valve in the region of the turbulent flow.

Effects of Blood Flow

Gius[28] has suggested that arteriovenous communications contribute to the pathogenesis of varicose veins, as did Piulachs and Vidal-Barraquer.[29] Gius based his findings on examination of vessels at operation combined with the histologic evidence of proliferating vessels obtained from the skin in some patients and the visual evidence that bright blood issues from varices at operation. Haimovici et al.,[30] using radiologic criteria, have also suggested that arteriovenous shunting has a role in the pathogenesis of varicose veins. However, subsequent investigation has failed to confirm the presence of such communications.

Etiologic Factors

Varicose veins may develop as a consequence of many factors, including age, sex, race, weight, height, pregnancy, diet, bowel habits, occupation, heredity, alcohol intake, clothing, and erect posture.

Varicose veins may occur at any age in adult life, but they appear to be more common with advancing years. A peak frequency between the ages of 50 and 60 years has been reported.[31] Large surveys have demonstrated that there is a female-to-male predominance of between 2:1 and 4:1 in the prevalence of varicose veins. These figures probably preclude the possibility that women present more frequently to their physicians for treatment of varicose veins.

Pregnancy. A number of studies have investigated the incidence of varicose veins developing during pregnancy. The incidence varies between 8% and 20%, depending on the study, and varicose veins appear to be more common in multiparous than in primiparous women.[32-34] The development of varicose veins during pregnancy may reflect the effect of estrogen and progesterone on the vein wall; alternatively, it has been suggested that compression of the iliac veins by the uterus may result in increased pressure in the lower veins.

Race. Foote[35] stated that varicose veins were uncommon in Africans, and Dodd[36] found only three cases of varicose veins in 11,000 inpatient admissions in a tribal reserve in Zululand. Burkitt has claimed that there may be a dietary link to this observation. He suggested that the high-fiber diets normally eaten by Africans resulted in relative ease of defecation and no rise in intra-abdominal pressure. Burkitt assumed that this diet was an important factor in the development of varicose veins, but his theory now seems doubtful.

Height and weight. The static foot vein pressure measured by manometry is undoubtedly related to the height of the subject. Therefore it has been suggested that tall subjects may be at greater risk for the development of varicose veins than shorter subjects. Widmer,[37] in a survey in Switzerland, found no association with height or weight. Myers[38] and Ludbrook[39] found that patients with varicose veins were heavier than age- and sex-matched controls without varicose veins. This association was not confirmed by Widmer in the Basel study.

Posture. The effect of posture on varicose veins has been investigated by a number of authors. In a study of department store employees, Lake et al.[40] found that 74% of employees who stood while working had varicose veins, compared with 57% who sat. Santler et al.[41] reviewed 2854 patients with varicose disease and found that 6.3% were required to walk in their occupation, 29.2% spent their time sitting, and 64.5% stood still at work. These data tend to suggest that occupations involving standing carry an increased risk of varicose veins.

Heredity. A large number of patients presenting with varicose veins recall having close relatives who also had varicose veins. However, since the prevalence of the condition is so high in Western countries, it is not surprising to find such a phenomenon. A number of studies have investigated the association between varicose veins in relatives. It has been shown that between 50% and 75% of the relatives of a person with varicose veins also may be affected by varicosities. In 1969 a study by Gunderson and Hauge[42] found that 43% of the relatives of the women and 19% of the relatives of the men had varicose veins. These figures are far higher than would be expected from the prevalence of the disease determined through epidemiologic studies. However, they are somewhat lower than would be expected if the inheritance were of a truly dominant nature. We conclude that the inheritance of varicose veins is polygenic.

■ ■ ■

The preceding data show that the question of how varicose veins develop is still unanswered. It is unlikely that the cause of this problem is related to the anatomic distribution of valves in the proximal venous system, and pressure effects alone are not the explanation. Distention of the vein at or below the level of the cusp may lead to valvular incompetence, or the valvular incompetence may precede and initiate distal distention of the vein. Insufficient data are available to decide which is the case. Both inherited and environmental factors are important in the pathogenesis of varicose veins, although the contribution of each to the disease awaits a full understanding of the processes that result in varicosities. We are impressed with how little is known of the pathologic mechanisms in this disease.

PATHOGENESIS OF VENOUS ULCERATION

Venous ulceration occurs when the muscle pumping mechanisms of the leg are impaired because of disease in the superficial or deep venous systems.[43] This condition may be simply a consequence of varicose veins, which account for 20% to 50% of venous leg ulcers,[44,45] or it may result from incompetence of the valves of the deep veins. Venous ulceration may arise from a previous deep vein thrombosis, or it may be caused by primary valve failure in a manner similar to that which results in incompetence of the superficial veins in patients with varicose veins.[46] The consequence of incompetent lower limb vein valves is that the pumping mechanism no longer reduces the pressure in the veins to low levels during walking. A cannula placed in the dorsal foot vein usually shows a reduction of the resting pressure from 80 to 100 mm Hg to 10 to 20 mm Hg in a physically fit person. Patients with severe calf muscle pump impairment may not be able to reduce the foot vein pressure below the resting level[47] (Figure 3-1). The presence of substantial venous reflux will result in rapid refilling of the veins of the calf after exercise, which is shown as a rapid rise in foot vein pressure after the end of exercise. These two components of foot venous pressure trace have been combined in a single term by some authors to facilitate analysis of the severity of venous impairment. A number of indexes of venous function have been described.[48-50] These

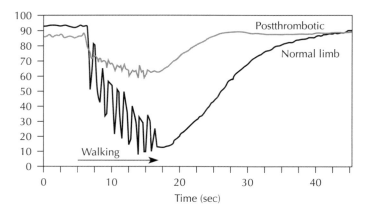

FIGURE 3-1. Ambulatory venous hypertension. This recording shows traces from a patient who had suffered a previous venous thrombosis in one limb. In the affected limb the ambulatory venous pressure is high and the refilling time is short.

indexes give an indication of the magnitude of the problem, but some patients seem to tolerate severe muscle pump impairment without ulceration and others suffer ulcers of the leg with only moderate venous impairment. Clearly, other factors are important in the pathogenesis of this disease, but what leads to increased or decreased susceptibility to ulcers of the leg remains unclear. Hypotheses have been proposed since the Middles Ages, but recently they have revolved around the theory that ulceration is attributable to skin hypoxia.[51]

Mechanisms of Ulceration

Homans[52] suggested that ulceration of the skin overlying large varicosities was caused by low oxygen levels in the stagnant blood of the varicosities, resulting in hypoxia of the skin. The oxygenation of blood in varicose veins has been the subject of several subsequent studies.[53,54] It is now clear that with the patient in a supine position the hemoglobin oxygen saturation in varicose veins is greater than in normal veins. In the standing position no difference is noted between normal subjects and patients with varicose veins. Therefore, even if venous blood were responsible for nutrition of the skin, there would be no difference in hemoglobin oxygen saturation between normal subjects and those with varicose veins.[55] Increased venous oxygen tension in patients with venous disease has led to the suggestion by some that arteriovenous fistulas were present, possibly depriving the skin of oxygen.[56,57] Research with microspheres and macroaggregates has failed to demonstrate an increase in arteriovenous shunting in the skin of patients with venous disease.[58]

Fibrin cuff theory. In 1982 Browse and Burnand[59] proposed that oxygen diffusion into cutaneous tissue was restricted by a pericapillary fibrin cuff, which they had observed histologically. They suggested that increased capillary pressure resulting from the elevated venous pressure produces an increased loss of plasma proteins through the capillary wall. This loss includes fibrinogen, which polymerizes to provide the "fibrin cuff" that can be seen around capillaries by both histochemical and immunohistochemical methods. Measurements of protein loss from capillaries by Browse and Burnand showed that fibrinogen was quantitatively the most important plasma protein leaking into tissue in patients with venous disease. Subsequent measurements of fibrinolysis have shown that patients with venous disease have reduced fibrinolytic activity in the blood and veins, which might explain why the fibrin cuff theory persists.[60]

The fibrin cuff theory has tended to perpetuate the suggestions of previous authors that the nature of venous ulceration is related to oxygen deprivation in tissues. Surprisingly, however, it is difficult to find satisfactory evidence that the skin and subcutaneous tissues are hypoxic in liposclerotic skin. There is no published evidence to prove that fibrin provides a barrier to oxygen diffusion. It seems probable from the composition of other human connective tissue that such a fibrin gel would comprise much water with a small amount of fibrin. Diffusion of small molecules through such a cuff might be expected to be similar to that of water in other human tissue. If the assumption is made that the fibrin layer contains

0.5% fibrin, similar to that of a fibrin blood clot, calculations reveal no impairment of oxygen delivery to the tissue. Even a cuff consisting of 100 times more fibrin than this would result in a reduction of oxygen delivery of only 50%.[61] The results of these calculations have not been confirmed by measurement. Browse and Burnand[59] employed a piece of commercial bovine fibrin from a suture manufacturer to assess the permeability of fibrin. They found that this material significantly impeded the passage of oxygen. It is unlikely that fibrin cuffs seen in humans are of the same composition.

The evidence advanced to support the assertion that the skin is hypoxic comes from data obtained by transcutaneous oximetry.[62,63] A Clark-type electrode equipped with an integral heater is applied to the skin to register oxygen availability at the skin surface. Such a device was originally designed for neonatal monitoring, in which skin heating was used so the resulting vasodilation would ensure that the measurement accurately reflected the arterial oxygen tension. In venous disease different findings have been obtained, depending on whether the transducer is heated to 43° or 37° C. At the higher temperatures used by most authors, it has been found that patients with venous disease tend to have lower transcutaneous oxygen tension ($tcPO_2$) readings than normal subjects (Figure 3-2). Measurements made with an electrode temperature of 37° C are even more paradoxical.[64] Under these circumstances the oxygenation of the skin is greater in patients with venous disease than in normal subjects. This technique has a number of limitations, and $tcPO_2$ may be influenced by many factors other than skin oxygenation.

Direct measurement of skin oxygen tension would be the most satisfactory method of investigation if it were not fraught with technical difficulties. For example, it would be necessary to advance a microelectrode through the skin and

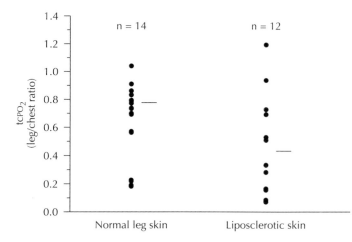

FIGURE 3-2. Reduced transcutaneous oxygen pressure ($tcPO_2$) of the leg skin in venous disease. These measurements were made at The Middlesex Hospital Vascular Laboratory. The results are expressed as the ratio of leg $tcPO_2$ to chest wall $tcPO_2$.

measure oxygen tension by polarography or one of the more recent fiberoptic methods that involve dye phosphorescence quenching. It is debatable whether this approach could be considered a reasonable investigation in skin prone to ulceration, but it is certainly within the capabilities of modern technology.

Consequently, some authors have tried to assess gas exchange in the skin microcirculation by alternative methods. Hopkins et al.[65] used positron emission tomography techniques to assess blood flow and oxygen extraction in the skin and subcutaneous tissue of patients with venous disease. He showed that the oxygen extraction ratio was reduced in such tissues but that cutaneous blood flow was increased by a substantial amount. Therefore it is unclear from these measurements whether oxygen delivery was increased or decreased.

We have measured the clearance of xenon 133 from the skin to assess the efficiency of the microcirculation in handling a molecule of similar size to oxygen. This gas has a molecular weight four times that of oxygen; therefore its diffusion rate would be half that of oxygen (if it is assumed that the solubility of oxygen and xenon in body fluids [water] is similar). We used Sjerson's technique,[66] in which the xenon gas is applied topically to the skin and diffuses through the skin to reach the dermis and subcutaneous fat readily. This method avoids direct injection of solutions of xenon, which might alter blood flow in the skin. Measurements were made in the liposclerotic skin of patients with venous disease and compared to those of control subjects under conditions of reactive hyperemia after 5 minutes of cuff occlusion of the arterial supply to the leg. No difference in xenon clearance was found between patients with venous disease and control subjects.[67] This finding was a considerable surprise to us and led us to assess further measurement of gas exchange in the skin.

The rate of recovery of the tcPO$_2$ after a period in which arterial blood supply has been interrupted is another measurement that may be used to determine whether a diffusion barrier to delivery of oxygen to the tissues exists. We measured the time taken for reoxygenation of the skin after a period of ischemia produced by inflating a leg cuff above systolic arterial pressure for 5 minutes. No difference was found between the control group and the venous disease group.[68] These results have led us to conclude that in patients with chronic venous insufficiency (CVI) it is unlikely that there is a substantial abnormality in the delivery of oxygen to tissues. Unfortunately, until a satisfactory method of measuring skin oxygenation in patients with venous disease is developed, it will not be possible to answer this question completely. The possibility remains that some elements in the skin may receive insufficient nutrition, which renders them susceptible to injury by mechanical or other factors.

White cell trapping theory. The search for alternative mechanisms of skin damage in venous disease has resulted in investigation of the blood itself. Moyses et al.[69] studied the limbs of normal subjects in response to increased venous pressure and measured hematologic parameters to assess the effect of venous hypertension. Their subjects sat on a bicycle saddle without moving and with their limbs dependent for 40 minutes. Blood samples were taken from the long saphenous vein at the ankle. Moyses et al. found that the hematocrit level and the red

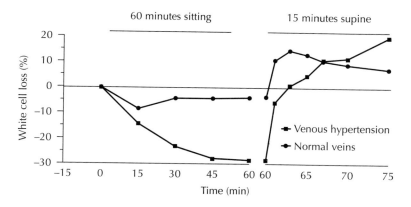

FIGURE 3-3. White cell trapping in patients compared to controls. (Modified from Scott HJ, Mc-Mullin GM, Coleridge Smith PD, Scurr JH. Venous ulceration and the role of the white blood cell. J Med Sci Tech 14:184-187, 1990.)

cell count increased in parallel, as expected. The white cell count remained unchanged, despite the increased hematocrit level. White cells were being "lost" from the circulation, which after 40 minutes amounted to a 25% change. Thomas et al.[70] performed a similar study in which they compared patients with normal lower limbs with patients with venous disease that resulted in lipodermatosclerosis and ulceration (Figure 3-3). Their patients were permitted to sit with their legs dependent, a less stringent requirement than that of Moyses. Blood sampling was again done from the long saphenous vein at the ankle. After 60 minutes the patients with venous disease were "trapping" 30% of the white cells and the control subjects were trapping 7%. This led us to examine the microcirculation through capillary microscopy. We found that venous hypertension appeared to reduce the number of visible capillary loops in patients with venous disease but not in control subjects,[71] which suggested that capillary damage may be occurring during venous hypertension.

Bollinger et al.[72] investigated the events in venous disease through fluorescence capillary videomicroscopy. They measured the rate of diffusion of fluorescein out of capillaries after an intravenous injection. These authors showed that in venous disease capillaries are much more permeable to this molecule than in normal veins, contrary to the suggestions made in the fibrin cuff hypothesis. Using fluorescence and light capillary microscopy simultaneously, Franzeck et al.[73] described the appearance of capillary loops, which were filled with red blood cells (RBCs) but did not appear to be perfused. They suggested that this appearance may be due to capillary "thrombosis."

White cell margination is a normal event in the arterioles, capillaries, and venules. This phenomenon is thought to be important in the mechanism that results in tissue injury following ischemia. White blood cells (WBCs) are substantially larger than RBCs and are responsible for many of the rheologic properties of blood. WBCs take 1000 times longer than RBCs to deform on entering a capillary bed, and they are responsible for about one half of the peripheral vascular

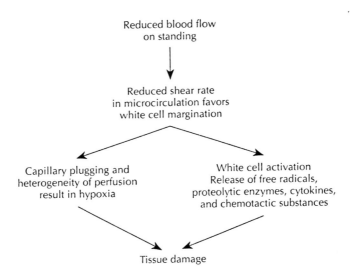

FIGURE 3-4. White cell "trapping" hypothesis. We now believe that if white cells cause occlusion of capillaries they probably do not cause local hypoxia. It seems more likely that the toxic products released by white cells are the mediators of tissue injury. (Modified from Coleridge Smith PD, Thomas P, Scurr JH, Dormandy JA. Causes of venous ulceration: A new hypothesis. BMJ 296:1726-1727, 1988.)

resistance, despite their small numbers in the circulation, compared to RBCs.[74] In myocardial infarction WBCs cause capillary occlusion, which can be prevented in experimental animals by first rendering the animal leukopenic.[75,76] WBCs have been implicated as the mediators of ischemia in many types of tissue, including myocardium, brain, lung, and kidneys.[77-80] Polymorphonuclear leukocytes, particularly those attached to capillary endothelium, may become "activated" when cytoplasmic granules containing proteolytic enzymes are released.[81] In addition, a nonmitochondrial "respiratory burst" permits these cells to release free radicals, including superoxide radicals, which have nonspecific destructive effects on lipid membranes, proteins, and many connective tissue compounds.[82] Leukocytotactic factors are also released, attracting more polymorphonuclear cells.

We published a hypothesis suggesting that white cell trapping resulted in neutrophil activation, causing damage to the tissues (Figure 3-4).[83] Based on the literature on myocardial ischemia, we proposed that WBCs might cause occlusion of capillaries, a suggestion originally made by Moyses.[69] If some of the capillaries were occluded, heterogeneous perfusion might result, causing tissue hypoxia and ischemia. This seemed to be a reasonable suggestion at the time, since it predated our attempts to measure the severity of the "diffusion block," and we included this factor in explaining the "hypoxia" observed by transcutaneous oximetry. Our conclusion from the data presented here is that tissue hypoxia is not the main cause of venous ulceration. In fact we have specifically investigated the response of the microcirculation to venous hypertension to determine whether this response causes degradation of microcirculatory function. Although we used laser Doppler fluxmetry and transcutaneous oximetry, we were unable to show any progressive microcirculatory deficit in patients with venous disease when they sat still with their lower limbs dependent for 30 minutes.[71] Subsequently we applied a more severe venous hypertensive insult to the normal circulation by placing a cuff around the leg and inflating it to 80 mm Hg for 15 minutes and measuring the hyperemic response. We were able to show a small reduction in microcirculatory function by this means, which suggests that microcirculatory injury may be produced in the short term (15 minutes) by increased venous pressure in the leg. Although white cell trapping occurs in the lower limb, it does not cause capillary occlusion to the extent that perfusion of the skin is impaired (this part of our original hypothesis was incorrect).

The second part of the theory suggested that white cell activation was part of the process, resulting in release of proteolytic enzymes, superoxide radicals, and chemotactic substances. All classes of WBCs appear to become trapped, so a wide range of phenomena is possible. Monocytes might become activated, releasing the cytokines interleukin-1 (IL-1) and TNFα.[84] These agents may produce many effects, including endothelial cell activation in which these metabolically active cells permit the passage of much larger molecules than would normally be possible.[85] Decreased fibrinolysis observed in patients with venous disease may be a result of the effects of IL-1.[86] IL-1 acts on endothelial cells to stimulate production of plasminogen activator inhibitor-1 (PAI-1) and decreases the production of tissue plasminogen activator (t-PA), producing a reduction in fibrinolysis.

To investigate the role of leukocytes in venous disease, we undertook a quantitative histologic study of skin from the limbs of patients with CVI and subjects with normal skin. Three groups of patients were studied. The first group included patients with no evidence of skin changes as a consequence of their venous disease. The next group exhibited lipodermatosclerosis without any ulceration of the limb. The third group had ulceration but were left with lipodermatosclerosis after healing of the ulcer.[87] Patients with normal skin had a low number of WBCs (4/mm^2) visible in the upper 0.5 mm of the skin. There were 8 times as many WBCs in patients with liposclerotic skin and 40 times as many in patients with healed venous ulcers. We have subsequently undertaken an immunohistologic study to determine the types of WBCs present in this infiltrate. The majority of cells are macrophages with a T-lymphocyte component but no excess of neutrophils compared with control sections taken from normal limbs. Therefore this infiltrate is a reflection of a chronic inflammatory process, which suggests that an investigation of the cell products of these leukocytes might indicate the mechanisms involved in venous ulceration. Using immunohistochemical methods, we have also been able to identify IL-1 as an inflammatory mediator in this process.

Leukocyte Activation

The effect of venous hypertension on leukocyte activation has been studied subsequently in our laboratory with a series of plasma and cellular markers. Control subjects exposed to lower limb venous hypertension produced by standing were studied by taking blood samples from hand and leg veins. Degranulation of neutrophils was studied by measuring plasma levels of neutrophil elastase (a primary neutrophil granule enzyme) and lactoferrin (a secondary neutrophil granule enzyme). After a 30-minute period of experimental venous hypertension, an increase in plasma lactoferrin concentration was observed in both the blood taken from the foot and from the arm.[88] When venous hypertension was produced by inflation of a cuff around one lower limb, a rise in lactoferrin was observed only in that limb. Subsequently expression of the surface neutrophil ligand, CD11b, has been investigated as a marker of neutrophil activation. The experiment was repeated as before on control subjects. Blood was taken from a dorsal foot vein. CD11b expression was assessed by fluorescent-labeled monoclonal antibody used to label neutrophils in whole blood that were counted by flow cytometry. During the period of ambulatory venous hypertension in control subjects, no rise in CD11b expression was seen in the lower limb blood.[89] Following return to the supine position, when neutrophils might be expected to leave the lower limb, according to the studies of Thomas et al.[70] increased levels of CD11b were observed. This increase indicates that neutrophils were up-regulated by their period of adhesion to normal endothelium. An increased white cell : red cell ratio was also observed during this phase, confirming white cell egress from the lower limb.

This study has also been conducted in patients with venous disease, including only subjects with nonulcerated skin to avoid the possibility that the inflammatory processes involved in the ulcer may result in up-regulation of inflammatory mediators in a way unrelated to the development of the ulcer. Two groups of patients were studied: one group with uncomplicated varicose veins and one with skin changes (lipodermatosclerosis) attributable to venous disease. The adhesion of neutrophils and monocytes to endothelium was investigated. This activity is a two-stage process. Initially these cells roll along the endothelium, binding in a loose manner, using a ligand on the leukocytes known as CD62L or L-selectin. When binding occurs, a fragment of L-selectin is released into the plasma (soluble L-selectin) and can be detected by ELISA. It was found that the concentration of soluble L-selectin increased during venous hypertension, confirming that endothelial : leukocyte binding had occurred. There was no major difference in magnitude between the two groups of patients.

Subsequently, firm binding of neutrophils and monocytes occurs with CD11b/CD18 ligands, which link to endothelial ICAM. This action is reflected in the peripheral blood by a decline in the cells expressing most CD11b (Figure 3-5). Such a decline was seen in the blood taken from the leg in both groups of patients. We had expected to see an egress of leukocytes expressing more CD11b in these patients when they returned to the supine position; however, in contrast to the studies on control subjects, this was not observed. In the time scale of this experiment (up to 10 minutes following venous hypertension), the more activated neutrophils and monocytes remained bound to the endothelium of the lower limb.

Plasma lactoferrin and elastase have been assessed in groups of patients with active venous disease. Blood was taken from the arm veins (not the lower limb veins) of patients with varicose veins, liposclerotic skin change, and active venous

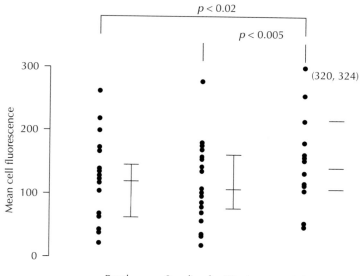

FIGURE 3-5. Neutrophil CD11b expression measured by flow cytometry in volunteers before and 10 minutes after a period of ambulatory venous hypertension produced by standing. Increased CD11b expression is noted on return to the supine position during the period of leukocyte efflux. Error bars show the median and interquartile range of data. Statistical significance was determined by the Mann-Whitney test.

ulceration.[90,91] In all samples the levels of lactoferrin and elastase were higher in the patients than in the age- and sex-matched control groups (Figures 3-6 and 3-7). However, it was found that the highest levels of plasma lactoferrin were present in patients with active varicose veins. Subsequently blood was taken from the arms of patients for measurement of neutrophil CD11b expression. This level was elevated in patients with varicose veins but depressed in patients with lipo-dermatosclerosis.[92] The explanation may be that the more active leukocytes are attracted to the region of the inflammatory process and do not circulate in the peripheral blood. Alternatively, such patients may have high circulating levels of neutrophil inhibitors.

Histology

The microcirculation of the skin has been investigated through histology[93] and capillary microscopy.[94] Both methods demonstrate capillary proliferation in patients with CVI: vast numbers of capillaries are visible by both techniques. However, capillary microscopy shows that these capillaries probably arise from a single capillary loop rather than from an increase in the numbers of capillaries, and appear as a glomerulus. Recent immunohistochemical investigations have shown that the pericapillary cuff contains far more than fibrin. The capillary endothelium is perturbed, expressing increased amounts of factor VIII–related anti-

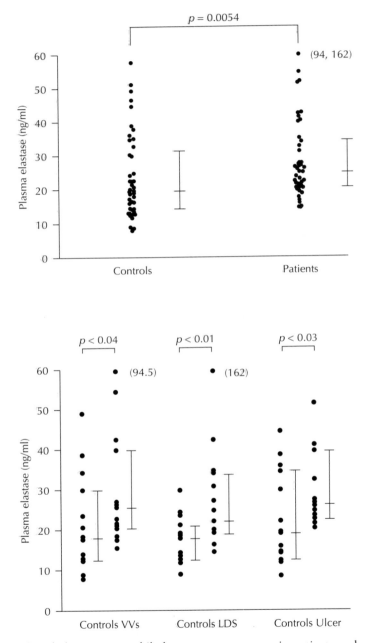

FIGURE 3-6. Results of plasma neutrophil elastase measurements in patients and control subjects. Error bars show the median and interquartile range of data. Statistical significance was determined by the Mann-Whitney test. *LDS*, Lipodermatosclerosis; *VVs*, skin change absent.

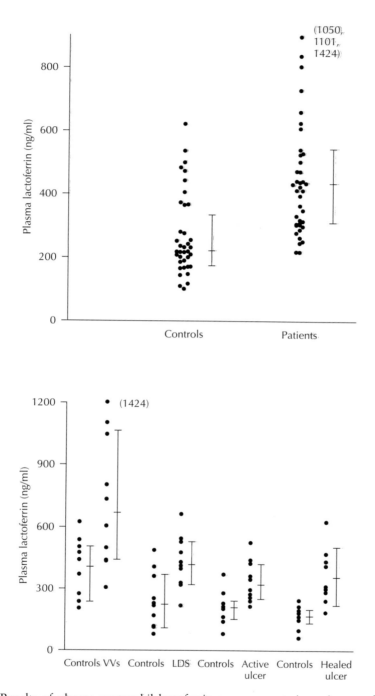

FIGURE 3-7. Results of plasma neutrophil lactoferrin measurements in patients and control subjects. Error bars show the median and interquartile range of data. *LDS*, Lipodermatosclerosis; *VVs*, skin change absent.

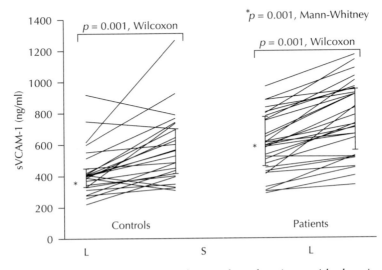

FIGURE 3-8. Plasma VCAM-1 levels in normal controls and patients with chronic venous disease (with and without skin changes) before and after venous hypertension. Descriptors: median and interquartile ranges; statistics; Wilcoxon and Mann-Whitney test for unpaired data. *L,* Lying; *S,* standing.

gen[95,96] and adhesion molecules, especially ICAM-1. ELAM-1 may be slightly up-regulated, but VCAM appears to be normal in patients without venous ulceration. Perturbed endothelium is more likely to attract the adhesion of leukocytes. The presence of the pericapillary fibrin cuff has been confirmed, but it also contains collagen IV, laminin, fibronectin, and tenascin.[97] A strong leukocyte infiltration has been measured in patients with venous disease.[98] These cells are macrophages and T lymphocytes. The cytokines involved include IL-1α and IL-1β. TNFα has not been detected in these histologic sections. The presence of the perivascular fibrin cuff (with other components) is a reflection of the inflammatory process and is seen in other chronic inflammatory conditions. In patients with venous disease increased plasma D-dimer levels have been observed, suggesting enhanced deposition of fibrin.[99] The perturbed state of the endothelium allows the passage of large molecules through the endothelium, permitting their perivascular accumulation, and explains the presence of the fibrin cuff.

In recent studies undertaken in the department of surgery at University College London (UCL), measurements of plasma levels of endothelial adhesion molecules have been performed along with those of von Willebrand factor. These levels may reflect endothelial injury in the microcirculation. Patients with chronic venous disease (a group with uncomplicated varicose veins and a group with skin changes) were studied again and compared to normal controls. The concentration of soluble VCAMs (vascular endothelial adhesion molecules) was elevated in both patient groups compared to control subjects and was highest in the group with skin changes (Figures 3-8 and 3-9). Smaller elevations of von Willebrand factor, soluble ICAM, and e-selectin were also observed. All subjects were then exposed

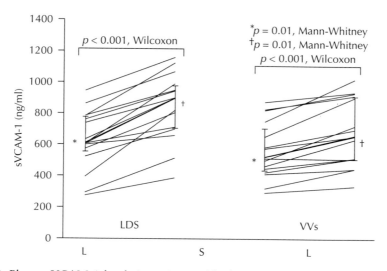

FIGURE 3-9. Plasma VCAM-1 levels in patients with chronic venous disease before and after venous hypertension. Descriptors: median and interquartile ranges; statistics: Wilcoxon and Mann-Whitney test. *L*, Lying; *S*, standing; *LDS*, lipodermatosclerosis; *VVs*, skin change absent.

to venous hypertension for 30 minutes, with the protocol described earlier used. Further increases in soluble adhesion molecules were noted, of which the rise in VCAMs was the most marked; this increase was greatest in the patients with skin changes attributable to venous disease. These elevations of soluble endothelial adhesion molecules probably reflect endothelial injury in response to short-term experimental venous hypertension, which occurs in both control subjects and patients with venous disease.

Search for Angiogenic Factors

The vascular proliferation seen in the skin of patients with venous disease has been known for many years[100] but has not been explained. In recent years many angiogenic factors that stimulate the growth of blood vessels have been recognized. In a further study conducted in the department of surgery at UCL, immunohistochemistry was used to evaluate the presence of a number of such factors in the skin of patients with venous disease.[101] At the time of surgery for varicose veins, skin biopsies were taken from the legs of patients with and without skin changes as well as of breast skin in patients without clinical evidence of venous disease for use as a control. Histologic examination demonstrated no evidence of up-regulation of transforming growth factor$_\beta$ (TGF$_\beta$) in the skin of patients with venous disease. In contrast, there was some increase in platelet-derived growth factor, subtype BB (PDGF-BB) in patients with venous disease. This increase was found in the capillary wall in vessels of the dermal papillae. Considerable up-regulation of the production of vascular endothelial growth factor

(VEGF) was also noted in the epidermis of patients with venous disease, being most marked in those with skin changes. It seems likely that VEGF may account for at least some of the vascular proliferation seen in the skin of patients with venous disease. This growth factor is also responsible for increased vascular permeability to large molecules, a feature of the skin microangiopathy that has been reported from capillary microscopy studies. The mechanism of stimulation of epidermal VEGF production is unclear at present.

DISCUSSION
Interpretation of Data

The studies conducted in our laboratory and those of the other small bands of researchers interested in this field have shown probable mechanisms by which endothelial injury is initiated in patients with venous disease, but so far these studies have failed to demonstrate why some patients develop skin changes and others do not.

Endothelial adhesion is a normal physiologic activity of neutrophils and monocytes. During venous hypertension the fall in blood flow to the lower limb and the increase in diameter of capillaries result in a decline in the shear rate in cutaneous capillaries. This decline favors leukocyte adhesion, which may be observed even in control subjects but is of greater magnitude in patients with venous disease, presumably because of the modifications that take place in the endothelium in chronic venous disease.

The indicators of leukocyte-endothelial interaction show that this activity occurs during short-term venous hypertension (within 30 minutes) and that during this period neutrophil degranulation may be detected, releasing primary and secondary granule enzymes into the region of the endothelium. At the same time an increase in von Willebrand factor and soluble endothelial adhesion molecules can be found in the leg blood. These arguments apply to control subjects as well as to patients, although the magnitude of change is always greater in the patients rather than in the control subjects. In fact, it is most unusual for a subject with normal veins to experience venous hypertension for a 30-minute period. Small movements of the calf result in rapid reduction of lower limb venous pressure in a normal subject, so the circumstances of our experiment are not usually experienced by individuals with normal lower limb veins. However, the experiments do show that when the venous system becomes deranged endothelial injury may result. We have also observed the egress of activated leukocytes from the lower limbs of control subjects following venous hypertension. In patients with venous disease these cells appear to remain in the lower limb, perhaps attached to the abnormal endothelium.

The chronic changes seen in liposclerotic skin may be the response to sustained low-grade assault on the endothelium by neutrophils and monocytes over many months or years. The perivascular infiltration of vessels in the papillary dermis by macrophages and T lymphocytes may simply be a tissue response to the chronic inflammatory processes referred to earlier. The vascular proliferation seen in this condition is also observed in patients with skin conditions such as psoriasis. A consistent pathologic feature in patients at risk of venous ulceration is the development of vascular proliferation in the skin and liposclerotic skin change. Whether these changes are simply associated phenomena or crucial to subsequent ulceration remains unclear at present.

The progression from chronic skin damage to actual ulceration also remains difficult to understand. Although many skin conditions are associated with inflammatory changes, few result in chronic nonhealing skin ulceration. Ulceration is clearly the cumulation of long-term skin injury attributable to all the processes already described. The progression from the chronic inflammatory state to ulceration is difficult to investigate, and no animal model is available. A possible answer is that an initiating stimulus causes massive activation of the perivascular macrophages, resulting in extensive tissue and blood vessel destruction. This activation may be a spontaneous event such as thrombosis of one of the capillary loops, which has been observed through capillary microscopy.[102] Alternatively, minor trauma to the region may set in motion the series of events that leads to ulcer formation.

One view commonly suggested is that venous ulcers fail to heal because of faulty wound-healing processes. This may be true, but it has long been known that rapid venous ulcer healing can be achieved if the precipitating factor (venous hypertension) can be corrected by a varicose vein operation. The ulcer heals within 1 or 2 weeks, and in many cases the skin may return to normal. We therefore believe that the main reason that a venous ulcer fails to heal is that the factors producing it are still present.

The data collected in the studies of neutrophil, monocyte, and endothelial cell activity have so far failed to identify major differences between those patients who develop skin changes and are at risk of ulceration and those who do not. Clearly a limited range of processes has been studied so far, and many areas have been left unexplored. We have concentrated on the processes that may cause damage and have not addressed the defense or response mechanism. Neither have inhibitors of leukocyte activation been studied. Searching each of these areas will take time and will require differing techniques. Unfortunately, few other authors have published research in this area, although increasing interest has been seen in Germany in recent years.

Other Systems Involved in Disease Process

Although we have described the events taking place in the microcirculation in CVI at length, several other skin structures become damaged in patients with CVI. The regulation of the microcirculation is dependent on intact innervation. It has been known for some time that the vasoconstrictor response of the microcirculation is impaired in the leg skin of patients with venous disease. We have assessed the presence of neuropathy in patients with venous disease to determine whether venous disease is associated with nerve injury. We found normal thresholds of sensation in the foot to vibration (A fiber) and cooling (A fiber) but substantially increased thresholds for skin warming (C fiber) (patients, median: 3.4° C, interquartile range: 2.4-5.8; control, median: 1.2° C, interquartile range 2.1-1.1). This finding suggests that this nerve fiber type is particularly susceptible to injury in patients with venous disease. The consequence for the microcirculation is unclear, but this finding implies a loss of external regulation. We have investigated this possibility by taking measurements of the vasomotion (cyclical fluctuations in flow assessed by laser Doppler fluxmetry) and performing frequency analysis by Fourier transform analysis. This approach revealed that the main vasomotion component was increased in magnitude and frequency in the patients with liposclerotic skin compared with control subjects.[103] This finding may also suggest a loss in neuronal regulation of the microcirculation.

Bollinger et al.[104] have elegantly demonstrated that the lymphatic capillaries in the skin are abnormal and damaged in venous disease, with dilatation and incompetence of their valves. Eventually the lymphatic vessels are destroyed and cannot be found in the most severely affected skin. This state may result in impairment of lymphatic drainage, which may account for some features of the leg in patients with CVI. It seems probable that the changes reported by Bollinger et al. are a consequence of the inflammatory and destructive mechanisms described in the preceding sections. However, the precise relationship of the lymphatic abnormality to the ulceration process is unclear and warrants further elucidation.

Implications for Pharmacologic Treatment

Although bandaging and stockings have been used effectively in the treatment of CVI for many years, modern pharmacologic science may provide assistance in healing venous ulcers. Enhancing fibrinolysis has been attempted to promote removal of the fibrin cuff.[105] This particular treatment did not improve ulcer healing. Drugs that reduce white cell activation may be useful in healing venous ulcers (assuming that this mechanism is important in the perpetuation of ulceration). Pentoxifylline (Trental, Hoechst AG, Germany) has already been evaluated. This drug reduces the likelihood of white cell activation by an effect that appears to be independent of other known activators of neutrophils such as TNF, resulting in much lower likelihood of endothelial adhesion.[106] In a multicenter study of 82 patients, pentoxifylline was shown to result in much better ulcer healing rates than did placebo.[107] It has been recommended that this drug may be useful for the treatment of resistant ulcers.[108] Prostaglandin E_1 inhibits the respiratory burst of neutrophils, preventing the release of superoxide radicals. A preliminary study has suggested that this agent is also effective in healing venous ulcers.[109] Other pharmacologic treatment strategies are possible and await evaluation. We think that adjuvant pharmacologic treatment will eventually become commonplace in the management of venous ulceration.

CONCLUSION

The precise mechanisms through which venous hypertension causes ulceration remain unclear. Abnormalities in several structures within the skin have been identified by research into the problem of venous ulceration, but it has been difficult to determine which are active participants and which are spectators. A better understanding of the initiating processes of this problem may lead to improvements in the management of patients with venous ulceration.

ACKNOWLEDGMENTS

Our grateful thanks are given to the following members of the department of surgery of University College London and Middlesex School of Medicine, who have undertaken much of the work described in this chapter and have made substantial intellectual contributions to our understanding of venous disease: Miss C. Butler, Mr. T.R. Cheatle, Dr. S. Chittenden, Mr. J. Farrah, Ms. G.M. McMullin, Miss H. Pardoe, Mr. S. Sarin, Mr. H.J. Scott, Mr. M. Saharay, Mr. S. Shami, and Mr. D. Shields. We are grateful to Miss L. Wilkinson for kindly summarizing the findings described in her M.Phil. thesis, presented here in connection with the inflammatory changes in varicose veins.

REFERENCES

1. Friedrich N. Über das Verhalten der Klappen in den Cruralvenen, sowie über das Verkommen von Klappen in den grossen Venenstämmen des Unterleibes. Morph Jahrb 7:323-325, 1882.
2. Barber RF, Shatara FI. The varicose disease. NY State J Med 25:162-166, 1925.
3. Fegan WG, Kline AL. The cause of varicosity in the superficial veins of the lower limb. Br J Surg 59:798-801, 1972.
4. Trendelenburg F. Über die Unterbindung der Vena saphena magna bei Unterschenkelvarizen. Beitr Klin Chir 7:195-210, 1891.
5. Eger SA, Casper SL. Etiology of varicose veins from an anatomic aspect based on a dissection of thirty-eight adult cadavers. JAMA 123:148-149, 1943.
6. Eger SA, Wagner FB. Etiology of varicose veins. Postgrad Med 6:234-238, 1949.
7. Basmajian JV. The distribution of valves in the femoral, external iliac, and common iliac veins and their relationship to varicose veins. Surg Gynecol Obstet 95:537-542, 1952.
8. Ludbrook J. Valvular defect in varicose veins. Cause or effect? Lancet 2:1289-1292, 1963.
9. Folse R. The influence of femoral vein dynamics on the development of varicose veins. Surgery 68:974-979, 1970.
10. Rose SS, Ahmed A. Some thoughts on the aetiology of varicose veins. J Cardiovasc Surg 27: 534-543, 1986.
11. Chant ADB, Jones HO, Townsend JCF, Edmund Williams J. Radiological demonstration of the relationship between calf varices and saphenofemoral incompetence. Clin Radiol 23:519-523, 1972.
12. Cockett FB, Elgan Jones DE. The ankle blow-out syndrome—A new approach to the varicose ulcer problem. Lancet 2:17-23, 1953.
13. Negus D. Prevention and treatment of venous ulceration. Ann R Coll Surg Engl 67:144-148, 1985.
14. Burnand KG, Lea Thomas M, O'Donnell T, Browse NL. The relative importance of incompetent communicating veins in the production of varicose veins and venous ulcers. Surgery 82: 9-14, 1977.

15. Burnand KG, Lea Thomas M, O'Donnell T, Browse NL. Relation between postphlebitic changes in deep veins and results of surgical treatment of venous ulcers. Lancet 1:936-938, 1976.
16. Zukowski AJ, Nicolaides AN, Szendro G, Irvine A, Lewis R, Malouf GM, Hobbs JT, Dudley HAF. Haemodynamic significance of incompetent calf perforating veins. Br J Surg 78:625-629, 1991.
17. McMullin GM, Coleridge Smith PD, Scurr JH. Which way does blood flow in the perforating veins of the leg? Phlebology 6:127-132, 1991.
18. King ESJ. The genesis of varicose veins. Aust N Z J Surg 20:126-133, 1950.
19. Cotton LT. Varicose veins: Gross anatomy and development. Br J Surg 48:589-598, 1961.
20. Svejcar J, Prerovsky I, Linhart J, Kruml J. Content of collagen, elastin and water in walls of the internal saphenous vein in man. Circ Res 11:296-300, 1962.
21. Andreotti L, Cammelli D, Banchi G, Guarnieri M, Serantoni C. Collagen, elastin, and sugar content in primary varicose veins. Rev Clin Lab 8:273-285, 1978.
22. Haardt B. Histochemistry of normal and varicose veins. Phlebology 2:135-158, 1987.
23. Obitsu Y, Ishimaru S, Furukawa K, Yoshihama I. Histopathological studies of varicose veins. Phlebology 5:245-254, 1990.
24. Wilkinson L. The presence of immune cells in vascular disease. M. Phil. thesis. London: University College London, 1987.
25. Layer GT, Pattison M, Evans B, Davies DR, Burnand KG. Tissue fibrinolytic activity is reduced in varicose veins. In Negus D, Jantet G, eds. Phlebology '85. London: John Libbey, 1986, pp 10-13.
26. Wolfe JHN, Morland M, Browse NL. The fibrinolytic activity of varicose veins. Br J Surg 66: 185-187, 1979.
27. Holman EF. Development of arterial aneurysms. Surg Gynecol Obstet 100:599-611, 1955.
28. Gius JA. Arteriovenous anastomoses and varicose veins. Arch Surg 81:299-310, 1960.
29. Piulachs P, Vidal-Barraquer E. Pathogenic study of varicose veins. Angiology 4:59-100, 1953.
30. Haimovici H, Steinman C, Caplan LH. Role of arteriovenous anastomoses in vascular diseases of the lower extremity. Ann Surg 164:990-1002, 1966.
31. DeSilva A, Widmer LK, Martin H, Mall TH, Glaus L, Schneider M. Varicose veins and chronic venous insufficiency. Vasa 3:118, 1974.
32. Dodd HJ, Wright HP. Vulval varices in pregnancy. Br Med J 1:831-832, 1959.
33. Kilbourne NJ. Varicose veins in pregnancy. Am J Obstet Gynecol 25:104-112, 1933.
34. Nabatoff RA. Varicose veins in pregnancy. JAMA 174:1712-1716, 1960.
35. Foote RR. Varicose veins. London: Butterworth, 1955.
36. Dodd HJ. The cause, prevention and arrest of varicose veins. Lancet 2:809-811, 1964.
37. Widmer LK. Peripheral venous disorders. Prevalence and socio-medical importance. Observations in 4529 healthy persons. Basel III Study. Berne: Hans Huber, 1978.
38. Myers TT. Varicose veins. In Barker NW, Hines EA, eds. Barker and Hines Peripheral Vascular Diseases, 3rd ed. Philadelphia: WB Saunders, 1962.
39. Ludbrook J. Obesity and varicose veins. Surg Gynecol Obstet 118:843-844, 1964.
40. Lake M, Pratt GH, Wright IS. Arteriosclerosis and varicose veins: Occupational activities and other factors. JAMA 119:696-701, 1942.
41. Santler R, Ernst G, Weiel B. Statistisches über der varikösen Symptomenkomplex. Hautarzt 10:460-463, 1956.
42. Gunderson J, Hauge M. Hereditary factors in venous insufficiency. Angiology 20:346-355, 1969.
43. Nicolaides AN, Zukowski A, Lewis R, Kyprianou P, Malouf GM. Venous pressure measurements in venous problems. In Bergan JJ, Yao JST, eds. Surgery of the Veins. Orlando, Fla.: Grune & Stratton, 1985, pp 111-118.
44. Dodd H, Cockett FB. The Pathology and Surgery of the Veins of the Lower Limb. Edinburgh: Churchill Livingstone, 1976.

45. Hoare MC, Nicolaides AN, Miles CR, Shull K, Jury RP, Needham T, Dudley HAF. The role of primary varicose veins in venous ulceration. Surgery 92:450-453, 1982.

46. Kistner RL. Primary venous valve incompetence of the leg. Am J Surg 140:218-224, 1980.

47. Pollack AA, Taylor BE, Myers TT, Wood EH. The effect of exercise and body position on the venous pressure at the ankle in patients having venous valvular defects. J Clin Invest 28:559-563, 1949.

48. Schanzer H, Converse Pierce E. Pathophysiologic evaluation of chronic venous stasis with ambulatory venous pressure studies. Angiology 33:183-191, 1982.

49. Psathakis ND, Psathakis DN. Investigation of the venous haemodynamics of the lower limb by venous pressure models. Angiology 37:499-507, 1986.

50. Christopoulos D, Nicolaides AN, Szendro G. Venous reflux: Quantification and correlation with the clinical severity of chronic venous disease. Br J Surg 75:352-356, 1988.

51. Browse NL. Venous ulceration. BMJ 286:1920-1922, 1984.

52. Homans J. The aetiology and treatment of varicose ulcers of the leg. Surg Gynecol Obstet 24:300-311, 1917.

53. Fontaine R. Remarks concerning venous thrombosis and sequelae. Surgery 41:6-24, 1957.

54. Blumhoff RL, Johnson G. Saphenous vein Po_2 in patients with varicose veins. J Surg Res 23:35-36, 1977.

55. Scott HJ, Cheatle TR, McMullin GM, Coleridge Smith PD, Scurr JH. A reappraisal of the oxygenation of the venous blood of varicose veins. Br J Surg 77:934-936, 1990.

56. Pratt GH. Arterial varices. A syndrome. Am J Surg 77:456-460, 1949.

57. Brewer AC. Arteriovenous shunts. BMJ 2:270, 1950.

58. Lindmayer W, Lofferer O, Mostbeck A, Partsch H. Arteriovenous shunts in primary varicosis: A critical essay. Vasc Surg 6:9-14, 1972.

59. Browse NL, Burnand KG. The cause of venous ulceration. Lancet 2:243-245, 1982.

60. Browse NL, Gray L, Jarrett PEM, Morland M. Blood and vein-wall fibrinolytic activity in health and vascular disease. BMJ 2:478-481, 1977.

61. Michel CC. Oxygen diffusion in edematous tissue and through pericapillary cuffs. Phlebology 5:223-230, 1990.

62. Stacey MC, Burnand KG, Layer GT, Pattison M. Transcutaneous oxygen tension as a prognostic indicator and measure of treatment of recurrent ulceration. Br J Surg 74:545, 1987.

63. Clyne CAC, Ramsden WH, Chant ADB, Wenster JHH. Oxygen tension in the skin of the gaiter area of limbs with venous ulceration. Br J Surg 72:644-647, 1985.

64. Dodd HJ, Gaylarde PM, Sarkany I. Skin oxygen tension in venous insufficiency of the lower leg. J R Soc Med 78:373-376, 1985.

65. Hopkins NFG, Spinks TJ, Rhodes CG, Ranicar ASOA, Jamieson CW. Positron emission tomography in venous ulceration and liposclerosis. BMJ 286:333-336, 1982.

66. Sjerson P. Blood flow in cutaneous tissue in man studied by washout of radioactive xenon. Circ Res 25:215-229, 1969.

67. Cheatle TR, McMullin GM, Farrah J, Coleridge Smith PD, Scurr JH. Three tests of microcirculatory function in the evaluation of treatment for chronic venous insufficiency. Phlebology 5:165-172, 1990.

68. Stibe ECL, Cheatle TR, Coleridge Smith PD, Scurr JH. Liposclerotic skin: A diffusion block or a perfusion problem? Phlebology 5:231-236, 1990.

69. Moyses C, Cederholm-Williams SA, Michel CC. Haemoconcentration and the accumulation of white cells in the feet during venous stasis. Int J Microcirc Clin Exp 5:311-320, 1987.

70. Thomas PRS, Nash GB, Dormandy JA. White cell accumulation in the dependent legs of patients with venous hypertension: A possible mechanism for trophic changes in the skin. BMJ 296:1693-1695, 1988.

71. Scott HJ, McMullin GM, Coleridge Smith PD, Scurr JH. Venous ulceration and the role of the white blood cell. J Med Sci Tech 14:184-187, 1990.

72. Bollinger A, Haselbach P, Schnewlin G, Junger M. Microangiopathy due to chronic venous incompetence evaluated by fluorescence videomicroscopy. In Negus D, Jantet G, eds. Phlebology '85. London: John Libbey, 1986.

73. Franzeck UK, Speiser D, Haselbach P, Bollinger A. Morphologic and dynamic microvascular abnormalities in chronic venous incompetence (CVI). In Davy A, Stemmer R, eds. Phlebologie '89. Montrouge, France: John Libbey Eurotext, 1989, pp 104-107.

74. Braide M, Amundson B, Chien S, Bagge U. Quantitative studies of leukocytes on the vascular resistance in a skeletal muscle preparation. Microvasc Res 27:331-352, 1984.

75. Engler RL, Dahlgren MD, Peterson MA, Dobbs A, Schmid-Schoenbein GW. Accumulation of polymorphonuclear leukocytes during three-hour myocardial ischemia. Am J Physiol 251:H93-100, 1986.

76. Romson JL, Hook BG, Kunkel SL, Abrams GD, Schork MA, Lucchesi BR. Reduction of the extent of ischemic myocardial injury by neutrophil depletion in the dog. Circulation 67:1016-1023, 1983.

77. Wilson JW. Leukocyte sequestration and morphologic augmentation in the pulmonary network following haemorrhagic shock and related forms of stress. Adv Microcirc 4:197-232, 1972.

78. Linas SL, Shanley PF, Whittenburg D, Berger E, Repine JE. Neutrophils accentuate ischemia-reperfusion injury in isolated perfused rat kidneys. Am J Physiol 255:F728-735, 1988.

79. Yamakawa T, Suguyama I, Niimi H. Behaviour of white blood cells in microcirculation of the cat brain cortex during hemorrhagic shock. Intravital microscopic study. Int J Microcirc Clin Exp 3:554, 1984.

80. Braide M, Blixt A, Bagge U. Leukocyte effects on the vascular resistance and glomerular filtration of the isolated rat kidney at normal and low-flow rates. Circ Shock 20:71-80, 1986.

81. Weissman G, Smolen JE, Korchak HM. Release of inflammatory mediators from stimulated neutrophils. N Engl J Med 303:27-34, 1980.

82. Babior BM. Oxidants from phagocytes: Agents of defense and destruction. Blood 64:959-966, 1984.

83. Coleridge Smith PD, Thomas P, Scurr JH, Dormandy JA. Causes of venous ulceration: A new hypothesis. BMJ 296:1726-1727, 1988.

84. Adams DO, Hamilton TA. The cell biology of macrophage activation. Ann Rev Immunol 2: 283-318, 1984.

85. Pober JS. Cytokine-mediated activation of vascular endothelium. Am J Pathol 133:426-433, 1988.

86. Schleef RR, Bevilaqua MP, Sawdey M, Gimbrone MA, Loskutoff DJ. Cytokine activation of vascular endothelium: Effects on tissue-type plasminogen activator and type 1 plasminogen activator inhibitor. J Biol Soc 263:5797-5803, 1988.

87. Scott HJ, McMullin GM, Coleridge Smith PD, Scurr JH. A histological study into white blood cells and their association with lipodermatosclerosis and ulceration. Br J Surg 78:210-211, 1990.

88. Shields DA, Andaz S, Abeysinghe RD, Porter JB, Scurr JH, Coleridge Smith PD. Neutrophil activation in experimental ambulatory venous hypertension. Phlebology 9:119-124, 1994.

89. Shields D, Andaz SK, Timothy-Antoine CA, Scurr JH, Porter JB. CD11b/CD18 as a marker of neutrophil adhesion in experimental ambulatory venous hypertension. Phlebology 1995 (Suppl) 1:108-109.

90. Shields DA, Andaz S, Abeysinghe RD, Porter JB, Scurr JH, Coleridge Smith PD. Plasma lactoferrin as a marker of white cell degranulation in venous disease. Phlebology 9:55-58, 1994.

91. Shields DA, Andaz SK, Sarin S, Scurr JH, Coleridge Smith PD. Plasma elastase in venous disease. Br J Surg 81:1496-1499, 1994.

92. Shields D, Saharay M, Timothy-Antoine CA, Porter JB, Scurr JH. Neutrophil CD11b expression in patients with venous disease. Phlebology 1995 (Suppl) 1:108-109.

93. Burnand KG, Whimster I, Naidoo A, Browse NL. Pericapillary fibrin in the ulcer-bearing skin of the leg: The cause of lipodermatosclerosis and venous ulceration. BMJ 285:1071-1072, 1982.
94. Haselbach P, Vollenweider U, Moneta G, Bollinger A. Microangiopathy in severe chronic venous insufficiency evaluated by fluorescence video-microscopy. Phlebology 1:159-169, 1986.
95. Wilkinson LS, Bunker C, Edwards JC, Scurr JH, Coleridge Smith PD. Leukocytes: Their role in the etiopathogenesis of skin damage in venous disease. J Vasc Surg 17:669-675, 1993.
96. Veraart JC, Verhaegh ME, Neumann HA, Hulsmans RF, Arends JW. Adhesion molecule expression in venous leg ulcers. Vasa 22:213-218, 1993.
97. Herrick SE, Sloan P, McGurk M, Freak L, McCollum CN, Ferguson MW. Sequential changes in histologic pattern and extracellular matrix deposition during the healing of chronic venous ulcers. Am J Pathol 141:1085-1095, 1992.
98. Scott HJ, McMullin GM, Coleridge Smith PD, Scurr JH. A histological study into white blood cells and their association with lipodermatosclerosis and ulceration. Br J Surg 78:210-211, 1990.
99. Falanga V, Kruskal J, Franks JJ. Fibrin- and fibrinogen-related antigens in patients with venous disease and venous ulceration. Arch Dermatol 127:75-78, 1991.
100. Burnand KG, Whimster I, Clemenson G, Thomas ML, Browse NL. The relationship between the number of capillaries in the skin of the venous ulcer-bearing area of the lower leg and the fall in foot vein pressure during exercise. Br J Surg 68:297-300, 1981.
101. Pardoe HD. The expression of angiogenic growth factors in the skin of patients with chronic venous disease of the lower limb. M. Sc. thesis. London: University College London, September, 1996, pp 1-61.
102. Franzeck UK, Speiser D, Haselbach P, Bollinger A. Morphologic and dynamic microvascular abnormalities in chronic venous incompetence (CVI). In Davy A, Stemmer R, eds. Phlebologie 1989. Montrouge, France: John Libbey Eurotext, 1989, pp 104-107.
103. Chittenden SJ, Shami SK, Scurr JH, Coleridge Smith PD. Vasomotion in the leg skin of patients with chronic venous insufficiency. Vasa 2:138-142, 1992.
104. Bollinger A, Isenring G, Franzeck UK. Lymphatic microangiopathy: A complication of severe chronic venous incompetence. Lymphology 15:60-65, 1982.
105. Layer GT, Stacey MJ, Burnand KG. Stanozolol and the treatment of venous ulceration—An interim report. Phlebology 1:197-203, 1986.
106. Sullivan GW, Carper HT, Novick WJ, Mandell GL. Inhibition of the inflammatory action of interleukin-1 and tumour necrosis factor (alpha) on neutrophil function of pentoxifylline. Infect and Immun 56:1722-1729, 1988.
107. Colgan M-P, Dormandy JA, Jones PW, Schraibman IG, Shanik DG. Oxpentifylline treatment of venous ulcers of the leg. BMJ 300:972-975, 1990.
108. Oxpentifylline for venous leg ulcers. Drug Ther Bull 29:59-60, 1991.
109. Rudovsky G. Intravenous prostaglandin E_1 in the treatment of venous ulcers—A double-blind, placebo-controlled trial. Vasa (Suppl) 28:39-43, 1989.

Chapter 4

Common Anatomic Patterns of Varicose Veins

John J. Bergan

A fundamental tenet in the treatment of any condition is that therapy must be directed at the cause. With varicose veins, the cause of the abnormality is multifactorial. Theories of causation of varicosities are many, and no unifying hypothesis has been offered.

The most important hypotheses of the pathogenesis of primary varicose veins are twofold. The first ascribes varicosities to incompetence of valves located above the saphenofemoral junction and exposure of the saphenofemoral valve rings to transient high pressures.[1] Such varicosities cause the valves to stretch and become incompetent. Repetition of the process ultimately results in dilation and elongation of the saphenous vein and its thin-walled tributaries. This gravitational reflux is aggravated by dynamic forces of intra-abdominal pressure. This theory of descending incompetence agrees with observation of long-standing varicosities in which the entire greater saphenous system, from thigh to midcalf, is involved with the varicose process.

The second hypothesis postulates that the initiating factor in varicose disease is a generalized or focal weakness of vein walls. According to this theory, the thin-walled tributaries to the greater saphenous vein become varicose when they are exposed to normal hydrostatic pressure. Support for this theory is demonstrated in patients with rather uniform and prominent reticular veins in the subcutaneous tissue, any of which have become varicose. Opposition to this hypothesis underlies the regular finding of focal saccular lateral wall blowouts in saphenous veins or tributary veins. A variation of the theory of generalized vein wall weakness is the hypothesis that the initial defect is valvular incompetence in communicating veins of the leg. Such valve failure allows the relatively unsupported subcutaneous veins to be subjected to high pressures generated during intercompartmental muscular exercise.

These hypotheses are not mutually exclusive. Therefore it is possible to bring

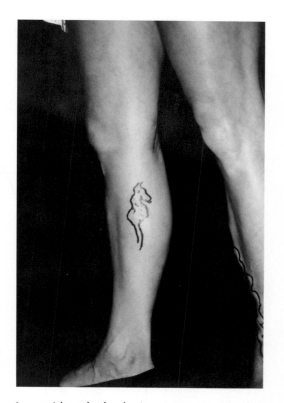

FIGURE 4-1. In some patients with early-developing varicosities, the first cluster appears in the anteromedial calf in association with a Boyd perforating vein, as shown here. Symptoms are aching, heaviness, and localized pain, which can be relieved by local pressure. Ultimate treatment with sclerotherapy or surgical removal of the varicose cluster and perforating vein will relieve the symptoms.

together these theories in order to recognize the patterns of varicosity formation, which is the objective of this chapter.

Observation of patients with varicose veins suggests that in some individuals perforator incompetence becomes the source of varicosities that form a distinctive and recognizable pattern (Figure 4-1). For example, the Boyd perforating vein in the anteromedial calf may become incompetent early in the varicose process. Then the anterior and posterior tributary veins of the greater saphenous system in that location may become varicose as the first finding in varicose disease.[2] Patients with this condition later may develop proximal or distal saphenous venous incompetence. Eventually this condition may lead to reflux in the entire greater saphenous vein (Figure 4-2). Secondary varicosities would appear wherever tributary veins are subjected to resultant high hydrostatic pressure. Furthermore, varicosities could develop from any of the other perforating vein sites and form patterns that are easily recognized or completely aberrant.

Recognition of patterns and relating them to specific perforating veins, many of which are identified by name, increase our familiarity with various types of pri-

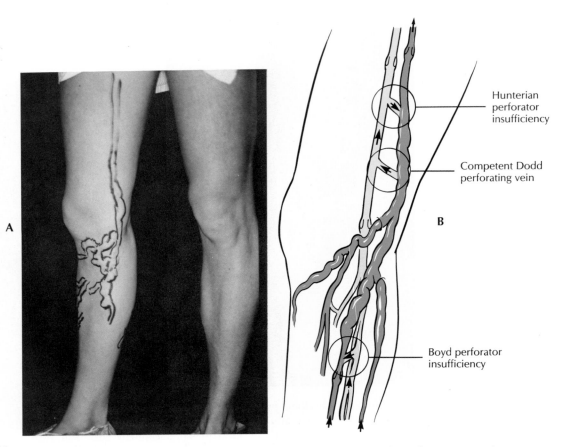

FIGURE 4-2. This photograph (**A**) and accompanying diagram (**B**) show the next stage in progression of varicosities that originate in the anteromedial calf. The refluxing greater saphenous vein in the distal thigh is seen to be dilated, whereas the refluxing greater saphenous vein in the middle third and proximal third of the thigh is less involved but still shows gross reflux.

mary venous stasis and allow for planning of operations and comparison of patients. Fundamental to recognition of the patterns is a knowledge of superficial venous anatomy and the location of important perforating veins.

NORMAL VENOUS ANATOMY OF LOWER EXTREMITY

Figures 4-3 and 4-4 show the main patterns of normal venous anatomy. Each named vein may be doubled (totally or partially) or absent (entirely or segmentally). This situation accounts for the wide variation in patterns observed in normal veins of the lower extremity.

Of greatest concern to the physician treating venous problems in the lower extremity is the greater saphenous vein (Figure 4-3). The term "saphenous" is derived from the Greek word for "visible."[3] The saphenous vein originates on the dorsum of the foot in the dorsal venous arch, passes anterior to the medial malleolus, progresses through the medial calf across the posteromedial aspect of the

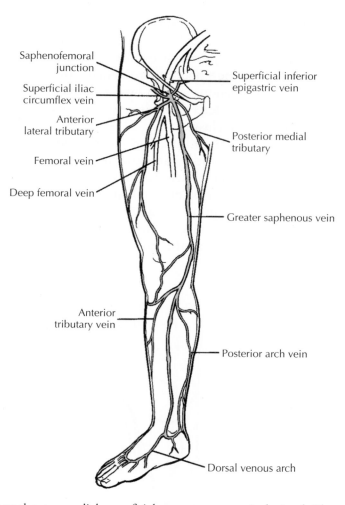

FIGURE 4-3. Normal anteromedial superficial venous anatomy is depicted. The greater saphenous vein ascends from the dorsal venous arch and dominates the anteromedial superficial drainage system. It receives the posterior arch vein (vein of Michelangelo). It also receives variable anterior and posterior tributary veins in the anteromedial calf just below the knee. As the saphenous vein reaches its termination, it receives important tributaries medially and laterally. These tributaries are commonly visualized in duplex ultrasound examinations, which may identify reflux in one or both of these vessels.

popliteal space, ascends in the medial thigh, and terminates in the femoral vein.

The anatomy of the greater saphenous vein is relatively constant. It is well appreciated that this vein lies on the deep fascia of the leg and thigh. However, it is less well recognized that it lies below or deep to the superficial fascia. Even contemporary descriptions of the anatomy of the veins of the lower extremity do not make this distinction.[4] Yet this fact is important to knowledge of the development of varicosities.

In varicose venous anatomy, the important tributaries to the greater saphenous vein extending upward from below are the posterior arch vein, which receives the three Cockett perforating veins; the anterior tributary vein to the saphenous system, which lies below the patella and collects blood from the anterior and lateral surface of the leg; and the posterior tributary vein, which also empties into the greater saphenous vein in the upper anteromedial calf. Other tributaries that may terminate high in the saphenous system near the groin are the posterior medial thigh vein and the anterior lateral thigh vein. Either or both of these veins may become the site of varicose clusters.

Less common in primary varicosities, and more important in recurrent varicose veins after surgery, are other tributaries to the greater saphenous vein as it terminates in the fossa ovalis. These include the superior external pudendal vein, the superior epigastric vein, and the superficial circumflex iliac vein.

Posteriorly, the most important of the axial veins is the lesser saphenous vein (Figure 4-4). This vein originates on the lateral aspect of the foot in the dorsal venous arch and ascends virtually in the midline of the calf. Unlike the greater

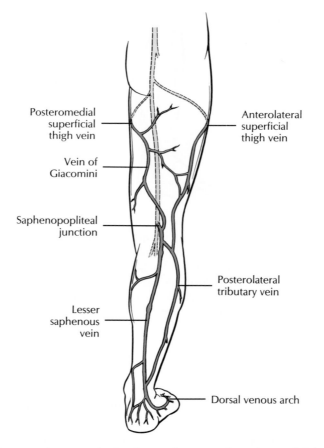

FIGURE 4-4. The lesser saphenous vein dominates the posterolateral superficial venous drainage. It originates in the dorsal venous arch; at the posterolateral ankle, it is intimately associated with the sural nerve. Note the important posterolateral tributary vein and the posterior thigh vein, which ascends and connects the lesser saphenous venous system with the greater saphenous venous system. The anterolateral superficial thigh vein and the posterolateral tributary vein can be very important in congenital venous anomalies such as Klippel-Trenaunay syndrome.

saphenous vein, the lesser saphenous vein may penetrate the deep fascia at any point from the middle third of the calf upward. This fact explains the segmental rather than total nature of reflux that is found in the lesser saphenous vein.

Important tributaries to the saphenous vein are inconstant but may include the posterolateral tributary vein. Superiorly, this tributary may be associated with a lateral thigh vein called the anterior lateral superficial thigh vein. Another important and frequently encountered vein is the ascending superficial vein, which leaves the popliteal space and progresses proximally to join the saphenous vein medially at a point high in the thigh. This vessel is the vein of Giacomini.

The importance of knowing the regular features of the gross anatomy of the superficial veins of the lower extremity is that any one of the systems may be the site of growth of clusters of varicosities. Such clusters can be referred to by the name of the normal vein in that location. All named tributaries to the greater and lesser saphenous system lie superficial to the membranous fascia and are relatively unsupported in comparison to the greater and lesser saphenous vein and the deep veins of the muscular compartments (Figure 4-5).

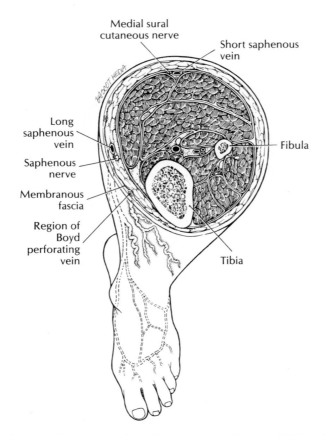

FIGURE 4-5. This diagram illustrates the fact that varicosities lie superficial to the membranous fascia while the saphenous vein lies on the deep fascia and is externally supported by the membranous fascia. Note the proximity of the saphenous nerve to the saphenous vein below the knee. (From Bergan JJ, Kistner RL, eds. Atlas of Venous Surgery. Philadelphia: WB Saunders, 1992, p 36.)

IMPORTANT PERFORATING VEINS

Veins that connect the superficial venous system to the deep venous system and penetrate the fascia are properly called perforating veins. Any one of these veins, or any combination of them, may be the source of the hydrodynamic forces of venous hypertension that produce superficial varicosities. It is the abnormally high pulses of hydrodynamic pressure transmitted through incompetent valves that affect relatively unsupported superficial veins. Such pulses of increased fluid force originate to some extent from increased abdominal pressure and to a greater extent from increased compartmental pressure during muscular contraction.

The best recognized connections between the superficial venous system and the deep venous system are the saphenofemoral and saphenopopliteal junctions. Incompetence of the check valves at their termination has been suggested as the cause of distal varicosities from gravitational reflux. This reverse flow is said to dilate more distal veins in a progressive fashion. As noted earlier, such reflux is neither always present nor is it the cause of highest hydrodynamic pressure.

Because it is frequently the site of the first varicose veins or the first reticular veins that become varicose, the Boyd perforating vein in the anteromedial calf (Figure 4-6) now receives great attention by physicians who treat venous problems.[5] Experience with the duplex scanner reveals that venous incompetence at this level may be isolated and may be the first reflux to appear. Such incompetence may be asymptomatic. However, when the incompetence is symptomatic, it produces aching pain, fatigue, and even a throbbing discomfort. These symptoms can be relieved by firm local pressure. In some patients the next perforator system to become incompetent is the distal thigh perforating vein(s) (Figure 4-7).

The frequency of varicosities in this location is documented in a graph by Cotton[6] that tabulates the number of varices in limbs from the monumental and informative study performed by him in 1957. It was Cotton who pointed out that the "most extreme degree of tortuosity is exhibited by small tributaries which are found close to, and draining into, communicating [perforating] veins." In the figures illustrating Cotton's thesis, one can see the normal deep veins and the abnormal communicating veins *receiving* blood from "intensely tortuous veins which are seen to be varicose tributaries entering the communicating veins."

Reversing this observation, one can visualize pulses of compartmental exercise pressure being delivered to unsupported superficial veins through incompetent perforators (Figure 4-8). Once it is realized that intercompartmental pressure can be transmitted through incompetent check valves of perforating veins to unsupported tributaries of these veins, it can easily be seen how the hydrostatic forces of gravitational reflux are additive to the hydrodynamic forces of muscular contraction. These very high pressures approach 100 mm Hg as they are generated within the muscular compartments. When transmitted outward, they produce localized blowouts or varicosities.

Progressing proximally from the Boyd communicating vein are the perforating veins in the distal third of the thigh. These veins, named for Harold Dodd,

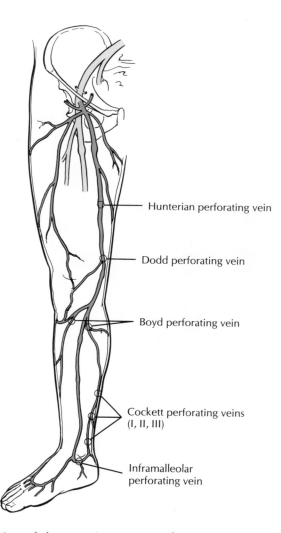

Hunterian perforating vein

Dodd perforating vein

Boyd perforating vein

Cockett perforating veins
(I, II, III)

Inframalleolar
perforating vein

FIGURE 4-6. The location of the most important perforating veins associated with the greater saphenous system are shown. Note that the Cockett and inframalleolar perforating veins are actually separate from the greater saphenous system. The Boyd perforating vein is constantly present, but it may drain the saphenous vein or its tributaries. Perforating veins in the distal third of the thigh are referred to as Dodd perforators, whereas those in the middle third of the thigh are referred to as hunterian perforators.

may be found in any location along the saphenous pathway in the distal third of the thigh.

The third important series of communicating veins, named for John Hunter, are found in the midthigh. Lea Thomas has surveyed phlebograms to study the anatomy of midthigh perforating veins.[7] He found that 61% of limbs had one or more communicating veins in the middle third of the thigh; in addition, he noted that 27% of the limbs had a perforating vein in the lower third of the thigh. Only 11% of the 100 phlebograms showed no evidence of communicating veins.

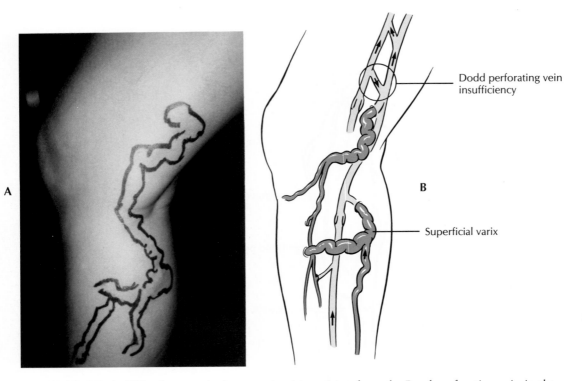

FIGURE 4-7. **A,** This photograph shows varicosities arising from the Boyd perforating vein in the posteromedial calf and the Dodd perforating vein in the distal third of the thigh. Doppler study and duplex confirmation failed to reveal greater saphenous reflux in any other locations. **B,** Depiction of the varicosities and their relationship to localized venous incompetence.

A concurrent study from St. Mary's Hospital in London revealed that the incompetent thigh perforating veins were found to occur anywhere in the thigh from the upper edge of the patella to a few centimeters below the saphenofemoral junction. Seventy-one percent were found in the middle third of the thigh, and 20% of the limbs had more than one perforating vein.[8] All the incompetent thigh perforating veins communicated directly with the long saphenous vein. It is interesting to note that five patients with incomplete saphenous stripping also demonstrated connections of thigh perforating veins to residual saphenous trunks. This observation emphasizes the need for removal of the entire refluxing saphenous vein in the thigh.

Another important perforating vein may be found on the anterior aspect of the thigh, usually in its middle third. This vein connects the deep venous system with superficial clusters of varicosities coursing laterally or medially across the thigh itself. This perforator and its clusters have no relationship to the saphenous veins.

In the leg the principal communicating veins have been named for Frank Cockett. Many surgeons incorrectly assume that the perforating veins on the me-

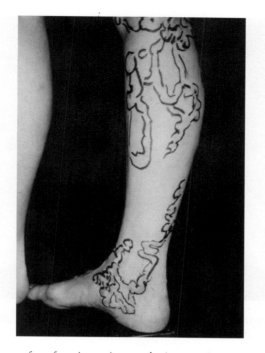

FIGURE 4-8. Combinations of perforating veins producing varying patterns of superficial varicosities present a confusing picture to the untrained eye. Yet a careful look illustrates that the inframalleolar perforating vein (perhaps a Cockett I), a posterior midcalf perforating vein, and the Boyd perforating vein contribute to the pattern seen here.

dial aspect of the ankle and calf connect the deep system to the greater saphenous vein. That concept is false. These perforating veins actually connect the posterior tibial deep venous system with the posterior arch vein (vein of Michelangelo). Posterior tibial veins are frequently paired, and phlebography may show their connection through perforating veins to the superficial system and the posterior arch vein.[9] Cockett has described the medial communicating veins as if they were relatively constant in location, but they are not. The location is commonly given as the distance from the medial malleolus or the sole of the foot. Figures given above the malleolus are 7, 12, and 18 cm from this point.

Other important perforating veins in the most distal part of the extremity are the inframalleolar perforating vein, frequently the site of a retromalleolar or an inframalleolar painful ulceration. A flare of intradermal telangiectasias below this perforating vein is called the corona phlebectatica (Figure 4-9).

Perforating veins on the posterior aspect of the lower extremity are much less well known. However, several are encountered frequently and are found to be the site of origin of varicose clusters. Among these are the lateral thigh perforating vein, which may be located in the middle third of the thigh on its lateral aspect, and the lateral leg perforating vein, also variably located in the middle or proximal third of the calf on its lateral aspect.

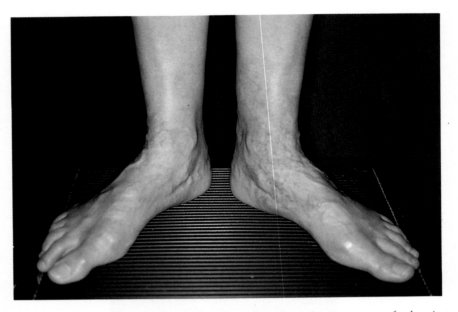

FIGURE 4-9. Below the inframalleolar perforating vein, a prominent pattern of telangiectasias is termed the corona phlebectatica.

PATTERNS OF VARICOSITIES

Recognizing the normal anatomy and the most common perforating vein sources of varicosities makes identification of patterns of varicosities relatively easy. As noted earlier, varicosities arising from the location of the Boyd perforating vein may be the first to appear and may occur in the absence of varicose veins elsewhere in the lower extremity. Such varicosities may consist of the anterior tributary vein varicose cluster or, more commonly, a posterior varicose cluster. Their first manifestations may be pain, aching, and heaviness. Relief may be obtained by applying local pressure and then by performing local excision of the cluster of varicosities and its perforating vein. Whether or not sclerotherapy for this pattern of varicosities will give long-term benefit is undetermined.

Of some importance is the relationship of the saphenous nerve to the Boyd perforating vein and its varicose clusters. In a study of this relationship, the most common vein-nerve pattern was found to be the saphenous vein and saphenous nerve, which meet a few centimeters below the knee.[10] Below this point the vein and the nerve were inseparable as far as the medial malleolus. This pattern was noted in 41 of 60 limbs studied. The next most common pattern seen in 10 limbs was the nerve joining the saphenous vein a few centimeters more proximally. Thus, in 50 of 60 limbs, nerve injury could be a problem in limbs in which the saphenous vein was dissected below the Boyd perforating vein. Clusters of varicosities may be isolated or connected with saphenous reflux. They may or may not empty into named perforating veins (Figure 4-10).

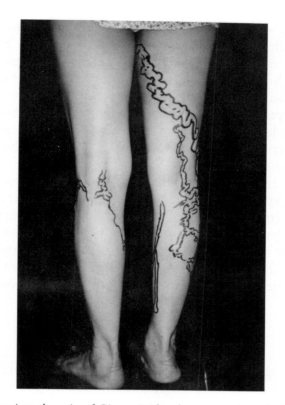

FIGURE 4-10. In this patient the vein of Giacomini has become varicose in its connection between the lesser saphenous system and the greater saphenous system.

Another isolated pattern of varicosities arises from the anterior thigh perforating vein and the anterior lateral tributary vein. These veins may form prominent, ropelike varicosities across the anterior surface of the thigh, coursing laterally and descending on the lateral aspect of the thigh. They may cross the popliteal space and arborize distally on the calf.

Other prominent varicose cluster patterns originate from the perforating veins of Hunter and of Dodd and are sometimes isolated clusters of varicosities. Usually they occur in association with greater saphenous reflux throughout its length. In fact, recognition that these clusters of varicosities are markers of saphenous reflux will alert the interested physician. The probable occurrence of greater saphenous insufficiency, when varicose clusters of the midthigh or the distal thigh are present, then can be confirmed by Doppler study.

In a study intended to classify the clinical appearance of uncomplicated varicose veins, Goren and Yellin[11] found that 71% of the limbs of patients studied demonstrated typical saphenous varicosities. Of the 164 limbs, 147 demonstrated greater saphenous incompetence, whereas only 17 limbs showed lesser saphenous incompetence. Twenty-two percent of the limbs did not show saphenous incompetence; instead they showed isolated perforator vein incompetence. The necessity of reconciling preservation of the saphenous vein for subsequent arterial surgery[12] to the needs of varicose vein surgery is considerably aided by recognizing that greater saphenous incompetence may not be present in some limbs with gross varicosities. In such instances (22% of the limbs in the study by Goren and Yellin), the greater saphenous can be spared, yet the operation can be done properly to remove symptomatic varicosities. The Doppler evaluation and duplex confirmation aid considerably in planning such surgical interventions. However, it also should be understood that in more than 75% of limbs the greater saphenous vein may need to be sacrificed.

Knowledge of the anatomy of the perforating veins, especially those in the medial thigh, has explained why the formerly advocated operation, high ligation of the greater saphenous vein, failed to achieve any of its objectives. Duplex ultrasound scanning has revealed that as many as 80% of these ligated saphenous veins remain patent and that more than half of those showing some thrombosis demonstrated a <10 cm occlusion.[13] Two other duplex ultrasound studies performed in limbs after high saphenous ligation also have confirmed these findings.[14,15]

CONCLUSION

Despite many abnormalities in superficial venous anatomy, patterns of varicose clusters can be recognized. These patterns usually are found in association with named perforating veins. Successful surgical treatment is dependent on removal of the varicosities without the absolute need for identification of the perforating vein itself (see Chapter 11).

REFERENCES

1. Ludbrook J. Primary great saphenous varicose veins revisited. World J Surg 10:954-958, 1986.
2. Thibault P, Bray A, Wlodarczyk J, Lewis W. Cosmetic leg veins: Evaluation using duplex venous imaging. J Dermatol Surg Oncol 16:612-618, 1990.
3. Goldman MP, Fronek A. Anatomy and pathophysiology of varicose veins. J Dermatol Surg Oncol 15:138-145, 1989.
4. Nehler MR, Moneta GL. The lower extremity venous system. I. Anatomy and normal physiology. Perspect Vasc Surg 4(2):104-116, 1991.
5. Boyd AM. Treatment of varicose veins. Proc R Soc Med 41:633-639, 1948.
6. Cotton LT. Varicose veins: Gross anatomy and development. Br J Surg 48:589-598, 1961.
7. Tung KT, Chan O, Lea Thomas M. The incidence and sites of medial thigh communicating veins: A phlebologic study. Clin Radiol 41:339-340, 1990.
8. Papadakis K, Christodoulou C, Christopoulos D, et al. Number and anatomical distribution of incompetent thigh perforating veins. Br J Surg 76:581-584, 1988.
9. O'Donnell TF Jr. Surgical treatment of incompetent communicating veins. In Bergan JJ, Kistner RL, eds. Atlas of Venous Surgery. Philadelphia: WB Saunders, 1992.
10. Holme JB, Holme K, Sorensen LS. The anatomic relationship between the long saphenous vein and the saphenous nerve. Acta Chir Scand 154:631-633, 1988.
11. Goren G, Yellin AE. Primary varicose veins: Topographic and hemodynamic correlations. J Cardiovasc Surg 31:672-677, 1990.

12. Mellière D, Cales B, Martin-Jonathan C, Schadeck M. Nécessité de concilier les objectifs du traitement des varices et de la chirurgie artérielle: Conséquences pratiques. Journal des Maladies Vasculaires 16:171-178, 1991.

13. Friedell ML, Samson RH, Cohen MJ, et al. High ligation of the greater saphenous vein for treatment of lower extremity varicosities: The fate of the vein and therapeutic results. Ann Vasc Surg 6:5-8, 1992.

14. Hammarsten J, Pedersen P, Cederlund C-G, et al. Long saphenous vein–saving surgery for varicose veins: A long-term follow-up. Eur J Vasc Surg 4:361-364, 1990.

15. Rutherford RB, Sawyer JD, Jones DN. The fate of residual saphenous vein after partial removal or ligation. J Vasc Surg 12:422-428, 1990.

PART TWO

Diagnostic Evaluation

Chapter 5

Classification of Venous Insufficiency

John J. Bergan

As treatment of varicose veins and telangiectasias becomes more scientifically based, it is important to classify these lesions. Advancement in the science of treatment of venous insufficiency depends upon an improved method of classification of the conditions treated. Kistner[1] has emphasized that if progress is to be made in the management of chronic venous disease, it is necessary to define the cause, location, and pathophysiology of the disease process in each case, as is done with the arterial system.

Attempts have been made to classify venous problems in general and venous insufficiency in particular. Widmer,[2] in his often quoted study, presented a clinical classification that related to the appearance of the limb. A more comprehensive approach, based on hemodynamic and phlebographic data, was proposed in Russia and published in English in *International Angiology,* but it did not gain universal acceptance.[3] In 1992 Enrici and Caldevilla[4] in Argentina described a classification based on clinical presentation of the patient, much as the ad hoc committee of the Joint Council of the Society for Vascular Surgery and the North American Chapter of the International Society for Cardiovascular Surgery (SVS/ISCVS) did by using anatomic regions, clinical severity, physical examination, and functional assessments.[5]

Hach et al.[6] in Germany classified greater saphenous reflux into four stages, ranging from reflux in the proximal thigh (stage 1) to reflux in the ankle and foot (stage 4), and were able to correlate increased deep vein diameter, elongation, and tortuosity with the progressive stages of reflux. Their classification has been used by many but has not achieved worldwide acceptance. Cornu-Thénard et al.[7] in France limited their contribution to venous classification to varicose veins and made no attempt to include more severe venous disorders. In contrast, Griton and Widmer[8] recognized that a modern view of chronic venous insufficiency must include both superficial and deep lesions, regardless of their cause or clinical presentation. They suggested a five-stage classification that shows thoughtfulness and wisdom but has not had any clinical impact. Others have also made attempts at classification of venous dysfunction.[9-11]

The most recent contribution to classification of venous insufficiency was drawn up by a large number of physicians and surgeons interested in venous problems. It is known as the Hawaii classification, in reference to its site of origin, the 1994 American Venous Forum meeting in Maui. This classification was approved by the Joint Councils of the American Vascular Societies, which published it in the *Journal of Vascular Surgery*.[12] Subsequently, it has received wide attention elsewhere.[13]

Attempts to use the initial SVS/ISCVS clinical classification with its three stages proved disappointing. Investigators found that in practice stages 1 and 2 would be considered together hemodynamically. Only then were they separable from the more advanced stage 3.[14]

The Hawaii classification has been well published. It is unfortunate that it was circulated before being tested in practice and perhaps modified. The classification is based on clinical presentation of the patient (C), etiology of the problem (E), anatomic abnormality(ies) found (A), and pathophysiology encountered (P). A clinical severity score was proposed, and a diagnostic process was suggested. This score was not an integral part of the classification. By February 1997 the classification had been published in 20 journals worldwide and in the American Venous Forum *Handbook of Venous Disorders*.[15]

EXPERIENCE WITH THE CEAP CLASSIFICATION

Labropoulos,[16] in publishing his application of the CEAP classification to 250 limbs examined in London at the St. Mary's Hospital and in Maywood, Illinois, at the Loyola University Medical Center, characterized the classification as "practical and useful owing to its simplicity." His display of experience in applying the classification clinically (Table 5-1) appeared elegant and informative. On closer inspection, however, the analysis was seen to be a documentation of the obvious. Included were more limbs with telangiectasias and varicose veins than with healed or open ulcers. More reflux than obstruction was present. In addition, more women than men were studied, a fact not given by the CEAP classification, and the finding that only 2% of the limbs had obstruction raised a serious question about the method used in making the diagnosis of obstruction. It is notable that this report made no mention of the anatomic segments that were afflicted; nor did it refer to the severity score. Ultimately, the vast amount of work that went into classification of each limb and the assembly of results yielded only the information that these limbs depicted the population referred to by the two laboratories named earlier.

My colleagues and I have used the consensus statement and the CEAP classification and its disability classification in three research efforts.[17-19] These are typical of the studies that the originators of the classification had in mind. Therefore

TABLE 5-1. Clinical classification of specimens*

Specimen No.	Sex	Age (yr)	Disability Score	CEAP Classification
1 R	M	48	$C_1A_2D_2$	$C_{2s}E_pA_{4R,5R}P_R$
1 L	M	48	$C_1A_2D_2$	$C_{2s}E_pA_{4R,5R}P_R$
2	F	39	$C_1A_3D_1$	$C_{2s}E_pA_{2R,17R,18R}P_R$
3	M	48	$C_5A_4D_6$	$C_{4s}E_sA_{13RO,14RO,16R,17R}P_{RO}$
4	M	67	$C_1A_2D_1$	$C_{2s}E_pA_{2R,3R}P_R$
5 R	M	48	$C_1A_3D_1$	$C_{3s}E_pA_{3R,17R,18R}P_R$
5 L	M	48	$C_1A_6D_1$	$C_{3s}E_pA_{1R,2R,3R,4R,17R,18R}P_R$
6	F	69	$C_1A_5D_2$	$C_{4s}E_pA_{1R,2R,3R,4R,5R}P_R$
7	F	53	$C_1A_2D_1$	$C_{2s}E_pA_{2R,3R,5R}P_R$
8	M	80	$C_1A_3D_1$	$C_{2s}E_pA_{2R,3R,5R}P_R$
9 R	F	60	$C_1A_2D_1$	$C_{2s}E_pA_{2R,3R}P_R$
9 L	F	60	$C_1A_2D_1$	$C_{2s}E_pA_{2R,3R}P_R$
10	F	71	$C_3A_5D_1$	$C_{4s}E_pA_{1R,2R,3R,17R,18R}P_R$
11 M	F	29	$C_1A_3D_1$	$C_{2s}E_pA_{2R,3R,17R}P_R$
11 ST	F	29	$C_1A_3D_1$	$C_{2s}E_pA_{2R,3R,17R}P_R$
12	F	33	$C_1A_2D_1$	$C_{2s}E_pA_{2R,3R}P_R$
13	F	63	$C_1A_2D_1$	$C_{2s}E_pA_{2R,3R}P_R$

L, Lesser saphenous vein; *M*, midsaphenous; *ST*, subterminal.
*From Labropoulos N. CEAP in clinical practice. Vasc Surg 31:224-225, 1997.

a description of our experience may predict what others will encounter if they attempt to use the classification in its present form.

We found that the CEAP classification was most valuable when the number of limbs under study was the fewest. For example, 17 surgical specimens were removed for detailed study of leukocyte infiltration into venous walls and valves.[17] When the findings were positive and the distribution of the CD68 monocytic infiltration was more concentrated on proximal endothelial surfaces, it was informative to know how each limb supplying the specimen had been classified (Figure 5-1). Each limb had been classified accurately according to the CEAP classification, and the exact sites of venous dysfunction were known (at least within the limitations of duplex testing).

It was found that a spectrum of venous dysfunction was present in the limbs that contributed the specimens. Only limbs with no venous disorder and those with only telangiectasias were absent. Therefore it was disappointing to find that no relationship existed between the magnitude of the infiltrates or the location of the monocytes on the endothelium (or the macrophages in the venous wall) and the severity or duration of the venous insufficiency. Thus the classification could be said to describe the clinical situation with some accuracy, but it did not correlate with histopathologic findings.

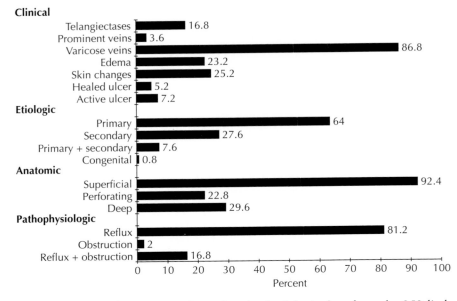

FIGURE 5-1. Clinical, etiologic, anatomic, and pathophysiologic data from the 250 limbs in this study. (From Ono T, Bergan JJ, Schmid-Schönbein GW, Takase S. Monocyte infiltration into venous valves. J Vasc Surg 27:158-167, 1998.)

ERRORS IN CEAP

In addition, the apparent accuracy of the pathophysiologic classification of each limb promoted a false sense of veracity. This point is also noted in the report by Labropoulos,[16] which indicated that venous obstruction must be underrepresented. Unfortunately, in the present clinical/economic milieu, all patients cannot be subjected to the diagnostic testing that would provide highly accurate anatomic information regarding the presence of obstruction versus reflux. In short, ascending phlebography that includes the vena cava and the iliac system cannot be done in every case. Similarly, descending phlebography cannot be applied to patients with relatively minor venous dysfunction. This limitation is not a great defect, however, because duplex evaluation has proven to be accurate with regard to reflux.

The anatomic portion of the CEAP classification provides for designation of reflux or obstruction in the inferior vena cava, the common, internal, and external iliac veins, and the pelvic, gonadal, and broad ligament veins; however, today's practice, even in a research setting, gives information only from the femoral vein distally. Some will say that duplex study will detect proximal iliac venous obstruction, but experience in clinical practice has shown that this is not true. Even in our research experience with a very limited number of specimens, a false element of accuracy of classification of venous dysfunction was present.

SIMPLIFYING CEAP

At the other end of the scale of experience with the CEAP classification is the report of the North American Registry on subfascial endoscopic perforator surgery (SEPS) to the Society for Vascular Surgery.[14] This registry seemed ideal for demonstrating the utility of the CEAP classification. By employing this classification to designate each limb being subjected to the operation, the experience derived from 17 institutions could theoretically be combined.

Ultimately, data from 151 patients having operations on 155 limbs from the 17 medical centers were submitted to the Registry office. The investigators used the Hawaii classification to the best of their ability. Quickly it was learned that the entire CEAP designation for each limb could not be included in the analyses. Even if complete accuracy were assumed, the anatomic segment designation of reflux or obstruction or both was simply too cumbersome as a working method.

Therefore only the simplest form of the CEAP classification was utilized. This version identified limbs as being in class 4, 5, or 6, and this approach was more precise than the former classification previously approved by the ad hoc committee of the Joint Councils of the American Vascular Societies. However, in reporting to the Registry, investigators listed the anatomic segments that were studied as having reflux or obstruction but did not note the incomplete nature of their preoperative investigations. Logically, not all limbs were subjected to complete phlebography; nor was it acknowledged that physiologically obstructing lesions are exceedingly difficult to detect. Therefore, although the classification of limbs was clinically accurate, the anatomic classification could not have been.

THE DISABILITY SCORE

Perhaps the most valuable contribution of the new classification was the use of the disability score. Although the mean follow-up of limbs in this report was only 5.4 months, the average preoperative clinical score decreased from 9.4 (range, 0-18) to 2.9 (range, 0-12) ($p < 0.0001$).[18]

Finally, in a recent experience from our group reporting the effects of subfascial perforator vein interruption on ulcer healing, it has been possible to use the clinical and disability score as assessed both preoperatively and postoperatively.[19] As in the Registry report, the pathophysiologic classification appeared to be entirely accurate. However, we know that it was flawed for the reasons indicated earlier. The lack of phlebologic evaluation of the abdominal and pelvic venous system results in an underestimation of the incidence of major venous obstruction in the limbs treated. Once again, however, the disability score as calculated preoperatively and postoperatively gave a clear indication of the results of the intervention. Preoperatively the average disability score was 9.3 (range, 0-18), and this decreased to a disability score of 3.5 postoperatively, with the follow-up extending to 24 months. This information gives subjective evaluation of the results of the intervention.

The CEAP classification is a step forward in precisely identifying the clinical states of limbs afflicted by venous dysfunction. Its use clarifies the stages of venous stasis that are being treated. As indicated in the experience cited earlier, flaws in the system do exist; however, this limitation was predicted by the committee that proposed the classification.

Perhaps the greatest contribution of the CEAP classification will be as a stimulus for a more sophisticated approach to the causes of venous valve and vein wall damage and an examination of the reasons for the cutaneous changes of severe chronic venous insufficiency so that these factors can be incorporated as an integral part of a better system. An example of the need for this incorporation is our finding that patient plasma, when reacted against a panel of naive leukocytes, causes neutrophil activation but that the activation strength is not proportional to the severity of venous insufficiency. Only when classes 1, 2, and 3 are combined and compared to classes 4, 5, and 6 is there a statistically significant difference in neutrophil activation. Similarly, the CD68 monocyte infiltrate concentration seen in the surgical specimens in the study described earlier is no greater in the advanced stages of venous stasis than in the less severe forms.

"The availability of accurate diagnoses and classification is basic to our understanding of the natural history of chronic venous disease and to its prognosis," said Kistner[20] in describing the classification of venous disease that was later termed the CEAP classification.

CONCLUSION

Difficulty with devising a useful classification may be inherent in the nature of severe venous insufficiency. It is possible that hemodynamic and hemostatic abnormalities act independently of leukocyte-induced skin damage and monocyte infiltration into venous valves and the venous wall. Perhaps only a better understanding of the effect of physiologic obstruction, as opposed to anatomic obstruction, or a discovery of the fundamental cause of primary venous dysfunction will allow a simple practical classification to be constructed.

REFERENCES

1. Kistner RL. Classification of chronic venous disease. Vasc Surg 3:217-218, 1997.
2. Widmer LK. Classification of venous disorders. In Peripheral Venous Disorders. Basel III. Bern: Hans Huber, 1978.
3. Sytchev GG. Classification of chronic venous disorders of the lower extremities and pelvis. Int Angiol 4:203-206, 1985.
4. Enrici EA, Caldevilla HS. Clasificación de la insuficiencia venosa crónica. In Enrici EA, Caldevilla HS, eds. Insuficiencia Venosa Crónica de los Miembros Inferiores. Editorial Celcius, 1992, pp 109-114.
5. Porter JM, Rutherford RB, Clagett CP, et al. Reporting standards in venous disease. J Vasc Surg 8:172-181, 1988.
6. Hach W, Schirmers U, Becker L. Veränderungen der tiefen Leitvenen bei either ner Stammvarikose der Vein saphena magna. In Müller Wiefel H, ed. Mikrozirkulation und Blutrheologie. Baden-Baden: Witzstrock, 1980.

7. Cornu-Thénard A, de Vincenzi I, Maraval M. Evaluation of different systems for clinical quantification of varicose veins. J Dermatol Surg Oncol 17:345-348, 1991.

8. Griton PH, Widmer LK. Classification des varices et de l'insuffiance veineuse. J Mal Vasc 17(Suppl B):102-108, 1992.

9. Partsch H. "Betterable" and "nonbetterable" chronic venous insufficiency: A proposal for a practice-oriented classification. Vasa 9:165-167, 1980.

10. Pierchalia P, Tronnier H. Diagnosis and classification of venous insufficiency of the leg. Dtsch Med Wochenschr 110:1700-1702, 1985.

11. Miranda C, Fabre M, Meyer P, Marescaux J. Evaluation of a reference anatomoclinical classification of varices of the lower limbs. Phlebologie 46:235-239, 1993.

12. Porter JM, Moneta GL. Reporting standards in venous disease: An update. J Vasc Surg 21:635-645, 1995.

13. Beebe HG, Bergan JJ, Bergqvist D, et al. Classification of chronic venous disease in the lower limbs. A consensus statement. Eur J Vasc Endovasc Surg 12:487-492, 1996.

14. Iafrati MD, Welch H, Belkin M, O'Donnell T. Correlation of venous noninvasive tests with the SVS/ISCVS clinical classification of chronic venous insufficiency. J Vasc Surg 19:1001-1007, 1994.

15. Gloviczki P, Yao JST. Handbook of Venous Disorders. London: Chapman & Hall, 1996.

16. Labropoulos N. CEAP in clinical practice. Vasc Surg 31:224-225, 1997.

17. Ono T, Bergan JJ, Schmid-Schönbein GW, Takase S. Monocyte infiltration into venous valves. J Vasc Surg 27:158-167, 1998.

18. Gloviczki P, Bergan JJ, Menawat SS, et al. Safety, feasibility, and early efficacy of subfascial endoscopic perforator surgery (SEPS): A preliminary report from the North American Registry. J Vasc Surg 25:94-106, 1997.

19. Bergan JJ, Ballard JL, Sparks S, Murray JS. Subfascial surgery of perforating veins: SEPS. Phlebologie 49:467-472, 1996.

20. Kistner RL. Clinical presentation and classification of chronic venous disease. In Gloviczki P, Bergan JJ, eds. Atlas of Endoscopic Perforator Vein Surgery. London: Springer-Verlag, 1997.

Chapter 6

Laboratory Evaluation of Varicose Veins

Paul S. van Bemmelen and David S. Sumner

Noninvasive evaluation of patients with varicose veins is used to detect or rule out valvular incompetence in venous segments that may be difficult to assess through physical examination. Accurate identification of incompetent superficial veins serves the dual purpose of ensuring complete treatment of all involved veins while preserving those that are normal. Such testing also helps to distinguish primary from secondary varicose veins by determining the status of the deep venous system. Ideally, objective methods can be used to replace the more subjective physical examination and offer quantitative information regarding the severity of venous reflux. Application of reliable methods ultimately may improve our understanding of venous pathophysiology and its therapy.

This chapter is concerned with the most useful tests for patients with varicose veins. Emphasis is placed on noninvasive tests that give the clinician information that affects therapeutic decisions. The tests are discussed in historical order, with invasive methods preceding noninvasive methods. In clinical practice noninvasive tests are done before invasive ones.

DIAGNOSTIC TESTS
Ambulatory Venous Pressure

Although measuring foot vein pressure after exercise may provide important physiologic information, this method is cumbersome and therefore is not routinely used. For two reasons ambulatory venous pressure (AVP) cannot be considered a preferred method for evaluating varicose veins: (1) venous puncture on the dorsal foot can be painful and technically demanding, and (2) interpretation of results may be difficult.[1]

When varicose veins are accompanied by changes in chronic cutaneous venous stasis, finding an elevated AVP merely confirms the clinical diagnosis of venous hypertension. Early studies of this method compared AVP with ascending venography. Patients were usually stratified on the basis of history and physical examination. Improvement of refilling time with application of a tourniquet was assumed to indicate uncomplicated superficial vein incompetence. These early AVP studies have not been repeated with varicography, saphenography, or descending venography, which would provide a more solid basis for topographic accuracy.

Theoretically, normalization of refilling time would not take place if proximal perforators connect the superficial hydrostatic column to the deep system. In practice, many patients have patterns of combined deep and superficial vein incompetence that are uncontrollable by tourniquet application even if selective occlusion of superficial veins were possible.[2] Based on a study of the highly variable (40 to 300 mm Hg) tourniquet pressures required to occlude incompetent superficial veins, it seems unlikely that tourniquets would provide reliable compression.[3] After it was suggested that similar information could be obtained noninvasively through the use of photoplethysmography, direct pressure measurements virtually disappeared from daily practice.[4]

Photoplethysmography

Photoplethysmography (PPG), like light reflection rheography, measures the reflection of infrared light by red blood cells in cutaneous capillaries. Dorsal or plantar flexion of the foot reduces the amount of blood in the dermal plexus. On cessation of exercise, a curve is obtained that is similar in shape to an AVP recording. Since this method is simple and inexpensive, it is a useful screening tool for initial assessment of venous disease.[5] The original validation of the method in 1979 compared PPG results to those of direct venous pressure measurements.[4] A high correlation coefficient was found when groups of patients with severe venous disease were compared to normal controls. The original patient group studied contained only 14 patients with uncomplicated varicose veins, and the expectation that PPG would be useful to localize incompetence in the greater saphenous system was never prospectively verified with an imaging technique. The claim was made that a tourniquet occluding an incompetent superficial vein would normalize an abnormally short refilling time.[5,6] A prospective study in 1990 compared the results of PPG to those of segmental duplex scanning in 151 symptomatic legs.[2] The kappa coefficient of overall agreement was 0.12 ± 0.06, a value approaching zero. When attention was focused on the calf segment of the greater saphenous vein (considered to be readily amenable to tourniquet occlusion), the greater saphenous vein was found to be incompetent more often when the PPG refilling time was normal than when the PPG indicated superficial incompetence. Thus the use of tourniquets represents a large source of error in the evaluation of venous insufficiency.[3]

When attention was turned to the results of PPG obtained without the use of a tourniquet, refilling times could not be used to discriminate between normal patients and those with venous incompetence at one, two, or three levels of the leg. Only in the most extensive degree of incompetence, level four, did PPG have a sensitivity greater than 49%; this group of patients is easily recognized clinically by ulceration or obvious skin changes. PPG offered no improvement over clinical inspection of gaiter area skin made prior to laboratory evaluation.

Since PPG recordings in different areas of the same leg have led to different results, it seems that PPG refilling time is more apt to reflect local superficial hemodynamics than the hemodynamics of the entire limb venous system.[7] PPG refilling time may be related to dermal microscopic valvular status.[8] It is likely that PPG and light reflection rheography measurements will continue to provide information regarding microcirculatory changes, but PPG should not play a role in the decision to treat saphenous veins.

Air Plethysmography

In the 1960s plethysmography was pioneered and applied to the study of varicose veins. Allan[9] described changes in leg vein volume that occur as a result of varicose disease. Recently, a new air plethysmograph has become available commercially. It differs from previous devices in that it has a larger chamber to surround the entire calf. A sensitive recorder makes possible volume readings as small as 2.5 ml. With this device quantitative measurements of reflux from above-knee to below-knee veins are feasible. The amount of reflux has been related to disease severity and incidence of ulceration.[10,11] The foot is not enclosed in the air cuff, and reflux from ankle to foot would, at least in theory, affect APG measurements paradoxically. Reduction of the volume of venous reflux after removal of varicosities has been documented.[12] Leg volume after exercise correlates to direct venous pressure measurements when legs of normal volunteers are compared to legs with active or healed ulceration reminiscent of those of the first PPG studies.[13]

To distinguish between superficial and deep reflux, the air plethysmography device relies on proper application of a tourniquet that occludes superficial veins. As noted previously, the tourniquet is a source of error: at times successful occlusion of a long saphenous vein is accomplished easily, but occlusion of the subfascial lesser saphenous vein may be impossible in the legs of obese individuals, leading to a false diagnosis of deep vein incompetence. Although air plethysmography equipment is less expensive than a duplex scanner, topographic information is paramount in the treatment of varicose veins.

Portable Doppler Ultrasound

The portable continuous-wave Doppler device is probably the single most helpful tool for experienced clinicians. It can quickly and noninvasively detect incompetent veins, even when these veins are not visible.[14,15]

The purpose of continuous-wave Doppler examination is to discern the relationship of existing varicose veins to the saphenous system, to assess the competency of the greater and lesser saphenous veins, and to determine if the deep venous system is obstructed. For optimal examination, the patient should be in a standing position. Standing allows for the filling of incompetent venous reservoirs so that when compression of these reservoirs is released, flow can be detected with the Doppler probe. Examination of the patient in a supine position may yield erroneous results since thin-walled accessory branches are often collapsed or will collapse with external pressure from the Doppler probe. The examination of venous segments distal to the groin is unreliable with regard to retrograde flow elicited by a Valsalva maneuver.[16] Proximal compression of the limb by hand is not a reliable way to promote retrograde flow and valve closure, although a qualitative, subjective impression often can be obtained through this approach.[17] The best method for examining the popliteal fossa and the rest of the leg is with the patient standing,[18] with his/her weight supported by the contralateral leg and the knee of the leg under study slightly flexed.[19,20] A systematic approach from top to bottom includes the venous confluence in the groin and the greater saphenous vein in the thigh, including its anterolateral and posteromedial branches. At the knee level the medial aspect is examined for both the main greater saphenous vein and the accessory or secondary saphenous vein. Often the greater saphenous vein runs posterior to the femoral condyle and connects to the deep or lesser saphenous system.

Examination is continued from the anterolateral aspect of the patella to the lateral aspect of the knee. Superficial veins in this area may be anterolateral branches of the greater saphenous vein,[21] or they may form part of a separate lateral system of dilated subdermal veins.[22] Examination of the popliteal fossa is most demanding. The examiner can best determine the location of the popliteal vein by first locating the popliteal arterial signal. It is possible, however, to mistake sural arteries for the popliteal artery in obese patients and, subsequently, to mistake the gastrocnemius vein or the lesser saphenous vein for the popliteal vein. The distinction between the lesser saphenous vein and more superficially located subcutaneous branches can be difficult. A prudent approach is to consider an all-negative examination of the popliteal fossa as constituting sufficient screening. With reflux at the popliteal fossa, additional study with an instrument that has imaging capabilities usually is necessary for accurate diagnosis.

Examination of the lower leg must be tailored to the individual patient since virtually all areas of the lower leg can be affected with varicosities. The anatomic relationship between superficial branches and the greater and lesser saphenous veins can be assessed by positioning the probe over the saphenous veins and listening during release of compression of the superficial convolutions. Pretibial branches usually are connected to the greater saphenous vein. Posterior tibial veins at the level of the ankle are located alongside the artery and are assessed by release of foot compression. Reflux at this level often occurs because superficial veins are located in the path of the ultrasound beam; it rarely is associated with the deep ankle veins themselves. Therefore the use of a portable Doppler to localize incompetent ankle perforators has limited accuracy.[23]

Failure to detect incompetent veins with the continuous-wave Doppler technique in clinical practice is possible when the patient is obese and superficial varicose veins are located at a depth of several centimeters. In this situation the use of a lower-frequency Doppler probe is indicated. Often only one portable probe is used (8 MHz), an approach that is less versatile than using separate low-frequency (5.4 MHz) and high-frequency (9.3 MHz) probes.

Duplex Scanning and Color-Flow Imaging

Some clinicians might question the need for the expensive equipment involved in duplex scanning and color-flow imaging to view simple varicosities. Certainly, many patients have adequate diagnosis and treatment of their varicose veins without duplex scanning. This argument depends in large part on the weight of the patient involved. Obesity is very common in the United States, with 25% of the population weighing in excess of 120% of their ideal body weight. In many of these patients the visible varicosities represent the tip of an "iceberg," with the "iceberg" itself not amenable to clinical examination. The consequences of incomplete therapy resulting from incomplete examination are often more troublesome than performing duplex scanning prior to therapy.

The basic principle of ultrasonic duplex scanning is the combination of B-mode echographic imaging and pulsed-wave Doppler ultrasound beams to allow examination of vessels at a specific depth. This approach is based on the principle that the amount of time between emission and reflection of the ultrasound beam is related to the distance that the ultrasound travels in tissue. The sample volume can be directed at the vein at a specific angle. With the newer color-flow machines, the Doppler signals are depicted as colored pixels in the B-mode image. The Doppler principle of maintaining an angle smaller than 90 degrees to the direction of blood flow is paramount in obtaining reliable data with these devices.

The automatic cuff inflator consists of an air compressor that inflates and deflates pneumatic cuffs within 0.3 seconds. This device is used instead of manual compression of the leg and has replaced the Valsalva maneuver, which can generate reflux only in proximal veins and depends on the variable presence of iliac vein valves.[17]

The patient is examined in the standing position as described for continuous-wave Doppler examination.[24] Since the patient needs to place his/her weight on the contralateral leg and keep the knee slightly flexed, a frame or walker is needed for balance. The reflux test maneuver can be standardized with pneumatic cuffs. This technique was originally devised for examination of deep veins[25] and may not be as important in the examination of superficial varicose veins, which often can be emptied by manual compression. Some authors, who subsequently adopted this method, also have used distal cuff deflation at multiple levels of the leg.[26] Since the status of deep veins is often unpredictable from clinical information alone, a complete examination is recommended.[27]

The examination begins at the groin, with the examiner directing the duplex probe at the confluence of the common femoral and greater saphenous veins. A pneumatic cuff (24 cm wide) placed around the thigh is inflated to 80 mm Hg for 3 seconds. Reflux then is measured as the cuff is rapidly deflated. The sample volume is placed in the common femoral vein, the greater saphenous vein, and the

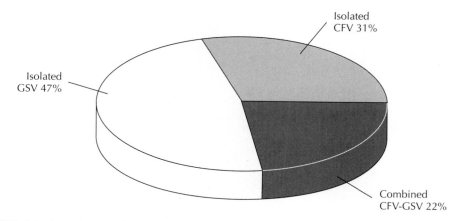

FIGURE 6-1. Association of deep and superficial incompetence near the inguinal ligament. Combined incompetence of the common femoral vein and the greater saphenous vein (true saphenofemoral incompetence) occurs in a minority of patients. N = 55 unoperated legs with reflux. *CFV*, Common femoral vein; *GSV*, greater saphenous vein.

proximal superficial femoral vein, in turn. In normal limbs reflux during closure of competent valves does not exceed 0.45 seconds. When the color-flow scanner is used, reflux is evident as persistent flow. In borderline incompetence the use of spectrum analysis is recommended for more precise timing.

Even though saphenofemoral incompetence is frequently noted in clinical practice, 78% of 55 unoperated legs with reflux in this area involved isolated incompetence of either the common femoral vein only or isolated incompetence of the proximal greater saphenous vein with a normal common femoral vein (Figure 6-1). This finding has important implications for the rationale of simple ligation: if no saphenofemoral incompetence is present initially, the hemodynamics will be unchanged after simple ligation of the proximal greater saphenous vein.

A quick screening test to evaluate outflow can be done at this point by rapidly inflating a cuff applied to the calf to a pressure of 100 mm Hg. If the antegrade velocity in the proximal superficial femoral vein reaches 143 ± 29 cm/sec during cuff inflation, significant obstruction in the popliteal–superficial femoral vein segments is unlikely.[28] This test adds only a few minutes to the study and helps to distinguish patients with primary varicose veins from those with secondary varicose veins.

The popliteal fossa is examined with a cuff placed below the knee. After inflation of the cuff for 3 seconds, reflux in the popliteal vein and lesser saphenous vein is measured as the cuff is deflated (Figure 6-2). Although the lesser saphenous vein usually enters the popliteal vein, the termination point is highly variable and must be accurately localized. Both atypical termination of the lesser saphenous vein into the greater saphenous vein and high termination into the superficial femoral vein or profunda vein have been described.[29] Continuation of the lesser saphenous vein as a sciatic vein is more common than the arterial counterpart of

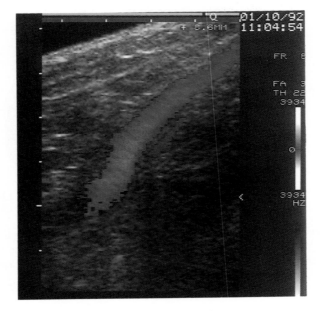

FIGURE 6-2. Incompetent lesser saphenous vein at back of knee. Incompetence of this vein was not evident clinically because of deep location of the vein in the subcutis. Head of patient is toward left. Flow toward the feet is depicted in red.

this anatomic variation. Multiple connections of the lesser saphenous vein to the gastrocnemial and popliteal veins also occur.

The medial side of the knee is examined to assess flow in the greater saphenous vein and additional accessory veins (Figure 6-3). Incompetent greater saphenous veins can present as straight dilated vessels (Figure 6-4). It is possible to calculate the volume of reflux flow from the diameter of incompetent veins and the velocity of retrograde flow.[30,31] In spite of previous stripping operations or sclerotherapy, incompetent veins are frequently present on the medial side of the knee.[32] After a previous stripping operation, recurrent or accessory saphenous veins can remain as straight vascular structures (Figure 6-5). In other cases the greater saphenous vein is replaced by a conglomerate of convoluted veins (Figure 6-6) in which it is impossible to identify the flow direction. The anterolateral branch of the greater saphenous vein can be identified only if significant dilatation has occurred. In one study scanning the anterolateral aspect of the thigh near the patella yielded incompetent anterolateral branches in 20% of referred patients.[2]

The calf level is examined with the cuff placed around the ankle. At this level the greater saphenous vein often consists of two branches. Evaluation of the deep calf veins, including the peroneal veins, is facilitated by color imaging.[33] The lesser saphenous vein can be identified at the midcalf level by its straight course and deep position in the posterior midline. Reflux within this segment of the lesser saphenous vein can occur without concomitant incompetence of the proximal part.

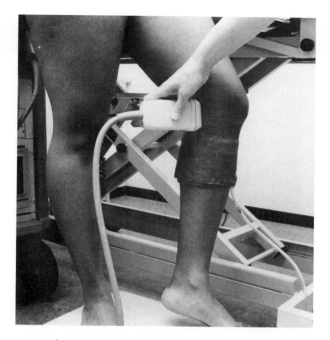

FIGURE 6-3. Examination of medial aspect of the knee. Reflux is measured during deflation of cuff.

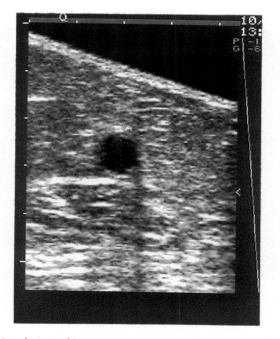

FIGURE 6-4. Cross-sectional view of incompetent greater saphenous vein of male patient presenting with severe weeping stasis dermatitis. Diameter at the knee is 8.3 mm. Depth from the skin is 13.8 mm.

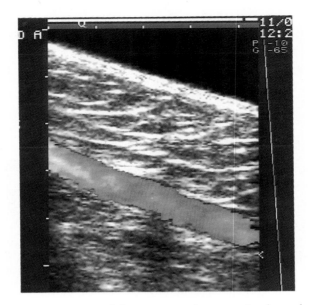

FIGURE 6-5. Recurrent incompetence of the greater saphenous vein above the knee, after previous stripping operation. Head of patient is toward left. Reflux is depicted in red.

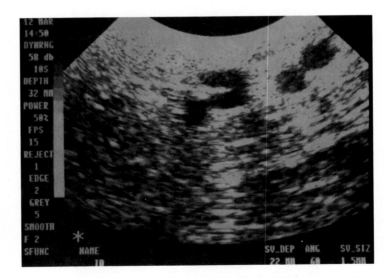

FIGURE 6-6. Typical tortuous varicosities are located in the subcutis at medial aspect of the knee.

Veins at the ankle level are examined with a small (7 cm wide) cuff placed around the foot. An inflation pressure of 120 mm Hg is used. The posterior tibial veins are easily located behind the medial malleolus and alongside the artery. Unless the greater saphenous vein has been previously removed, it can be examined at its premalleolar site. Anterior branches of the greater saphenous vein can be identified in the pretibial area in 13% of subjects. Further imaging of the posterior arch veins and gaiter area can be done if changes in chronic venous stasis complicate the picture. Using duplex scanning, certain authors have confirmed the high incidence of superficial disease in patients with stasis ulceration.[34] A detailed search of the gaiter area for incompetent perforating veins has been described,[35] but the hemodynamic significance of small perforating veins near the ankle is unclear.

The recent advent of endoscopic perforator ligation has stimulated interest in the duplex imaging of medial calf perforators. However, several important observations have been reported by Sarin et al.[36] Their study noted that flow in the medial calf perforators can be inward or outward in limbs without evidence of venous disease. Outward flow was demonstrated in 21% of perforators in normal limbs. Therefore it would be inappropriate to call all these veins pathologic "incompetent perforating veins." On release of a distal cuff (pressure 60 mm Hg, with leg in dangling position), perforator flow was found in 33% to 44% of limbs with objective evidence of venous disease, and this finding was considered to be of pathologic significance. Hanrahan et al.[35] found that perforators of more than 4 mm diameter can occur, with unidirectional-inward flow in patients with ulceration.

CLASSIFICATION OF REFLUX IN SPECIAL AREAS
Groin Area: Saphenofemoral Incompetence

The term "saphenofemoral incompetence" has become a buzzword to describe patients with varicose veins who are candidates for surgery. Most insurance companies require the presence of saphenofemoral incompetence (SFI) to give preapproval for surgical procedures such as ligation-stripping. The term "SFI" seems to have originated in the era of continuous-wave Doppler ultrasound examination of this area. SFI refers to reflux at the level of the uppermost valve of the greater saphenous vein during Valsalva maneuvers. It implies reflux from the common femoral vein into the greater saphenous vein (Figure 6-7, A).

With the use of color imaging in the groin area, we now recognize other patterns of reflux that do not fit the category of SFI. Frequently the proximal saphenous vein is completely normal, but an incompetent anterolateral branch enters the saphenofemoral junction (SFJ) and is responsible for reflux in the region (Figure 6-7, B). Another pattern is reflux from enlarged superficial epigastric branches on the lower abdomen, feeding into the greater saphenous vein below a normal competent SFJ (Figure 6-7, C). In many of these cases a complete dissection of the SFJ is necessary to appreciate the anatomy and ligate the origin of the incompe-

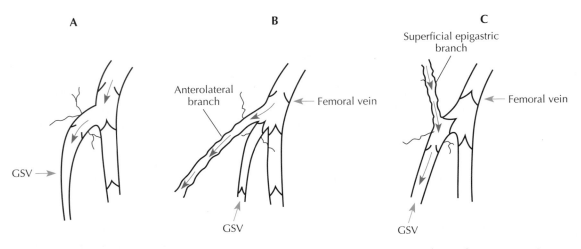

FIGURE 6-7. A, Saphenofemoral incompetence: reflux from an incompetent femoral vein into an incompetent greater saphenous vein *(GSV)*. "Femorosaphenous reflux" might be a more appropriate term. **B,** Reflux into an incompetent anterolateral branch, with intact valve in the proximal greater saphenous vein. There is no indication to ligate or remove the saphenous vein in this situation. **C,** Reflux from enlarged superficial epigastric branches into the proximal greater saphenous vein, with intact valve at the junction of the saphenous vein and the femoral vein.

tent veins. A normal SFJ should not be ligated around the intact proximal saphenous vein, which would cause bothersome phlebitis and unnecessary loss of vein segments.

Therefore it may be necessary to explore the SFJ in cases where the reflux does not pass from the femoral vein into the proximal saphenous vein. A more accurate description should be used whenever possible. If the preoperative anatomy is somewhat unclear, more general terminology, such as "reflux in the region of the saphenofemoral junction," should be used.

Popliteal Fossa

The anatomy of the veins in the popliteal fossa is highly variable. On one hand, this variability makes duplex scanning extremely useful; however, an accurate description often defies the simple term "saphenopopliteal incompetence." Combined incompetence of both the short saphenous vein and the popliteal vein was noted in 45% of cases with reflux behind the knee.[37] A common finding is the popliteal area vein, a superficially located vein named by Dodd.[38] The short saphenous vein can be recognized by its subfascial position, as shown in Figure 6-8, and its often close proximity to a small arterial branch. The point where the lesser saphenous vein perforates the fascia is variable: the most common location (52%) is the middle third of the leg.[39] Entry of the lesser saphenous vein at the popliteal fossa fascia has been found in 9%. No termination of the lesser saphenous vein in

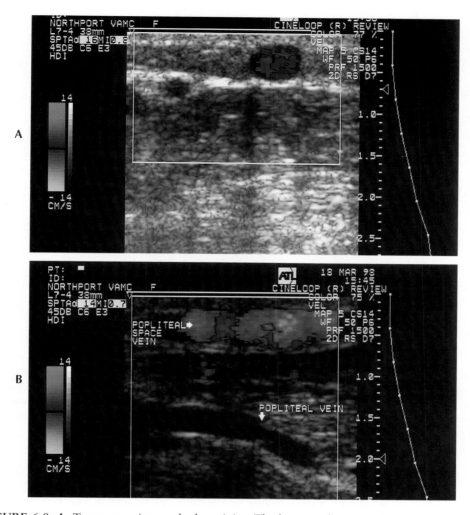

FIGURE 6-8. A, Transverse view at the knee-joint. The lesser saphenous vein is shown on the left, with echogenic fascia over it. On the right is the larger incompetent popliteal area vein. **B,** Longitudinal view showing the incompetent superficial popliteal area vein lying on top of the fascia (in red on cuff deflation). Normal popliteal vein is black because of the absence of reflux flow.

the popliteal vein was found in 25% of 200 cadaver limbs. In another study[40] two thirds of the cases had a popliteal vein consisting of two trunks at the level of the knee-joint, with one usually being much larger than the other.

The lesser saphenous vein often joins the gastrocnemius vein prior to joining the popliteal vein (Figure 6-9, *A*). A "flush" ligation at the popliteal vein could result in obstruction of the gastrocnemic vein. Leaving a stump of lesser saphenous vein not only increases the risk of recurrent varicosities; in our experience it also increases the risk that a thrombus may develop and propagate into the popliteal

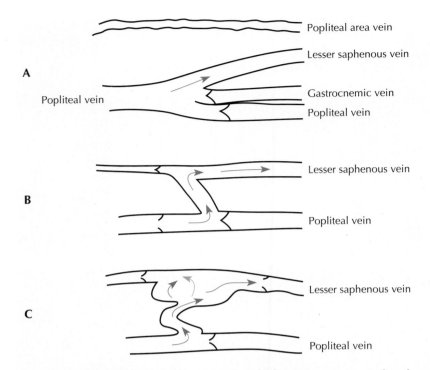

FIGURE 6-9. A, Incompetent lesser saphenous vein, which joins a gastrocnemic vein and popliteal vein. Popliteal area vein is not connected to the deep system in this case. **B,** Incompetent lesser saphenous vein, which continues as a smaller competent vein on the posterior thigh, combined with an incompetent popliteal vein. **C,** Incompetent lesser saphenous vein, with "blowout" of the fascia and large varix of the proximal lesser saphenous vein.

vein. Figure 6-9, *B* and *C,* shows more possible ways in which the lesser saphenous vein may join the popliteal vein in the popliteal fossa.[41]

DISCUSSION

Laboratory evaluation of patients with varicose veins is useful if it makes a difference with regard to the modality or extent of treatment. For example, on clinical examination accessory veins on the medial side of the leg are easily mistaken for the greater saphenous vein (Figure 6-10), a problem that may account for some of the controversy regarding the relative efficacy of sclerotherapy and surgery. Comparison of treatment results is possible only if identification of the saphenous vein and measurement of its diameter are done with a reliable method, that is, duplex scanning. Accurate stratification of patients with reflux in the groin area requires more than a single category of saphenofemoral incompetence, as explained earlier. Duplex scanning can also provide reliable follow-up data after surgery or sclerotherapy.

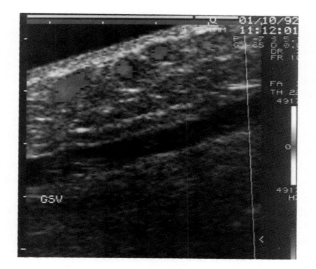

FIGURE 6-10. Longitudinal view at medial side of the knee. Incompetence of superficially located tortuous accessory vein is noted. Reflux is depicted in red and blue because of tortuosity with varying Doppler angles. Absence of reflux in the normal, more deeply located greater saphenous vein is shown in black. This absence was noted during deflation of a cuff placed around the calf.

Recurrent varicose veins may be either residual varicose veins caused by incomplete removal during the first operation, or they may represent true recurrences. With early recurrences the possibility of secondary varicose veins caused by deep venous disease must be considered. A duplex scan examination that includes the deep veins can help identify this situation prior to treatment. For this purpose using the standardized reflux-provoking maneuver by deflating a distally placed cuff, with the patient in a standing position, gives the most consistent results.[42] Reducing the extent of surgery by limiting treatment to incompetent venous segments ensures the preservation of normal veins and reduces the incidence of inadvertent damage to saphenous and sural nerves. The distinction between multiple recurrences of primary varicose veins and chronic venous insufficiency is often unclear in clinical practice; evaluation of calf pump function with an air plethysmograph can be helpful in complicated situations.

CONCLUSION

For lean patients with readily visible varicosities, examination of the popliteal fossa and the saphenofemoral area with a portable Doppler device may be all that is needed. If, however, reflux is noted at the back of the knee or if patency of the popliteal vein is in question, duplex examination is recommended. Duplex scanning also is indicated for obese patients with varicose veins, patients with recurrent varicose veins, and those with complaints of severe stasis or ulceration.

REFERENCES

1. Randhawa K, Dhillon S, Kistner RL, Ferris EB. Assessment of chronic venous insufficiency using dynamic venous pressure studies. Am J Surg 148:203-209, 1984.

2. van Bemmelen PS, van Ramshorst B, Eikelboom BC. Photoplethysmography reexamined: The lack of correlation with duplex in venous insufficiency. Surgery 112:544-548, 1992.

3. McMullin GM, Coleridge Smith PD, Scurr JH. A study of tourniquets in the investigation of venous insufficiency. Phlebology 6:133-139, 1991.

4. Abramowitz HB, Queral LA, Flinn WR, Nora PF, Peterson L, Bergan JJ, Yao JST. The use of photoplethysmography in the assessment of venous insufficiency: A comparison to venous pressure measurements. Surgery 86:434-441, 1979.

5. Flinn WR, Queral LA, Abramowitz HB, Yao JST. Photoplethysmography in the assessment of chronic venous insufficiency. In Nicolaides AN, Yao JST, eds. Investigations of Vascular Disorders. New York: Churchill Livingstone, 1981, Chapter 32.

6. Barnes RW. Noninvasive techniques in chronic venous insufficiency. In Bernstein EF, ed. Noninvasive Diagnostic Techniques in Vascular Disease. St. Louis: Mosby, 1985, Chapter 84.

7. Rosfors S. Venous photoplethysmography: Relationship between transducer position and regional distribution of venous insufficiency. J Vasc Surg 11:436-440, 1990.

8. Braverman IM, Keh-Yen A. Ultrastructure of the human dermal microcirculation. IV. Valve containing collecting veins at the dermal-subcutaneous junction. J Invest Dermatol 81:438-442, 1983.

9. Allan JC. Volume changes in the lower limb in response to postural alterations and muscular exercise. S Afr J Surg 2:75-90, 1964.

10. Christopoulos D, Nicolaides AN, Szendro G. Venous reflux: Quantification and correlation with the clinical severity of chronic venous disease. Br J Surg 75:352-356, 1988.

11. Christopoulos D, Nicolaides AN, Cook A, Irvine A, Galloway JMD, Wilkinson A. Pathogenesis of venous ulceration in relation to the calf muscle pump function. Surgery 106:829-835, 1989.

12. Christopoulos D, Nicolaides AN, Galloway JMD, Wilkinson A. Objective noninvasive evaluation of venous surgical results. J Vasc Surg 8:683-687, 1988.

13. Welkie JF, Kerr RP, Katz ML, Comerota AJ. Can noninvasive venous volume determinations accurately predict ambulatory venous pressure? J Vasc Technol 15:186-190, 1991.

14. Sumner DS. Evaluation of the venous circulation using the ultrasonic Doppler velocity detector. In Rutherford RB, ed. Vascular Surgery. Philadelphia: WB Saunders, 1977.

15. Folse R, Alexander RH. Directional flow detection for localizing venous valvular incompetency. Surgery 67:114-121, 1970.

16. van Bemmelen PS, Beach K, Bedford G, Strandness DE. The mechanism of venous valve closure. Arch Surg 125:617-619, 1990.

17. van Bemmelen PS, Bedford G, Beach K, Isaac CA, Strandness DE. Evaluation of tests used to document venous valve incompetence. J Vasc Technol 14:87-90, 1990.

18. Mitchell DC, Darke SG. The assessment of primary varicose veins by Doppler ultrasound—The role of saphenopopliteal incompetence and the short saphenous systems in calf varicosities. Eur J Vasc Surg 1:113-115, 1987.

19. Nicolaides AN, Fernandes é Fernandes J, Zimmerman H. Doppler ultrasound in the investigation of venous insufficiency. In Nicolaides AN, Yao JST, eds. Investigation of Vascular Disorders. New York: Churchill Livingstone, 1981, Chapter 28.

20. Schull KC, Nicolaides AN, Fernandes é Fernandes J, Miles C, Horner J, Needham T, Cooke ED, Eastcott FHG. Significance of popliteal reflux in relation to ambulatory venous pressure and ulceration. Arch Surg 114:1304-1306, 1979.

21. Goren G, Yellin AE. Primary varicose veins: Topographic and hemodynamic correlations. J Cardiovasc Surg 31:672-677, 1990.

22. Albanese AR, Albanese AM, Albanese EF. Lateral subdermic varicose vein system of the legs. Vasc Surg 3:81-89, 1969.

23. O'Donnell TF, Burnand KG, Clemenson G, Lea Thomas M, Browse NL. Doppler examination vs. clinical and phlebographic detection of the location of incompetent perforating veins. Arch Surg 112:31-35, 1977.
24. Szendro G, Nicolaides AN, Zukowski AJ, Christopoulos D, Malouf GM, Christodoulou C, Myers K. Duplex scanning in the assessment of deep venous incompetence. J Vasc Surg 4:237-242, 1986.
25. van Bemmelen PS, Bedford G, Beach K, Strandness DE. Quantitative segmental evaluation of venous valvular reflux with duplex ultrasound scanning. J Vasc Surg 10:425-431, 1989.
26. Czeredarzuk M, Branas CC, Weingarten MS. Duplex imaging and distal cuff deflation to measure venous reflux time. J Vasc Technol 15:196-208, 1991.
27. van Bemmelen PS, Bedford G, Beach K, Strandness DE. Status of the valves in the superficial and deep venous system in chronic venous disease. Surgery 109:730-734, 1991.
28. van Bemmelen PS, Bedford G, Beach K, Strandness DE. Functional status of the deep venous system after an episode of deep venous thrombosis. Ann Vasc Surg 5:455-459, 1990.
29. Franco G, Nguyen Khac G, Nguyen Morere MC. Intérêt de l'écho Doppler de la saphène externe. Confrontation clinique. Phlebologie 43:135-145, 1990.
30. Vasdekis SN, Clarke GH, Nicolaides AN. Quantification of venous reflux by means of duplex scanning. J Vasc Surg 10:670-677, 1989.
31. Bergan JJ, Beeman S, Poppiti R. Quantitative segmental evaluation of venous valve reflux: Impact on clinical practice. Vienna, Vascular European-American Symposium on Venous Diseases. Nov 7-10, 1990.
32. Bishop CRC, Fronek HS, Fronek A, Dilley RB, Bernstein EF. Real-time color duplex scanning after sclerotherapy of the great saphenous vein. J Vasc Surg 14:505-510, 1991.
33. van Bemmelen PS, Bedford G, Strandness DE. Visualization of calf veins by color flow imaging. Ultrasound Med Biol 16:15-17, 1990.
34. Hanrahan LM, Araki CT, Rodriguez AA, Kechejian GJ, LaMorte WW, Menzoian JO. Distribution of valvular incompetence in patients with stasis ulceration. J Vasc Surg 13:805-812, 1991.
35. Hanrahan LM, Araki CT, Fisher JB, Rodriguez AA, Walker TG, Woodson J, LaMorte WW, Menzoian JO. Evaluation of the perforating veins of the lower extremity using high-resolution duplex imaging. J Cardiovasc Surg 32:87-97, 1991.
36. Sarin S, Scurr JH, Coleridge Smith PD. Medial calf perforators in venous disease: The significance of outward flow. J Vasc Surg 16:40-46, 1992.
37. van Bemmelen PS, Bergan JJ. Quantitative measurement of venous incompetence. Austin: RG Landes, 1992.
38. Dodd H. The varicose tributaries of the popliteal vein. Br J Surg 52:350, 1965.
39. Moosman DA, Hartwell SW. The surgical significance of the subfascial course of the lesser saphenous vein. Surg Gynecol Obstet 113:761, 1964.
40. Williams AF. The formation of the popliteal vein. Surg Gynecol Obstet 97:769, 1953.
41. Baud JM. Echo-Doppler du creux poplite et du mollet-préalable à la phlebectomie ambulatoire. Phlebologie 43:319, 1990.
42. Evers EJ, Wuppermann TH. Die Charakterisierung des postthrombotischen Refluxes mittels farbcodierter Duplexsonographie. Vasa 26:190-193, 1997.

Chapter 7

Pretreatment Testing of Patients With Varicose Veins and Telangiectatic Blemishes

Ulrich Schultz-Ehrenburg

A physical examination is conducted before sclerotherapy or surgical treatment of varicose veins for many different reasons. These reasons are related to the therapeutic indications and contraindications, anatomic and functional venous findings, treatment plans, and prospects for lasting results.

The contraindications for sclerotherapy include (1) deep vein thrombosis, (2) lymphedema, (3) arterial occlusive disease, (4) immobility, and (5) severe general disease. A deep vein thrombosis is an absolute contraindication. The induced phlebitis triggered by sclerotherapy can impair venous hemodynamics and lead to unpredictable thrombotic reactions. In cases of chronic lymphedema, injections involving the affected leg, as well as surgical measures, are usually inadvisable. The iatrogenic inflammation can further damage the defective lymphatic system, causing further deterioration of lymphatic flow.[1]

Arterial occlusive disease is a relative contraindication to sclerotherapy. Combinations of arterial occlusive disease and varices are encountered particularly after 50 years of age. In these cases the pathophysiologic state is such that negative interactions occur among the various therapeutic measures. At an advanced stage, arterial occlusive disease can interfere with all effective forms of therapy for chronic venous insufficiency (CVI). Patients with this type of mixed vascular disease are unable to elevate their legs, wear compression stockings, or walk with bandaged legs to improve the impaired venous return. For this reason, measuring systolic pressure of the malleolar arteries with the Doppler probe is the first diagnostic measure undertaken before sclerotherapy for patients older than 50 years. This approach also applies to younger patients with corresponding clinical symptoms. If a decrease in systolic blood pressure relative to systemic pressure can be demonstrated, it is advisable to proceed with extreme caution. The hyperemia induced by sclerotherapy can increase the disproportion between blood supply and blood requirements. Poorly healing ulcerations may result.

The following figures serve as a rule of thumb: at pressures <100 mm Hg, varix operations and injections of the lower leg should not be considered; at pressures <80 mm Hg, compression treatment generally is not tolerated since compression may cause the arterial perfusion pressure to decrease to critical values.[2]

Additional contraindications include immobility and severe general diseases. As a general rule, it is stipulated that patients should walk for 30 minutes after sclerotherapy. Otherwise there is a danger that the sclerosing agent will drain poorly and pass into the deep veins, causing a deep vein thrombosis.

CLINICAL EXAMINATION

The medical history provides information about the patient's past and present complaints and his/her motives for seeking consultation. Visual inspection and palpation permit clinical classification with respect to many different factors, especially the type of varix and the clinical stage of CVI.

Varices can be subdivided clinically into two groups comprising the five types of genuine varicose veins:
1. Large varicose veins
   a. Trunk varicosities
   b. Branch varicosities
   c. Incompetent perforators
2. Small varicose veins
   a. Reticular varicosities
   b. Telangiectasias

Refluxes play a decisive role in the pathogenesis of large varices. They are usually detected over the saphenofemoral junction or the saphenopopliteal junction. Identification of these refluxes represents an important area of application for Doppler ultrasonographic techniques. When perforators become incompetent, they may become an additional source of refluxes. Such refluxes are called "blowouts." Usually a protrusion in the area of the blowout is detected by visual examination, and palpation reveals an enlarged fascial gap.

The second important clinical objective is to correctly assess the degree of CVI. Not all varices meet the requirements for CVI. For example, telangiectasias and reticular veins do not represent a disturbance of venous function. Likewise, mild forms of trunk and branch varices (and even incompetent perforators) do not necessarily trigger functional disturbances. Not until these major varices exert a hemodynamic effect do they meet the requirements for venous insufficiency, which is naturally chronic (i.e., a CVI). Approximately 80% of all cases of CVI are caused by a decompensation of varicose veins, whereas the remainder are caused by a postthrombotic syndrome. Functionally, CVI is characterized by a deterioration of venous function. Another name for CVI is calf pump insufficiency.

CVI can be divided into three clinical stages (see box, p. 112).[3] Edema and corona phlebectatica characterize stage I. Stage II is distinguished by various cutaneous complications occurring below the level of a leg ulcer. I believe that

CLINICAL STAGES OF CHRONIC VENOUS INSUFFICIENCY*

Stage I
  Edema
  Corona phlebectatica
Stage II
  (Eczema, dermatitis)
  (Purpura, pigmentation)
  Fibrosing panniculitis
  Lipodermatosclerosis
  White atrophy (atrophie blanche)
  Stasis papillomatosis
Stage III
  Venous ulcer
  Ulcer scar

*Modified from Widmer LK, Stähelin HB, Nissen C, dáSilva A. Venen-, Arterienkrankheiten, koronare Herzkrankheit bei Berufstätigen. Prospektiv-epidemiologische Untersuchung. Basel Study I-III, 1959-1978. Berne: Hans Huber, 1981.

eczema and pigmentation are not linked to any particular clinical stage. They may appear during stage I and may be missing at more advanced stages. Stage III is manifested by a healed or current venous ulcer. These three clinical stages do not correspond to the division into three degrees of venous insufficiency that can be done on the basis of photoplethysmography.

DIAGNOSTIC METHODS

Highly effective noninvasive examination methods are available for further evaluation of varicose veins. A distinction must be made between anatomic and functional methods. For routine diagnostic purposes, venous Doppler ultrasonography is the most important anatomic method, and photoplethysmography is the most important functional examination method. Further developments of the Doppler technique, such as duplex scanning or color-coded duplex devices (described in the preceding chapter) represent expensive equipment that is not necessary for a correct diagnosis and treatment of varicose veins in most straightforward cases. This chapter is limited to the use of conventional venous Doppler examinations and photoplethysmographic measures, which are described with detailed comments. Concerning the older clinical examination tests, such as the Perthes' test, the Linton test, and Trendelenburg's test, that are frequently recommended in textbooks, I think that they can be dispensed with entirely because they are imprecise by modern diagnostic standards.

Photoplethysmography

Photoplethysmography is a method of quantitatively evaluating venous function. The devices used measure changes in the blood volume of the skin brought about by calf pump activity. These devices include an optical sensor that emits infrared light. The infrared light penetrates the skin to a depth of approximately 3 mm; the light is partly absorbed and partly reflected. Blood vessels reflect about 10 times less infrared light than does cutaneous tissue. If the blood volume in the area being measured is decreased—for example, by muscular activity—the average skin reflection rises.

During measurement the patient needs to perform 8 or 10 dorsiflexions while sitting. The probe usually is located 10 cm above the inner ankle. During muscle exercise a curve is produced similar to that obtained by invasive measurement of venous pressure. Muscle movement causes a change in the degree of filling of cutaneous blood vessels and thus in the degree of light reflection, until the maximum amount of blood has been pumped out of the leg. In the subsequent resting phase, the vessels of a healthy person refill slowly by arterial inflow. In patients with varices the vessels refill more quickly by means of venous refluxes. This action leads to a shortening of the refilling time.

The refilling time thus provides a quantitative measure of the capability of the calf muscle pump. According to a generally accepted system of classification, there are three degrees of insufficiency.[4] Degree III corresponds to a refilling time of <10 seconds; degree II, to a refilling time of 10 to 20 seconds. Degree I corresponds to a refilling time of 20 to 25 seconds; values >25 seconds are considered normal (Figure 7-1). Although only these refilling time values (T_0) could be evaluated with older devices, modern quantitative digital photoplethysmographic devices also enable a determination of amplitude of venous pump power (V_0).[5] Further details of photoplethysmography are described in other sources.[6-10]

The muscle pump test measures venous function as a whole. A more detailed picture of the underlying CVI can be obtained with the aid of a tourniquet test. The examination distinguishes between improvable and nonimprovable CVI, which will be explained later in this chapter.

Doppler Ultrasonography

Venous Doppler ultrasonography is the second important diagnostic method for evaluating venous function. This examination provides information about the competence or incompetence of an individual vein. During examination, S sounds must be differentiated from A sounds. S sounds represent spontaneous flow sounds and are important in the diagnosis of a thrombosis. A sounds, or augmented sounds, represent artificial accelerations of flow caused by manual compression. In combination with Valsalva's maneuver, A sounds are used to diagnose reflux in the varicosis.

Doppler ultrasonography is most frequently used for examination of the

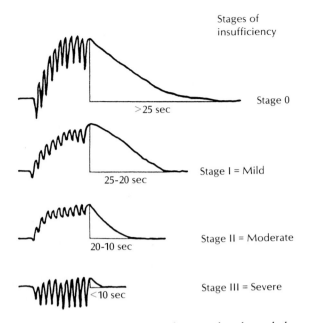

FIGURE 7-1. Assessment of calf pump function by photoplethysmography.

long saphenous vein, which is verified by Valsalva's maneuver. By means of abdominal pressure, blood is forced in a retrograde direction. Retrograde blood flow is not possible, however, if the venous valves of the long saphenous vein are intact. When valvular incompetence of the saphenofemoral junction exists, reflux occurs and is registered by the Doppler probe as a sharp flow sound. With the Doppler probe the reflux can be followed along its entire length; therefore this device can be used to determine the origin and course of a varicose reflux.

Valsalva's maneuver is not suitable for examining the short saphenous vein since this vein does not have a connection of its own to the pelvic region. For this reason manual compression and decompression are performed in the lower part of the vein while the Doppler probe is positioned above the saphenopopliteal junction. The decompression phase is decisive for diagnosis. In the event of valvular incompetence, the pull exerted by the decompression leads to a reflux that can be heard with the Doppler probe. If the valves are intact, no reflux sound is heard.

The Doppler probe is suitable not only for examining the superficial veins but also for diagnosing refluxes of the deep veins.[11] By using five test methods, it is possible to accurately detect refluxes of the deep venous system. These methods are calf compression, calf decompression, thigh compression, thigh decompression, and Valsalva's maneuver. Two examples are provided here to illustrate the use of these methods.

Refluxes in the ankle region play an important role in the pathogenesis of CVI. They can be examined by means of calf compression (Figure 7-2). The

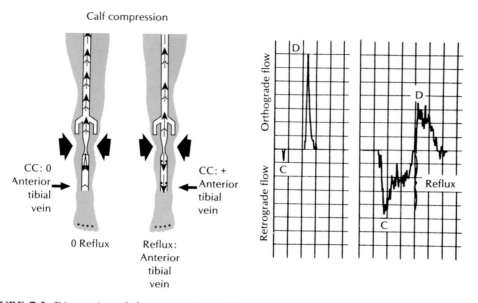

FIGURE 7-2. Diagnosis and documentation of deep refluxes in ankle region. *CC,* Compression of calf; *C,* compression; *D,* decompression.

Doppler probe is placed in the ankle region above the anterior or posterior tibial veins, and a deep calf compression is performed. In the event of incompetent valves a loud reflux sound is heard over the malleolar vein; this sound is absent if the valves are intact.

The popliteal vein can be tested by means of calf decompression, thigh compression, and Valsalva's maneuver (Figure 7-3). During the entire examination the Doppler probe is positioned above the popliteal vein. A Doppler sound heard during calf decompression is evidence of reflux extending from the hollow of the knee downward, whereas a Doppler sound noted during thigh compression is evidence of reflux extending from the thigh downward to the hollow of the knee. A Doppler sound heard during Valsalva's maneuver indicates reflux extending from the pelvis to the hollow of the knee.

By systematically applying the diagnostic methods available for detecting superficial and deep venous refluxes, it is possible to obtain a detailed picture of the superficial and deep veins in the leg. This approach plays an important role in formulating an accurate treatment plan.

The efficiency of the Doppler probe can be seen, in particular, in cases of atypical saphenous varices. These are trunk varices of the long saphenous vein with a negative Valsalva segment proximally and a positive Valsalva segment distally. This condition also is called a paradoxical reflux. In reality, the reflux is not paradoxical; the intact proximal venous segment is circumvented via collateral veins. In this context two types of atypical refluxes can be differentiated: (1) simple atypical refluxes with a superficial collateral circulation, and (2) hidden atypical refluxes with a deep collateral circulation (see box, p. 120). Additional methodologic details and exact instructions regarding examination techniques have been described.[11]

The benefits of noninvasive diagnostic methods make them an indispensable part of the routine diagnostic workup. The examination methods provide a great deal of information without placing a burden on the patient; consequently they can be repeated as often as desired. Today photoplethysmography and Doppler

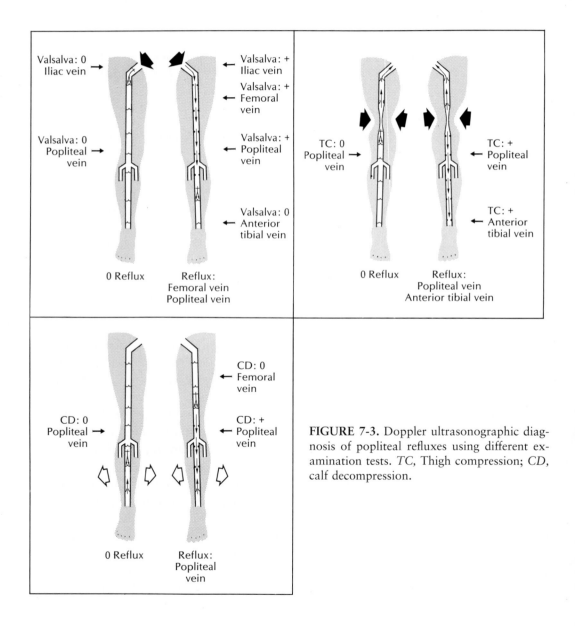

FIGURE 7-3. Doppler ultrasonographic diagnosis of popliteal refluxes using different examination tests. *TC,* Thigh compression; *CD,* calf decompression.

ultrasonography are part of the basic phlebologic diagnostic arsenal. They represent the examination methods of choice and in most cases obviate the necessity for resorting to invasive methods. There is no reason to deny photoplethysmographic or Doppler ultrasonographic examination to a patient with a genuine varicosis or more severe phlebological findings. In the event of contradictory results, however, the diagnosis should be confirmed with invasive methods (e.g., direct venous pressure measurement, phlebography, or duplex ultrasonography).

CHRONIC VENOUS INSUFFICIENCY

The results of the photoplethysmographic examination do not provide information as to whether the underlying vein incompetence is superficial or deep. For this reason the examination is repeated with the tourniquet test, in which a cuff placed below the knee occludes varicose refluxes in the long and short saphenous veins. Two different results can be obtained: improvement or nonimprovement of venous function, referred to as improvable or nonimprovable CVI (Figure 7-4).

Improvable CVI generally indicates superficial vein incompetence, whereas nonimprovable CVI most often indicates deep vein incompetence, usually in connection with a postthrombotic syndrome. Incompetent perforators also can simulate nonimprovable CVI within the scope of a genuine varicosis; this condition is called falsely nonimprovable CVI (see Figure 7-4). Finally, deep vein thrombosis also can result in nonimprovable CVI. Therefore several explanations are possible for a tourniquet test result of nonimprovable CVI.

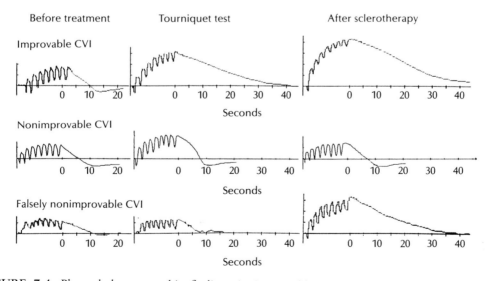

FIGURE 7-4. Photoplethysmographic findings in improvable, nonimprovable, and falsely nonimprovable chronic venous insufficiency (pretherapeutic tourniquet test and findings after complete varix elimination).

Improvable Chronic Venous Insufficiency

Improvable CVI constitutes a clear indication for invasive varix treatment (i.e., surgery and/or sclerotherapy). In these cases the tourniquet test has clearly demonstrated that calf pump insufficiency can be improved by eliminating the varices. The foremost value of photoplethysmographic examination thus lies in this objective identification of an indication. Consequently this technique also should be used after the treatment has been completed and to detect recurrences at follow-up examinations.

Nonimprovable Chronic Venous Insufficiency

The management of nonimprovable CVI is quite different. Since the majority of cases are caused by deep vein incompetence, eliminating the varices makes little sense. In this situation the dominant pathologic condition is the deep venous disturbance, which cannot be corrected by treating the superficial varicose veins. Patients must wear medical compression stockings their entire lives, especially when they exhibit cutaneous complications or edema or have subjective complaints. This kind of treatment cannot cure CVI; however, it can compensate for the condition. Complete varix elimination is no longer necessary and, in fact, is not advisable. Such therapy would not eliminate the need for compression therapy, which the patient may be tempted to discontinue because of the improved cosmetic results.

The Doppler probe should be used in every case to confirm whether a nonimprovable venous function is actually caused by a deep venous incompetence. In many cases Doppler ultrasonography reveals a completely normal deep venous system. In the clinical setting patients thus affected regularly show multiple incompetent perforators of the lower leg, so that the missing improvement during the tourniquet test can be explained by the blowout refluxes. In these cases the result of the Doppler examination of the deep veins is of prime importance for deciding on therapy.

Falsely Nonimprovable Chronic Venous Insufficiency

If Doppler ultrasonographic examination shows competent deep veins, I do not base a treatment plan on the tourniquet test result. Instead, I perform a complete varix treatment for these patients, with preference given to sclerotherapy. After completion of therapy, the functional result is checked with photoplethysmography. In most cases a normalization of venous function is observed, confirming the diagnosis of falsely nonimprovable CVI retrospectively.

In such situations the incompetent perforators are probably the reason for the negative result of the tourniquet test. This theory presupposes that the incompetent perforators are located below the tourniquet and that they have a hemodynamic effect, which appears to be the case in only a minority of patients with clinically incompetent-appearing perforating veins. The question arises whether the effect of these perforating veins can be excluded by lowering the tourniquet. Since the photoplethysmographic sensor normally should be placed 10 cm above the inner ankle, the advantages gained by lowering the tourniquet are limited. Even when the tourniquet is lowered, perforating veins often remain more distally.

Combined Photoplethysmography and Doppler Ultrasonography

The diagnostic possibilities of photoplethysmography increase when this method is used in conjunction with Doppler ultrasonography. With the Doppler method the competence of the deep veins can be checked directly rather than indirectly. In this way contradictions can be discovered quickly and the conclusions can be used to determine the most effective treatment for the patient. It is necessary only to correlate the findings from photoplethysmography with those from Doppler ultrasonography to differentiate among improvable CVI, nonimprovable CVI, and falsely nonimprovable CVI (Figure 7-5).

Determination of Need for Duplex Ultrasonography

The question may arise about whether it is necessary to use duplex ultrasonography in every case of CVI. Figure 7-5 provides guidelines for making such a determination. If photoplethysmography reveals improvable venous function, the results are clear-cut. In such situations duplex ultrasonography can be dispensed with since the indication for an invasive treatment (i.e., stripping and/or sclerotherapy) is unquestionable. If photoplethysmographic examination shows nonimprovable venous function, duplex ultrasonographic examination of the deep veins of the leg is required to distinguish between truly and falsely nonimprovable venous function. Patients with falsely nonimprovable CVI also should receive complete treatment of varicose veins. Since venous function can be completely normalized in many cases, the phlebologist should not "shy away" from

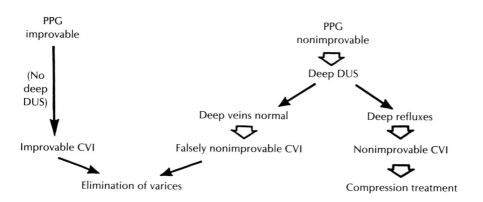

FIGURE 7-5. Flow chart of noninvasive checkup before invasive varix treatment for chronic venous insufficiency. *PPG,* Photoplethysmography; *DUS,* duplex ultrasonography.

this indication. I prefer successive sclerotherapy to one-time surgical treatment because injection treatments can be followed up step by step, both clinically and photoplethysmographically.

SAPHENOUS VARICES

One of the greatest mistakes made by physicians who are performing sclerotherapy is that they limit injections to those venous segments that can be recognized by the naked eye as varicose veins. A comparable mistake made by surgeons performing vein surgery is that they often prefer standard operations, even when the actual findings call for a modified procedure. The pitfalls accompanying both of these frequently observed modes of behavior are seen, in particular, in connection with atypical saphenous varices.

Atypical Saphenous Varices

Atypical saphenous varices are characterized by atypical reflux paths, whereas typical saphenous varices are distinguished by typical reflux paths. Typical saphenous refluxes exhibit junctional valvular incompetence, with reflux passing through the proximal trunk. Visible varices may affect the trunk and branches. Atypical refluxes circumvent proximal venous segments via collateral circulation. A distinction can be made between simple and hidden atypical refluxes (see box), as illustrated by the two examples presented here.

One well-known example is incomplete trunk varicosis of the perforator type. Doppler examination reveals a negative Valsalva segment in the junctional region and the proximal long saphenous vein; a clear reflux sound is noted in the distal truncal segment. For purposes of classification, a deep reflux examination of

---

ATYPICAL SAPHENOUS VARICOSE VEINS

Simple Atypical Refluxes
Reflux in long saphenous vein transmitted by a lateral branch
Reflux in double long saphenous vein
Reflux in long saphenous vein transmitted by external pudendal veins
High-ending, incompetent long saphenous vein
Reflux in short saphenous vein transmitted by long saphenous vein

Hidden Atypical Refluxes
Reflux in long saphenous vein transmitted by perforating veins
Reflux in lateral veins transmitted by perforating veins
Reflux in short saphenous vein transmitted by femoropopliteal vein
Reflux in short saphenous vein transmitted by a high-ending femoropopliteal vein

the external iliac vein and the femoral vein is necessary. The reflux runs from the external iliac vein and the femoral vein across one or more perforating veins into the long saphenous vein (Figure 7-6).

This type of reflux belongs to a group of hidden atypical refluxes that consist of a combination of superficial and deep venous segments. The proximal trunk of the long saphenous vein is sufficient and is circumvented by deep venous reflux. A complete ankle-to-groin stripping should not be done because it would sacrifice an intact venous segment. The most proximal location for surgery or sclerotherapy is the uppermost incompetent perforator, which must be ligated or injected before treatment is directed toward the dependent insufficient segments.

In contrast to hidden atypical refluxes, simple atypical refluxes consist of superficial venous segments along their entire length. The most well known example is a branch type of incomplete trunk varicosis in which the proximal trunk of the long saphenous vein is circumvented by an insufficient tributary and a connecting vein (Figure 7-7). The entire length of the reflux can be followed by the Doppler probe, even if there is no visible varicose dilatation.

Atypical saphenous varices occur in 20% of all genuine varices.[12] In addition to the two reflux paths described, seven types of atypical refluxes can be differentiated. Because of the diversity exhibited by these refluxes, clinical examination alone is not sufficient for establishing an optimal treatment plan. Frequently it is not possible to determine the origin of reflux during clinical examination. For this

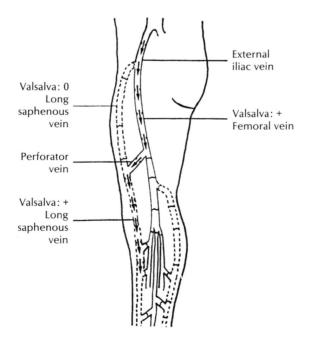

FIGURE 7-6. Doppler findings with hidden atypical reflux of long saphenous vein transmitted by perforating veins.

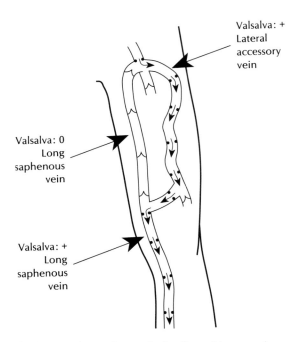

Valsalva: +
Lateral
accessory
vein

Valsalva: 0
Long
saphenous
vein

Valsalva: +
Long
saphenous
vein

FIGURE 7-7. Doppler findings with simple atypical reflux of long saphenous vein transmitted by a lateral branch.

reason Doppler examination of the superficial venous system is essential in every case of genuine varicosis. This type of examination is the best way to determine the origin, length, and course of venous reflux.

The trend in modern phlebology is clearly away from sacrificing competent venous segments. The long saphenous vein is a valuable "spare part" used in arterial bypass surgery. For this reason routine stripping of the long saphenous vein cannot be accepted as a treatment for atypical saphenous varices. It is necessary to exclude the most proximal escape point and the pathologic reflux path and to occlude or remove the varicose segments via surgery and/or sclerotherapy. In cases of hidden atypical refluxes the uppermost incompetent perforating vein of the long saphenous vein is the uppermost therapeutic location. In cases involving simple atypical refluxes the superficial collateral reflux path located "upstream" also must be eliminated.

Atypical saphenous varices constitute an excellent indication for sclerotherapy. The disappearance of collateral refluxes can be demonstrated by normalization of Valsalva reflux from positive to negative.

Typical Saphenous Varices

For typical saphenous varices high ligature and stripping of the long saphenous vein are now considered the treatment of choice. The remaining branches lend themselves to sclerotherapy. Thus the patient is spared unnecessary (and often disfiguring) scars. Nevertheless, there are patients, probably more in Europe than in the United States, who would prefer no treatment rather than undergo surgery. In these cases sclerotherapy with injection of the saphenous junction is an alternative treatment that is particularly recommended for the short saphenous vein. Although all trunk varices can be treated surgically, patients eligible for sclerotherapy must be selected carefully.

The risk associated with sclerotherapy that is not associated with varix surgery is recanalization. However, the recanalization rate is not the same for all patients. A decisive factor is whether the patient has reflux of the popliteal or femoral vein in addition to saphenous reflux. Five years after successful primary junction obliteration of the short saphenous vein, my associates and I observed recanalization in 73% of patients with reflux of the popliteal and femoral veins. In those patients with only saphenous reflux, the recanalization rate was only 27%.[11] A similar situation exists with respect to the long saphenous vein. These Doppler-controlled long-term observations show that lasting saphenous junction obliteration can be achieved in a high percentage of patients who have trunk and branch varicosis but no deep refluxes. Thus a precise Doppler diagnosis offers at least some patients the possibility of receiving conservative treatment.

To select suitable patients, Doppler examination of the superficial and deep venous system is necessary. Investigation of the deep venous system can be limited to examining the femoral and popliteal veins by means of Valsalva's maneuver. Those patients in whom a deep reflux is demonstrated at these locations should be advised of the high risk of recanalization and referred for surgery.

INJECTION SCLEROTHERAPY FOR TELANGIECTATIC BLEMISHES

In contrast to large varices, small varices represent a condition in which refluxes and hemodynamic factors do not play an important role. If no contraindications are known, in principle no impediment to injection treatment of telangiectatic blemishes and reticular varices exists. Sclerotherapy is the treatment of choice, one for which there is no surgical alternative. The injections are performed according to cosmetic visual criteria, with sclerotherapy always being started with the vessel in front of the branching. Apart from this requirement, no hierarchic treatment plan is required.

In their pure form small varices do not require any apparative diagnostic measures. However, they may occur in combination with large varicose veins. Therefore I recommend that, even for these two types of varices, photoplethysmography and Doppler ultrasonography be performed to measure venous function and to detect refluxes of the saphenous veins. This approach ensures that medically relevant findings are not overlooked.

SUMMARY

Examinations performed before an invasive varix treatment have different objectives. These objectives are related to indications and contraindications, anatomic and functional findings, and the treatment plan. A schematic stripping of the entire saphenous trunk in all cases should be rejected. Likewise, blinded sclerotherapy that involves injection of only the visible varices should not be done. The operative diagnostic measures should consist of an anatomic and a functional test. Two noninvasive examination methods are now available for this purpose: Doppler ultrasonography (diagnosis of superficial and deep venous refluxes) and photoplethysmography (venous function test with tourniquet test).

An improvable CVI can be distinguished from a nonimprovable CVI by means of photoplethysmography. Truly nonimprovable CVI can be distinguished from falsely nonimprovable CVI by means of an additional deep Doppler examination. Improvable and falsely nonimprovable CVI constitute indications for invasive varix therapy (i.e., surgery and/or sclerotherapy).

Before formulating a treatment plan, the physician should perform an exact Doppler examination of the saphenous system and the deep venous system. Surgery is the treatment of choice for typical saphenous varices. Atypical saphenous varices are highly suitable for sclerotherapy. Reticular varices and telangiectatic blemishes can be injected, regardless of location, according to visual and cosmetic criteria. Complete elimination of large varices is not advisable in patients with nonimprovable CVI. In such cases treatment with medical compression stockings is indicated as soon as cutaneous complications, edema, or subjective complaints develop.

REFERENCES

1. Földi M, Casley-Smith JA, eds. Lymphangiology. Stuttgart: Schattauer, 1983.
2. Schultz-Ehrenburg U, Weindorf N. Problemsituation Ulcus mixtum. Swiss Med 6(9a):41-44, 1984.
3. Widmer LK, Stähelin HB, Nissen C, daSilva A. Venen-, Arterienkrankheiten, koronare Herzkrankheit bei Berufstätigen. Prospektiv-epidemiologische Untersuchung. Basel Study I-III, 1959-1978. Berne: Hans Huber, 1981.
4. Blazek V, May R, Stemmer R, Wienert V. Die Standardisierung der LRR-Untersuchung. In May R, Stemmer R, eds. Die Licht-Reflexions-Rheographie (LRR). Erlangen: Perimed, 1984, pp 151-155.
5. Blazek V, Schmitt HJ, Schultz-Ehrenburg U, Kerner J. Digitale Photoplethysmographie (D-PPG) für die Beinvenendiagnostik. Medizinisch-technische Grundlagen. Phlebol Proktol 18:91-97, 1989.
6. Blazek V, Wienert V. Licht-Reflexions-Rheographie: Eine nichtinvasive Technik zur Beurteilung chronisch-venöser Insuffizienz. Wiss. Berichte d. Österr. Ges. f. Biomed Tech 261-277, 1981.
7. Blazek V, Schmitt HJ, Schultz-Ehrenburg U. Digitale Photoplethysmographie: Ein neues mikroprozessorgesteuertes Meßsystem für die Beinvenendiagnostik. Biomed Tech 33 (Suppl 2):307-308, 1988.
8. Fronek A. Noninvasive Diagnostics in Vascular Disease. New York: McGraw-Hill, 1989.
9. Weindorf N, Schultz-Ehrenburg U. Der Wert der Photoplethysmographie (Lichtreflexionsrheographie) in der Phlebologie. Vasa 15:397-406, 1986.
10. Blazek V, Schultz-Ehrenburg U. Quantitative photoplethysmography—Basic facts and examination tests for evaluating peripheral vascular functions. Fortschr.-Ber. VDI series 20: Rechnerunterstützte Verfahren, vol 192, Düsseldorf: VDI, 1996.
11. Schultz-Ehrenburg U, Hübner HJ. Reflux Diagnosis With Doppler Ultrasound. Significance for Diagnosis, Indication and Objective Follow-up in Phlebology. Stuttgart: Schattauer, 1989.
12. Goren G, Yellin AE. Primary varicose veins: Topographic and hemodynamic correlations. J Cardiovasc Surg 31:672-677, 1990.

PART THREE

Treatment Options

Chapter 8

Compression Therapy

H.A. Martino Neumann and Dig J. Tazelaar

Compression therapy is one of the most powerful instruments of the phlebologist, and it is the one most commonly used. In the treatment of venous diseases this therapy plays a role both when used alone and as an adjunct to other forms of therapy.

Compression techniques are used to improve venous and lymphatic circulation. Different techniques of compression include the following types: (1) bandages: elastic, half-elastic, and nonelastic; (2) medical compression hosiery: elastic; (3) mechanical: pneumatic (intermittent).[1]

Although compression therapy is usually used for leg disorders, it also can be used for arm problems with great success. In daily practice compression therapy is often called "ambulant compression therapy" because the interaction between the bandage and the muscular contraction associated with walking is important in accomplishing the aims of treatment. Mechanical techniques, such as intermittent pneumatic compression, however, are not performed in association with ambulation.

Compression therapy is divided into two phases: (1) initial therapy and (2) maintenance therapy. The first phase usually involves the use of nonelastic bandages until total reduction of edema or healing of ulceration has been achieved. Since compression is not a permanent solution, it is necessary to assess and correct the pathologic alterations of venous flow (if possible). To be effective, compression must be maintained during the daytime. The maintenance phase involves use of medical compression hosiery. This type of hosiery is indicated when pathologic hemodynamics cannot be permanently corrected by interventional treatment, surgery, or the use of drugs.

Chronic venous insufficiency (CVI) refers to all late results of nonoptimal venous system function. CVI can develop from superficial, deep, and perforator venous insufficiency (Figure 8-1). The clinical picture is well known and consists of pitting edema, cutaneous pigmentation, abnormal keratosis, lipodermato-

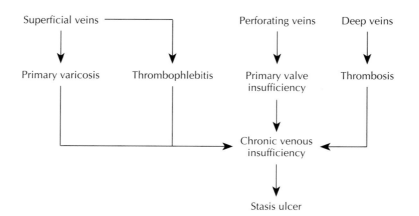

FIGURE 8-1. Development of chronic venous insufficiency.

sclerosis, atrophie blanche, and corona phlebectatica. CVI may develop into leg ulceration.

The human circulation is a closed system characterized by high pressure in the arteries and low pressure in the veins. Capillaries separate one type of pressure from the other. Pressure, especially in the veins, also is influenced by gravity. In the standing position hydrostatic pressure is added to resting pressure (as measured in the supine position). This fact explains why pressure in the posterior tibial vein is only 20 mm Hg when an individual is in the supine position but is approximately 90 mm Hg in the standing position. Since venous valves are open in the standing position, they cannot close the blood column. Thus they do not reduce the foot venous pressure. In other words, the valves will not influence the hydrostatic pressure when the patient is standing (properly, this hydrostatic pressure is often called standing venous pressure). The implication is that patients suffering from CVI, those with only varicose veins, and nonpatients will have the same standing venous pressure, which is influenced only by the length of the blood column (right atrium–to–foot distance).

Since the pumping action of the heart is much more like that of a pressure pump than a suction pump, other mechanisms are needed to obtain an adequate venous return and thus a reduction of venous pressure. The mechanisms for venous return are (1) vis a tergo (force from behind), (2) vis a fronte (force from in front), (3) venous tonus, and (4) muscle pump. The muscle pump, which is the most important mechanism for venous return to the heart, reduces standing venous pressure to ±20 mm Hg during walking (walking venous pressure). With insufficient valve function or reduced muscle activity (dependency), this degree of pressure reduction will not occur. The leg blood volume is increased and the Starling equilibrium is disturbed because of rising transmural pressure (intracapillary pressure reduced by tissue pressure). Decompensation of the venous and lymphatic system occurs, which, in turn, adversely affects the microcirculation.[2]

Most clinical signs of CVI directly reflect this failure of the microcirculation.

In 1956 Charpy and Audier[3] stated that "all problems start when the patient leaves the hospital after a deep venous thrombosis in a so-called healed condition." Good compression therapy is an inexpensive and effective method of preventing serious sequelae, including leg ulcers, in such patients.

There is no doubt about the effectiveness of compression therapy. Recently, the effectiveness of compression therapy after deep venous thrombosis was proven.[4] However, much attention to detail is necessary to obtain good results. Poor compression and inadequate support can lead to serious side effects and disappointing results. In a 5-year follow-up, Callam et al.[5] reported 147 cases of ulcers and necroses caused by inadequate compression therapy.

Compression as therapy has a long history. In Ancient Egypt compression bandages were used for treatment of leg ulcers. The Bible (Isaiah) also indicates that compression therapy was used for venous disease. Hippocrates used linen bandages for compression. The first modern report of compression therapy dates from 1768, when Wieseman used dog-skin "hosiery" around the leg. William Brown introduced rubber-inlaid threads for hosiery in 1848. Jonathan Sparks made these rubber threads more comfortable by surrounding them with cotton.[6]

Today synthetic elastomers are used for making therapeutic medical compression hosiery. The European Economic Community plans to introduce a European standard for medical compression hosiery. This standard will include different compression classes and requirements for factors such as compression gradation and maintenance.[7]

Compression therapy influences deranged venous flow in CVI at different levels. With phlebography, Fischer[8] proved that the diameter of both epifascial and subfascial veins diminishes under compression. More recently phlebography and Doppler ultrasound have been used to confirm that reflux in deep veins is decreased by external compression.[9,10] Extra pressure from special padding used as a compression aid may make incompetent valves become competent,[11-13] and insufficient perforating veins will resume their function.[14]

Compressing the veins of the legs reduces the blood volume. Bandages decrease this volume by 72% in the standing position.[14] Furthermore, the mild compression (6 to 10 mm Hg) produced by antithrombosis hosiery reduces blood volume in the sitting position in comparison to the volume in the supine position.[15] A reduction in blood volume combined with more competent valves enables the muscle pump to increase venous return.[16]

INDICATIONS FOR TREATMENT

It is essential to emphasize that compression therapy plays an important role in the treatment of CVI. Since CVI is already a substantial socioeconomic problem, increased mean life expectancy of an aging population will increase its impact in the future. Compression therapy is an inexpensive and effective treatment for a large number of patients. In addition, this therapy is used not only for CVI but also for a variety of other conditions (see box on p. 130).

INDICATIONS FOR COMPRESSION THERAPY

Chronic venous insufficiency
Therapy phase of varicose vein treatment with sclerotherapy or surgery
Superficial venous thrombosis (thrombophlebitis)
Deep venous thrombosis
Angiodysplasia
Lymphedema: Primary, secondary
Other edemas: Posttraumatic, postinflammatory, postsurgery, dependent, diabetic angiopathy, erysipelas/cellulitis, cardiac or renal
Some dermatologic diseases: Vasculitis, erythema nodosum, Schamberg's disease

Chronic Venous Insufficiency

All the stages and clinical manifestations of CVI benefit from compression therapy. Therefore this therapy is the basic treatment for all patients with CVI (including those with postthrombotic syndrome). Edema, induration, stasis dermatitis, lipodermatosclerosis, and venous leg ulcer all should be treated with compression therapy. Today, with the more frequently encountered mixed ulcer (a combination of CVI and diminished arterial influx), special care must be given to the technique of compression.

In cases of primary varicosis without hemodynamic disturbances (normal venous refill time, normal ambulatory venous pressure), treatment is not needed from a medical point of view. However, in patients with this condition it is wise to prescribe the use of medical compression hosiery during pregnancy or for extended periods of sitting or standing.[17] Treatment of this condition by sclerotherapy is a good possibility. The effectiveness of compression in CVI is mainly the result of improving venous drainage through a more competent muscle pump and by increasing lymphatic drainage.

A substantial correlation exists between CVI and microcirculation. Most clinical signs (e.g., pigmentation, edema, and leg ulcer) are the visible results of decompensated microcirculation. Although the effect of compression therapy on microcirculation is not yet fully understood, compression does increase venous refill time and expelled blood volume.[18] However, it is unclear whether or not venous hypertension is influenced by compression. A decreased pressure can be observed by direct venous pressure measurements.[19,20] Unfortunately, most investigations have not proved any influence on ambulatory venous pressure.[21,22] Therefore, on the venous side of the microcirculation, pressure remains high. As a result, physiologic recovery of microcirculation is not possible. The Starling equilibrium shifts toward a decrease in capillary filtration and an increase in reabsorption. Thus the capillary filtration rate diminishes. This reduction is mainly caused by a loss of water rather than protein.[23] When compression is discontinued, edema will quickly recur. Therefore compression therapy must be a continuous therapy modality.

One technique for evaluation of microcirculation is transcutaneous oxygen tension ($tcPO_2$) measurement. This measurement is performed with a modified Clark electrode.[24] In patients with CVI, $tcPO_2$ is diminished[25,26] and there seems to be a direct correlation between morphologic factors and the severity of CVI.[6] Partsch[27] found very low $tcPO_2$ values (12.9 ± 12.5 mm Hg) in the borders of venous leg ulcers. Through positron emission tomography, Gowland Hopkins et al.[28] studied the borders of venous leg ulcers in areas with lipodermatosclerosis. Blood flow was increased, and diminished fractional oxygen extraction was noted.

With reduction of edema during compression therapy, capillary density increases[29]; blood flow increases[28,30]; and $tcPO_2$ rises.[31-33] It is interesting to note, however, that pneumatic compression does not increase $tcPO_2$.[34]

Fibrin plays a special role in CVI. Burnand et al.[35] found that perivascular fibrin cuffs were present in lipodermatosclerosis. This finding was confirmed by others.[36,37] Fibrin cuffs may lead to an increase in the collagen layer of the capillaries.[38] The initial presumption that fibrin cuffs are a barrier for oxygen is not true.[39] Compression therapy has no influence on fibrin cuffs,[36] although fibrinolytic activity increases during compression.[40,41] For example, intermittent compression of an arm leads to increased fibrinolytic activity.[42] This observation is of interest for the prevention of venous thrombosis.

The fibrin cuffs are a sign of a decompensated microcirculation.[39] Besides fibrin, α_2-macroglobulin is found in the pericapillary halos. It has been hypothesized that macromolecules, like α_2-macroglobulin,[43] accumulate around the capillaries and "trap" growth factors and matrix proteins.[44,45] Higley et al.[44] found extravasated factor VIIIa and α_2-macroglobulin in the fibrin cuffs. The distribution within fibrin cuffs and co-localization with extravasated plasmaproteins, particularly α_2-macroglobulin, which is a recognized scavenger for transforming growth factor-beta (TGF-β) and other growth factors, provides evidence for a possible trapping of growth factors in CVI, especially with leg ulceration.

Adjunctive Compression Therapy

Immediately after varicose vein surgery, harvesting of vein grafts, or sclerotherapy for varicosity, the use of a compression bandage is effective in reducing and minimizing side effects and complications. The compression bandage prevents edema formation and enhances wound healing. For sclerotherapy it is essential to apply compression immediately after injection.[46,47] Compressing superficially injected veins is helpful, especially when pads are placed over the veins to achieve extra local compression. This method may prevent intravascular thrombus formation. Thrombi that occur after sclerotherapy may cause early recanalization, pigmentation, and inflammation.[47]

Although there is no consensus about the duration of compression after sclerotherapy, a period of 3 to 6 weeks is usually sufficient, depending on vein size and extent of reflux.[47] Compression done immediately after the treatment of telangiectasias is also recommended.[48] The duration of compression in this particular situation can be limited to 3 to 7 days.

Superficial Venous Thrombosis (Thrombophlebitis)

Treatment of superficial venous thrombosis comprises incision and expression of the thrombus. This approach relieves pain and discomfort for the patient. After the thrombus has been removed, a compression bandage is applied and an extra pressure pad is placed over the treated vein to avoid refilling.

In the upper leg, incision and expression of the thrombus are not always advisable because of technical difficulties and the danger that an embolus may slip off. Ligation of the saphenous vein at the saphenofemoral cross is recommended when the thrombus is located very close to this transition.[49,50] Superficial venous thrombosis after sclerotherapy is sparse. Clots, however, frequently occur after sclerotherapy. Local compression with firm, long cotton wool rolls placed over the injected veins are effective in preventing intravasal clotting and superficial venous thrombosis.[51]

Deep Venous Thrombosis

Although limited to patients with sufficient arterial circulation, deep vein thrombosis (DVT) is a very good indication for compression therapy. Such therapy is the treatment of choice for thrombosis that is limited to calf veins.[52] Compression therapy can be performed without bedrest when it is combined with the administration of anticoagulants.

Compression as a part of the late therapy of DVT has been used for many years by European phlebologists to prevent postthrombotic syndrome. Since deep veins can be compressed to narrow cords,[8] blood velocity increases in these veins after compression therapy.[14,53] Thrombi are thought to be fixed to the vein wall, and various enzymes and mediators are released from endothelial cells, which results in an immediate relief of pain and a reduction of edema. The transcapillary filtration is reduced, and it is suggested that collaterals are stimulated to develop.[54]

In patients with a first episode of proximal DVT, custom-made, flat-woven class III elastic medical compression hosiery reduces the rate of postthrombotic syndrome by about 50%. DVT was defined as thrombi involving the popliteal vein or above, irrespective of concomitant calf vein thrombosis. Patients started to wear the hosiery 2 to 3 weeks after the thrombosis and continued to do so for at least 2 years during the daytime. Recurrence of venous thromboembolism was not influenced by the hosiery.[4]

DVT of the legs, extending to the pelvis, does not have a higher risk of pulmonary embolism when treatment involves anticoagulation and ambulatory compression.[55] The possibilities for anticoagulation treatment of DVT have been increased recently. Two large studies demonstrated the effectiveness and safety of treatment with subcutaneous low-molecular-weight heparin (LMWH) administered at home in patients with proximal vein thrombosis.[56,57] The rates of recurrent thromboembolism and major bleeding were as low as in the standard hospital treatment with intravenous unfractionated heparin. In the Columbus Investigators Study the full spectrum of patients with venous thromboembolism was included: all patients with symptomatic venous thromboembolism, regardless of whether the patients had pulmonary embolism or a history of venous thrombo-embolism. Unmonitored use of subcutaneous LMWH is an effective and safe treatment for these patients too.[58] As a consequence, many patients with thromboembolism may be treated as outpatients in the very near future, or they may be discharged early from the hospital. It seems logical to start compression therapy as soon as possible to express edema, to relieve pain, and to prevent post-thrombotic syndrome. In the initial phase compression bandages are often necessary (Figure 8-2). After 1 or 2 weeks custom-made, flat-knitted (or, less frequently, circular-knitted) medical compression hosiery will keep the leg edema-free. AD-hosiery will often be sufficient, even after proximal DVT. It is hard to predict how long the medical compression hosiery must be worn. The clinical signs—the appearance of complaints or symptoms of CVI—are still the most important. In the near future function tests may offer more information about the development of CVI or otherwise.[59,60]

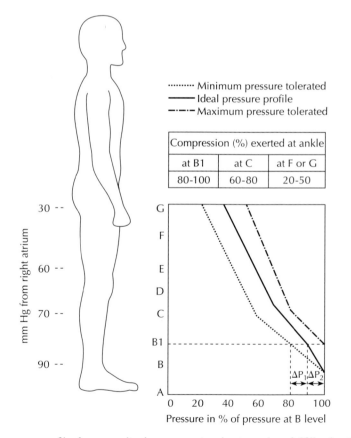

FIGURE 8-2. Pressure profile for a medical compression hosiery that fulfills the CEN criteria for class III hosiery. (From Neumann HAM. When therapy can only be . . . a stocking: Prescription requirements for medical compression stockings. Scripta Phlebologica 4:30-35, 1996.)

Angiodysplasia

Conditions such as Klippel-Trenaunay syndrome, Servelle-Martorell syndrome, and Parkes-Weber syndrome can be complicated by varicose veins. Apart from possible arteriovenous anastomoses, it is wise to take a conservative attitude regarding intervention in treatment of these varicose veins. Therefore maintenance of compression therapy with medical compression hosiery is of great value.

Lymphedema

Compression therapy is the most important type of treatment for all types of lymphedema. For best results a high degree of compression is needed. Initially, long mechanical pneumatic compression should be used, and it should be followed by maintenance compression with a high-compression medical compression hosiery (Table 8-1). Such treatment requires experience in fitting hosiery since the condition requires precision in measurements. Custom-made, flat-woven, high-gradient medical compression hosiery with closed toes is best for treatment of lymphedema.

Other Edemas

In principle, all forms of edema—posttraumatic, postinflammatory, and postrevascularization—can be treated with compression. In addition, compression therapy can be used for posttraumatic and postsurgical hematomas. Furthermore, dependency edema caused by a deficient muscle pump resulting from paralysis or joint deviations responds to compression; in this situation the therapy is helpful even though pump function is not influenced. Treatment of cardiac and renal ede-

TABLE 8-1. Indications for elastic hosiery correlated with compression class

Indication	Class*
Prevention of thrombosis in hospitalized patient	A
Minor complaints with normal venous refill time	I
Prevention of thrombosis during pregnancy	II-III
Prevention of complications in postthrombotic syndrome	(II)-III-(IV)
Sclerotherapy	II-(III)
Edema (nonvenous)	II-III
Varicose veins	II-III
Angiodysplasia	III-IV
Lymphedema, grade II	III-IV
Lymphedema, grade III	IV
Lymphedema, grade IV	Maximum in class IV

*See Table 8-2.

mas also can be diminished by compression therapy as long as overfilling of the circulation does not occur. Prevention of congestive heart failure remains a prime consideration in patients with these conditions.

Diabetic neuropathy, when associated with microangiopathy, can lead to edema. In such cases compression therapy is effective.[61] Only light compression should be applied since the patient will not experience pain because of the neuropathy. Severely diminished arterial inflow must be ruled out through appropriate noninvasive examinations (see Requirements for Compression Bandages).

Other Dermatologic Diseases

It is well known that some vascular-mediated cutaneous disorders, such as vasculitis and erythema nodosum, are likely to occur on the lower legs. This occurrence can be explained by induction of flow in capillaries so that immune complexes, antigens, antibodies, and other agents adhere more easily to the vessel wall. Also, CVI will exacerbate some skin diseases, such as progressive pigmental purpura and Schamberg's disease. Vasculitis, especially leukocytoclastic vasculitis and erythema nodosum, are typical examples of conditions that resolve quickly with good compression bandaging (Figure 8-3). The underlying cause of the disease, of course, also must be treated.

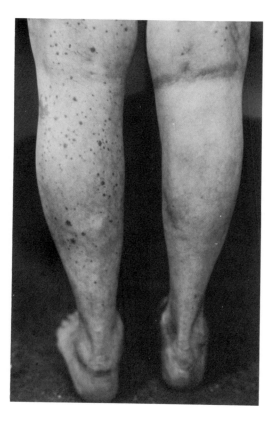

FIGURE 8-3. Leukocytoclastic vasculitis. Right leg has been treated with a compression bandage. Note that total absence of eruptions because of compression applied in the lower right leg.

PHYSICAL AND PATHOLOGIC ASPECTS OF COMPRESSION

The extent to which the intended effects of compression are achieved depends largely on the pressure with which the bandage is applied.[62] This pressure (P) is directly correlated with bandage tension (S) and indirectly correlated with the radius (R) of the surface (P = S/R). This relationship is known as Laplace's law. Pressure on the leg can vary according to the surface curvature. On areas of decreased radius, for example, the malleolus, over the distal Achilles tendon, and at the sharp edge of the tibia, there is a danger of producing excessive pressure. The curvature must be flattened with padding to avoid pressure necrosis.[12,13,63] On the other hand, pressure may be insufficient over areas in which the convex curvature is naturally low, such as the retromalleolar sulci, or convex areas, such as the dorsum of the foot. Therefore the radius needs to be altered artificially in these areas by means of prominent pads. From Laplace's law it can be concluded that less pressure is needed to achieve the same amount of pressure on a thin leg than on one of larger circumference. In an experimental study this conclusion was proven for compression therapy.[12]

Bandage pressure changes during walking. Working pressure develops during muscle contraction, and a resting pressure is obtained during muscle relaxation. The extent of the variation in pressure is determined to a considerable extent by the bandage material.[63,64] Nonelastic fibers have a large working pressure because they do not stretch during muscle contraction. Also, the resting pressure they produce is low because the material does not shrink during muscle relaxation. For these reasons nonelastic bandages can be worn at night. The large pressure differences induced by walking augment the muscle pump, providing a strong anti-edema effect.[65-67] Nonelastic and short-stretch bandages are preferable for use in cases of lymphedema and deep venous insufficiency.

Long-stretch elastic material is used in patients without edema but with superficial reflux. The pressure differences with such material are less than those of nonelastic materials. The working pressure is less because of the stretching bandage. The resting pressure is high because the bandage must be applied with a certain amount of tension. In the supine position, when the influence of gravity on the circulation is absent, high resting pressure can cause ischemia, especially if arterial circulation is impaired. Similarly, an elastic bandage or medical compression hosiery with pressure of ~25 mm Hg around the ankle must be removed at night.[68,69] The question arises about whether the high rate of ulceration and necrosis in patients with compression bandages and medical compression hosiery, as reported by certain Scottish surgeons, correlates with this bandaging technique.[5]

Compression Bandages

Application of a compression bandage is not easy. Experience is necessary to develop a good technique. Although it is not possible to learn this application from a book, the main problems of bandaging are illustrated in Figures 8-4 through 8-10 and will be helpful in training.

Text continued on p. 141.

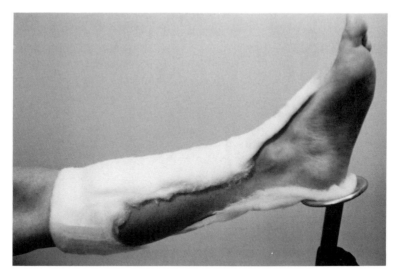

FIGURE 8-4. Leveling of all areas with a strong curvature, such as the ankles, Achilles tendon, instep, and sharp edges of the tibia.

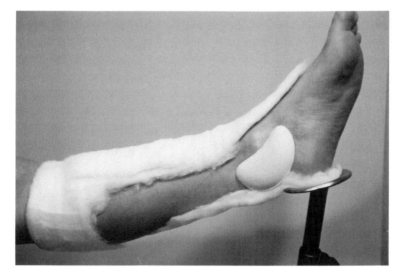

FIGURE 8-5. Raising the retromalleolar space with pads to achieve a good bend with the Achilles tendon.

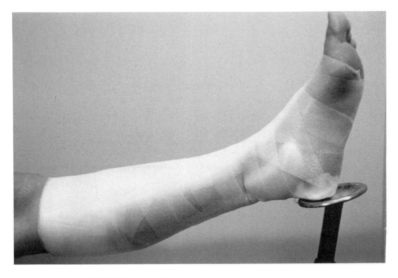

FIGURE 8-6. Fixing cotton wool and pads.

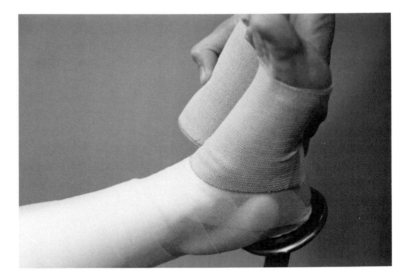

FIGURE 8-7. Bandaging is begun at the median dorsal area with the foot in dorsiflexion.

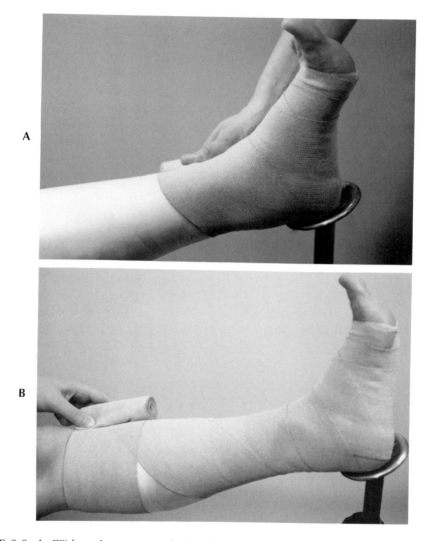

FIGURE 8-8. A, With each turn, two thirds of the bandage is covered, except for a circular turn done under the knee. **B,** The other bandage turns are not circular. The bandage turns across the leg and follows the natural contour of the leg. This method produces no constriction and eliminates slippage.

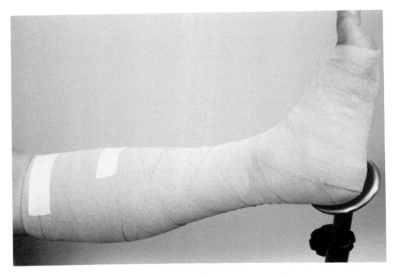

FIGURE 8-9. First bandage is applied.

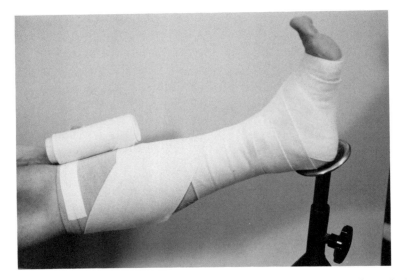

FIGURE 8-10. Second bandage is applied, from the opposite direction, starting from the lateral dorsal area.

Requirements for compression bandages. Pressure needs to be modified for the type of underlying disease. We believe that in primary varicosis or mild CVI a pressure of 25 to 35 mm Hg is sufficient. With severe CVI or in the postthrombotic state, we recommend at least 40 mm Hg. Lymphedema and indurated edema can be treated successfully only with bandages that produce a working pressure of 60 to 80 mm Hg in the ankle region.[70-74] However, some authorities use less pressure.[75,76] We must recognize the importance of arterial circulation in every patient. In patients with nonpalpable arteries a determination of the ankle systolic pressure through Doppler ultrasound is necessary before any compression bandage is applied. In diabetes mellitus it is important to realize that the ankle-arm index may be very high because of the impossibility of using compression and the condition of the arterial walls because of mediasclerosis (see accompanying box). When a bandage is applied, the amount of pressure depends on the person who applies the bandage. The individual will usually bandage within the same pressure range each time. However, the amount of pressure applied can be increased or decreased. It should be noted that the pressure does decrease quickly after application of the bandage.[77] As long as there are no practice objective methods for measuring the pressure applied, physician experience is the most important factor for successful treatment.

For optimal support of muscle pump function, a gradient of pressure reduction from distal to proximal is needed.[78,79] Laplace's law states that in cases of bandage stretch the pressure located distally on the leg will be higher than that found proximally.

The retromalleolar sulci must be filled with cotton wool, and the tibial area must be protected with the same material to avoid overpressure and underpressure.[12] Above indurated tissue, increased pressure is necessary for identifiable insufficient perforators or ulcers.[58,63]

The bandage must not constrict the skin. When the bandage is applied, circular turns must be avoided. The use of oblique turns avoids constriction and leads to a bandage that crosses over to a firm but flexible tube, thereby fitting the leg like an external fascia.[11,80]

Muscle pump function is possible only when the patient is able to walk. For this reason the bandage must not be too thick since the patient will need to wear shoes. Bandage materials must be nonallergic to avoid the development of dermatitis.

CONTRAINDICATIONS FOR COMPRESSION THERAPY

Diminished arterial inflow (arterial pressure <70 mm Hg)
Acute deep venous thrombosis without sufficient collaterals
Severe congestive heart disease
Undefined ulcers (e.g., carcinoma cutis, leishmaniasis)

Medical Compression Hosiery

Medical compression (or elastic) hosiery is very effective in maintaining compression. When no cure is possible (e.g., in postthrombotic syndrome or angiodysplasia), medical compression hosiery is the treatment of choice.[19,81]

Patient education is the key to good maintenance of compression. In The Netherlands half of the prescribed medical compression hosiery is not worn by patients.[81] In such cases the hosiery often is poorly fitted, inconvenient, or ugly.

Medical compression hosiery also can be used in the therapeutic phase of compression, such as when varicose veins are being treated with sclerotherapy. In such instances the hosiery is not intended to reduce edema, only to keep the leg edema-free.[47] In some cases medical compression hosiery is successfully used for the treatment of venous leg ulcers.[82]

The classification of medical compression hosiery is summarized in Table 8-2. Since the effect of compression on deep veins occurs above 30 mm Hg of pressure, and since in postthrombotic syndrome the mean pressure in the calf veins is approximately 60 mm Hg, elastic hosiery of class III or IV is recommended (see Table 8-2).[13,83] A patient with a relatively large leg circumference and long-standing high pressure also will need a high level of pressure for compression.

Requirements for elastic hosiery. Methods for obtaining exact pressure, independent of hosiery size, are possible.[84,85] The hosiery must remain durable for at least 6 months without demonstrating a significant decrease in pressure.[86] After 6 to 12 months pressures usually decrease.[64,87,88] Therefore it is best to replace hosiery every 6 months. For proper hygiene it is advisable to prescribe two hosiery units at a time for each leg requiring therapy so that compression can be continued while one hosiery is being washed.

Taking accurate measurements for medical compression hosiery is a key to proper fit. Such measurement is possible only when the patient's legs are edema-

---

TABLE 8-2. Compression classes, based on European norm

Class	Pressure* (hPa)†	Pressure* (mm Hg)	Effect
A (very mild)	13-19	10-14	
I (mild)	20-28	15-21	Small effect on superficial veins
II (moderate)	31-43	23-32	Clear effect on superficial veins; small effect on deep venous system
III (strong)	45-61	34-46	Effect on superficial and deep superficial venous system
IV (very strong)	>65	>49	Clear effect on deep venous system

*The values indicate the compression exerted by the hosiery at a hypothetical cylindrical ankle.
†1 mm Hg = 1333 hPa (hydrostatic arterial pressure).
From Nonactive medical devices—Medical compression hosiery. Document No. CEN-TC205/WG205. N190, Draft prEN 12718. Delft: NNI, European Committee for Standardization, 1998.

free. Therefore, if edema is present, a compression bandage is used until the edema has disappeared totally. Leg circumference is measured at defined locations[7] (see Figure 8-2).

Two types of medical compression hosiery are available: flat-knit and circular-knit. Both kinds can be ready-made or custom-made, but the most exact medical compression hosiery can be made only by using the flat-knit technique. With this technique the exact number of stitches can be decreased and/or increased at each turn. In circular-knit hosiery the circumference can be influenced only by increasing or decreasing the tension of the inlaid thread. For this reason the pressure produced by circular-knit hosiery will never be as precise as that of the flat-knit type. Because of the constant tension of the inlaid thread, circular-knit hosiery also is more difficult to apply. Most of the worldwide prescribed medical compression hosiery is the circular-knit type.

Manufacturers try to select their compression value from the center of the compression curve (see Figure 8-2). In this case the manufacturer avoids a relatively high compression within the determined compression class and has enough space for the decrease of compression during the use of the hosiery. Because manufacturers need a certain tolerance (at least 5% because of manufacturing problems), they focus on the middle of the pressure curve to be on the safe side. This tolerance can be detected easily in Figure 8-2: ΔP_1 is the lower limit and ΔP_2 is the upper limit for a certain hosiery. The given tolerance ($\Delta P_1 + \Delta P_2$) is defined in the upcoming CEN-norm.[7] The manufacturer makes a pressure-circumference curve for the elastic materials used (Figure 8-11). In this figure two different ma-

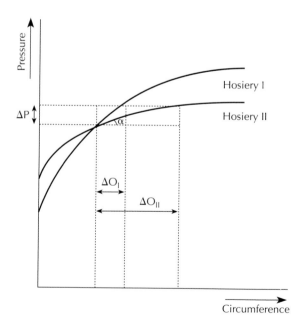

FIGURE 8-11. Pressure circumference relation. Hosiery I: high EC; hosiery II: low EC; tan α = EC = $\Delta P/\Delta O$. *EC*, External compression; ΔO, maximal circumference tolerance; ΔP, pressure. (From Neumann HAM. When therapy can only be . . . a stocking: Prescription requirements for medical compression stockings. Scripta Phlebologica 4:30-35, 1996.)

terials are shown, one with low external compression (EC) and one with high EC. The maximal possible circumference tolerance (ΔO) is related to the pressure tolerance and the EC: $\Delta P : \Delta O = \tan \alpha$.

To minimize the sizes that they must produce, manufacturers use elastic materials with a low EC, leading to high circumference tolerance and a pressure within the limits of the compression class.

As shown in Figure 8-11, ΔO_2 is much greater than ΔO_1. Therefore low EC leads to a high tolerance in circumference with stable pressure. In a broad study de Mooy et al.[89] showed the wide variability of the sizes at point B_1. With the forthcoming CEN-norm, it can be calculated, regarding the variety of B_1-sizes, that in case the B size is stable, hosiery with a medium EC will not fulfill the pressure profile in the B-B_1 stretch. This fact is illustrated by considering compression hosiery in class II with a pressure of 30 mm Hg at B (ankle)-level. At measuring point B_1 a pressure equal to 90% of 30 mm Hg is needed (27 mm Hg). Tolerance is accepted 3 mm Hg downward (ΔP_1) and upward (ΔP_2). With an assumption of an average EC of 2.5, the circumference possibilities at B_1 with a given size of B can be calculated. From a Hohenstein study done in 1991, the spread range of 2850 legs is known.[90] With a B-size of 21 cm, the average size of B_1 is 26.5 cm. The estimated standard deviation is 2 cm. With the tolerance of 3 mm Hg and an EC of 2.5, the size spread is 3:2.5 = 1.2 cm. The normal distribution table shows that the change of size at B_1 >26.5 + 1.2 is equal to 27.4%, and the same is true for the size at B_1 <26.5 − 1.2. So for 55% of the patients the use of standard-sized hosiery (confection) must be rejected on the basis of the size at B_1. Manufacturers can decrease this percentage by diminishing the EC. Therefore the individual sizes, especially at B and B_1, together with the desired EC will contribute to answering the question of choosing confection or tailor-made hosiery. It would be beneficial to patients if insurance companies would keep this matter in mind when they are defining the requirements for reimbursement of the cost of elastic hosiery.

The prescriber needs to choose between ready-made and custom-made hosiery. He/she realizes that all patients with significant CVI and all patients with lymphedema do much better with custom-made hosiery. In contrast, when sclerotherapy is done, ready-made hosiery nearly always suffices.

Ready-made hosiery never will fit (1) when there is a difference between the A and B circumference value, or (2) when the D value is equal to or higher than the C value[91] (see Figure 8-2).

In many patients there is a difference in the relation between leg length and girth. Ready-made hosiery is knitted for the average leg. Prescription is possible only when the leg circumference corresponds to the manufacturer's size table. If the leg circumference does not agree with the size table, good compression is not possible. In such cases prescription of custom-made hosiery is the best solution.[92]

Compression with hosiery has the same contraindications as compression therapy in general (see box on p. 141), but there are also some specific contraindications related to the use of hosiery. The risk of diminishing the arterial flow increases in elderly patients, who may not be able to remove the compression hosiery themselves because of the accentuated vessel recoil when the patient is supine. This issue is of special interest for arteriosclerotic vessels, as in hypertension and diabetes. For most maintenance therapy in patients with below-knee symptoms, AD-hosiery will meet therapeutic demands. This short hosiery will be more comfortable for the patient than the long above-knee AF or AG type (see Figure 8-2).

To determine the effectiveness of medical compression hosiery, the absence of edema is considered the major indicator. An experienced physician and a well-motivated patient are necessary to ensure successful ongoing therapy. If either of these two factors is inadequate, treatment with elastic hosiery will lead to disappointing results.[93]

To maintain the desired effect of compression and to ensure patient compliance with therapy, it is essential for the patient to visit the physician at least twice a year. During these visits the best objective parameter for determining the effectiveness of compression is edema formation. Measuring the circumference at point B (see Figure 8-2) generally gives sufficient information about compression. However, from time to time the circumference of the leg at all levels needs to be measured.

If pressure must be increased, such as when edema formation occurs during treatment with medical compression hosiery, either of the following steps should be taken:

1. Medical compression hosiery from a higher compression class should be chosen (see Table 8-2).
2. Two units of medical compression hosiery should be worn together, one over the other on the same leg. Pressure is then complementary. For example, two units of hosiery that produce an ankle pressure of 25 mm Hg will have the same effect as one with a pressure of 50 mm Hg. The use of two units of hosiery will enable many elderly patients to obtain the correct compression because one strong medical compression hosiery is too difficult for them to apply. In practice the so-called antithrombosis stocking (13 to 17 mm Hg) is often used as a primary hosiery.

Only stronger compression class III medical compression hosiery (>40 mm Hg at the ankle) increases the pressure in the deep venous system in the supine position.[83] Because of this effect, this type of medical compression hosiery will have a positive influence on the condition of patients with a deep venous insufficiency, such as occurs after a deep venous thrombosis.

Medical compression hosiery is of great value for many patients. They will derive the greatest benefit from this aid when their physician understands how medical compression hosiery is produced and how it works.

REFERENCES

1. Molen van der HR. Physikalische Therapie im Rahmen der Lymphödembehandlung mit Extubatio. Actuel Probl Angiol 35:58-64, 1977.
2. Neumann HAM. Measurement of microcirculation. In Altmeyer P, et al., eds. Wound Healing and Skin Physiology. Berlin: Springer Verlag, 1995, pp 115-126.

3. Charpy J, Audier M. Les troubles trophiques des membres inférieurs d'origine veineuse. Paris: Masson, 1956.

4. Brandjes DPM, Büller HR, Heyboer H, Huisman MV, de Rijk M, Jagt H, ten Cate JW. Randomised trial of the effect of medical compression hosiery in patients with symptomatic proximal-vein thrombosis. Lancet 349:759-762, 1997.

5. Callam MJ, Ruckley CV, Dale JJ, Harper DR. Hazards of compression treatment of the leg: An estimate from Scottish surgeons. BMJ 295:1382, 1987.

6. Hohlbaum GG. Zur Geschichte der Kompressionstherapie (Part I). Phlebol Proktol 16:241-255, 1987.

7. Non-active medical devices—Medical compression hosiery. Document No. CEN-TC205/WG205.N190, Draft prEN 12718. Delft: NNI, European Committee for Standardization, 1998.

8. Fischer H. Action de la compression sur les veines. Phlebologie 32:171-178, 1979.

9. Christopoulos D, Nicolaides AN, Szendro G. Venous reflux: Quantification and correlation with the clinical severity of chronic venous disease. Br J Surg 75:352-356, 1988.

10. Partsch H. Reduktion der venösen ambulatorischen Hypertonie durch Veneneinengung. Z Arztl Fortbild (Jena) 80:123-126, 1986.

11. Tazelaar DJ. Het compressieverband: Keuze en techniek van aanleggen. The Practitioner (NL uitgave) 231:973-978, 1987.

12. Veraart JCJM, Neumann HAM. Effects of medical elastic compression stockings on interface pressure and edema prevention. Dermatol Surg 22:867-871, 1996.

13. Veraart JCJM, Pronk G, Neumann HAM. Pressure differences of elastic medical compression hosiery at the ankle region. Dermatol Surg 23:935-939, 1997.

14. Lofferer O. Kompressionstherapie—Wirkungsweise und Anwendungsgebiet. Z Hautkr 57:633-642, 1982.

15. Partsch H, Rigal K. Reduktion des venösen Pooling in der Wade durch Antithrombosestrumpf und Beinhochlagerung. Phlebol Proktol 12:58-62, 1983.

16. Christopoulos D, Nicolaides AN, Belcaro G, Duffy P. The effect of elastic compression on calf muscle pump function. Phlebology 5:13-19, 1990.

17. Norgren L, Austrell C, Nilson L. The effect of graduated elastic medical compression hosiery on femoral blood flow velocity during late pregnancy. Vasa 24:282-285, 1995.

18. Kuiper JP. Venous pressure determination (direct method). Dermatologica 132:206-217, 1966.

19. Somerville JJF, Brow GO, Byrne PJ, Quill RD, Fegan WG. The effect of elastic hosiery on superficial venous pressures in patients with venous insufficiency. Br J Surg 61:979-981, 1974.

20. Kuiper JP, Brakkee AJM. Über die haemodynamischen Auswirkungen von Kompressionsstrumpfen. Phlebol Proktol 17:202-207, 1988.

21. O'Donnell TF, Rosenthal DA, Callow AD, et al. Effect of elastic compression on venous haemodynamics in postphlebitic limbs. JAMA 242:2766-2768, 1979.

22. Mayberry JC, Moneta GL, DeFrang RD, Porter JM. The influence of elastic medical compression hosiery on deep venous hemodynamics. J Vasc Surg 13:91-100, 1991.

23. Partsch H, Mostbeck A, Leitner G. Experimentelle Untersuchungen zur Wirkung einer Druckwellenmassage (Lymphapress) beim Lymphodem. Phlebol Proktol 9:124-128, 1980.

24. Huch R, Huch A, Albani M, et al. Transcutaneous P_{O_2} monitoring in routine management of infants and children with cardiorespiratory problems. Pediatrics 57:681-690, 1976.

25. Neumann HAM, van Leeuwen M, van den Broek MJThB, Berretty PJM. Transcutaneous oxygen tension in chronic venous insufficiency syndrome. Vasa 13:213-218, 1984.

26. Franzeck UK, Bollinger A, Huch R, Huch A. Transcutaneous oxygen tension, capillary morphology, and the density in patients with chronic venous incompetence (CVI). Circulation 70:806-811, 1984.

27. Partsch H. Hyperaemic hypoxia in venous ulceration. Br J Dermatol 110:249-250, 1984.

28. Gowland Hopkins NF, Spimks TJ, Rhodes GC, et al. Positron emission tomography in venous ulceration and liposclerosis: Study of regional tissue function. BMJ 286:333-336, 1983.

29. Mahler F, Chen D. Intracavital microscopy for evaluation of chronic venous incompetence. Int J Microcirc Clin Exp (Suppl) 106:1, 1990.

30. Partsch H, Lofferer O, Mostbeck A. Zur Beurteilung der Lymph- und Venenzirkulation am Bein mit und ohne Kompression. In Zeiter E, ed. Diagnostik mit Isotopen bei arteriellen und venösen Durchblutungsstorungen der Extremitäten. Wien: Hans Huber, 1973.

31. Neumann HAM. Transcutaneous PO_2 measurements in chronic venous insufficiency syndrome. In Merlin NJ, ed. Phlebologie 1983. Brussels: Medical Media International, 1984, pp 199-200.

32. Neumann HAM. Possibilities and limitations of transcutaneous oxygen tension measurements in chronic venous insufficiency. Int J Microcirc Clin Exp (Suppl) 105:1, 1990.

33. Kolani PJ, Pekan Muki K. Effects of intermittent compression treatment on skin perfusion and oxygenation in lower legs with venous ulcers. Vasa 16:312-317, 1986.

34. Nemeth AJ, Falanga V, Alstadt SA, Eaglestein WH. Ulcerated edematous limbs: Effect of edema removal on transcutaneous oxygen measurements. J Am Acad Dermatol 120:191-197, 1989.

35. Burnand GK, Whimster I, Naidoo A, Browse NL. Pericapillary fibrin in the ulcer-bearing skin of the leg. The cause of lipodermatosclerosis and venous ulceration. BMJ 285:1071-1072, 1982.

36. Neumann HAM, van den Broek MJThB. Stanozolol and the treatment of severe chronic venous insufficiency. Phlebology 3:237-246, 1988.

37. Falanga V, Moosa HH, Nemeth AJ, Alstadt SP, Eaglestein WH. Dermal pericapillary fibrin in venous disease and venous ulceration. Arch Dermatol 123:620-623, 1987.

38. Neumann HAM, van den Broek MJThB. Increased collagen IV layer in the basal membrane area of the capillaries in severe chronic venous insufficiency. Vasa 1:26-29, 1991.

39. Neumann HAM, van den Broek MJThB, Boersma IH, Veraart JCJM. Transcutaneous oxygen tension in patients with and without pericapillary fibrin cuffs in chronic venous insufficiency, porphyria cutanea tarda and non-venous leg ulcers. Vasa 25:127-133, 1996.

40. Clarke RL, Orandi A, Cliffton EE. Tourniquet induction of fibrinolysis. Angiology 11:367-370, 1960.

41. Haas S, Altenkamper H, Lill G, et al. Einfluss der intermittierenden pneumatischen Kompression auf die fibrinolytische Aktivität der Venenwand. Phlebol Proktol 16:107-111, 1987.

42. Knight MTN, Dawson R. Effect of intermittent compression of the arms on deep thrombosis in the legs. Lancet 1:1265-1267, 1976.

43. Grinnell F, Zhu M. Fibronectin degradation in chronic wounds depends on the relative levels of elastasis, α1-proteinase inhibitor, and α2-macroglobulin. J Invest Dermatol 106:335-341, 1996.

44. Higley HR, Ksander GA, Gerhardt CO, Falanga V. Extravasation of macromolecules and possible trapping of transforming growth factor-β in venous ulceration. Br J Dermatol 132:79-85, 1995.

45. Falanga V, Eaglestein WH. The "trap" hypothesis of venous ulceration. Lancet 341:1006-1008, 1993.

46. Fegan WC, Fitzgerald DE, Milliken JC. The results of simultaneous pressure recordings from the superficial and deep veins of the leg. Ir J Med Sci 6:363, 1964.

47. Tazelaar DJ, Neumann HAM. Macrosclerotherapy and compression. In Goldman MP, Bergan JJ, eds. Ambulatory Treatment of Venous Disease. St. Louis: Mosby, 1996, pp 105-112.

48. Goldman MP. Compression in the treatment of leg telangiectasias: Theoretical considerations. J Dermatol Surg Oncol 15:184-188, 1989.

49. Blanken R, Mackaay AJC, Dur AHM, Rauwerda JA. Ascenderende flebothrombose. Ned Tijdschr Geneeskd 137:1568-1570, 1993.

50. Plate G, Eklöf R, Jensen R, Ohlin P. Deep venous thrombosis, pulmonary embolism and acute surgery in thrombophlebitis of the long saphenous vein. Acta Chir Scand 151:241-244, 1985.

51. Tazelaar DJ, Neumann HAM, de Roos K-P. Long cotton wool rolls as compression enhancers in macrosclerotherapy for varicose veins. Dermatol Surg 1999 [in press].

52. Voorhoeve J, Bruyninckx CMA. Het thrombosebeen, een bedrieglijk ziektebeeld. Ned Tijdschr Geneeskd 128:2289-2292, 1989.

53. Mostbeck A, Partsch H, Hahn P, Tham B. Nuklearmedizinische Untersuchungen zur Beurteilung von regionalem Blutvolumen und venösen Stromungsgeschwindigkeit. Phlebol Proktol 13: 111-115, 1984.

54. Brakkee AJM, Kuiper JP. The influence of compressive hosiery on the haemodynamics in the lower extremities. Phlebology 3:147-153, 1988.

55. Partsch H, Oburger K, Mostbeck A. Häufigkeit von Longembolien bei Bein/Becken Venenthrombosen unter Antikoagulation, Kompressionsverband und Gehen. Phlebologie 20:205-209, 1991.

56. Koopman MNW, Prandovi P, Piovella F, et al. (The Tasman Study Group). Treatment of venous thrombosis with intravenous unfractionated heparin administered in the hospital as compared with subcutaneous low-molecular-weight heparin administered at home. N Engl J Med 334: 682-687, 1996.

57. Levine M, Gent M, Hirsch J, et al. A comparison of low-molecular-weight heparin administered primarily at home with unfractionated heparin administered in the hospital for proximal vein thrombosis. N Engl J Med 334:677-681, 1996.

58. The Columbus Investigators. Low-molecular-weight heparin in the treatment of patients with venous thromboembolism. N Engl J Med 337:657-662, 1997.

59. van Gerwen JHL, Brakkee AJM, Kuiper JP. Non-invasive measurement of venous muscle pump function in the supine position. Phlebology 7:146-149, 1992.

60. Janssen MCH, Claassen JAHR, van Asten WNJC, Wollersheim H, de Rooy MJM, Thien TH. Validation of the supine venous pump function test: A new non-invasive tool in the assessment of deep venous insufficiency. Clin Sci 91:483-488, 1996.

61. Belcaro G, Laurora G, Cesarone MR, Pomante P. Elastic hosiery in diabetic microangiopathy. Vasa 21:193-197, 1992.

62. van der Molen H, Kuiper J. Mesure de la compression en thérapeutique phlébologie et notamment de la pression permanente efficace après reduction de l'oedème. Phlebologie 2:105-112, 1960.

63. Stemmer R. Konzentrische und exzentrische Kompression. Phlebol Proktol 13:53-57, 1984.

64. von Gregory R. Eigenschaften des elastischen Binden. Phlebol Proktol 7:171-182, 1978.

65. Hargens AR, Millard RW, Petterson K, Johansen K. Gravitation haemodynamics and oedema prevention in the giraffe. Nature 329:59-60, 1987.

66. Wupperman TH, Pretschner DP, Holm I, Emter M. Nuklearmedizinische Messung des Intravasal- und Extravasalraumes an Wade und Fuss beim Gehen und Sitzen zum Vergleich zweier Arten der Kompressionstherapie. Phlebol Proktol 16:175-183, 1987.

67. Ohlert P, Wienert V. Zum Wirkungsnachweis von Kompressionsverbanden. Vasa 17:262-266, 1988.

68. Berg van den F, Wupperman TH. Plethysmographische Ermittlung des Andruckes elastischer Kompressionsstrumpf—"Anti-Thrombose-Strumpfe." Swiss Med 2:4a, 1980.

69. Callam MJ, Haiart D, Farouk M, et al. Effect of time and posture on pressure profiles obtained by three different types of compression. Phlebology 6:79-84, 1991.

70. Orbach EJ. Compression therapy and lymph vessel disease of the lower extremities. Angiology 3:95-103, 1979.

71. Jones NAG, Webb PJ, Rees RI, Kakkar VV. A physiological study of elastic medical compression hosiery in venous disorders of the leg. Br J Surg 67:569-572, 1980.

72. Stemmer R, Marescaux J, Furderer CH. Die Kompressionsbehandlung der unteren Extremitäten speziell durch Kompressionsstrümpfe. Hautarzt 31:355-365, 1980.

73. Blair SD, Wright DDI, Backhouse ChM, Riddle E, McCollum CN. Sustained compression and healing of chronic venous ulcers. BMJ 297:1159-1161, 1988.

74. Stoberl CH, Gabler S, Partsch H. Indikationsgerechte Bestrumpfung—Messung der venösen Pumpfunktion. Vasa 18:35-39, 1989.

75. Fentem PH. Claims about compression treatment for venous disease. BMJ 285:61, 1982.

76. Struckmann J. Low-compression, high-gradient hosiery in patients with venous insufficiency: Effect on the musculovenous pump evaluated by strain gauge plethysmography. Phlebology 1:189-196, 1986.

77. Rai TB, Goddard M, Makin GS. How long do compression bandages maintain their pressure during ambulatory treatment of varicose veins? Br J Surg 67:122-124, 1980.

78. Sigel B, Edelstein AL, Savitch L, et al. Type of compression for reducing venous stasis. Arch Surg 110:171-175, 1975.
79. Horner J, Fernandes E, Fernandes J, Nicolaides AN. Value of graduated medical compression hosiery in deep venous insufficiency. BMJ 297:820-821, 1980.
80. Schneider W, Fischer H. Die chronisch-venöse Insuffizienz. Stuttgart: Enke, 1969.
81. Korstanje MJ, Neumann HAM. Compressietherapie door middel van elastische kousen. Ned Tijdschr Geneeskd 134:799-802, 1990.
82. Partsch H, Horakova MA. Kompressionsstrümpfe zur Behandlung venöser Unterschenkelgeschwüre. Wien Med Wochenschr 144:242-249, 1994.
83. Veraart JCJM, Oei TK, Neumann HAM. Compression therapy and pressure in the deep venous system. Thesis: Veraart JCJM. Clinical aspects of compression therapy. Maastricht: Unigraphic, University of Maastricht, 1997, pp 99-109.
84. Stolk R. Ein pneumatisches Druckmessgerat für direktes Messen von Druckwerten bei Kompressionsstrümpfen. Phlebol Proktol 9:176-182, 1980.
85. Weber G, Gohr O. Eine neuartige Methode zur Ermittlung der Druckeigenschaften von Kompressionsstrümpfen. Phlebol Proktol 11:34, 1982.
86. Bernink BP. Elastische Strümpfe und ihre Qualitäts-Beurteilung. Medita 8:152-157, 1978.
87. Stemmer R. Vorschläge zur Verbesserung der Kompressionsstrümpfe. Phlebol Proktol 9:129-137, 1980.
88. Veraart JCJM, Daamen E, Vet HCW de, Neumann HAM. Elastic compression stockings: Durability of pressure in daily practice. Vasa 26:282-286, 1997.
89. de Mooy MC, Oosterwal SH. Confectiekousen? Maat houden! Scripta Phlebologica 4:14-19, 1996.
90. German study into leg measurements and proposal of an improved size system for medical compression hosiery. Document No.: CEN-TC205/WG2. N199; Draft prEN 12718. Delft (NL): European Committee for Standardization, NNI, 1998.
91. Olsen G. Zur Praxis der Versorgung von Beinkranken mit Gummistrümpfen. Fortschr Med 83:697-699, 1965.
92. Hohlbaum GG. Mass- oder Konfektionsstrumpf. Phlebol Proktol 11:42-49, 1982.
93. Ellerbroek U. Arzt und Kompressionsstrumpfverordnung. Therapiewoche 26:2376, 1976.

Chapter 9

Historical Development of Varicose Vein Surgery

Sidney S. Rose

The treatment of varicose veins has developed over a period of more than 2000 years (Figure 9-1) and includes a wide variety of methods. Most surgical treatments for varicose veins that were used in the past failed to give satisfactory results. Even when the results seemed reasonable in the short term, they did not prove to be successful in long-term follow-up. Many of the operations failed from both a functional and a cosmetic point of view. Some surgeons, in an attempt at radical vein removal, produced disfiguring scars. One example is the horrifying result of the Rindfleisch-Friedel operation of 1908. After ligation of the internal saphenous vein in the thigh, a spiral gutter was cut into the leg, encircling the leg four to seven times, down to deep fascia, with superficial veins being tied as they came into view. The wound was left open to granulate in an attempt to prevent infection!

The disregard for cosmetic result that typified early attempts at surgical treatment was unfortunate since leg appearance has been in the past, and remains today, the most common patient complaint and reason for referral. Throughout the years many family practitioners probably have dismissed women who were genuinely distressed by their ugly but asymptomatic varicose veins because the surgical results would be unsatisfactory and would not produce a good cosmetic appearance. In general, varicose vein surgery has been relegated to the junior members of a surgical team, and this practice has been reflected in the results.

In the past the approach to treatment of varicose veins focused on the mechanical effect of back pressure on the varicosity. Such pressure was perceived to be its underlying cause. A modern trend toward the additional removal of varicosities has developed because of better results with this modification. This trend is more in accord with the weak vein wall theory, which explains the basic cause of venous dilatation. In light of that theory, back pressure is viewed as a secondary effect. Only recently has the cause of varicosities begun to become clear.

In the following discussion we will look backward throughout history to fol-

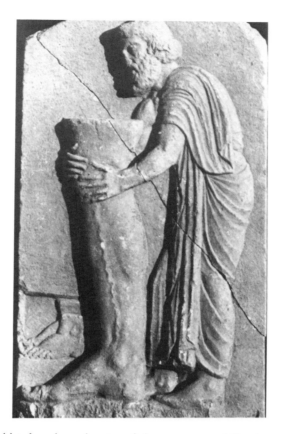

FIGURE 9-1. Votive tablet found on the site of the sanctuary of Dr. Amynos near the Acropolis dates from the fourth century. It is the earliest known depiction of varicose veins. (From Browse NL, Burnand K, Lea Thomas M, eds. Diseases of the Veins. London: Edward Arnold, 1988.)

low the evolution of medical and surgical techniques used in the treatment of varicose veins. After a summary of three important periods of progress, the discussion turns to the nineteenth century and goes back through the preceding centuries, ending with the Greco-Roman era.

PERIODS OF PROGRESS
The War Years and Postwar Trends: 1941-1953

The opinions expressed in this chapter are the result of experience gained throughout almost 50 years of my practice of varicose vein surgery. This experience included the personal treatment and follow-up of approximately 15,000 patients. It began in 1941, just 50 years after Trendelenburg's classic paper on varicose vein surgery, when this type of surgery was beginning to escape the domination of his teaching. The operation that my associates and I practiced then was called the Trendelenburg procedure, but our approach involved two important

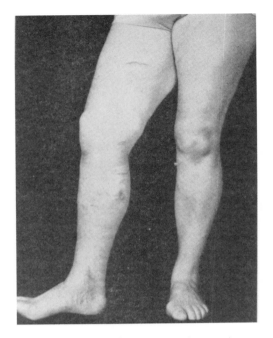

FIGURE 9-2. At the turn of the century the dominant varicose vein operation was the Trendelenburg procedure, in which the upper incision was placed in the midthigh, as shown here. After World War I the modified Trendelenburg procedure, which involved the groin incision and a high saphenous ligature, became increasingly popular. (From Foote RR. Varicose Veins. London: Butterworth, 1952.)

differences from Trendelenburg's classic description. First, the uppermost incision and ligation was done in the groin, not in the middle third of the thigh (Figure 9-2). Second, the operation included adjunctive sclerotherapy done simultaneously.

In 1941 there was no shortage of patients with varicose veins in either civilian or military practice in Great Britain. The notable frequent occurrence of varicose veins among members of the armed forces demonstrated that this complaint was by no means limited to women. However, varicosities in men were largely asymptomatic and usually were discovered on routine medical examination. The worst cases had been identified earlier, at the original military medical examination. Nevertheless, the complaint of varicose veins was exceedingly common. Perhaps the appeal of a few days in hospital, light duty, excused drill, and sick leave made the complaint of an aching leg seem an attractive alternative to many. Whatever the reason, the highest surgical admission rate to the Emergency Medical Service hospitals during World War II was for treatment of varicose veins. In fact, this type of high admission rate is a common experience in wartime. In 1811 Sir Everard Home, brother-in-law of John Hunter, wrote, "No surgical complaint, incident to the soldier, has deprived His Majesty's Service of so many men as that of ulcers of the leg due to varicose veins."

The operation I performed in 1941 was high ligation at the saphenofemoral junction, ligation of tributaries, and retrograde passage of a ureteric catheter down the cut end of the vein until it would go no further. About 6 to 8 ml of 5% to 10% sodium morrhuate was injected down the catheter as it was slowly withdrawn. The entire procedure was carried out with the patient under local anesthesia and done on an outpatient basis. The result was an immediate massive reaction along the line of the saphenous vein from ankle to groin. A chemical thrombophlebitis was produced that required heavy bandaging and caused considerable disability. The patients were painfully incapacitated during the 2 to 4 weeks it took for the condition to resolve. The ultimate fate of the thrombosed vein was recanalization, which took place sooner than expected.

The differences from the classic Trendelenburg operation did not seem to make much difference in regard to the results. A follow-up of cases operated on in the war years was impractical. However, the inadequacies of that surgery became apparent because large numbers of patients returned for further treatment. Recurrences were largely the result of the recanalized saphenous vein.

Use of the ureteric catheter was discontinued in 1945, and the practice of simultaneous sclerotherapy was ended in 1946. The operation performed with the patient under general anesthesia was simplified in 1947. The simplified version involved high ligation of the internal saphenous vein in the groin and low ligation in the distal third of the thigh and just below the knee. The main benefit of this approach was early ambulation, but the patient was kept in hospital for a week. The results of the operation were not noticeably different from those of the more complicated method.

Turn-of-the-Century Contributions

In 1896 William Moore, a Melbourne surgeon, advocated groin ligation performed with the patient under local anesthesia and done on an outpatient basis. In those days communications from Australia took a long time to reach the West, which may account for the fact that Moore's work did not arouse much attention in the surgical world at the time. There was no such excuse for the work of Thelwall Thomas of Liverpool, also published in 1896, which passed almost unnoticed. Thomas also described ligation of the internal saphenous vein at the saphenous opening. Despite this publication, 20 years later, in 1916, credit for suggesting the flush ligation of the internal saphenous vein in the groin was given to John Homans of San Francisco. In 1930 credit for carrying out the operation as an outpatient procedure with the patient being administered a local anesthetic went to Geza de Takats of Chicago.

To discover the origin of simultaneous use of a sclerosant at operation, one must go back to 1908, when this method was practiced by Beniamino Schiassi in Bologna (Figure 9-3). Schiassi used an iodide solution of unpredictable action. Fifteen years later E. Unger introduced the modification of injecting a sclerosant down a ureteric catheter. He used sodium salicylate, the first of the "safe" sclerosant agents.

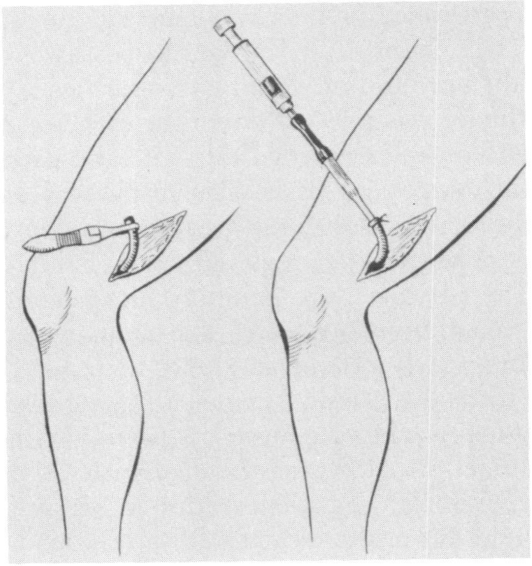

FIGURE 9-3. Simultaneous use of sclerosants and surgery was introduced by Schiassi in 1908 with the technique demonstrated here. Fifteen years later Unger developed a technique that consisted of injection of a sclerosant down a ureteral catheter from the groin. (From Foote RR. Varicose Veins. London: Butterworth, 1952.)

Sclerotherapy. Sclerotherapy as a treatment for varicose veins once was practiced by nonsurgeons as an alternative to surgery. However, more recently sclerotherapy has assumed the role of an adjunct to surgery.

For accuracy, sclerosants should be divided into two categories, thrombosants and true sclerosants. This categorization should be done in accordance with the agent's method of action, whether it causes (1) clotting of blood or (2) an inflammatory action in the vein wall. In the latter situation, if the vein is compressed, its walls will adhere to each other and produce luminal occlusion. Salicylates, quinine urethan, hypertonic saline, and sodium morrhuate all are thrombosant agents. Ethamoline (monoethanolamine oleate) is closer to being a true sclerosant. Ideally, a true sclerosant is required since intraluminal thrombosis usually leads to recanalization. Such thrombotic recanalization was the reason for introduction of the empty vein injection technique and pressure sclerotherapy.

The sclerosants in general use in 1941 were ethamoline and sodium morrhuate. Ethamoline, introduced into the United States in 1937 by H. Biegeleisen, was not widely used because of a long-standing antipathy to injection therapy. This agent was not in general use in England until the later years of World War II. Sodium morrhuate was widely used both in England and in the United States in 1941. In Europe, where centers of sclerotherapy arose and became increasingly popular after the war, the perceived need for a true sclerosant led to the decline of sodium morrhuate. Reports of unpleasant side reactions, such as allergy and skin necrosis, also contributed to the unpopularity of this agent.

A cycle of popularity follows the introduction of every sclerosant and thrombosant. In the nineteenth century perivenous injection was practiced by the influential Viennese school, sometimes with disastrous effects. The Surgical Congress of Lyons of 1894 condemned this technique as unsafe, and this censure was probably the cause of this method's traditional unpopularity in the United States. Later, Paul Ehrlich, whose world stature as a chemist commanded attention, was able to show that, when properly injected, some agents could produce a thrombosis safely. This demonstration by Ehrlich led to Professor L. Sicard's successful introduction of the first "safe thrombosant," sodium salicylate, in 1911. For the next 30 years arguments for and against sclerotherapy raged. However, in 1947 N. Garber of Johannesburg wrote a very convincing paper arguing against the use of sclerosants. Garber advocated high resection of the saphenous vein followed by multiple resection of varices. This approach is basically what is practiced today, although techniques differ and sclerotherapy is used as an adjunct to surgery. Sclerosants in general use today include polidecanol, sodium tetradecyl sulfate, and chromated glycerin.

Introduction of the stripper. The introduction of the stripper has been attributed to William Keller in 1905, Charles Mayo in 1906, and Stephen Babcock in 1907. The Keller instrument was a flexible intraluminal wire that turned the vein inside out. The Mayo instrument was an external ring that was passed along the vein, cutting the tributaries as it went. Babcock used an intraluminal stripper with an acorn-shaped head that pleated the vein along its length, as do strippers in use today. The Keller operation was given up because it was ill conceived; the Mayo, because of severe hemorrhage; and the Babcock, probably because the instrument was too short, too straight, and inflexible.

The Trendelenburg Years: 1841-1891

Friedrich Trendelenburg (Figure 9-4) described a transverse incision at the junction of the upper and middle third of the thigh. He could not have attempted to carry out a groin dissection through this incision, and he believed that step was not necessary. Since Trendelenburg simply ligated the vein in the midthigh, it seems strange that his operation won worldwide acclaim. Probably this acclaim was the result of his reputation for manual dexterity and the general tenor of his presentation. In his paper describing the operation, Trendelenburg paid tribute to those who had gone before him. He singled out Sir Benjamin Brodie for recommending midthigh ligation of the saphenous vein. Trendelenburg felt that such ligation was a logical procedure to relieve the effects of proximal valvular incompetence. It was, however, practiced before the discovery of blood circulation, when it was believed that the blood drained down the leg under its own weight. In fact, it would have been illogical to those who followed the teaching of Harvey to tie the saphenous vein if the blood were flowing in the opposite direction. Trendelenburg pointed out that after his operation the blood during exercise would flow through competent perforators and thus alleviate back pressure. He also created a stir by claiming that he could do the operation so quickly that no anesthetic was required. The operation required only a 3 cm incision, an aneurysm

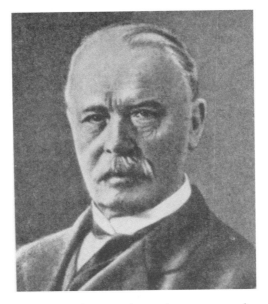

FIGURE 9-4. Friedrich Trendelenburg dominated vascular surgery at the end of the nineteenth century. His technique of ligation of the greater saphenous vein in the upper third of the thigh was a logical development from his observations of greater saphenous vein reflux as a powerful influence on varicosities and venous ulceration. (From Foote RR. Varicose Veins. London: Butterworth, 1952.)

needle, and division between ligatures. Therefore one wonders why the patient was kept in hospital for 5 weeks after so minor a procedure.

When Trendelenburg published the results of patients he operated on and personally followed 4 years later, he admitted a 22% recurrence rate. This rate was probably an optimistic assessment. In those halcyon days no one would have the temerity to suggest an independent audit to a distinguished professor of surgery. In fact, Trendelenburg's work was followed up 4 years later by his disciple Georg Perthes, who advocated a much higher level of saphenous vein ligation and gave a glowing account of success with varicose ulcers, with a recurrence rate of 18% in 41 cases. In his paper Perthes introduced his extension of what would later be known as the Trendelenburg test, first described by Sir Benjamin Brodie in 1846. The "Trendelenburg" operation was practiced in the Bonn Surgical Clinic in Germany for the next 35 years.

HISTORICAL APPROACHES TO TREATMENT
Nineteenth Century

If one goes back to the nineteenth century, one would expect that lack of anesthesia in the first half of that century would have severely inhibited surgical practice. However, such was not the situation. Instead, the battle against the varix was unabated, and in some instances the action was remarkably modern. For ex-

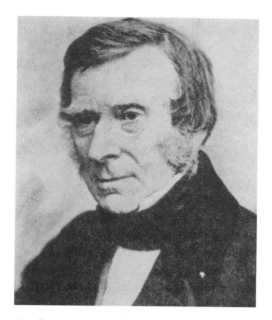

FIGURE 9-5. Sir Benjamin Brodie is shown at the height of his career at St. George's Hospital in the early nineteenth century. (From Foote RR. Varicose Veins. London: Butterworth, 1952.)

ample, a little-known Italian surgeon, Giovanni Rima (1777-1843), not only advocated but practiced midthigh ligation of the saphenous vein without inducing anesthesia. In Rima's operation, done almost 100 years before the time of Trendelenburg, speed was of the essence.

Sir Benjamin Brodie (1783-1862) (Figure 9-5), of St. George's Hospital in London, was the first to demonstrate reflux in the saphenous vein; in 1846 he described in great detail what later was to be known as the Trendelenburg test. Actually Trendelenburg was inspired by work done in the previous century, and he admired Brodie. Brodie was a distinguished surgeon and clinician who made valuable contributions to the literature on venous disease. Toward the end of his life, disillusioned by his operative results, Brodie disagreed with his colleague Sir Everard Home about varicose vein surgery. This disagreement was based largely on the matter of sepsis. Brodie eventually advocated conservative treatment for all but the most severe cases. Therefore he developed a system of double bandaging with flannel for treatment of varicose ulcers and instructed patients on how to apply the bandages. The patients were taught to include the foot in the bandage to prevent swelling and to apply the pressure from below in an upward direction. Although Brodie's treatment was ambulatory, he recommended elevation of the limb whenever possible and especially in bed at night. Brodie knew the value of calf muscle exercises, was aware of skin allergies to various medicaments, and was especially averse to sticky bandages.

Brodie was at the height of his fame when Queen Victoria came to the throne

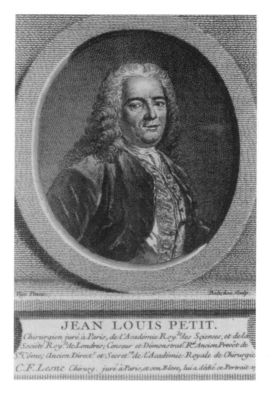

FIGURE 9-6. Jean Louis Petit performed radical excision of varices without inducing anesthesia. (From Haeger K, ed. The Illustrated History of Surgery. Gothenburg, Sweden: AB Nordbok, 1988.)

of England in 1837. She promptly knighted him for his services to medicine. At that time Brodie was reputed to be earning £10,000 a year, and, on hearing of his honor, he was quoted as saying to his entourage, "Gentlemen, there is more in veins than just blue blood."

Eighteenth Century

In the early eighteenth century the leading phlebologists were in France. Jean Louis Petit (1674-1750) (Figure 9-6), first director of the Academy of Surgery of Paris, taught that the cause of varicose veins was "anything that obstructed the rising of blood in the veins." Petit practiced radical excision of varices. We know nothing of his use of anesthesia, if he used it at all. Petit's distinguished predecessor, Pierre Dionis (1668-1718), Surgeon-in-Ordinary to the Queen of France and the Empress Maria Theresa, believed that the cause of varicosity was "gross blood that caused the vein to make a small purse to allow blood both space and liberty." Dionis's poetic description of a varicose blowout was equaled by his allegorical reference to venous valves. "These [valves]," he said "form steps to help the ascension of the blood and so facilitate its return to its source." Dionis strongly advocated the use of compression bandages on the leg and the use of support hose

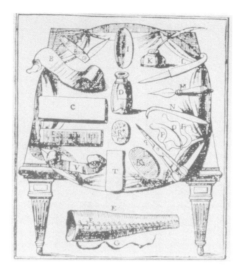

FIGURE 9-7. Instruments used by Pierre Dionis for treatment of venous stasis in the eighteenth century. Note the tapered legging fashioned of linen or canine skin to effect compression therapy. (From Foote RR. Varicose Veins. London: Butterworth, 1952.)

fashioned of linen or dog skin. In surgical treatment he made multiple longitudinal incisions over the veins and used cautery to destroy the veins (Figure 9-7). Like Sir Benjamin Brodie, Dionis became disillusioned with varicose vein surgery. Several of his works, which influenced many generations of surgeons to come, were even translated into Chinese as footnotes to the *Nei Ching* (*Canon of Medicine*), which had been handed down verbally for many centuries until it was first recorded in the third century and updated thereafter. The other writings of Dionis received the accolade of highest quality when they were burned during the French Revolution as a symbol of aristocratic decadence.

The French Revolution and the rise to prominence of John Hunter moved the center of excellence from Paris to London. John Hunter (1728-1793) offered his most important contribution to vein surgery in his work on thrombophlebitis and pulmonary embolus. He emphasized differentiation between septic phlebitis, which was a frequent occurrence requiring drainage, and spontaneous (traumatic) thrombophlebitis, which did not require surgical treatment.

Seventeenth Century

The seventeenth century was one of the most turbulent periods in history. It was the century of the pilgrim fathers, the civil war in England, Cromwell's protectorate, the Great Plague, the Great Fire, the restoration of the monarchy, and, most dramatically, the execution of King Charles I. In attendance was the man who had made one of the greatest medical discoveries of all time, the royal physician, William Harvey (1578-1657) (Figure 9-8). After publication of his *De Motu Cordis* in 1628, Harvey endured a 20-year struggle for acceptance against the

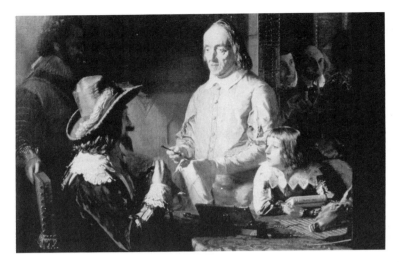

FIGURE 9-8. William Harvey formulated his theory of circulation of the blood through a study of venous valves and valves in the heart. He is seen demonstrating a point of anatomy to his royal patron and patient, the ill-fated Charles I of England *(left)*. The future Charles II *(right)* is an interested onlooker. (From Haeger K, ed. The Illustrated History of Surgery. Gothenburg, Sweden: AB Nordbok, 1988.)

prevalent humeral theory of Galen, which had held sway for almost 1400 years. Harvey was attacked by members of the medical profession and by such distinguished philosophers as Descartes and Bacon. Harvey's theory of circulation was formulated through his study of venous valves and heart valves. Through this approach, Harvey came to two conclusions that had escaped all other investigators: (1) that blood could flow only one way in blood vessels, and (2) that blood was pumped throughout the body by the heart. Strangely enough, Harvey still subscribed to Galen's teaching that the vital spirit dwelt in the heart. Descartes accused Harvey of being obsessed with the Aristotelian principle that true perfection lay in the completion of the circle.

As Trendelenburg pointed out, discovery of the function of valves in assisting return of blood to the heart meant a complete reversal of attitude toward surgery of varicose veins. It could no longer be maintained that blood moved downward under its own weight. Although treatment remained much the same, the rationale changed.

Venous stagnation must have been in the mind of Richard Wiseman, sergeant surgeon to King Charles II, in 1666, the year of the Great Fire, when he treated leg ulcers by a "rowled up compress and bandage from foot to gartering." When healed, the leg was supported by a "laced up stocking." Thus Wiseman demonstrated that he was a man ahead of his time.

Sixteenth Century

The subject of varicose veins was exercising the great surgical minds of the sixteenth century, as evidenced by the writings of Ambroise Paré (1510-1590) (Fig-

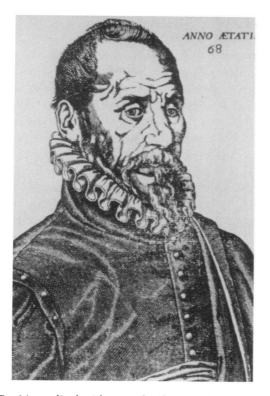

FIGURE 9-9. Ambroise Paré is credited with several milestones in surgery, including reintroduction of the ligature, which he used in midthigh ligation for treatment of varicose disease. (Courtesy New York Academy of Medicine.)

ure 9-9). It must be remembered, however, that at this time medical thinkers did not understand how blood circulated. Galenical theory prevailed, and it was believed that blood in the heart oscillated back and forth through fine pores in the interventricular septum to produce a pulse. It was Harvey's denial of this idea that provoked so much opposition.

Paré wrote concerning varicose veins: "The matter of them is usually melancholy blood, for varices often grow in men of a melancholy temper, who usually feed on gross meats, or such as breed and grow melancholy humors. Also women with child are commonly troubled with them by reason of the heaping together of their suppressed menstrual evacuation. It is best not to meddle with them."

The breadth of Paré's surgical experience was demonstrated by the sophistication of his operative treatment of varicose veins. His approach should not surprise us. Once again, it was midthigh ligation.

To appreciate the level of Paré's surgical skill in the context of his time, one must recall that it was during his period of preeminence in Europe that King Henry VIII granted the charter to the barber-surgeons in England to found the Royal College of Surgeons.

Middle Ages

In the centuries from the Renaissance back to the fall of the Roman Empire, there are few accounts of advances in surgery. This period comprised the Dark Ages, when most records were destroyed from time to time by the barbaric hordes that swept across Europe in waves. Nevertheless, some illustrious names survive. In fourteenth-century France, Guy de Chauliac, the physician to three popes, produced his great book on surgery, *La Grande Chirurgie*. In this work he wrote extensively about varicose veins and influenced teaching on many surgical subjects for the next 300 years. De Chauliac treated varicose veins by opening the vein and cauterizing the bleeding ends. If this method was not successful, he advised avulsion. We do not know about de Chauliac's success rate, but since he practiced long before the advent of blood transfusion, it might be just as pertinent to ask about his patient survival.

When the Moors conquered Spain toward the end of the seventh century, they brought with them the cultures of the eastern Mediterranean. From Greece, Persia, Cyprus, Egypt, the Holy Land, and Byzantium came the culture that, when wedded to Spanish subculture, flowered to create great centers of learning in the cities of the Iberian peninsula. Among these centers was Cordova, where a mixture of Arabic, Hebraic, and European knowledge formed the basis for establishing an eminent center of medical excellence in the eleventh century. The famous Maimonides (1135-1204) was born here. However, the most illustrious surgeon of this academy was Albucasis of Cordova (936-1013), who bore the medical tradition of his Arabic forebears with great distinction. In raising the standards of surgery, he deplored the fact that it "had passed into the hands of vulgar and uncultivated minds and had fallen into contempt." By this statement, Albucasis showed his disapproval of those colleagues whose ignorance and malpractice had given support to the ancient fallacy of the intellectual supremacy of the physician, an attitude that has stayed with us throughout the ages. Albucasis was an extremely cautious surgeon. However, he described the operation of multiple vein ligation and stripping with an external vein stripper 900 years before it was advocated by Charles Mayo.

In the tenth century another Arabic surgeon, Haly Abbas (d. 994), who also subscribed to the humoral theory of varicosity, described the clinical picture of varicose veins most vividly. He said that the dilated veins were caused by "overloading with viscous blood that sinks into the legs under its own weight. It therefore happens mostly in peasants, porters and sailors, and women with child . . . and these veins become tortuous and thick and inclined to become green or black in colour." Abbas advised multiple puncture, bleeding, and cautery, which constituted standard practice at the time.

Approximately 300 years earlier in Byzantium, Paul of Aegina (607-690), who trained in Alexandria, seems to have been not only a competent surgeon but also one who adopted a very modern approach. He described in great detail his sophisticated operation for varicose veins. He made novel use of tourniquets, applied above and below the knee, and then made the patient walk until the appropriate vein was filled with blood. The veins were marked with a special ink. The patient was then positioned on a table with legs extended, and an incision was made over the vein. The vein was quickly mobilized, and double sutures were passed around the upper and lower ends. The sutures were tied and cut, with a length of vein left between them that was removed. The wound was left open and was packed with an "oblong compress soaked in wine and oil." The vein removed was the internal saphenous vein in the midthigh.

After a search of fourteen centuries, we have found the originator of the midthigh ligation in Paul of Aegina. He demonstrated not only impeccable technique but also removal of a length of vein; moreover, he was aware that the way to avoid sepsis was to pack the wound open and leave it to granulate.

Greco-Roman Era

The great men of surgery who were regarded by Paul of Aegina and his distinguished Byzantine colleague Aetius of Amida as their source of inspiration were two Greeks and a Roman. The Greeks were Galen and Hippocrates, and the Roman was Celsus.

Galen (c. 130–c. 200), born in Pergamon in Asia Minor, was groomed in medicine and surgery from a very early age. It was his father who recognized his aptitude. Galen started his surgical career as physician to the gladiators. He was the first to realize that if a gladiator could be saved to fight again, it would be a great advantage to all concerned, especially the gladiator. Too many gladiators had been left to die of their wounds. Galen soon gained great renown and was invited to Rome, where he set up what now would be called a casualty and intensive care center at the Colosseum. There his skill came to the attention of Emperor Marcus Aurelius, who appointed Galen as his personal surgeon. Galen became a great expert in trauma and is credited with inventing the ligature, without which most surgery would be impossible. He removed varicose veins through three to six incisions with a hook that has been reinvented several times since its introduction. In addition, Galen developed a method of bandaging that held the wound edges together, and occasionally he was known to use a needle to transfix the wound edges to keep them in apposition. As noted earlier, Galen's theory of circulation was to remain standard theory for the next 1400 years. His voluminous works became a medical bible that dominated the Western World for the next 1500 years, even though only a third of them escaped destruction after the fall of Rome.

Cornelius Celsus (53 BC–AD 7), born a year after Julius Caesar invaded Britain for the second time, had no formal medical training. Being a physician in early Roman times was an arbitrary status. There is no record of Celsus's surgical apprenticeship, but there is no doubt that he became a very skillful operator. He questioned everything he saw and soon developed his own opinions, which he recorded most assiduously. Celsus was an inveterate chronicler of events who established himself as an authority in a vast number of medical fields. He became a legend in his own lifetime, and his opinions were sought on a great variety of matters both within and outside the field of medicine. Celsus developed a method of operating on varicose veins in which he made multiple incisions along the varicosity four fingerbreadths apart and touched the vein with a cautery through each incision. He then grasped the ends of the vein and extracted as much vein as he could. Those who practice multiple avulsion today will derive great comfort from the fact that this method was highly recommended by so great an authority as Celsus.

Greek civilization reached its height in the fourth century BC. The island of Cos was the center of medical learning, and there Hippocrates reigned supreme. His advice on the subject of varicose veins consisted of making multiple punctures in the varicosities and then bandaging the limb firmly. This practice was intended to let out blood along with whatever "evil" it contained. Hippocrates was opposed to excision because of the possibility of ulceration and infection. A great believer in cautery, he was quoted as saying, "What cannot be cured by medicaments is cured by the knife, what cannot be cured by the knife is cured by the searing iron, whatever this cannot cure must be considered incurable."

Long before the Hippocratic era, Greeks were treated by the priests of the god Asclepios, who were known as Asclepiads. To be treated, the patient brought a votive offering to the altar. Figure 9-1 shows such an offering, a tablet that dates from 350 BC. The slab was found near the Acropolis in Athens at the shrine of a physician named Amynos. The tablet, showing a sculptured leg with a large varicose vein, was placed on the altar presumably as an offering for a cure. It shows that the ancient Greeks had knowledge of varicose veins and that they considered there to be a need for treatment of varicosities. Since the Greeks of this time believed that evil humors were present in the thickened blood, they were adverse to bandaging. They thought that bandaging would drive the humors back into the body and produce dire results. Faith healing for varicose veins, which was popular 2000 years ago, is currently exemplified by the miracle cures offered in the popular press.

History therefore teaches that the common denominator of treatment throughout the years has been midthigh ligation and venous excision, often with the addition of venous sclerosis by one means or another. Thus we are reminded that there is nothing new under the sun.

MODERN SURGICAL TECHNIQUES—A PERSONAL VIEW: 1941-1991

The Trendelenburg operation described at the beginning of this chapter technically should have been called the Moore-Unger modification, a somewhat different procedure. In the Moore-Unger modification, sclerotherapy, considered a fundamental part of the operation, was done postoperatively. However, from approximately 1945 to 1948, sclerotherapy was deliberately avoided because of concern about sodium morrhuate. Radiologic evidence had helped to establish the fact that material injected into the thigh could find its way into the deep veins with all the consequences implied. The recommended method of treatment was changed to include an even more meticulous groin ligation and a midthigh and below-knee ligation plus, if necessary, short saphenous exploration and ligation. No veins were removed, and simultaneous sclerotherapy was not performed. The number of residual veins that accumulated postoperatively, however, required another look at sclerotherapy. Since ethamoline had become increasingly acceptable, being viewed as a safer and more appropriate sclerosant, this agent began to be used for residual veins and as definitive treatment for veins not considered large enough to warrant surgery. This method became standard practice from 1949 to 1952. In regard to development these were somewhat unproductive years because the method in common use was a mere modification of the prewar practice.

In order to trace the modern development of surgery of veins, a personal history can be used for demonstration.

The Stripping Technique

In the course of a visit to the Mayo Clinic in 1952, I learned the stripping technique. The use of a modified Babcock technique of vein stripping by Thomas T. Myers at the clinic in the late 1940s had led to a revival of the stripping operation, which had been abandoned in 1907. A newly designed, long, flexible stripper that pleated up the vein along its length proved to be immensely popular. The worldwide prestige of the Mayo Clinic coupled with Tom Myers's personal charm and hospitality contributed much to the widespread and immediate acceptance of the procedure.

The essence of the operation was a careful groin dissection followed by high ligation of the internal saphenous vein just distal to the saphenofemoral junction. Tributaries of the saphenous vein at the junction were ligated and divided. Stripping was carried out in the following way. An incision large enough to accommodate the sizable stripper head was made over the medial malleolus. The saphenous vein was isolated at the ankle, with care taken not to damage the saphenous nerve. The vein was supported by two untied ligatures. An incision was made into the lumen of the vein, and the guide end of the stripper was inserted into the vein. The distal ligature was tied, and the stripper was passed from below upward so that it would not catch in a valve. The stripper was extracted from the saphenous vein at the upper incision. The lower end of the vein was then tied firmly with a ligature around the neck of the stripper, and the vein was divided in front of the ligatures. The stripper head was eased into the malleolar incision with continuing firm traction that moved the stripper up the leg until it emerged from the groin incision with the vein pleated upward behind the head of the stripper.

I was surprised to find that the stripping technique sometimes demanded a blood transfusion because of bleeding along the stripper track. Such bleeding was the result of an attempt to avoid a hematoma by dragging a roll of gauze along the track by a length of ligature previously attached to the stripper. As would be expected, this method only caused further bleeding. Subsequently this practice was abandoned and substituted by the use of aspiration combined with manual pressure along the stripper track and firm bandaging from toe to groin as the vein was stripped.

Experience With Instrumentation

On returning to England in 1953, I began performing the operation with guarded optimism. Groin dissection and high ligation at the saphenofemoral junction were carried out as before. All tributaries of the saphenous vein at the junction were divided and ligated.

I began by using the stripper presented to me by Dr. Tom Myers. This instrument had a fixed head and guide. It soon became apparent that it would be advantageous to have detachable heads of various sizes and a detachable guide and handle. Thus the Rose stripper (Down Brothers, London) was developed. As I gained experience through the use of this stripper, I modified my technique. First, this stripper allowed me to gauge which head seemed to be least traumatic at the ankle and yet large enough to perform efficient stripping. Further, the stripper could be used in reverse if necessary. The ankle incision, in this situation somewhat smaller, was made in the submalleolar hollow and not over the malleolus so that it was safely away from the pressure point over the bone. The ankle dissection of the saphenous vein was done as before. The use of a smaller ankle acorn exposed the saphenous nerve to less trauma. The limb was compressed along the stripper track and firmly bandaged as the stripper was taken slowly up the leg in a series of short lengths.

At first, lengths of sponge rubber were laid along the track of the stripper to enhance the local pressure, but this practice was discontinued when careful bandaging proved to be equally effective. Peripheral varices were ignored since most were expected to disappear after they had been cut off from the main saphenous veins. One of the obvious attractions of the operation was the speed with which it could be performed.

Those who advocated stripping believed that the technique would achieve three main objectives. First, it would remove the main saphenous vein, which was always thought to be incompetent, in most (if not all) of its length. Second, it would isolate the varicose tributaries that would then thrombose. Third, it would interrupt any incompetent deep perforators that might feed the varicose clusters. It soon became obvious that only the first objective was being achieved. The most important observation that emerged was that all the tributaries of the saphenous vein that were interrupted by the stripper could be prevented from bleeding by the use of firm pressure. This was a well-known surgical fact concerning blood vessels that had not been applied before in this situation. Ligation was still necessary at the main saphenofemoral and saphenopopliteal junction, but the fact that broken ends of the smaller tributaries would seal off spontaneously made it apparent that varicosities could be removed without the need to tie the ruptured ends, especially if the varicosities were removed by traction rather than after clean division.

As experience with this procedure grew, three very interesting facts emerged. First, the stripper often passed unhindered under a scar at the site of a supposed previous ligation, and second, the peripheral varicosities had survived unchanged. The latter was the usual source of concern to the patient and constituted the indication for repeat surgery. Third, and most important, it became apparent from examination of the stripped vein that whole lengths of the vein were normal. This observation did not arouse much comment at that time since there was no stimulus to preserve the vein; arterial bypass surgery was not yet a common part of practice.

Coincidentally, from approximately 1956 to 1957, a revival of interest in sclerotherapy was spearheaded by Fegan's compression injection technique, which was soon rigorously practiced in the follow-up clinics. The immediate results of Fegan's procedure were satisfactory, but in the long term they proved to be disappointing. Such, however, was the volume of cases in postoperative clinics that, when limited to 50 cases per session twice a week, the caseload soon became unmanageable. By 1957 it was decided that stripping, as practiced at that time, was only a partial answer. It was thought that the only way to avoid overcrowded postoperative outpatient clinics was to excise the larger peripheral varicosities at the time of the original stripping.

Development and Experimentation: 1957-1964

The years from 1957 to 1964 were a period of further experimentation. The operations that my associates and I performed were based on stripping, with other procedures added as appropriate. In late 1957 we adopted a policy of making incisions over larger peripheral varicosities and excising them. At first it was thought prudent to ligate larger veins with fine catgut sutures. We were still not confident that blind avulsion would not give rise to difficult bleeding. This approach considerably lengthened the operation but gave a much more acceptable result to the patient. Coincidentally, the number of postoperative injections declined. Later we became bold enough to rely on pressure applied to smaller veins as a means of stopping bleeding. This practice was extended to larger veins provided that they were at a safe distance from a main junction. From 1963 onward, the trend in surgery turned further away from routine stripping and increasingly toward multiple avulsion. This trend marked the development of the currently accepted operative technique, limited axial stripping with the addition of extensive multiple avulsion.

Incompetent Perforating Veins

At this point we began to reconsider the role of perforating veins in relation to varicose clusters. Supposedly these clusters were caused by underlying incompetent deep perforators. When it was possible to demonstrate such perforators through phlebography, it was thought that cause and effect had been established. Some surgeons went further and considered these perforators to be the main cause of many mainline varicosities as well as the outlying varicose clusters. They thought these perforators were the explanation for all varicosities that occurred below a competent valve. Therefore it seemed logical to identify and ligate incompetent perforators. So strong was belief in this doctrine that eventually ligation of these veins alone was advocated and practiced by many. Even eminent surgeons followed this practice. Prior to operation incompetent perforators were identified by Doppler ultrasonography, thermography, and/or phlebography. Though the phlebogram was the gold standard, even with a practiced eye there was difficulty in interpretation. Although some perforators were found and ligated in relation to the varicosities, many explorations were tedious and carried out in vain. Even when these perforators were identified, simple ligation alone failed to produce the desired effect, and many varicosities remained. Worse still, the operation could be a cosmetic disaster because of the length of the incisions required. Such a result was particularly unfortunate when the complaint was cosmetic in the first place. Therefore the majority of surgeons preferred to both strip and ligate perforators, but results of this treatment were marginally better, although they did not justify widespread acceptance of the procedure.

My colleagues and I decided to investigate the role of incompetent deep perforators, and we started a lengthy but unrewarding period of searching for and ligating them. When the technical difficulties of locating the perforator in relation to the varicosity became apparent, and when these perforators could not be found through cosmetically acceptable incisions, we restricted this approach to limbs where such a result was a secondary consideration. One could justify this procedure only for operations for varicose ulcer.

The stripping operation demonstrated that many peripheral varicosities were independent of the main saphenous system. Also, in many cases the main systems themselves were either not involved or only partially involved. This fact has been confirmed recently by several centers using duplex ultrasonography. This technique has shown that the relationship between saphenofemoral incompetence and peripheral varicosities can be inconsistent. In fact, some varicose clusters were completely isolated without demonstrable deep connection.

If incompetence of perforating veins is not exclusively caused by back pressure, loss of valvular competence can be explained if the perforator itself becomes dilated as the result of the varicose process (Figure 9-10). In such a case it might be argued that ligation is still necessary. However, ligation by itself would not cause the overlying varicosity to regress. On the other hand, if the overlying varicosity were removed, this action would not only solve that problem but also would divide any connecting perforator by traction. Pressure hemostasis then would occlude it. Even if it were theoretically possible for such perforators to remain patent, there would be no superficial varicosity into which to feed (Figure 9-11). These observations caused us to abandon the search for incompetent perforators. In addition, general enthusiasm for the procedure by others has diminished.

The evolution of this theory of incompetent perforating veins has made us concentrate on removing the outlying varicosities ever more thoroughly. Also, it has caused us to refocus on the vein wall and in particular to review the weak

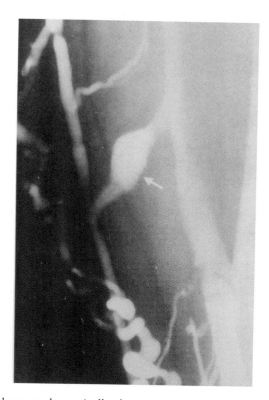

FIGURE 9-10. This phlebogram dramatically shows involvement of a perforating vein in the varicose process. Note the grossly varicose greater saphenous vein *(arrow)*. (From Browse NL, Burnand K, Lea Thomas M, eds. Diseases of the Veins. London: Edward Arnold, 1988.)

vein wall theory more seriously. This line of thought started an investigation, the development and conclusions of which are fully described in Chapter 2.

Currently we avulse all irregular varicosities through much smaller incisions because we are confident of hemostasis achieved by firm pressure. The immediate results of this approach are far superior to those obtained earlier. It is obvious that the improvement is the result of removal of the varicose veins themselves.

Careful clinical examination and Doppler insonation have revealed that saphenous dilatation may begin in the lower third of the thigh approximately at the site of the Hunter perforator or further down below the knee at the site of the Boyd perforator. It was through this vein that Boyd was concerned that sclerosants injected around the knee could gain access to the deep venous system, an effect that he demonstrated by phlebography. In the early 1960s we began to do less stripping and more avulsion. This approach has meant that we are able to perform more outpatient and day-case procedures with the patient under a local anesthetic when a full groin exploration is not considered necessary. This practice has helped to lessen the demand for hospital beds and to shorten waiting lists. It was this approach, in fact, that had made compression sclerotherapy so popular

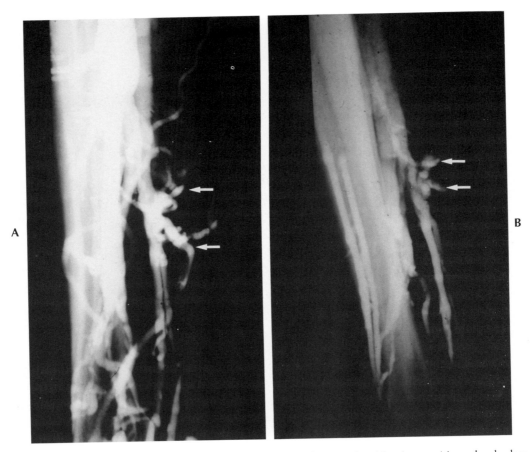

FIGURE 9-11. A, Preoperative phlebogram shows below-knee varicosities *(arrows)* in a clearly demonstrated perforating vein. A large communication exists between the greater and the lesser saphenous systems. **B,** After multiple avulsion of the superficial varicosities without any stripping, the perforating vein is still patent but there is no superficial varicosity into which the vein can feed *(arrows)*. Considerable improvement in the varicose condition is noted.

in the early 1960s in a time of financial stringency. As we began to strip the internal saphenous vein less often, the question arose whether we should strip the internal saphenous vein at all.

ISSUES IN SURGERY
Stripping the Internal Saphenous Vein

The relevance of saphenofemoral incompetence to the occurrence and development of peripheral varicosities needs to be examined. In particular, the pros and cons of stripping the internal saphenous vein must be elucidated.

Let us consider some technical objections. First, it is recognized that reflux in the groin is not present in all cases of varicose veins. Second, there is always the possibility of sural or saphenous nerve damage during stripping. Third, increased postoperative morbidity is associated with stripping. Although stripping is a comparatively painless procedure, it often involves postoperative bruising, tenderness, and induration along the line of the stripped vein. Certainly there is more discomfort after stripping than after simple local avulsion. Fourth, and perhaps the most potent argument for not removing the main saphenous vein, is the possibility of future arterial bypass requirements. However, an obviously dilated varicose vein is not likely to be suitable for such a purpose. Nor is it certain that a normal section of a saphenous vein that is only moderately dilated should be used as an arterial bypass. It could be argued that this section might become varicose at some future time. Yet cases have been described in which no extension of the varicosity develops. Some arterial surgeons have reported success in using borderline veins for arterial repair. However, this method must be considered as a calculated gamble.

The main argument in favor of stripping the saphenous vein is that it will further the aims of treatment. Therefore one must ask whether this approach will contribute to the eradication of varicose veins and the prevention of recurrence. With regard to the first objective, the answer must be that stripping alone does not seem to be sufficient. As already described, many of the offending varicosities remain after stripping.

In order to assess the part played by removal of the internal saphenous vein, it is necessary to consider the incidence of recurrence with and without stripping of this vein. These investigations are now taking place at numerous surgical centers, but a significant period of time must elapse before meaningful results can be obtained.

Indications for Surgery

Not all patients with varicose veins require treatment. Many are asymptomatic and remain so for most of their lives. On the other hand, some patients complain of aching pain that varies from mild to severe. Pain in the leg and varicose veins are both common conditions. However, the important point is to establish whether the symptom and the cause are related. Pain of skeletal and arterial origin always must be eliminated. Male patients often present with severe varicose veins with well-developed skin pigmentation, eczema, and ulceration. They may have surprisingly little pain from the varicose veins themselves, but the ulcers become painful if infected. Often these patients have evidence of tinea pedis, which may predispose them to superficial phlebitis. Varicose veins are not confined to those individuals in an occupation that involves long periods of standing, but naturally the symptoms are more likely to be noted under these conditions. A history of a sudden hemorrhage or a dilated vein in a site vulnerable to trauma, such as the shin, the ankle, or the dorsum of the foot, is often an urgent indication for surgery. Athletes often have large asymptomatic veins, and many of those involved in track and team sports must undergo surgery because of the risk of large traumatic hematomas or superficial phlebitis. Superficial phlebitis also can arise spontaneously or after a local or general infection. This condition usually foretells morbidity, especially if it is repeated.

A history of previous deep phlebitis is not a contraindication to surgery if no evidence of persisting deep vein obstruction exists. Since such obstruction occurs in only 10% of cases, most patients will have some degree of deep venous reflux. Venous return from the leg will be hampered if superficial reflux also is present. With exercise, venous pressures show that if the superficial veins are dealt with, the fall in pressure associated with exercise is improved and in some instances will return to normal. If deep venous occlusion is present and persists, the patient will complain that firm bandaging makes the condition worse, even to the point of venous claudication. In such patients superficial veins are part of the collateral venous return.

Last, but by no means least, is the cosmetic problem. Many women complain of varicose veins for purely cosmetic reasons. Such complaints are often not considered seriously by physicians. Women who make these complaints constitute a wide age group. They may be multiparous and are drawn from all social classes and occupations. Despite such disparity, these patients all have one thing in common. They regard their veins as unacceptable disfigurements. Their complaint is as distressing to them as any painful affliction would be, and it is often less well tolerated. When fashion decrees that skirts are to be worn shorter, these women seek treatment at once. I think that they are entitled to our attention and that no surgeon should turn them away if he or she can assure them of a good cosmetic result.

Finally, some patients have no symptoms but are driven to seek advice because of some drastic happening to other members of their family who had varicose veins. Each such case needs to be treated on its own merits.

Contraindications to Surgery

Varicose veins should not be operated on during pregnancy; nor should such surgery be done in the presence of peripheral arterial disease, any contraindication to general anesthesia, any bleeding diathesis, or active skin infection in the lower limb. In addition, surgery for varicose veins should not be performed in association with lymphedema or in the presence of venous claudication. In any case of unusual presentation, a congenital malformation should be considered. The contraceptive pill should be discontinued 1 month before and 1 month after this type of surgery.

Preparation for Surgery

As stated in our goals, the only practical way of eradicating varicose veins is by a meticulous and radical removal of all the varicosities, with the addition of ligation, if necessary, at the saphenofemoral and saphenopopliteal junction and/or localized stripping of the main saphenous veins.

Veins are carefully charted after the patient has been standing for 10 minutes. The extent of varicosity is estimated by palpation, propagation of the cough impulse, and Doppler ultrasound. This approach establishes connections with the long saphenous vein. The short saphenous vein should be examined in the same way, but palpation is easier to do with the patient's knee slightly flexed to relax the deep fascia. A full abdominal examination is performed, and the peripheral pulses are palpated. Sciatic pain is eliminated by using the straight leg–raising test. The conditions of the ankle, knee, and hip are estimated. It is important to note any existing blemishes on the limb. The patient must be told that the veins can be removed but the tendency to varicosity is inborn and cannot be eliminated. Therefore maintenance treatment, consisting of injections or surgical removal done on an outpatient basis, may be necessary from time to time. An instruction sheet outlining the preoperative and postoperative routine is helpful. Great emphasis is placed on postoperative walking exercise of six 10-minute brisk bursts rather than a 60-minute walk since the latter tends to be more time-consuming and not as efficient in stimulating venous return.

SUMMARY

The history of the development of varicose vein surgery throughout the ages has been described, and the evolution of the modern operation has been followed over the last 50 years. The time-honored attitude to surgery that has been directed toward the doctrine of primary valvular incompetence has been questioned because it has been shown that varicose veins can develop in the absence of incompetence in the feeding veins. It has been postulated that the answer must lie in weakness of the vein wall and that, on examination, this theory will readily explain the anomalies described. Evidence for this theory is presented in Chapter 2.

As the modern trend in varicose vein surgery turns away from routine stripping and toward multiple avulsion, results have improved. There are, however, a number of circumstances in which limited stripping of the internal saphenous vein is indicated. Our approach to this problem is to combine limited stripping with multiple avulsion.

We suggest an operative technique that places great emphasis on elimination of varicosities wherever they occur while also achieving a good cosmetic result. Although we believe that a specialist clinic could achieve the best results from the patient's point of view, one of the most important functions of medicine is the training of young people in appropriate varicose vein surgery. This training must include an indoctrination that sees the high attainment of good results as a challenge. This challenge is to be met in a much neglected but most important branch of surgical art.

BIBLIOGRAPHY

Babcock WW. A Textbook of Surgery, 2nd ed. Philadelphia: WB Saunders, 1935.
Barros D'Sa Aires AB, Bell PRF, Darke SG, Harris PL. Vascular Surgery—Current Questions. Oxford: Butterworth Heinemann, 1991.

Bernsten A. Des varices du membre inférieur, spécialement au point de vue de l'étiologie et du traitement chirurgical. Acta Chir Scand 62:61, 1927.

Browse NL, Burnand K, Lea Thomas M, eds. Diseases of the Veins. London: Edward Arnold, 1988.

Buck AH. The Growth of Medicine. New Haven, Conn.: Yale University Press, 1917.

Edwards EA. The treatment of varicose veins: Anatomical features of ligation of the great saphenous vein. Surg Gynecol Obstet 59:916, 1934.

Foote RR. Varicose Veins, 2nd ed. London: Butterworth, 1954.

Garrison FH. Introduction to the History of Medicine, 4th ed. Philadelphia: WB Saunders, 1929.

Genevrier M. Soc de Med Mil Franc 15:169, 1921.

Greenhalgh RM. Vascular Surgical Techniques. An Atlas, 2nd ed. Philadelphia: WB Saunders, 1989.

Haeger K. The Illustrated History of Surgery. Gothenburg, Sweden: AB Nordbok, 1988.

Higgins TT, Kittel AB. The use of sodium morrhuate in treatment of varicose veins by injection. Lancet 1:68, 1930.

Homans J. The operative treatment of varicose veins and ulcers based upon a classification of these lesions. Surg Gynecol Obstet 22:143, 1916.

Homans J. Varicose veins and ulcer: Methods of diagnosis and treatment. Boston Med Surg J 187: 258, 1922.

Keller WL. A new method of extirpating the internal saphenous and similar veins in varicose conditions: A preliminary report. NY Med J 82:385, 1905.

Keller WL. Combined extirpation and obliteration in the treatment of varicose veins. Ann Surg 79: 907, 1924.

Lyons AS, Petrucelli RJ. Medicine: An Illustrated History. New York: Harry N. Abrams, 1978.

Maingot RH, Carlton CH. The injection treatment of varicose veins. An estimate of its place in practice. Lancet 1:806, 1928.

Mayo CH. Treatment of varicose veins. Surg Gynecol Obstet 2:385, 1906.

McPheeters HO, Anderson JK. The Injection Treatment of Varicose Veins, 2nd ed. Philadelphia: Davis, 1939.

Nicolaides AN, Sumner DS. Investigation of Patients With Deep Vein Thrombosis and Chronic Venous Insufficiency. London: Med Orion, 1991.

Ochsner A, Mahorner H. Varicose Veins. St. Louis: Mosby, 1939.

Paré A. Journeys in Diverse Places. Translated by S. Paget. New York: Collier, 1910.

Perthes G. Über die Operation der Unterschenkelvaricen nach Trendelenburg. Dtsch Med Wochenschr 21:253, 1895.

Schiassi B. Sem Med Paris 28:601, 1908.

Sicard JA, Gaugier L. Les Traitements des Varices par les Injections Locale Sclérosantes. Paris: Masson, 1927.

de Takats G. Ambulatory ligation of the saphenous vein. JAMA 94:1194, 1930.

de Takats G, Quillin L. Ligation of the saphenous vein. A report on two hundred ambulatory operations. Arch Surg 26:72-88, 1933.

de Takats G, Quint H. The injection treatment of varicose veins. Surg Gynecol Obstet 50:545, 1930.

Trendelenburg F. Beitr Klin Chir 7:195, 1891.

Warwick WT. The Rational Treatment of Varicose Veins and Varicocoele. London: Faber & Faber, 1931.

Chapter 10

Treatment of Varicosities of Saphenous Origin: Comparison of Ligation, Selective Excision, and Sclerotherapy

Peter Neglén

Patients suffering from varicose veins have many complaints. Some may be concerned about minute localized varicosities for cosmetic reasons, whereas others do not seek medical advice until they have major varicose veins with swelling, aching, and eczema. Naturally, the treatment expectations of the two groups differ. This chapter focuses on the treatment of varicose veins with main-stem insufficiency.

Several different treatments have been recommended for patients with long (greater) saphenous vein or short (lesser) saphenous vein reflux. Flush ligation combined with stripping, avulsion of local varicosities, and perforator interruption is still the most common operation. An alternative is to spare the long saphenous vein by performing proximal ligation with excision of local visible varices and ligation of incompetent perforators. Sclerotherapy, accomplished by injecting the visible vein perforators and/or the main stem, performed alone or in combination with flush ligation of the long saphenous vein at the saphenofemoral junction, has been advocated.

Since venous varicosity is a progressive, incurable disease, the treatment is only palliative without guarantee of a cure. Therefore the objectives should be the same for all modes of treatment, that is, to provide a satisfactory cosmetic result, relieve symptoms, avoid complications, and prevent recurrences.

GENERAL ASPECTS OF SURGICAL TREATMENT

Treatment of insufficiency of the long saphenous stem by ligation of the vein's termination was described in the late 1800s. The importance of performing flush ligation of the main stem and its tributaries close to the femoral vein to prevent recurrences was pointed out by Homans[1] in 1916. In the early 1900s, Mayo[2] introduced stripping of the long saphenous vein with the technique refined by Babcock[3] and later by Myers and Cooley.[4] In addition, proper excision of local

175

varicosities with meticulous disconnection of all incompetent perforators is the "classic" surgery of varicose veins. Very low recurrence rates have been claimed for this type of radical surgery.[5,6]

Several arguments have been made for restricting the removal of saphenous veins, either to avoid any stripping of the vein or to limit it to the thigh portion. With a limited operation the patient may not require hospitalization and will have a shorter convalescence. Increased morbidity, pain, bleeding, and wound infection, although minimal, are associated with complete stripping. A well-recognized complication of ankle-to-groin stripping of the long saphenous vein is damage to the distal portion of the saphenous nerve, resulting in skin anesthesia of the medial ankle and foot.[7] Stripping the vein in a distal direction (groin-to-ankle) decreases the incidence of nerve injury.[8] Thus it appears to be advisable to strip the long saphenous vein below the knee in a distal direction. If stripping the main stem is limited from the groin to just below the knee, nerve injury is markedly reduced from 39% to 4% to 7%.[9,10] In addition, the remaining distal portion may be used later for arterial reconstructive surgery.

The greater demand for arterial reconstructive surgery has accentuated the fact that unnecessary stripping of the long saphenous vein removes the most favorable graft conduit. On the other hand, a grossly dilated, tortuous, incompetent main stem is a poor arterial substitute. Nevertheless, the main reason for limited saphenous vein surgery is that the long saphenous vein is spared for future arterial surgery. The important issues are whether saphenous vein–saving surgery compromises the objectives of varicose vein treatment and whether the remaining veins can be used as grafts.

FLUSH LIGATION OF LONG SAPHENOUS VEIN

Flush ligation done without stripping of the long saphenous vein was the first operation recommended for saphenous vein incompetence. It has definite advantages because it is a simple operation that can be performed with the patient under local anesthesia; it involves little or no postoperative sick leave. An example of the utility of saphenous ligation has been described from the Naval Hospital San Diego.[11] There the objective was control of the symptoms of varicose veins. Proximal ligation and selective point ligation of perforating veins and varicose clusters was used in conjunction with sclerotherapy so that time away from duty could be minimized. Although the patient is initially relieved of symptoms, the recurrence rate is significantly reduced if removal of the long saphenous vein also is performed.[12]

Inappropriate flush ligation without interruption of all tributaries invites recurrence of varicose veins. If proper ligation of the saphenofemoral junction has been done, another explanation for recurrence is incompetence of the superficial and deep communicating veins of the leg and thigh, often called perforators. Although numerous perforators are present in the calf, three or four medial calf perforators are fairly constant in position. It is important to note that they do not communicate directly with the distal long saphenous vein but with the posterior

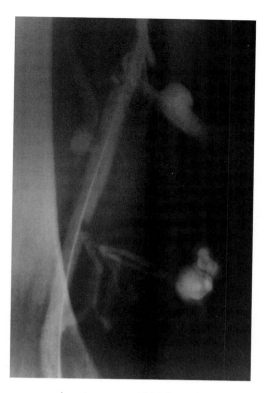

FIGURE 10-1. Popliteal venogram showing two midthigh perforators filling a distally incompetent long saphenous vein. (Courtesy Professor Bo Eklöf.)

arch vein. Therefore stripping the long saphenous vein below the knee does not correct all perforator incompetence. This is a valid argument for abandoning stripping of the distal long saphenous vein unless the vein is tortuous, dilated, and incompetent.

In contrast to calf perforator veins, thigh perforators drain the long saphenous vein directly to the superficial femoral vein (Figure 10-1). Retrograde saphenography has demonstrated at least one thigh perforator in 87% of patients.[13] Incompetent thigh perforating veins may be multiple and have been shown to occur anywhere in the thigh. However, in the majority of patients (80%) only one perforator is identified, with two thirds of them found in the middle third of the thigh.[14] Stripping the long saphenous vein at the thigh usually, but not invariably, disrupts these communications. Thus recurrence caused by dilatation of Hunter's thigh perforators and reflux into a preserved, patent long saphenous vein is prevented.[15]

What happens to the vein after simple ligation? It does not seem to be occluded completely by thrombosis. The long saphenous vein of the thigh remains patent in more than 85% of operated legs.[16] Presumably, the vein stays open to the point of the most proximal perforating vein, with thrombosis likely above this

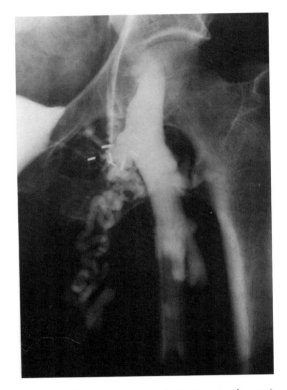

FIGURE 10-2. Popliteal venogram showing neovascularization in the groin after previous high ligation of the long saphenous vein. (Courtesy Professor Bo Eklöf.)

level. If this perforating vein becomes insufficient, the entire saphenous system again may undergo reflux and varicosities are likely to recur.

Another explanation for recurrence after a properly performed flush ligation of the saphenofemoral confluence has been suggested by Sheppard.[17] He found that connections between the long saphenous stump and the remaining saphenous vein or its tributaries may be reestablished by neovascularization of granulation tissue at the site of the flush ligation. Recurrence develops from reflux into the remaining incompetent saphenous vein (Figure 10-2).

Varicography of recurrent varicose veins was performed in 41 lower limbs 2 to 33 years after proximal ligation of the saphenous vein without stripping.[18] On examination, continuous-wave ultrasound indicated a source of reflux from above the knee. The varicogram revealed midthigh perforator incompetence in 34% of the lower limbs and a patent portion of the saphenous vein in the thigh in 54%. The most common cause of recurrence (80%), however, was a residual or recurrent communication between the femoral vein and the remaining long saphenous vein.

In one prospective study, 54 patients had long saphenous vein incompetence verified by duplex ultrasound prior to flush ligation of the long saphenous vein.[19]

At follow-up 6 to 12 months later, scanning of the saphenofemoral junction was repeated. The surprising finding was that two patients still had a patent and incompetent saphenofemoral junction. In addition, 46% of the remaining long saphenous veins were present and incompetent. In two patients reflux stemmed from a demonstrable midthigh perforator, with the remaining saphenous veins fed by small veins branching from the femoral vein. This observation supports the concept of collateral formation by neovascularization.

Regardless of whether recurrence is most commonly caused by remaining perforating thigh veins or by reestablishment of communication at the saphenofemoral confluence, stripping of the long saphenous vein of the thigh appears to be crucial in minimizing recurrence. A prospective trial in which limbs with saphenofemoral incompetence were randomly selected for saphenofemoral flush ligation alone or ligation combined with stripping of the long saphenous vein has been performed by Munn et al.[12] At follow-up 2.5 to 3.5 years later, an independent objective assessment revealed that stripping the vein conferred significantly greater protection against recurrence. Based on these observations, I strongly believe that it is inadequate to restrict surgery to proximal flush ligation of the incompetent long saphenous vein, and I firmly advocate stripping of the thigh portion of the long saphenous vein.

SELECTIVE EXCISION: LONG SAPHENOUS VEIN–SAVING SURGERY

Removal of the long saphenous vein from the groin to the knee leaves the distal portion of the vein for potential use as an arterial graft and avoids injury to the saphenous nerve. If the distal long saphenous vein is normal and since the calf perforating veins do not join the main stem, this limited stripping does not endanger the objectives of the operation. Negus[10] has reported a low recurrence rate (12.5%) in 96 limbs, with an average follow-up of 3.7 years.

Attempts have been made to limit surgery to flush ligation of the saphenofemoral/popliteal veins with avulsions of obvious varicosities through multiple stab incisions and the incompetent saphenous vein left in situ. Large[20] has reported excellent results in a retrospective follow-up done 3 years after this procedure in a randomly selected group of 171 from a total of 1000 patients with 295 affected limbs. A satisfactory result was observed in 90% of patients. Whether or not the remaining saphenous vein was useful for arterial grafting was not indicated.

Hammarsten et al.[21] have reported the results following random allocation of 42 patients to either "classic" operation, including ankle-groin stripping of the saphenous vein, or flush ligation of the saphenous vein at the saphenofemoral junction. Both procedures were combined with local excision of varicosities and ligation of incompetent perforators. Perforators were visualized by phlebography or were noted clinically. It is not clear whether thigh perforators were interrupted. At follow-up done more than 4 years later, the recurrence rate was low in both groups (12%). This finding was supported by a significant increase in venous return time as measured by strain-gauge plethysmography. Ultrasound scanning of the remaining long saphenous veins showed that 78% of these veins could be used for arterial grafting. This observation contradicts the findings of Sutton and Drake.[13] On retrograde saphenography performed during varicose vein surgery, 65% of long saphenous veins were found to be varicose with an average length of normal-appearing vein <16 cm, which made them unsuitable for arterial grafts.

Koyano and Sakaguchi[22] chose to remove only those segments of the long saphenous vein that involved reflux detected by Doppler ultrasound in 337 lower limbs with primary varicose veins. These authors found incompetence of the saphenofemoral junction and long saphenous vein from groin to at least knee level in 91% of limbs. An additional 7% of limbs had reflux of the saphenofemoral junction with limited or no incompetence of the long saphenous vein, whereas only 2% had segmental incompetence with no reflux at the junction. Almost 50% of the patients with varicosities of short saphenous vein origin had no reverse flow in the distal saphenous vein. The distribution of incompetence is probably different in another catchment area, but there is no doubt that most patients who complain of varicose veins have saphenofemoral or saphenopopliteal insufficiency with varying degrees of trunk involvement.

Selective stripping of incompetent veins was performed in 80 patients. The results were compared to those of 189 limbs in which standard stripping was done during the same time period, after an average follow-up of 3.2 years. Plethysmographic measurement of venous reflux volume in a limited number of the limbs and clinical examination of 80% of them at follow-up revealed no difference between the two groups. Whether the remaining veins were adequate for use as vascular grafts is not clear. As expected, a reduction in the rate of saphenous and sural nerve injury was observed.

Use of noninvasive modalities such as duplex scanning will undoubtedly facilitate the investigation of each segment of superficial and deep veins with detection of incompetent perforators. The ability to map superficial incompetence will make it possible to perform selective, directed surgery of incompetent segments. However, preservation of a diseased segment is of no proven value and may jeopardize the objectives of varicose vein surgery. The intention still must be to remove diseased incompetent superficial veins and to control reflux.

SURGERY VS. SCLEROTHERAPY

Sclerotherapy has been used in central Europe for decades. However, the method had its true revival when Fegan[23] published his basic studies on the effects of the sclerosant and stressed the necessity of effective elastic compression after injection. Having become firmly established in Great Britain and Scandinavia, sclerotherapy is now declining in acceptance in North America. The advantages of compression sclerotherapy are obvious: no anesthesia, no hospitalization, and no loss of work are required. These factors substantially decrease the cost to the patient and the community.[24] Advocates of sclerotherapy treatment also maintain that the cosmetic results are better. The advantages are real, however, only if sclerotherapy done alone or in combination with saphenofemoral flush ligation produces results equivalent to those of surgery. The initial economic advantage is greatly eroded if regular follow-up examinations and repeated treatments are necessary.

The results of "adequate" initial surgery, including stripping of the saphenous vein with flush ligation of the proximal vein, meticulous avulsion of all tributaries, and interruption of all perforating veins, have been reported to be extremely good in some reviews, with very low 10-year recurrence rates (<15%) noted.[6,25] Enthusiastic sclerotherapists have reported similar excellent results, 80% to 90% success following sclerotherapy performed alone.[23,26,27]

These studies probably exaggerate the results of both surgery and sclerotherapy. It is well known that varicose vein disease is a chronic condition and that intervention is palliative. With a long observation time, new varicosities invariably develop. Objective assessment of any treatment for varicose veins is extremely difficult because of the varying definition of what a recurrence is and how to measure it. This lack of uniformity also makes comparisons of studies difficult. In studies it is vital that the follow-up be long enough (at least 5 years) and that results be assessed as objectively as possible, preferably by someone who is not involved in treatment. In most studies treatment outcome is described by patients as a subjective opinion, with the objective findings reported by a surgeon. It is well known that agreement is oftentimes poor between what the surgeon and the patient consider a good result. Physiologic tests of calf pump function following the two forms of treatment are most valuable. From a socioeconomic viewpoint, the need for additional treatment is of greatest importance.

Despite the fact that modern compression sclerotherapy was introduced 25 years ago, controversy still exists as to whether sclerotherapy or surgery is the most effective treatment for varicose veins involving long saphenous vein or short saphenous vein insufficiency. Several studies have attempted to compare the two treatments in prospective controlled random trials.[28-33]

In 1972 Chant et al.[28] reported no significant difference in results between injection compression sclerotherapy in which Fegan's technique was used and radical surgery for varicose veins 3 years after initial treatment. However, by 5 years 40% of patients who initially received sclerotherapy had further treatment compared with 24% of those treated surgically[29] (Figure 10-3). This difference was statistically significant. Patients more than 35 years of age and those with signs of chronic venous insufficiency, such as edema and ankle flare, fared better with surgery than with sclerotherapy.

In 1975 Doran and White[30] described the results of another controlled study in favor of compression sclerotherapy over surgery after 1 year (24% vs. 45% failures). After 2 years the difference was not significant (21% vs. 16.4% failures). These two trials found no contraindications to sclerosis of primary saphenofemoral incompetence, but neither study identified the type of superficial insufficiency. Both studies can be criticized for being short-term or for having an unclear endpoint, which was set as the need for further treatment (e.g., prescription of stockings). In addition, patients who underwent retreatment were included in

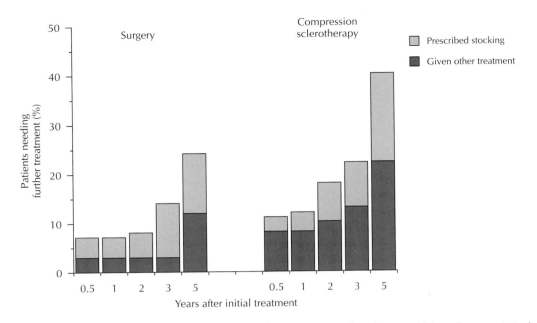

FIGURE 10-3. Chant's comparison of surgery and compression sclerotherapy. Although no statistical difference was noted after 3 years, at 5-year follow-up significantly more patients who had initial treatment with sclerotherapy needed further treatment. (Data from Chant ADB, Jones HO, Weddell JM. Varicose veins: A comparison of surgery and injection/compression sclerotherapy. Lancet 2: 1188-1191, 1972; Beresford SAA, Chant ADB, Jones HO, Piachaud D, Weddell JM. Varicose veins: A comparison of surgery and injection/sclerotherapy. Five-year follow-up. Lancet 1:921-924, 1978.)

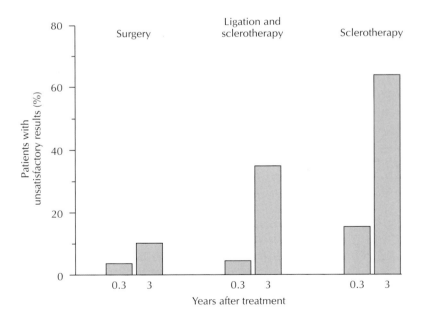

FIGURE 10-4. Recurrence rate was significantly lower for surgery compared to ligation combined with sclerotherapy. At 3 years after treatment, recurrence rate was significantly lower for combined treatment than for sclerotherapy alone. (Data from Jakobsen B. The value of different forms of treatment for varicose veins. Br J Surg 66:182-184, 1979.)

2- and 5-year follow-up studies, which rendered judgment of the initial treatment impossible.

In 1979 Jakobsen[31] studied 483 patients with incompetence of the long saphenous vein or the short saphenous vein or a combination of the two types. Patients were randomized into three comparable groups. Radical surgery was performed in 161 patients, and 167 patients received compression sclerotherapy. The third group of 165 patients had a combination of these treatment approaches. Objective success after 3 years was 90% for surgery and 37% for sclerotherapy alone (Figure 10-4). Injection sclerotherapy was performed according to Sigg.[32]

In 1974 and 1984 Hobbs[33,34] reported the results of the most comprehensive randomized long-term study done to date, comparing sclerotherapy and surgery for varicose veins in 500 patients. The large number of patients permitted stratification into defined groups according to short saphenous vein or long saphenous vein insufficiency, isolated perforator incompetence, or dilated local varicose veins. Although compression sclerotherapy initially seemed effective even when proximal incompetence was present, later objective results were substantially better with surgery (surgery vs. compression sclerotherapy at 5 years, 79% vs. 30% [excellent], and at 10 years, 71% vs. 6% [good], respectively) (Figure 10-5). Patients with main-stem insufficiency had a higher recurrence rate than the others. Hobbs[33,34] concluded that saphenous vein insufficiency is best managed by radical operation but that compression sclerotherapy is superior for treatment of local varicosities, isolated leg perforator incompetence, and residual or recurrent veins after appropriate surgery.

In a prospective study done by our group, 152 lower limbs with primary varicose veins and long saphenous vein incompetence were studied closely.[35] Of these, 78 limbs had been randomized for compression sclerotherapy and 74 limbs for radical stripping. Injection therapy was performed according to Hobbs's modification of the Fegan technique,[33] and surgery was performed as previously described. These patients were followed up not only for rate of recurrence after 5 years but also for assessment by foot volumetry. Expelled volume, which expresses calf muscle pump function, and refilling flow ratio, which is directly related to the amount of venous reflux, were estimated before and after treatment.

At follow-up, three groups were defined through inspection and palpation by the surgeon: (1) cured, in which no true varicose veins were seen or palpated (except for minor reticular veins); (2) improved, in which limited residual or recurrent varicosities or a long saphenous vein was palpable as recanalized at the injection site (even if no varicosities were seen); and (3) failed, in which large varicosities with incompetent perforators or retrograde flow in the long saphenous vein were noted. When treatment failed according to objective assessment, these limbs were considered failures throughout the study and were not reevaluated by foot volumetry.

As early as 6 months after treatment, the surgeon's findings showed a smaller cure rate with compression sclerotherapy compared to surgery, although the failure rate was minimal in both groups. After 5 years, a striking difference was found between the surgically treated patients (60% "cured" and 35% improved) and the sclerotherapy group (51% failure rate) (Figure 10-6).

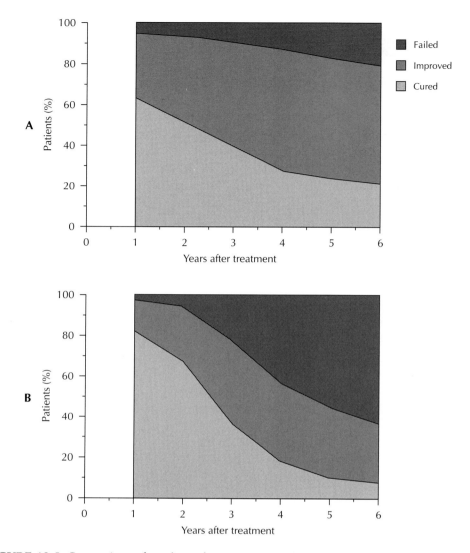

FIGURE 10-5. Comparison of results with surgery (A) and sclerotherapy (B). Early failure rates are similar, but after 6 years more patients were cured or improved with surgery. (Redrawn from Hobbs JT. Surgery and sclerotherapy in the treatment of varicose veins. Arch Surg 109:793-796, 1974. Copyright 1974, American Medical Association.)

FIGURE 10-6. Results with surgery (A), ligation combined with sclerotherapy (B), and sclerotherapy alone (C) in patients with incompetent long saphenous vein. After 5 years more cured and improved patients were found among the groups that had surgery or combined treatment than in the group that had sclerotherapy alone. (Data from Einarsson E. Compression sclerotherapy of varicose veins. In Eklöf B, Gjöres JE, Thulesius O, Bergqvist D, eds. Controversies in the Management of Venous Disorders. London: Butterworth, 1989, pp 203-211; Neglén P, Einarsson E, Eklöf B. High tie with sclerotherapy for saphenous vein insufficiency. Phlebologie 1:105-111, 1986.)

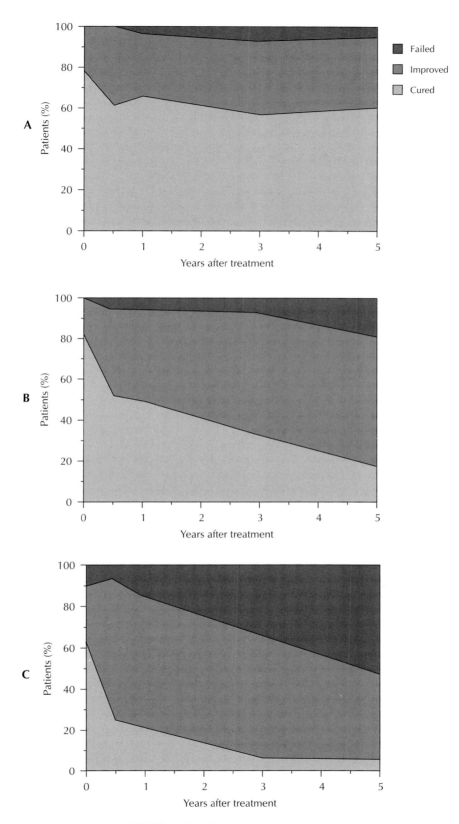

FIGURE 10-6. For legend see opposite page.

TABLE 10-1. Results of foot volumetric measurements compared to baseline values in patients having three different modes of varicose vein treatment

Treatment	Foot Volumetric Measurement	Baseline Value	Best Result	5-Year Result
Compression sclerotherapy	EV	10.0 ± 0.5	13.2 ± 0.9*	10.0 ± 0.7ns
	Q/EV_{rel}	5.1 ± 0.4	4.2 ± 0.3†	5.3 ± 0.7ns
		(n = 78)	(n = 58)	(n = 39)
Combined ligation and compression sclerotherapy	EV	9.5 ± 0.7	13.3 ± 0.9*	10.7 ± 0.7ns
	Q/EV_{rel}	4.8 ± 0.4	3.5 ± 0.2*	4.6 ± 0.4ns
		(n = 63)	(n = 60)	(n = 47)
Radical surgery	EV	10.4 ± 0.6	14.9 ± 0.8*	14.0 ± 0.8*
	Q/EV_{rel}	4.4 ± 0.3	2.3 ± 0.2*	3.2 ± 0.3‡
		(n = 74)	(n = 57)	(n = 57)

EV, Ejection volume (ml); Q/EV_{rel}, refilling flow ratio (1/min).
*$p < 0.05$.
†$p < 0.01$.
‡$p < 0.001$.
NOTE: Mean ± SEM; *ns*, not significant.

Foot volumetric results are shown in Table 10-1 and Figure 10-7. Throughout the study period of 5 years, the radical surgery group showed significantly greater functional improvement than did the sclerotherapy group (i.e., higher expelled volume and lower refilling flow). At 5 years, foot volumetric results had returned to pretreatment levels in the injected limbs, despite the fact that failures, which involved additional treatment, were not included. This study firmly supports previous reports in concluding that compression sclerotherapy cannot replace radical surgery for varicose vein disease that involves saphenous vein incompetence.

COMBINED SCLEROTHERAPY AND LIGATION OF LONG SAPHENOUS VEIN

The concept of combining ligation of the long saphenous vein with distal sclerotherapy had been discussed by the turn of the century, but it was popularized in the 1930s by de Takats and Quillin.[36] However, the early sclerotherapy technique differed from present methods. At the time of high ligation, sclerosant was injected distally in the vein without compression. Lofgren[37] reported poor results in 60% of patients assessed objectively after 5 years. Sladen[38] found that patients with main-stem insufficiency prior to treatment with injection sclerotherapy alone invariably developed saphenous vein incompetence 2 to 3 years later. If sclerotherapy was combined with ligation of the main stem, there were few recurrences.

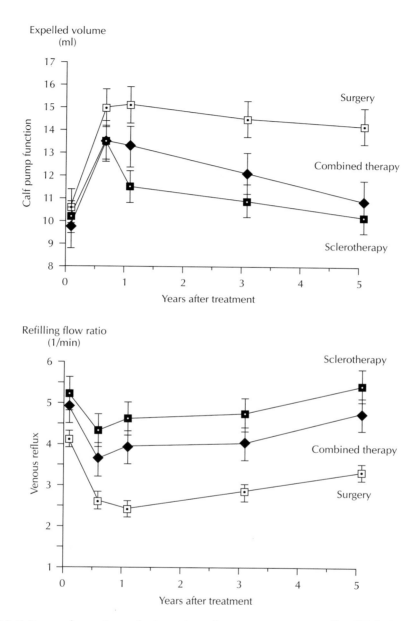

FIGURE 10-7. Foot volumetric results in patients from two separate studies. With the exception at 6 months, expelled volume was significantly higher following surgery compared to combined treatment or sclerotherapy alone. Refilling flow ratio was significantly lower for surgically treated patients throughout the observation period. (Data from Einarsson E. Compression sclerotherapy of varicose veins. In Eklöf B, Gjöres JE, Thulesius O, Bergqvist D, eds. Controversies in the Management of Venous Disorders. London: Butterworth, 1989, pp 203-211; Neglén P, Einarsson E, Eklöf B. High tie with sclerotherapy for saphenous vein insufficiency. Phlebologie 1:105-111, 1986.)

Jakobsen[31] not only randomized patients with main-stem vein insufficiency for surgery or compression sclerotherapy alone but also had a third group of 165 patients who received combined treatment. With the patient under local anesthesia, he performed flush ligation of the long saphenous vein or the short saphenous vein and ligation of incompetent perforators. This procedure was followed by injection sclerotherapy done with Sigg's technique. Jakobsen found that after 3 years 65% of patients had a satisfactory result. Although this finding was significantly better than the results following sclerotherapy alone (37%), it did not attain the level of that following surgery (90%) (see Figure 10-4).

Our group studied 63 lower limbs in 60 patients with long saphenous varicose vein incompetence.[39] Half of these patients had varicosities in the thigh. Injection treatment was performed as described by Hobbs, and the whole lower limb was firmly bandaged. After all tributaries were divided, flush ligation was performed at the saphenofemoral junction with the patient under local anesthesia. As in the previously described randomized study, patients were followed up for 5 years and assessed clinically and functionally by foot volumetry at regular intervals.

Although the initial results were good, a steady deterioration occurred throughout the study period, with only 16% of patients cured after 5 years. All limbs with treatment failure had recurrent insufficiency of the saphenous vein despite a properly performed high tie. Among the improved patients, almost half had a patent palpable (although not obviously insufficient) long saphenous vein. When the results for limbs with only minor local recurrent varicosities were combined with those of the cured legs, 67% were noted as satisfactory after 3 years and 40% after 5 years (Figure 10-8). Although combined therapy produced better results than sclerotherapy alone, the results were not comparable to those of radical surgery and appeared to deteriorate rapidly with time (see Figure 10-6).

Through foot volumetry measurements, the function of calf muscle was demonstrated to be improved with a decrease in venous reflux (see Figure 10-7). After 3 years venous reflux decreased considerably, and after 5 years the values had returned to pretreatment levels (see Table 10-1). Although the average best physiologic value in each group is similar, the deterioration in patients having sclerotherapy and those having the combined treatment is striking after 5 years. Recanalization of the main stem seems to precede complete treatment failure.

The aim of sclerotherapy is to produce an inflammation of the vein wall, which obliterates the lumen and eventually results in a fibrosed cord. Pressing the vein walls together is thought to facilitate this development. Swelling of the vein caused by induced inflammation may create the same situation. However, the thigh portion of the long saphenous vein may be more difficult to sclerose because it has a large diameter with a higher flow rate; it is more difficult to compress effectively during and after injection. If the injection of sclerosant results in intraluminal red thrombus alone, recanalization will commonly occur later and the vein will become incompetent. With reopening of the saphenous vein, a situation similar to that described for flush ligation of the saphenofemoral confluence alone may occur. Reflux may recur through thigh perforators or newly formed collater-

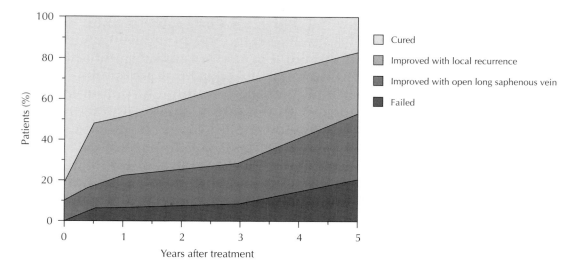

FIGURE 10-8. Results of combined high ligation and sclerotherapy in patients with varicose veins and long saphenous vein incompetence. After 3 years the number of recanalized long saphenous veins increased significantly and appeared to precede complete failure. (Modified from Neglén P, Einarsson E, Eklöf B. High tie with sclerotherapy for saphenous vein insufficiency. Phlebologie 1: 105-111, 1986.)

als between the saphenous stump and the remaining vein, and varicosities may return.

Both clinical and functional results after combined treatment indicate that it is a better method for patients with varicose veins and long saphenous vein incompetence compared to compression sclerotherapy alone. However, combined therapy does not appear to be as efficient as radical surgery, and results indicate that with longer follow-up further deterioration may occur with combined therapy. Combined therapy should be the treatment of choice for patients who are unwilling to undergo complete surgery and for those who are old, unfit, or in whom general or epidural anesthesia is contraindicated.

SELECTIVE TREATMENT FOR MAIN-STEM INSUFFICIENCY

Despite the availability of sclerotherapy and surgery for decades, the controversy regarding which patient to treat with a particular method still exists. The results of long-term prospective randomized studies strongly suggest that compression sclerotherapy as practiced during the 1970s and the early 1980s is a poor treatment for varicose veins involving short saphenous vein or long saphenous vein incompetence. On the other hand, sclerotherapy is the ideal treatment for patients with isolated primary varicosities and residual or recurrent varicosities following adequate main-stem surgery. Its role in the treatment of perforator insufficiency has not been clarified.

In recent years new methods for injecting the long saphenous vein and its junction with the femoral vein have been described.[40] Directed injection done under the guidance of ultrasound, modified compression bandaging, and new sclerosants may have greater efficacy in closing saphenous veins permanently. However, long-term randomized studies that include these recent developments have not been published. Until such studies appear, surgery remains the treatment of choice for main-stem insufficiency.

New diagnostic techniques also will influence surgical technique. Not every patient with varicose veins of saphenous origin needs a complete ankle-groin stripping of the saphenous vein. Segmental incompetence can be identified by Doppler ultrasound or duplex scanning, and insufficiency of the superficial venous system can be mapped. Therefore surgery can be directed toward ligation of main-stem confluences involving reflux, thereby limiting the stripping of the trunk to incompetent segments. With more emphasis on atraumatic technique and minimal incisions, cosmetic results are excellent even after radical surgery.

As the end of the century approaches, it is possible to look back on the various trials that compared alternative methods of treating varicosities surgically. The consensus of opinion favors saphenous stripping from groin to knee if axial reflux is present and detected preoperatively.

In a report from the Scripps Clinic in La Jolla, California, postoperative duplex studies were performed in 66 limbs of 54 patients who had undergone saphenofemoral ligation and subsequent sclerotherapy. Only one limb showed a persistence of saphenofemoral reflux. In the 59 limbs with a residual saphenous vein available for examination, the above-knee greater saphenous vein was patent in 56 (95%); of these, 52 (88%) showed incompetence. The below-knee greater saphenous vein was patent in 53 limbs (90%), of which 52 (88%) were incompetent.[41] Since persistent incompetence of the greater saphenous vein is associated with recurrent varices, it is clear that saphenofemoral junction ligation and subsequent sclerotherapy was inadequate treatment in this group of patients.

In a randomized trial of stripping versus high ligation combined with sclerotherapy in The Netherlands, clinical and Doppler ultrasound evidence of reverse flow in the saphenous vein was significantly less after the stripping procedure.[42] The authors concluded that the results of treatment of isolated saphenous vein insufficiency by stripping therefore was superior to results obtained by high ligation combined with sclerotherapy.

A dissenting vote is cast by the group from Cardiff.[43] They have emphasized that the greater saphenous vein itself is frequently not varicose and that it is the thin-wall tributaries that should be removed by careful stab avulsion. They term these multiple cosmetic stabs phlebectomies. They make a plea for accurate preoperative duplex ultrasonography and emphasize that selective stripping limited to affected greater saphenous vein segments should be done. Although these authors are firm that residual saphenous vein can be used for arterial bypass, they do admit that there is residual local reflux in segments of the greater saphenous vein that they stress is without symptoms or cosmetic abnormality. Most other authors think that residual saphenous vein reflux results in recurrent varicose veins.

CONCLUSION

It appears that stripping to the knee can be performed with few late recurrences in the majority of patients and without involvement of distal portions of the saphenous vein. The chronicity of varicose vein disease and the frequent presence of direct deep-to-superficial perforating veins in the thigh have been thoroughly discussed here. Leaving the thigh portion of a long saphenous vein, even though it is competent, may invite long-term recurrences. However, it is desirable to save the long saphenous vein for future use as a vascular graft. Therefore competent portions of saphenous trunks may be saved. There is no proven value in preservation of incompetent dilated saphenous trunks. The aim of varicose vein surgery still should be the removal of diseased incompetent vein segments and the control of reflux.

REFERENCES

1. Homans J. Operative treatment of varicose veins and ulcers. Surg Gynecol Obstet 22:143-158, 1916.
2. Mayo CH. Treatment of varicose veins. Surg Gynecol Obstet 2:385-388, 1906.
3. Babcock WW. A new operation for the extirpation of varicose veins of the leg. N Y Med J 86:153, 1907.
4. Myers TT, Cooley JC. Varicose vein surgery in the management of the post-phlebitic limb. Surg Gynecol Obstet 99:733-744, 1954.
5. Lofgren KA. Management of varicose veins: Mayo Clinic experience. In Bergan JJ, Yao JST, eds. Venous Problems. Chicago: Year Book, 1978.
6. Rivlin S. The surgical cure of primary varicose veins. Br J Surg 62:913-917, 1975.
7. Cox SJ, Wellwood JM, Martin A. Saphenous nerve injury caused by stripping of the long saphenous vein. Br Med J 1:415-417, 1974.
8. Jakobsen BH, Wallin L. Proximal or distal extraction of the internal saphenous vein? Vasa 4: 240-242, 1975.
9. Holme JB, Skajaa K, Holme K. Incidence of lesions of the saphenous nerve after partial or complete stripping of the long saphenous vein. Acta Chir Scand 156:145-148, 1990.
10. Negus D. Should the incompetent saphenous vein be stripped to the ankle? Phlebologie 1:33-36, 1986.
11. Greason KL, Murray JD. Outpatient management of superficial venous insufficiency at a Naval Medical facility. Ann Vasc Surg 10:524-529, 1996.
12. Munn SR, Morton JB, Macbeth WA, McLeish AR. To strip or not to strip the long saphenous vein? A varicose vein trial. Br J Surg 68:426-428, 1981.
13. Sutton R, Drake SG. Stripping the long saphenous vein: Preoperative retrograde saphenography in patients with and without venous ulceration. Br J Surg 73:305-307, 1986.
14. Papadakis K, Christodoulou C, Christopoulos D, Hobbs J, Malouf GM, Grigg M, Irvine A, Nicolaides A. Number and anatomical distribution of incompetent thigh perforating veins. Br J Surg 76:581-584, 1989.
15. Lofgren EP, Lofgren KA. Recurrence of varicose veins after the stripping operation. Arch Surg 102:111-114, 1971.
16. Rutherford RB, Sawyer JD, Jones DN. The fate of residual saphenous vein after partial removal or ligation. J Vasc Surg 12:422-428, 1990.
17. Sheppard M. A procedure for the prevention of recurrent saphenofemoral incompetence. Aust N Z J Surg 48:322-326, 1978.
18. Corbett CR, Runcie IJ, Thomas ML, Jamieson CW. Reasons to strip the long saphenous vein. Phlebologie 41:766-769, 1988.

19. McMullin GM, Coleridge Smith PD, Scurr JH. Objective assessment of high ligation without stripping of the long saphenous vein. Br J Surg 78:1139-1142, 1991.

20. Large J. Surgical treatment of saphenous varices, with preservation of the main great saphenous trunk. J Vasc Surg 2:886-891, 1985.

21. Hammarsten J, Pedersen P, Cederlund CG, Campanello M. Long saphenous vein–saving surgery for varicose veins. A long-term follow-up. Eur J Vasc Surg 4:361-364, 1990.

22. Koyano K, Sakaguchi S. Selective stripping operation based on Doppler ultrasonic findings for primary varicose veins of the lower extremities. Surgery 103:615-619, 1988.

23. Fegan G. Varicose veins. Compression sclerotherapy. London: Heineman Medical, 1967.

24. Neglén P, Jönsson B, Einarsson E, Eklöf B. Socio-economic benefits of ambulatory surgery and compression sclerotherapy for varicose veins. Phlebologie 1:225-230, 1986.

25. Larsson RH, Lofgren E, Myers TT, Lofgren KA. Long-term results after vein surgery: Study of 1000 cases after 10 years. Mayo Clin Proc 49:114-117, 1974.

26. Reid RG, Rothnie NG. Treatment of varicose veins by compression sclerotherapy. Br J Surg 55:889-895, 1968.

27. Dejode LR. Injection compression treatment for varicose veins. Br J Surg 57:285-286, 1970.

28. Chant ADB, Jones HO, Weddell JM. Varicose veins: A comparison of surgery and injection/compression sclerotherapy. Lancet 2:1188-1191, 1972.

29. Beresford SAA, Chant ADB, Jones HO, Piachaud D, Weddell JM. Varicose veins: A comparison of surgery and injection/sclerotherapy. Five-year follow-up. Lancet 1:921-924, 1978.

30. Doran FSA, White M. A clinical trial designed to discover if the primary treatment of varicose veins should be Fegan's method or by an operation. Br J Surg 62:72-76, 1975.

31. Jakobsen B. The value of different forms of treatment for varicose veins. Br J Surg 66:182-184, 1979.

32. Sigg K. Treatment of varicosities and accompanying complications (ambulatory treatment of phlebitis with compression bandage). Angiology 3:355-379, 1952.

33. Hobbs JT. Surgery and sclerotherapy in the treatment of varicose veins. Arch Surg 109:793-796, 1974.

34. Hobbs JT. Surgery or sclerotherapy for varicose veins; 10-year results of a random study. In Tesi M, Dormandy J, eds. Superficial and Deep Venous Diseases of the Lower Limbs. Turin: Edizione Minerva Medica, 1984, pp 243-246.

35. Einarsson E. Compression sclerotherapy of varicose veins. In Eklöf B, Gjöres JE, Thulesius O, Bergqvist D, eds. Controversies in the Management of Venous Disorders. London: Butterworth, 1989, pp 203-211.

36. de Takats G, Quillin L. Ligation of the saphenous vein. A report on two hundred ambulatory operations. Arch Surg 26:72-88, 1933.

37. Lofgren KA. Management of varicose veins: Mayo Clinic experience. In Bergan JJ, Yao JS, eds. Venous Problems. Chicago: Year Book, 1978, pp 71-83.

38. Sladen JG. Flush ligation and compression sclerotherapy for the control of venous disease. Am J Surg 152:535-538, 1986.

39. Neglén P, Einarsson E, Eklöf B. High tie with sclerotherapy for saphenous vein insufficiency. Phlebologie 1:105-111, 1986.

40. Raymond-Martimbeau P. Two different techniques for sclerosing the incompetent saphenofemoral junction: A comparative study. J Dermatol Surg Oncol 16:626-631, 1990.

41. Fitridge RA, Fronek HS, Dilley RB, Bernstein EF, Benveniste GI. Assessment of reflux in the greater saphenous vein (GSV) two years following high ligation. Cardiovasc Surg 3:71, 1995.

42. Rutgers PH, Kistlaar PJEHM. Randomized trial of stripping versus high ligation combined with sclerotherapy in the treatment of the incompetent greater saphenous vein. Am J Surg 168:311-315, 1994.

43. Fligelstone LJ, Salaman RA, Oshodi TO, Wright I, Pugh N, Shandall AA, Lane IF. Flush saphenofemoral ligation and multiple stab phlebectomy preserve a useful greater saphenous vein four years after surgery. J Vasc Surg 22:588-592, 1995.

Chapter 11

Treatment of Varicosities of Saphenous Origin: A Dialogue

Ralph G. DePalma, Sidney S. Rose, and John J. Bergan

Whenever a surgical condition is common, a plethora of operations is applied. Contrary opinions abound, and no single method becomes standard. Yet our constant objective is to improve surgery so that results are optimized, complications are minimized, and patient satisfaction is maximized. To achieve these goals, we have established the following dialogue among experienced vascular surgeons who bring a variety of background experiences and observations to one focal point, surgery of varicose veins.

Dr. Bergan: In practice, four goals must be kept in mind when planning the treatment of varicose veins.[1] Although the treatment needs to be individualized, the following objectives remain: (1) permanent removal of the varicosities, (2) determination and ablation of the source of venous hypertension, (3) achievement of the best cosmetic result possible, and (4) minimization of complications. Mr. Rose, what is your opinion about the indications for surgery?

Mr. Rose: First, not all patients with varicose veins require treatment. Many are asymptomatic and remain so for most of their lives.[2] On the other hand, it must be noted that aching pain from varicose veins can vary from mild to severe, any pain of skeletal or arterial origin must be eliminated in the differential diagnosis, and many patients, especially women, complain of varicosities for purely cosmetic reasons. Male patients may have surprisingly little pain from the veins and may encounter severe discomfort only when superficial ulceration occurs. In regard to female patients, in Chapter 2 of this book, I have described the hormonal relationship of varicose vein pain during pregnancy and menstrual cycles.

Dr. DePalma: I would agree. In my practice, about five times as many women as men present with primary varicose veins in the saphenous system distribution. Characteristically, symptoms of aching and fullness worsen during the day, particularly after periods of standing and activity. Recumbency and leg elevation relieve these symptoms and help to differentiate them from musculoskeletal and arterial causes. The severity of complaints of aching, fullness, pain, easy fatigability, and tiredness do not necessarily relate to the gross appearance of the varicosities. This situation is especially relevant to men who have gross, protuberant saccular varicosities but no symptoms. In women, the symptoms are clearly related to the progesterone phase of the menstrual cycle and appear maximally during the first or second day of a menstrual period, paradoxically when the predominant progesterone hormone level decreases and the estrogen level increases.

Prominence or protuberance of the varicosities appears to depend more on subcutaneous tissue thickness and venectasia rather than on the hemodynamic or physiologic effect from the varices.

Although women often seek consultation for the cosmetic appearance of tortuous varicosities related to the saphenous system or for microvarices or telangiectasias, in fact, these abnormalities also may be the source of symptoms. The telangiectasias especially can cause a burning or bursting discomfort and frequently, but not always, are associated with truncal or saphenous vein branch varicosities. The authors of Chapter 23 have described the symptom complex associated with telangiectasias, and they have pointed out the similarities of their pathophysiologic origin to gross varicosities and truncal or perforating venous reflux.

Dr. Bergan: It is clear that we agree that symptoms of aching pain, easy fatigability, tiredness, and even the appearance of gross, protuberant saccular varicosities are indications for surgical intervention. Are there other indications for surgery?

Dr. DePalma: Superficial thrombophlebitis of varices or of the saphenous trunk is another indication for surgery. Surgery may be required in the acute situation in which thrombophlebitis of the saphenous vein may propagate upward and encroach on the saphenofemoral junction. Furthermore, a cluster of varicosities may remain acutely inflamed for a long time, even with good conservative care. In such a situation, I recommend surgical intervention. When surgery is necessary, I use perioperative anticoagulant therapy with heparin and always examine the patient with the color-flow duplex scanner to investigate the deep venous system. When deep venous thrombosis is not present, I would proceed with saphenous vein ligation and retrograde stripping to remove the foci of inflamed varicose clusters.

Mr. Rose: To this I must add that a history of external bleeding or sudden hemorrhage from a dilated vein in a site vulnerable to trauma, such as the shin, ankle, or dorsum of the foot, is often an urgent indication for intervention.

I must emphasize that women who complain of varicosities for purely cosmetic reasons should be considered seriously. They regard their varicose veins as unacceptable disfigurements, and their complaint is as distressing to them as any painful affliction and it is often less well tolerated. When fashion decrees that skirts be shorter, such patients rush to the physician's door. I think that these patients are equally entitled to our attention and that no surgeon should turn them away, providing that he or she can assure them of a good cosmetic result.

With regard to external bleeding, this occurrence results from intracutaneous blue blebs and often appears in the aged patient. I believe that the varix hemorrhage is caused by venous hypertension. This hypertension is produced by steep increases in pressure caused by muscular contractions transmitted through failed perforating vein valves. Such external bleeding can be fatal, as has been reported. Treatment should be given by external pressure and not by cutaneous suture because cutaneous suture leads to venous ulceration in this situation.[3] Dr. DePalma, tell us about your preoperative evaluation of the patient.

Dr. DePalma: We have discussed the patient's history, which will elucidate the indications for surgical intervention for varicose veins or sclerotherapy for telangiectasias. In addition, the comprehensive consultation must include inquiry about possible risk factors for arterial disease, which might later require the saphenous vein to be used in peripheral or coronary artery revascularization. The intensity and duration of each of the risk factors that predispose the patient to atherosclerosis should be recorded. These factors include a history of cigarette smoking with an estimate of pack-years. Inquiry should be made into familial predispositions, such as hypercholesterolemia, diabetes, and hypertension. It is also important to record any familial pattern of varicose veins and to note whether deep venous thrombosis has occurred in the patient or his or her siblings. In addition, investigations into coagulopathy, including evaluation of protein C, protein S, antithrombin III, anticardiolipin antibodies, and lupus anticoagulant, should be done. Examination of the arterial system should be performed, with ankle-to-arm pressure indices recorded and peripheral pulses palpated. The saphenous vein should not be routinely removed in patients who have major risk factors for arterial occlusive disease (except when severely varicose), such as a male with an excess of 20 pack-years of smoking history in conjunction with another risk factor.

Mr. Rose: What Dr. DePalma has described is a complete evaluation of the patient. Such an evaluation is certainly necessary in every case involving a history of phlebitis, especially the recurrent type, and any situation in which arteriosclerotic disease is a risk factor. Of course, this type of evaluation is essential if basic research is being undertaken. Many clinics, however, are not equipped for such evaluations and are not research oriented. In addition, it must be recognized that many cases do not require this type of full investigation. It is a matter of clinical experience to separate those that do deserve such attention from those that do not. Initially, we rely heavily on the physical examination in evaluating patients for surgical intervention. After the patient has been standing for 10 minutes, the varicose vein pattern is carefully charted. The extent of varicosities is estimated by palpation, propagation of the cough impulse, and examination with the continuous-wave, hand-held Doppler instrument. The Doppler device establishes connection with the greater saphenous vein, and the short saphenous system should be examined similarly with the knee slightly flexed to relax the deep fascia. The patient undergoes a full abdominal examination, after which the peripheral pulses are palpated. The presence of sciatic pain is eliminated through the straight leg–raising test, and the condition of the ankle, knee, and hip are estimated through flexion, abduction, and external rotation. All these findings are duly recorded.

Dr. Bergan: Dr. DePalma, would you tell us about your preoperative testing routine?

Dr. DePalma: Rational treatment of saphenous varicosities requires delineation of points of reflux from the deep venous system as well as delineation of specific areas of truncal incompetence.[4] The patient is examined while standing, and the examiner is seated.

Palpation should include inspection; use of the tap, cough, and thrill tests; and insonation of the saphenofemoral and popliteal regions and the major trunks with use of a hand-held continuous-wave Doppler pencil probe (Figure 11-1). While the patient is standing, careful inspection is done to detect major perforating vein reflux. The most common area of deep-to-superficial connection is the anteromedial aspect of the upper calf in the region of the Boyd perforating vein. The next most common important perforating vein connection is located in the

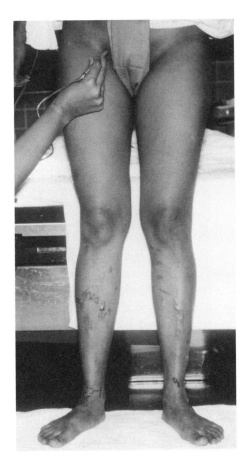

FIGURE 11-1. This photograph shows Doppler venous examination as part of preoperative evaluation of this 28-year-old woman with symptomatic below-knee varicosities, which are easily seen. The patient demonstrated severe truncal reflux on Doppler evaluation, and it was later confirmed through duplex scanning. Note the absence of visible thigh varices despite greater saphenous reflux found bilaterally.

midthigh in the region of Hunter's canal.[5,6] The third most common and important perforating vein is the one named for Dodd, which is located in the distal third of the thigh.[6] It should be noted that the Boyd perforating vein may be the first to give rise to primary varicosities in the anterior tributary group or the posterior tributary group or in both. Furthermore, this vein may be connected to the greater saphenous system, the lesser saphenous system, or even the popliteal vein. Appropriate superficial-to-deep disconnection will be required.

Dr. Bergan: What about the classic tourniquet tests that are taught in surgical services and medical schools?

Dr. DePalma: The classic tourniquet tests have been taught and are currently receiving attention. However, in my experience, I have found the tourniquet tests to be disappointing. Figure 11-2 illustrates some of the problems encountered with tourniquet application.

Dr. Bergan: What about use of the color-flow duplex scanner?

Dr. DePalma: After the results of physical examination and Doppler study have been recorded on the patient's chart, duplex scans are routinely obtained in our surgical service. We have completed a study in which we prospectively evaluated 80 limbs in 40 symptomatic patients prior to treatment of primary saphenous varicosities. We compared sensitivity, specificity, positive and negative predictive values of physical examination, and Doppler insonation with color-flow duplex scanning. When color-flow duplex scanning was used as a standard, physical examination had a sensitivity of only 48%. Its specificity was 73%, and there

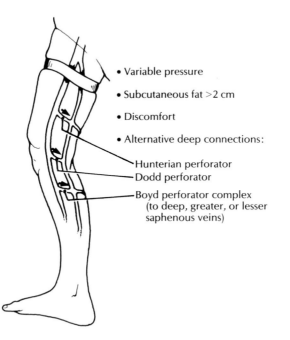

- Variable pressure
- Subcutaneous fat >2 cm
- Discomfort
- Alternative deep connections:
  - Hunterian perforator
  - Dodd perforator
  - Boyd perforator complex
    (to deep, greater, or lesser
    saphenous veins)

FIGURE 11-2. Limitations of tourniquet application are shown here. Duplex reflux evaluation has replaced tourniquet testing in the care of varicose veins at most institutions.

was a positive predictive value of 75% and a negative predictive value of 46%. The addition of Doppler insonation improved specificity and positive predictive values. Its sensitivity was 48%; specificity, 83%; and positive predictive value, 83%. The negative predictive value remained 49%.

As a result of this study, and with further experience, I recommend that a color-flow duplex scan be done prior to surgical intervention for varicose veins involving the saphenous system.[7] The color-flow scanning is particularly effective at the saphenofemoral junction. I have not yet recommended or practiced selective ligation at the saphenofemoral junction.[8,9] With major or gross saphenous reflux, I think that surgical intervention and removal of the saphenous trunk are needed. Others have practiced proximal ligation and distal sclerotherapy with success, but that approach is not our practice.[10,11]

Duplex scanning is particularly useful in patients with prior operations; in fact, it is invaluable. We have discovered retained lateral or medial saphenous trunks and missed groin communicating veins in 14 of 18 limbs in which groin scars existed and symptoms of primary varicosities continued.[12] Of equal importance is the fact that when saphenofemoral incompetence is not present the main saphenous trunk can be spared.[13] Surgery then will consist of selective ligation and removal of specific branches and deep disconnections.[14]

Mr. Rose: I would support what Dr. DePalma says about duplex scanning. It is the most valuable noninvasive technique for venous and arterial investigation thus far developed. However, although most major clinics have this equipment, it is not yet universally available, and many clinics will need to rely on the older methods of assessment. However, as Dr. DePalma has said, when our experience with duplex scanning offers us more information about the pros and cons of selective groin ligation, surgery then may consist of selective ligation and removal of specific branches and deep disconnections.

Dr. Bergan: In summary, the hand-held Doppler probe used as a screening test in patients with primary varicose veins has proven to be very useful. When the results of its use are compared to standard physical findings, it has been found that axial reflux in the greater saphenous vein is detected in 91% of cases. Missed cases are those with a competent saphenofemoral junction or very low–velocity reflux. Similar findings are also true in the popliteal fossa.[15] The duplex examination has proven to be invaluable where it has been applied.[16] Because of the 10% inaccuracies of the hand-held Doppler probe, the vascular group at the Sheffield Vascular Institute compared clinical examination to Doppler insonation and duplex scanning and found that ". . . cogent arguments can be made for the routine use of color duplex scanning in the preoperative assessment of varicose veins in order to reduce the possibility of recurrence. However, the resources required to implement this are not insignificant." Mr. Rose, when should operations for lower extremity varicosities *not* be done?

Mr. Rose: Patients with varicose veins should not be operated on during pregnancy, in very old age, or when peripheral arterial occlusive disease is present. Furthermore, if a patient has any contraindication to general anesthesia, a history of bleeding diathesis, or active skin infection in the limb, the operation should not be done until the condition is investigated or rectified. When varices are present in a limb with lymphedema, surgery should not be performed. Also, surgery should not be done when venous claudication is present; instead, extensive investigation should be undertaken.

Dr. DePalma: Actually, effective symptomatic treatment can be achieved through the use of prescription lightweight support pantyhose or below-knee support hosiery. It is important that these aids be obtained from a supplier who can be relied on for accuracy in specific fitting and will make adjustments to correct a poor "fit." Prescription of elastic support hosiery with less than 20 mm Hg pressure usually will suffice. Higher pressures must be prescribed if lipodermatosclerosis or dermatitis complicates primary saphenous varicosities. In patients who are not surgical candidates because of their age or medical condition, or for those who wish to delay therapy for any reason, the consistent use of elastic support hosiery can be quite satisfactory.

Sclerotherapy is an alternative to surgery or compression therapy. I use sclerotherapy for treatment of veins that do not communicate directly with the main trunks and for those that are less than 3 to 4 mm in diameter. In fact, I use sclerotherapy during surgery to identify small varices and telangiectasias. At the time of surgery, I introduce 11.7% or 23.4% saline solution while the patient is anesthetized.

Mr. Rose: We use the same criteria that Dr. DePalma does for sclerotherapy, but we tend not to use it perioperatively. The small varicosities and telangiectasias are not as easy to identify during surgery, and I worry that the sclerosant will leak into the tiny incised areas and cause an intradermal inflammatory response. It is probably true, however, that the use of hypertonic saline is less likely to cause any harm under these circumstances than is the detergent class of sclerosing agents. With regard to surgical technique, it is important to recognize that the only practical way of eradicating varicose veins is by meticulous and radical removal of all the varicosities with, if necessary, the addition of ligation at the saphenofemoral and saphenopopliteal junction and/or localized stripping of the main saphenous veins.[17] The operation can be performed as an outpatient procedure, a day-stay case, or an inpatient procedure with an overnight stay. A two-night stay is rarely necessary. Prior to surgery, the patient is examined while standing and the veins are marked very carefully. Particular attention must be paid to any localized painful areas or varicosities that cause special discomfort since these are the focal points of the patient's complaint and must not be missed.

Dr. Bergan: I think that there are two principles that should be used as a guide to successful varicose vein surgery. The first is ablation of reflux from the deep to the superficial venous system. The second is removal or destruction of all varicosities existing at the time of surgical intervention.[18] Ablation of reflux from the deep system should be done at the points indicated by Dr. DePalma. Detection of such reflux is obtained by physical examination and inspection and by use of the Doppler instrument; its presence is verified with the duplex scanner.[19] When gross saphenous reflux is present, the saphenous vein should be removed to encompass the perforating veins of Hunter, Dodd, and Boyd. Simple proximal ligation without segmental stripping has proven to be unsatisfactory.[20-22] Adherence to the second principle of varicose vein surgery allows correction of any errors made in preoperative detection of deep to superficial reflux; that is, if all varicose veins and varicose clusters are excised, the end organs of perforator reflux are removed. Thus missed identification of perforating veins is corrected by thorough removal of all varicosities.

Mr. Rose: To follow what Dr. Bergan was saying, if the principle of meticulous removal of isolated clusters is adhered to, the time-consuming search for elusive perforators is eliminated and a satisfactory operation can be carried out, even when a duplex scanner is not available.

The important points to observe in the groin dissection are as follows. The femoral pulse is palpated so that the position of the saphenous vein opening medial to that pulse is identified. The incision should be long enough to gain good access to the saphenous vein opening; the length will vary somewhat, depending on the obesity of the patient and the experience of the surgeon.

Dr. Bergan: All incisions must be carefully placed in the exact skin lines of the individual patient.[23,24] The most common error in saphenous vein surgery is placement of the upper incision too far distally. In the past it was taught that the incision should be placed distal to the groin crease, but that method is distinctly erroneous. At present, advocacy of placement of the incision in the groin crease also seems to be erroneous. In general, the transverse incision should be placed 1 to 2 cm proximal to the oblique groin crease (Figure 11-3). The incision should extend medially from the palpable femoral pulse, and every tributary to the saphenous vein should be sought and divided. Stanley Rivlin[18] has said:

> Attempts have been made to list the variations in so-called normal venous anatomy at the saphenofemoral junction. In fact, there is no normal. The arrangements of the venous tributaries are seemingly infinite and the ways in which they join the long saphenous or femoral vein seem to be decided only by the laws of chance.

Mr. Rose: At first sight it may appear that the anatomic abnormalities occur by chance, but in fact they are merely variations on a basic theme that is described as the normal anatomy. Either a high or a low insertion of the internal saphenous vein in the groin is possible, and accordingly variations occur in the path followed by the main tributaries, which generally enter the main saphenous vein. The anterolateral and posteromedial saphenous veins are similarly displaced according to their site of entry; when either one is enlarged alone, it constitutes an accessory saphenous vein that is sometimes referred to as a twin saphenous vein. Therefore the main patterns actually can be drawn without reference to an anatomy textbook and with a basic knowledge of what to expect. To obtain an adequate exposure of the operative field, I believe that it is best to use the oblique incision parallel to the groin crease. This incision is easy to enlarge to give better access, if necessary, without leaving an ugly scar. At operation, once the saphenofemoral junction has been dissected, with the understanding that it may be located above or below the normal position, the disposition of the tributaries then can be determined easily. The only troublesome variation is when an accessory saphenous vein opens posteromedially. I think that the mystique of the saphenofemoral junction

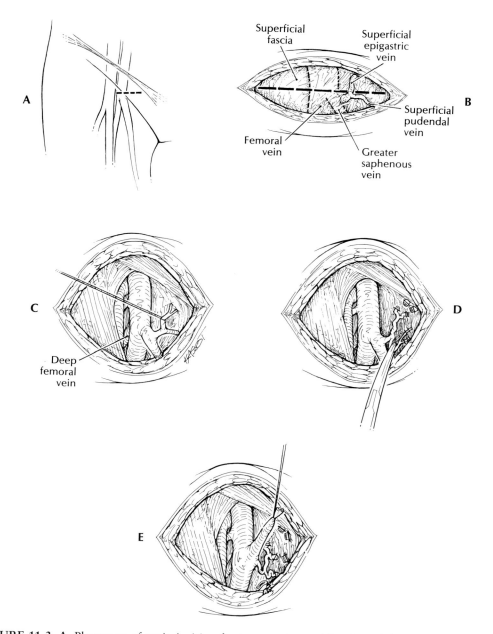

FIGURE 11-3. A, Placement of groin incision for interruption and ligation of the greater saphenous vein is shown. Incision is placed proximal to the inguinal crease in appropriate skin lines, depending on the physiognomy of the particular patient. **B,** With skin and subcutaneous tissues divided, the superficial fascia comes into view. Frequently, medial and superior tributaries to the saphenous vein are seen lying on this fascia. Fascia is incised transversely. **C,** Division of the fascia will expose saphenous vein at its termination with a variable number of tributaries entering the saphenous vein or femoral vein. Complete exposure of 2 cm of femoral vein is necessary to ensure division of all tributaries in this location. **D,** Each tributary to the saphenous vein and femoral vein is pulled into the incision and ligated or clipped; the tributary is divided beyond its bifurcation, as shown here. **E,** Saphenous vein is divided and lifted into view so that suture ligature can be placed carefully, obliterating any cul-de-sac that might form. Suture ligature should not impinge on femoral vein. (From Bergan JJ, Kistner RL. Atlas of Venous Surgery. Philadelphia: WB Saunders, 1992, p 66.)

has been overemphasized. It must be understood that, no matter how variable, the tributaries must not be allowed to escape ligation. Nevertheless, young surgeons should be closely supervised throughout their training course.

Recent experience at Leeds has shown that with accurate identification of sites of reflux preoperatively and with appropriate training by a consultant vascular surgeon, a junior surgical house officer can be instructed to perform varicose vein surgery successfully.[25]

Dr. Bergan: With regard to the surgical technique, one must pay attention to the recent reports of recurrent varicose veins studied by duplex ultrasound. Ruckley's group has provided a clear analysis that guides the performance of primary surgery.[26] One of the primary causes of recurrent varicose veins had to do with a new network of veins forming in the groin. Clearly, that network is caused by the flush ligation of tributary veins at their junction with the saphenous vein, thus leaving the primary and secondary tributaries to interanastomose and form a new network that can reflux distally to form new varicosities.

Therefore, after an appropriate groin incision has been made in the skin lines, the wound edges should be retracted atraumatically and the layers of superficial fascia divided. The saphenous vein lies beneath the superficial fascia, which must be incised. As each of the tributaries comes into view, it should be dissected back beyond its primary and even secondary tributaries so that the tributary vein is actually divided remote from the saphenous vein and not flush with it. In practice, we have found that the tributaries can be drawn into the wound with firm traction. As each tributary appears, it can be coagulated and divided, thus allowing long lengths of tributary veins to be excised. Although this is true of the epigastric and circumflex iliac vein, it is particularly true of the lateral anterior tributary vein, which, when drawn into the wound and with its tributaries electrocoagulated, can be excised for a distance often exceeding 15 cm. The medial posterior tributary vein must also be sought because it is often a very large communicator in direct continuity with the lesser saphenous system. Although that technique may sound somewhat unconventional, in fact, it is most effective in decreasing recurrence.

Finally, if very large tributary veins appear, such as the lateral anterior tributary, they should be divided and cannulated with an endoluminal stripper. Often, either the medial posterior or lateral anterior tributary vein can be stripped from above downward almost to the knee. Variations in the anatomy are common, but all tributaries should be identified and dealt with as described here.

Dr. DePalma: In the groin the main trunk at the saphenofemoral junction is carefully dissected. All collateral branches and the lateral tributary are divided, with care taken to spare lymphatic trunks. A stripper usually can be passed from the groin distally, easily traversing the incompetent valves that have been detected by color-flow Doppler imaging (Figure 11-4). The stripper is recovered through a microincision at a point near the knee. Stripping then is carried out over a period of 5 to 10 minutes. The procedure is done from the groin to the distal microincision with the operating table placed in 15 degrees of foot elevation prior to vein removal. Ultimately, the stripper is recovered through the groin incision by means

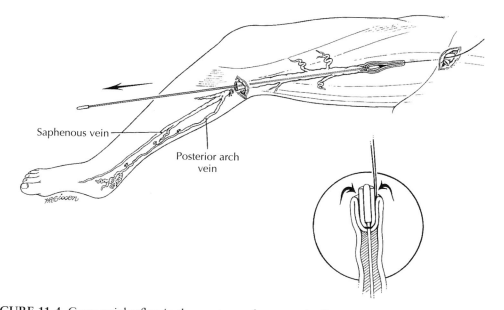

FIGURE 11-4. Gross axial reflux in the greater saphenous vein dictates removal of that vein, at least to the distal thigh or proximal calf. This illustration shows the principles of modern inversion stripping of the greater saphenous vein. The objective is to detach the perforating veins that enter the saphenous vein at the midthigh (hunterian perforators) and the distal thigh (Dodd perforators). The incisions shown here are larger than actual size, but the method is shown clearly: the saphenous vein is tied to the intraluminal stripper so that distal traction will invert the vein into itself and minimize trauma to soft tissues in the thigh. Communicating veins are detached from the saphenous vein so that a network of veins will not be left behind, which could cause recurrent varicosities. Note that stripping the greater saphenous vein from ankle to knee would not detach the perforating veins that enter the posterior arch circulation.

of an attached umbilical tape (Figure 11-5). This adds considerably to the cosmetic efficacy of the procedure.

Mr. Rose: We also strip the vein in a retrograde manner but do not pull the head of the stripper through the lower skin incision. Instead, the stripper is removed by upward traction on a long thread attached to the stripper head. We have developed a stripper with a drilled head that facilitates attachment of a ligature. Pressure is applied along the path of the stripper as it is pulled proximally, and the stripped vein is removed through the groin incision. The method avoids enlarging the lower incision, which would be necessary if one were to pull the stripper head through that opening. We have used this technique for the past 35 years without a single complication.

Dr. Bergan: We also introduce the stripper from above, attach a narrow umbilical tape to the stripper head, and then tie in a length of roller gauze that is 5 to 10 cm in width and use two to four layers of such gauze as a pack (Figure 11-6). The pack follows the stripper head distally and is left in place during the stab avulsion portion of the operation. We remove the saphenous vein through

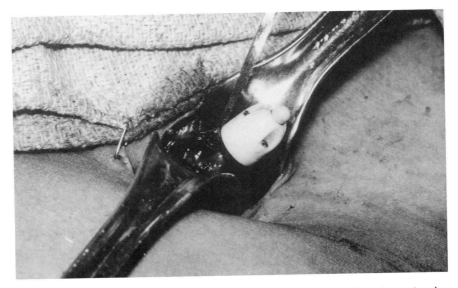

FIGURE 11-5. This photograph illustrates a proximal groin incision with stripper in place within the saphenous vein and umbilical tape tied to the stripper so that the stripper can be retrieved. Umbilical tape may be placed into the groove of the stripper head, where friction will hold it in contact with the plastic stripper.

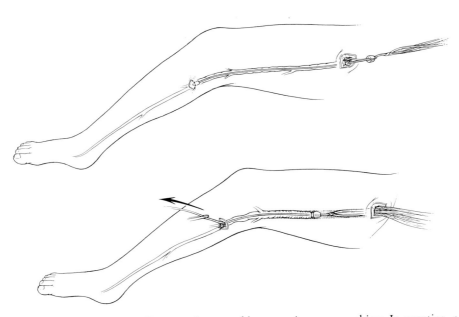

FIGURE 11-6. These drawings illustrate the use of hemostatic gauze packing. In practice, a 2-inch gauze roll soaked in 0.5% lidocaine with added adrenaline 1:1000 is attached by ligature to the intraluminal stripper. As the stripper inverts the saphenous vein, the gauze pack is drawn into the vein so that traction is placed on the gauze pack rather than on the saphenous vein. As the vein is inverted and the gauze pack follows, tearing of the vein is avoided and the gauze pack can be left for hemostasis during the stab avulsion. The end of the pack can be tucked into the deep recesses of the groin wound while the groin wound is closed in layers. This method allows the pack to be left in place a maximum amount of time because it can be removed and the distal incision can be closed just before the pressure dressing is applied. (From Bergan JJ, Kistner RL. Atlas of Venous Surgery. Philadelphia: WB Saunders, 1992, p 67.)

the distal incision to ensure that the distal tributaries are divided. This approach is especially necessary when the stripper exits below the knee in the region of the Boyd perforating vein tributaries.

In order to reduce hematoma formation, we do the entire operation with the patient's feet elevated on a picket fence or rack so that the entire limb is extended in a 30-degree elevated position while the table is kept flat. After all other steps of the procedure have been completed, the entire gauze pack, stripper head, and stripper are removed through the proximal incision.

Dr. DePalma: The groin incision is closed with fine subcuticular chromic catgut, and the extremity incisions used for stab avulsion also are closed with subcuticular absorbable sutures. Steri-Strips are applied to all these incisions.

Mr. Rose: Prior to closure of the groin incision, any hematoma that may have developed is squeezed out of the track of the stripper. We prefer not to use the sucker or gauze pack for this step because it can cause rebleeding. It is important to use manual pressure along the line of the strip, as described earlier. The groin incision is closed with subcuticular continuous 3-0 catgut sutures, and the skin edges are opposed with Steri-Strips. We leave this step to the end of the operation so that all oozing has stopped.

Dr. Bergan: Our own choice is for 3-0 Vicryl absorbable sutures for the superficial fascia and 5-0 Vicryl sutures for the subcuticular closure, but we also apply Steri-Strips.

Dr. DePalma: For stab avulsion, we use small distal skin-line incisions not greater than 2 to 3 mm in length. The underlying varicosities are best elevated by capturing the vein with a skin hook (Figure 11-7). This method permits smaller access than does a crochet hook, which must be inserted beneath the skin. Alternatively, veins can be grasped with hemostats, and a flexible vein grasper can be inserted through microincisions for removal of the remaining varices by avulsion.

Mr. Rose: We believe that the instruments used for multiple avulsion should be kept as simple as possible (Figure 11-8). We agree with Dr. DePalma about the crochet hook. We do not find it necessary to use a skin hook or a flexible vein grasper. We use a miniknife (Beaver 1600-B), mosquito forceps, heavier curved forceps, and toothed dissecting forceps. The multiple tiny incisions are made with the Beaver blade at intervals over the veins so that the maximal length of vein can be removed with the minimum number of incisions. The incisions are 2 to 3 mm but are not always of the stab incision type. They are made with much more care than a stab incision would imply. Stretching the skin in the line of the vein allows the incision to be made more easily and naturally. The incisions are stab type only when sufficient subcutaneous adipose tissue is present to prevent perforation of the vein. Otherwise the dissection is hampered by bleeding. The incisions are made precisely in the skin lines, and they disappear almost completely in time.[27] It is convenient to make the incisions where the veins are most easily palpable and can be grasped more easily. Incisions should not be made over indurated areas because it will be impossible to avulse the vein where indurated and inflamed subcutaneous tissue is present.

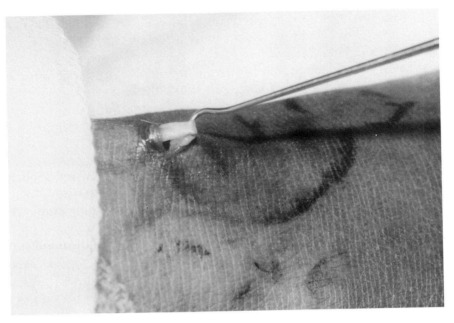

FIGURE 11-7. Use of a skin hook in grasping the anterior surface of the incompetent greater saphenous vein through an oblique microincision at the ankle. Note the complete skeletonization of the saphenous vein so that terminal filaments of saphenous nerve can be eliminated from the trauma of venous stripping.

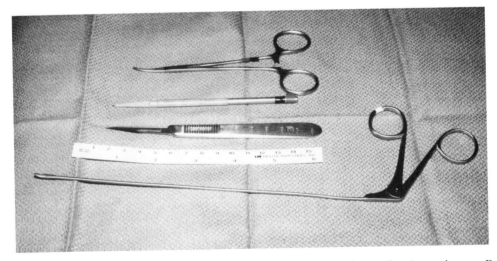

FIGURE 11-8. Instruments used for microincision as well as stab avulsion of varicose clusters. From above to downward, one sees a fine-pointed hemostat used for grasping varices and a Beaver blade used for creating microincisions. Below is a No. 11 Bard-Parker blade used for slightly larger incisions. Below the ruler is a flexible vein grasper made to specifications by the Pilling Corporation (Philadelphia).

The skin incision should penetrate the dermis. The skin edges are separated, the vein is identified, and the vein is picked up by grasping its adventitia (Figure 11-9). The hold on the vein is consolidated, and the vein is drawn through the surface. When the loop of vein emerges from the incision, a forceps can be passed under it so that the loop can be divided. Each end of the vein is now gradually drawn out by means of an alternate traction and twisting motion. A forceps is reapplied closer to the skin as the vein is avulsed. Care is taken not to pull the vein back across the incision because if the skin has lost its elasticity, the incision will become stretched. This caution applies especially to the posterior aspect of the leg. Ultimately, the vein breaks and hemostasis is secured by application of firm pressure, which is continued until the next incision is explored.

The process is repeated down the leg until all offending and previously marked veins have been removed. It has been postulated that any perforating veins will be automatically interrupted. Care must be taken to distinguish between fine cutaneous nerves and small veins. Avulsion of nerve filaments may produce significant hyperesthesia and sudden stabs of pain.

The leg is cleansed after avulsion of all the marked veins has been accomplished, and the wounds are sealed with Steri-Strips. The Steri-Strips must be simply laid in the line of the wound, and the skin edges must not be opposed under tension since this method may produce blistering of the skin. Careful bandaging is done firmly to complete the procedure.

A number of specialized instruments have been advocated by others, but they are not necessary if the technique described here is followed.[28-30]

Dr. DePalma: Although we have been discussing the usual removal of grossly refluxing saphenous vein and clusters of varicosities, there are situations in which specific and unnamed perforating veins must be treated. We have not been satisfied in defining posterior arch tributaries or delineating the detailed anatomy of the infracrural zone with color-flow duplex scanning. Therefore our approach is to expose the perforating vein near the knee and to perform intraoperative varicography with 60% Renografin, which is inserted into the varix through a blunt cannula. Control of infracrural incompetence can involve ligation of a deep direct perforating vein from the popliteal vein, excision and ligation of a contribution from the lesser saphenous vein, or division of a main contribution from an otherwise competent greater saphenous vein. Selective intraoperative venography makes possible the precise application of microincisions and rational ligation and excision for disconnection from the deep venous system in the popliteal area.

Mr. Rose: The short saphenous vein is dealt with according to the same principles as the long saphenous vein, but the dissection of the popliteal fossa is a much more complicated procedure. First, there is great variability in the location of the saphenopopliteal junction. Second, the short saphenous vein is deep to the deep fascia. Third, the gastrocnemius veins may be involved. The proximity of the medial popliteal nerve provides an additional hazard. Therefore the patient is operated on in the prone position so that vascular access is unhindered and the anat-

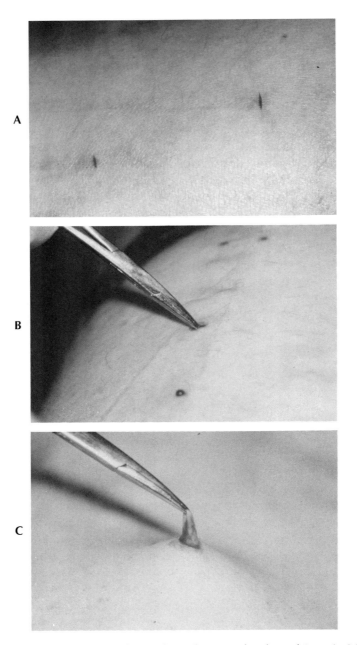

FIGURE 11-9. This operative series shows the technique of stab avulsion. **A,** Microincisions are made with a Beaver blade, with careful attention given to skin lines. **B,** Underlying varicosity can be grasped with a fine-pointed hemostat. **C,** Varix is raised above skin level.

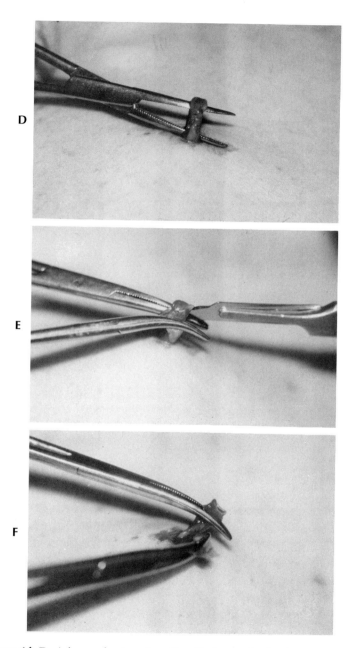

FIGURE 11-9, cont'd. D, A loop of vein, when identified completely, shows a proximal and a distal portion of varix. E, After the varix has been doubly clamped, it is divided sharply, as shown. F, Each end of the divided vein is winkled out of its subcutaneous position.   *Continued.*

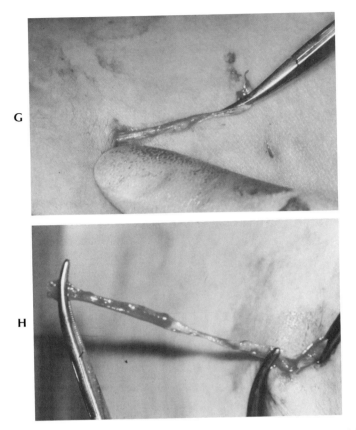

FIGURE 11-9, cont'd. G, Firm traction with a hemostat and countertraction with the finger allow maximum removal of varicosity in a proximal and distal direction. H, Frequently, great lengths of varicosity can be removed, thus minimizing the number of microincisions made in the skin.

omy can be easily visualized (Figure 11-10). The incision is placed where the saphenopopliteal junction has been identified preoperatively or through varicography, and the incision is not compromised by cosmetic considerations.

A natural skin line is identified for placement of the incision, and the incision is deepened through the subcutaneous fascia until the deep fascia is reached. The fascia is then incised (Figure 11-11). When the saphenous vein has been identified, the sural nerve should be sought and carefully protected. Proximal dissection allows identification of the saphenopopliteal junction. Frequently, a tributary that runs upward and medially can be identified. This tributary, which joins the internal saphenous system, is the so-called vein of Giacomini. This vessel is an important conduit for superficial blood flow if the deep connection of the saphenous vein to the popliteal vein is abnormally small. All other tributaries that may be varicose and that arise from the gastrocnemius muscle must be divided. Such tributaries may cause troublesome bleeding if they are not carefully ligated. They should never be avulsed. In surgery of the short saphenous vein, we often find

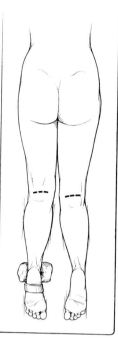

FIGURE 11-10. Surgery to interrupt the lesser saphenous vein in the popliteal space must allow adequate exposure. Such exposure can be achieved as shown here when the operation is done bilaterally. When bilateral operations are planned, the patient should be placed in a prone position on the operating table and exposure should not be compromised.

varicography to be most useful for identifying anatomic abnormalities and determining the extent of involvement of the gastrocnemius and soleal veins.

Proximal ligation is performed as close to the popliteal vein as is feasible with safety. The deep fascia is closed with absorbable sutures. We prefer not to strip the short saphenous vein for two reasons. First, the short saphenous vein is usually not varicose throughout most of its length. Second, damage to the sural nerve is possible. Damage to the sural nerve may occur with incisions lateral to the Achilles tendon and behind the lateral malleolus. Such damage can produce a very persistent sensory change on the outer side of the foot that is occasionally accompanied by distressing paresthesia. In general, operations on the upper end of the short saphenous vein are not recommended for the inexperienced surgeon because of the anatomic variability.

Dr. DePalma: The ideal goals of varicose vein surgery include minimum scarring, precise ablation of all varices, and interruption of points of deep venous connection. These goals are accomplished by using well-planned, minimally invasive incisions. Carefully considered, meticulously accomplished, and anatomically sound surgery will produce physiologically and cosmetically acceptable results in almost all patients. Effective treatment relieves aching discomfort and manifestations of dermatitis. Even after these goals have been accomplished, an intrinsic in-

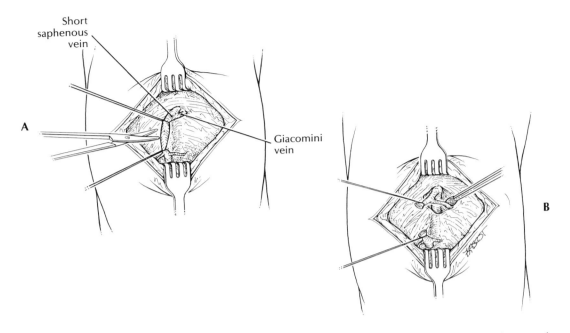

Short
saphenous
vein

Giacomini
vein

A

B

FIGURE 11-11. Short saphenous vein and its termination should be identified by duplex ultrasound or intraoperative varicography. Skin incision placement depends on the location of the termination of the short saphenous vein. Note exposure of tributaries to the short saphenous vein, including the vein of Giacomini (**A**). All these tributaries should be drawn into the wound and divided so that the short saphenous vein can be exposed at its termination in the popliteal vein (**B**). All tributaries should be removed, and a segment of short saphenous vein should be excised.

dividual recurrence rate can be noted, even though precise and comprehensive treatment has been done. We recommend annual follow-up for interval treatment of recurrent varices. Such treatment may include sclerotherapy or even minor surgical intervention.

Mr. Rose: Although sclerotherapy has always been popular on the European continent for the treatment of truncal and tributary varicosities, it has fallen into almost total disuse elsewhere. Truncal and tributary varicosities can be treated so simply by the surgical means described here that such sclerotherapy is justifiably reserved for patients who cannot be operated on because of age, general physical condition, or local skin complications such as refractory lipodermatosclerosis. Sclerotherapy can be used for postoperative recurrences of varicosities or new varicosities developing because of genetic or hormonal considerations. Furthermore, sclerotherapy is very effective for ablation of venous telangiectasias.

When Dr. DePalma spoke of minor surgical intervention, he made a very important point. Of course, we all aim for perfection in our results, but if saving the saphenous vein as a possible conduit results in having a few minor outpatient surgical interventions, it is a small price to pay. In any event, a patient with an inherent tendency to varicose veins is always a candidate for further procedures, even with the best of surgical treatment, and should be told at the outset that he or she may require therapeutic maintenance from time to time.

Dr. Bergan: No discussion of a surgical procedure would be complete without a description of complications. Who would like to address that subject?

Mr. Rose: Remarkably few complications occur with the procedure we have described. I can recall only one groin hemorrhage in our entire series. This complication resulted from an anterolateral saphenous tributary. It was memorable not only because of its uniqueness but also because it occurred on the day of President John F. Kennedy's assassination. As in other surgery, sepsis may occur, but it is extremely rare. We have seen no more than a case of minor wound infection once in 5 years. Curiously, such infections are found in small incisions and not in the groin. Other complications specific to the procedure include superficial phlebitis, which is often due to a residual hematoma in the path of the stripped vein. Theoretically, deep venous thrombosis should occur, but it is our practice to give one unit of low-molecular-weight dextran to obese patients or patients older than 50 during anesthesia and to firmly advise the patient to take brisk walking spells postoperatively. The last recorded case in our experience occurred years ago and involved a somewhat overweight 55-year-old woman.

Dr. Bergan: We have paid careful attention to deep venous thrombosis following superficial venous surgery and can only record two instances of this complication. The first occurred in a physician's wife, a 35-year-old woman who experienced dyspnea, tachycardia, and pleuritic pain of a transient nature 3 weeks after varicose vein surgery. Investigations were not performed, and the patient had no other manifestations. The second case involved an extremely tall male patient who experienced idiopathic atrial arrhythmia 48 hours following saphenous vein stripping. The patient was hospitalized, digitalis therapy was begun, and a normal sinus rhythm was restored. The ventilation/perfusion pulmonary scan was negative, but it was presumed that a small embolus had triggered the atrial arrhythmia.

Mr. Rose: In our surgical service we have had five minor pulmonary emboli cases after surgery in the last 40 years. Two of these situations were similar to your case and even involved a physician's wife. We have had no instance of pulmonary embolus in recent memory. I attribute these low figures to the comparatively atraumatic procedure, early ambulation, and the use of low-molecular-weight dextran in patients at risk. I think antiembolus stockings are at their most effective where there is no risk of embolus!

Dr. Bergan: We have noted two instances of lymphocele in which a fluid collection did transilluminate easily. Both lymphoceles were in the pathway of saphenous vein stripping.

Mr. Rose: Occasionally a collection of lymph develops under the groin scar because of damage to the lymphatics during the course of dissection in that area. Such a fluid collection usually resolves spontaneously and rarely requires aspiration. Antibiotics should be given if aspiration is necessary.

Dr. Bergan: Mr. Rose, with your long experience, what would you say are the most important changes that have occurred in varicose vein surgery in recent years?

Mr. Rose: The modern trend in varicose vein surgery has been away from routine stripping of truncal veins and toward multiple avulsion and removal of varicose clusters. As this change has occurred, the results have improved considerably. This improvement is what one would expect if the basic cause of varicosities was weakness in the vein wall.[31] Admittedly, there are still a number of circumstances in which limited stripping of the greater saphenous vein is indicated. Our approach to the problem has been outlined here, and we think that such stripping should be combined with multiple avulsions. Such an operation places great emphasis on elimination of all varicosities, wherever they occur, while also achieving the most cosmetic result.

We think that one of the most important functions of surgical teaching is the training of young surgeons in varicose vein surgery. This training must include indoctrination that focuses on the high attainment of good results as a challenge to be met in a much neglected but most important branch of the surgical art.

Dr. Bergan: Mr. Rose, that statement reminds us that all venous surgery is cyclic. Those techniques that were used and abandoned in the past later return repetitively and are used until better treatments are found to replace them. Your advice recalls the admonitions of Benjamin Brodie. Would you conclude this dialogue by repeating that story for us?

Mr. Rose: In 1846, while lecturing at the bedside of a patient suffering from a varicose ulceration, Benjamin Brodie said:

> . . . this is a case in which there is no question about the patient's life or death. I think it very probable that many among you may pass by the bedside of such a patient without thinking it worthy of attention. But I am not disposed to regard it in this manner. Although the patient will probably not die of this disease, without great care it will render her miserable. The disease may be very much relieved by art, and it is of very common occurrence. Such a case, as may meet you at every turn of practice, and your reputation in early life will depend more upon your understanding a case of this kind than upon your knowledge of one of more rare occurrence.

That story, which was quoted in the monograph by Rowden Foote[32] in 1949, is an appropriate conclusion for this dialogue.

REFERENCES

1. Bergan JJ. The veins. In Nora PF, ed. Operative Surgery. Philadelphia: Lea & Febiger, 1990, pp 991-997.
2. Samuels PB. Technique of varicose vein surgery. Am J Surg 142:239-244, 1981.
3. Bergan JJ. Management of external hemorrhage from varicose veins. Vasc Surg 31:413-418, 1997.
4. Goren G, Yellin AE. Primary varicose veins: Topographic and hemodynamic correlations. J Cardiovasc Surg 31:672-677, 1990.

5. Papadakis K, Christodoulou C, Christopoulos D, et al. Number and anatomical distribution of incompetent thigh perforating veins. Br J Surg 76:581-584, 1989.

6. Tung KT, Chan O, Lea Thomas M. The incidence and sites of medial thigh communicating veins: A phlebologic study. Clin Radiol 41:339-340, 1990.

7. Koyano K, Sagaguchi S. Selective stripping operation based on Doppler ultrasonic findings for varicose veins of the lower extremities. Surgery 103:615-619, 1988.

8. de Takats G. Ambulatory ligation of the saphenous vein. JAMA 94:1194, 1930.

9. de Takats G, Quillin L. Ligation of the saphenous vein. A report on two hundred ambulatory operations. Arch Surg 26:72-88, 1933.

10. Kistner RL, Ferris EB III, Randhawa G, et al. The evolving management of varicose veins: Straub Clinic experience. Postgrad Med J 80:51-59, 1986.

11. Sladen JC. Flush ligation and compression sclerotherapy for the control of venous disease. Am J Surg 152:535-538, 1986.

12. Lofgren EP, Lofgren KA. Recurrence of varicose veins after the stripping operation. Arch Surg 102:111-114, 1971.

13. Large J. Surgical treatment of saphenous varices with preservation of the main greater saphenous trunk. J Vasc Surg 2:886-891, 1985.

14. Mellière D, Cales B, Martin-Jonathan C, Schadeck M. Nécessité de concilier les objectifs du traitement des varices et de la chirurgie artérielle: Conséquences pratiques. J des Maladies Vasc 16:171-178, 1991.

15. Campbell WB, Niblett PG, Ridler BMF, Peters AS, Thompson JF. Hand-held Doppler as a screening test in primary varicose veins. Br J Surg 84:1541-1543, 1997.

16. Singh S, Lees TA, Donlon M, Harris N, Beard JD. Improving the preoperative assessment of varicose veins. Br J Surg 84:801-802, 1997.

17. Rose SS. Surgical techniques in the treatment of varicose veins. In Greenhalgh RM, ed. Vascular Surgical Techniques: An Atlas. Philadelphia: WB Saunders, 1989, pp 374-382.

18. Rivlin S. The surgical cure of primary varicose veins. Br J Surg 62:913-917, 1975.

19. Semroe CM, Laborde A, Buchbinder D, et al. Preoperative mapping of varicosities and perforating veins. J Vasc Tech 14:72-74, 1990.

20. Friedell ML, Samson RH, Cohen MJ, et al. High ligation of the greater saphenous vein for treatment of lower extremity varicosities: The fate of the vein and therapeutic results. Ann Vasc Surg 6:5-8, 1992.

21. Jakobsen BH. The value of different forms of treatment for varicose veins. Br J Surg 66:182-184, 1979.

22. McMullen GM, Scott HJ, Coleridge-Smith PD, et al. An investigation of the effect of ligation without stripping of the long saphenous vein. Surg Res Soc, Jan. 1990.

23. Cox HT. The cleavage lines of the skin. Br J Surg 29:234-240, 1941.

24. Flint MH. Langer's lines: A commentary. Surg Ann 8:25-46, 1976.

25. Turton EPL, Berridge DC, McKenzie S, Scott DJA, Weston MJ. Optimizing a varicose vein service to reduce recurrence. Ann R Coll Surg Engl 79:451-454, 1997.

26. Bradbury AW, Stonebridge PA, Callam MJ, Walter AJ, Beggs AI, Ruckley CV. Recurrent varicose veins: Assessment of the saphenofemoral junction. Br J Surg 81:373-375, 1994.

27. Chester JF, Taylor RS. Hookers and French strippers: A technique for varicose vein surgery. Br J Surg 77:560-561, 1990.

28. Ramelet AA. Muller phlebectomy: A new phlebotomy hook. J Dermatol Surg Oncol 17:814-816, 1991.

29. Ramelet AA. La phlébectomie ambulatoire selon Müller: Technique, avantages, désavantages. J Mal Vasc 16:119-122, 1991.

30. Ricci S, Georgiev M. Office varicose vein surgery under local anesthesia. J Dermatol Surg Oncol 18:55-58, 1992.

31. Rose SS, Ahmed A. Some thoughts on the aetiology of varicose veins. J Cardiovasc Surg 27:534-543, 1986.

32. Foote RR. Varicose Veins. London: Butterworth, 1949.

SUGGESTED READINGS

Bergan JJ. Saphenous stripping and quality of outcome. Br J Surg 83:1025-1027, 1996.

Darke SG, Vetrievel S, Foy DMA, Smith S, Baker S. A comparison of duplex scanning and continuous-wave Doppler in the assessment of primary and uncomplicated varicose veins. Eur J Vasc Endovasc Surg 14:457-461, 1997.

Georgiev M. The preoperative duplex examination. Dermatol Surg 24:433-440, 1998.

McMullin GM, Coleridge Smith PD, Scurr JH. Objective assessment of high ligation without stripping the long saphenous vein. Br J Surg 78:1139-1142, 1991.

Rutgers PH, Kistlaar PJEHM. Randomized trial of stripping versus high ligation combined with sclerotherapy in the treatment of the incompetent greater saphenous vein. Am J Surg 168:311-315, 1994.

Sarin S, Scurr JH, Coleridge Smith PD. Assessment of stripping the long saphenous vein in temperature treatment of primary varicose veins. Br J Surg 79:889-893, 1992.

Wilson S, Pryke S, Scott R, Walsh M, Barker SGE. "Inversion" stripping of the long saphenous vein. Phlebology 12:91-95, 1997.

Chapter 12

Controlled Radiofrequency–Mediated Endovenous Shrinkage and Occlusion

Robert A. Weiss and Mitchel P. Goldman

Endovenous shrinkage or occlusion by contraction of venous wall collagen through heat generated by radiofrequency (RF) is among the less invasive methods of treatment for axial reflux. This method approaches the problem of saphenofemoral reflux by obliterating a long segment of vein from within the lumen or restoring valvular competence in lieu of ligation and stripping. With a properly designed electrode, RF may be introduced through an intraluminal catheter to heat and shrink the vein wall in a controlled manner, restoring valvular competence. For conditions simulating ligation and stripping, maximal contraction of vein diameter is achieved through a specific electrode array by an endovenous technique with the vein destroyed over an extended length.

Although the concept of endovenous elimination of reflux is not new, previous approaches have relied on electrocoagulation of blood, causing thrombus to occlude the vein. The potential for recanalization of the thrombus is high. Historically, application of RF directly to tissue, not blood, has been used effectively in cardiology for ablation of abnormal conduction pathways in treatment of arrhythmias.[1] Venous occlusion using RF by the mechanism of venous blood coagulation has been previously reported.[2,3] It has also been termed endovascular diathermic vessel occlusion, a technique in which a spider-shaped intravascular electrode produces venous occlusion by electrocoagulation with minimal perivascular damage.[4]

MECHANISM OF ACTION

Directing RF energy into tissue to cause its destruction is safer and more controllable than other mechanisms used for this purpose. With RF energy delivered in continuous- or sinusoidal-wave mode, there is no stimulation of neuromuscular cells when a high frequency (between 200 and 3000 kHz) is used. The mechanism by which RF current heats tissue is resistive (or ohmic) heating of a narrow

217

rim (<1 mm) of tissue that is in direct contact with the electrode. Deeper tissue planes are then slowly heated by conduction from the small region of volume heating. Heat is dissipated from the region by further heat conduction into normothermic tissue.[5] By regulating the degree of heating, subtle gradations of either controlled collagen contraction or total thermocoagulation of the vein wall can be achieved.

This method is a relatively safe process because the temperature increase remains localized around the active electrode provided that close, stable contact between the active electrode and the vessel wall is maintained. By limiting temperature to 85° C, boiling, vaporization, and carbonization of the tissues are avoided.[6] With the system described here, electrode-mediated RF vessel wall ablation is a self-limiting process. As coagulation of tissue occurs, a marked rise in impedance occurs, limiting heat generation. Alternatively, if blood is heated instead of tissue, the impedance markedly decreases. This ensures efficient heating of the vein wall.[7]

REPRESENTATIVE SYSTEMS

Technologic advances of RF delivery to tissue include introduction of specific application electrodes and accompanying systems to monitor the electrical and thermal effects precisely. One such system is the VNUS Restore vein treatment system and the Closure catheter (VNUS Medical Technologies, Sunnyvale,

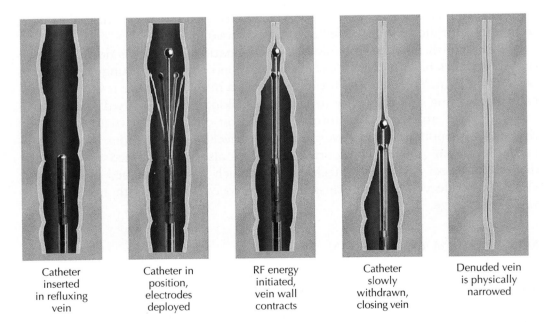

| Catheter inserted in refluxing vein | Catheter in position, electrodes deployed | RF energy initiated, vein wall contracts | Catheter slowly withdrawn, closing vein | Denuded vein is physically narrowed |

FIGURE 12-1. Schematic of Closure catheter. *RF*, Radiofrequency. (Courtesy of VNUS Medical Technologies, Sunnyvale, Calif.)

Calif.) (Figure 12-1). These devices produce precise tissue destruction with a reduction in the frequency of undesirable effects such as the formation of coagulum. Immediate evaluation of the anatomic lesional effect is performed through duplex ultrasound. With the Closure catheter system, bipolar electrodes heat the vein wall, which then collapses when the vein shrinks, allowing maximal physical contraction. The selective insulation of the electrodes results in a preferential delivery of the RF energy to the vein wall and minimal heating of the blood within the vessel. Acute elimination of spontaneous venous flow from vein diameter reduction can also occur following the application of RF energy. Animal experiments (described here) demonstrate endothelial denudation along with denaturing of media and intramural collagen with a subsequent fibrotic seal of vein lumen.

The catheter design for delivery of controlled RF to shrink vein wall collagen includes collapsible catheter electrodes, around which the vein may shrink, and a central lumen to allow a guidewire and/or fluid delivery structured within a 5 Fr (1.7 mm) catheter. This design permits treatment of veins as small as 2 mm and as large as 8 mm. A thermocouple on the electrode measures temperature and provides feedback to the RF generator. The control unit (Figure 12-2) displays power, impedance, temperature, and elapsed time so that precise temperature control is obtained. The unit delivers the minimum power necessary to maintain the desired electrode temperature.

CLINICAL FINDINGS

Initial animal studies comparing the effects of a potent sclerosing solution were performed on the rear limb saphenous veins of goats. Thirteen adult goats were treated by the endovenous RF occlusion device. The pretreatment mean vein diameter was 5.3 mm (4 to 8 mm). Percutaneous access obtained through a 5 Fr introducer sheath permits introduction of the RF catheter positioned at the treatment site under fluoroscopic guidance. Blood flow is impeded; as RF is applied, the catheter is moved distally along the vein, causing immediate contraction and

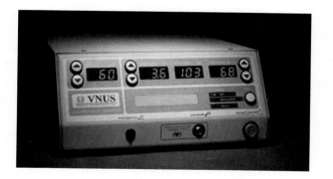

FIGURE 12-2. Control unit of controlled radiofrequency delivery. (Courtesy of VNUS Medical Technologies, Sunnyvale, Calif.)

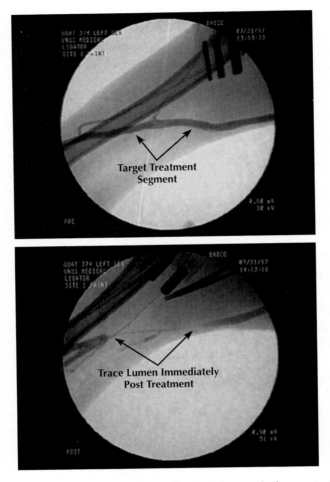

FIGURE 12-3. Greater saphenous vein seen immediately before and after controlled radiofrequency occlusion performed under fluoroscopic guidance.

cessation of flow (Figure 12-3). The electrodes maintain direct contact with the vein wall to maximize vein wall heating and minimize blood coagulation.

Acute observations indicate that 92% of the limbs treated resulted in significant reduction of vein diameter, with a mean diameter reduction of 5.3 mm to 1.1 mm. At 6 weeks persistent occlusion was maintained with no flow through the treatment site. Collateral flow was visible with high-pressure venography. Those veins that did not immediately occlude demonstrated total occlusion within 1 week. Figure 12-4 summarizes the treatment results of RF vein occlusion of goat saphenous vein.

In contrast, sclerotherapy of the posterior limb saphenous vein from five goats, with 0.5 to 1 ml of 3% sodium tetradecyl sulfate delivered under duplex ultrasound guidance, showed no evidence of occlusion. This result occurred despite

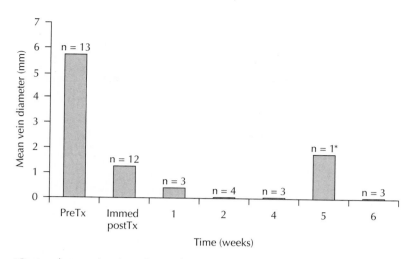

*Goat undertreated at time of procedure.

FIGURE 12-4. Graph of vein diameter reduction as measured by venography results in 13 goat saphenous veins. Complete closure is maintained at the conclusion of follow-up at 6 weeks except in one undertreated saphenous vein.

compressing the limb for 72 hours (compared with no compression following RF occlusion). Mean diameter change for sclerotherapy was from 5 mm (pretreatment) to 4 mm (posttreatment) with almost no change at 5 weeks' follow-up. Since the saphenous vein of the goat is a high-flow vessel, sclerotherapy is not predicted to be effective because sclerosing solutions require time to interact with the vessel wall to effect sufficient damage.[8,9]

HISTOLOGY

Histologic changes confirm the clinical findings. With sclerotherapy, limited endothelial denudation accompanied by some loss of birefringence in the vessel wall and 1 mm of surrounding tissue can be seen. No differences between acute and follow-up specimens are noted. For RF occlusion the acute changes show a 65% reduction in vessel lumen. Acute histologic features include denudation of endothelium, some thrombus formation, thickened vessel wall, denaturation of tissue with loss of collagen birefringence, and neutrophil (PMN) inflammation (Figure 12-5, A). The depth of vein wall damage is limited to 1 to 2 mm.

Chronic histologic changes 6 weeks following RF occlusion show further reduction in lumen diameter to complete occlusion (Figure 12-5, B). A small residual lumen may be recognized, but it is occluded by organized fibrous thrombi throughout the length of treated vein. Thrombus extension did not occur beyond the treatment site. Birefringence is almost fully restored, with new collagen growth detected. Electron microscopic findings confirm the light microscopic findings: marked endothelial damage and loss of the endothelium, neutrophils in the

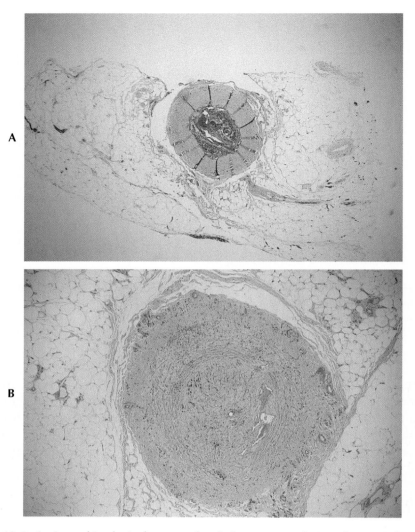

FIGURE 12-5. **A,** Acute histologic features of radiofrequency occlusion (hematoxylin-eosin stain, ×100). **B,** Histologic changes of controlled radiofreqency–occluded saphenous vein at 6 weeks (hematoxylin-eosin stain, ×100).

vessel lumen, and thickened, bulbous collagen fibrils. These findings indicate heat-induced contraction of collagen fibers and are indistinguishable from those changes seen with CO_2 laser resurfacing–induced collagen contraction. At 6 weeks electron microscopy shows a normal endothelium and normal amounts and location of vein wall myocytes, but with an apparent increase in collagen (Figure 12-6).

From these histologic findings it is concluded that acute contraction of myocytes and fibroblasts occurs from thermal denaturation. This change is accompanied by acute constriction and folding of intercellular matrix and collagen bun-

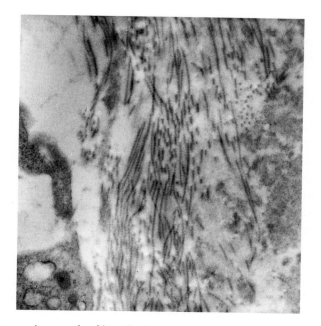

FIGURE 12-6. Electron micrograph of histologic appearance at 6 weeks following controlled radio-frequency occlusion of saphenous vein. Note new collagen bundles.

dles. Abundant new collagen and intercellular matrix formation appear within several weeks following RF occlusion. The result is a thickened vein wall with further constriction of lumen diameter.

The safety of this technique is evidenced by no thrombus extension and a limited zone of thermal damage, which appears no more than 2 mm beyond the targeted vessel. The high acute success rate of 92% is followed by long-term vessel occlusion.

INDICATIONS

Potential indications for this presently experimental technique include occlusion of segments of the greater saphenous vein, lesser saphenous vein, major saphenous tributaries, perforating veins, and recurrent varicosities following surgery. We predict that many surgical procedures may be replaced or supplemented by this technique. Application of a similar technology to restore valve competence in patients with early venous reflux is also undergoing worldwide clinical trials. This procedure, named Restore (VNUS Medical Technologies, Sunnyvale, Calif.), involves a slightly modified electrode, placed at the end of a catheter, that is designed to reduce vein diameter precisely at the base of a vein valve in order to restore valve competence.

Patients who have early disease with slight axial reflux are candidates for this procedure. Potential participants for clinical studies are screened by applying external pressure to reduce vein lumen diameter while measuring the effects on reflux by using duplex ultrasound. Those subjects in whom reflux is abolished through apposition of visible valve leaflets are ideal.

CONCLUSION

The targeted area of RF application heats and shrinks the vein wall in a controlled manner immediately below the valve annulus. The vein is therefore diminished in size, allowing previously incompetent valve leaflets to meet. Expandable insulated electrodes deliver bipolar RF energy to the vein wall, causing controlled diameter reduction. Thermal penetration is limited to 1 to 2 mm because of the bipolar electrode design. Our early clinical studies have shown no direct heating of blood, avoidance of heating valve leaflets, and shrinkage of vein wall components. The design of the catheter is such that the electrodes stent the vein and mechanically limit shrinkage. The physician performing the procedure has complete control over electrode expansion and degree of vein shrinkage.

In our limited clinical experience, restoration of valve function has persisted in the majority of patients during 2 months of follow-up. Potential indications for this procedure include restoration of competence at the saphenofemoral junction (particularly early disease with involvement of the subterminal valve/saphenopopliteal junction in which surgery is of higher risk), preservation of the saphenous vein for bypass while reducing reflux, and elimination of truncal vein reflux to enhance the efficacy of phlebectomy or sclerotherapy. Future applications may also include the restoration of deep vein valve competence.

REFERENCES

1. Olgin JE, Kalman JM, Chin M, Stillson C, Maguire M, Ursel P, et al. Electrophysiological effects of long, linear atrial lesions placed under intracardiac ultrasound guidance. Circulation 96:2715-2721, 1997.
2. Van Cleef JF. La "nouvelle electrocoagulation" en phlébologie. Phlebologie 40:423-426, 1987.
3. Gradman WS. Venoscopic obliteration of variceal tributaries using monopolar electrocautery. Preliminary report. J Dermatol Surg Oncol 20:482-485, 1994.
4. Cragg AH, Galliani CA, Rysavy JA, Castaneda-Zuniga WR, Amplatz K. Endovascular diathermic vessel occlusion. Radiology 144:303-308, 1982.
5. Haines DE. The biophysics of radiofrequency catheter ablation in the heart: The importance of temperature monitoring. Pacing Clin Electrophysiol 16:586-591, 1993.
6. Haines DE, Verow AF. Observations on electrode-tissue interface temperature and effect on electrical impedance during radiofrequency ablation of ventricular myocardium. Circulation 82:1034-1038, 1990.
7. Lavergne T, Sebag C, Ollitrault J, Chouari S, Copie X, Le HJ, et al. Radiofrequency ablation: Physical bases and principles. Arch Mal Coeur Vaiss 89 (Spec No 1):57-63, 1996.
8. Goldman MP, Sadick NS, Weiss RA. Cutaneous necrosis, telangiectatic matting, and hyperpigmentation following sclerotherapy. Etiology, prevention, and treatment [review]. Dermatol Surg 21:19-29, 1995.
9. Green D. Mechanism of action of sclerotherapy. Semin Dermatol 12:88-97, 1993.

Chapter 13

Treatment of Varicose Veins by Sclerotherapy: An Overview

André Cornu-Thénard and Pierre Boivin

Treatment of varicose veins by injection of a sclerosing agent is a very old method.[1-3] Its long history reflects the efficacy of this technique. However, sclerotherapy has evolved over the years, and this method is currently undergoing rapid progress. Clinical experience and controlled studies have defined indications for the technique. Development of new sclerosing agents has made this method more effective, and studies concerning the relationships between the diameter of varicose veins and the concentration of the sclerosant suggest the possibility of standardization of care. Use of Doppler and duplex ultrasound techniques provides better hemodynamic and anatomic precision, which also improves treatment efficacy.

The primary objective of sclerotherapy is to destroy the varicose vein with at least the same degree of efficacy achieved with surgical stripping. To maintain lasting aesthetic and functional results, it is essential to be guided by certain basic principles, comply with indications and contraindications, perform a complete pretreatment assessment, use optimal sclerosing solutions, and adopt a rigorous technique.

Sclerotherapy can be used for treatment of all pathologic superficial venous dilatations. However, this chapter focuses on the treatment of varicose veins >3 mm in diameter.

MECHANISM OF ACTION

When all the necessary conditions are combined—adequate sclerosant, effective dose, and sufficient compression—the intravaricose injection of a sclerosing agent results in sclerosis of the injected segment, followed by its resorption. The process that occurs between the time of injection and resorption can be divided into several stages.

First, injection of a sclerosing agent induces an endothelial and a mural lesion, followed by three phenomena that evolve simultaneously: spasm, inflammatory reaction in the vessel wall, and formation of an adherent thrombus. Spasm is induced by both needle trauma and sclerosing solution. It occurs immediately and may interfere with injections in adjacent sites.

The inflammatory reaction causes thickening of the vessel wall, which then is transformed into indurated scar tissue. The more effective the sclerosing agent, the greater the thickness of the vessel wall caused by this reaction. Ideally, the density of the scar tissue is sufficient to completely occlude the lumen, ensuring complete fibrous transformation of the varicose vein. The fibrous cord is subsequently transformed into a fine network that is totally resorbed. Occasionally venous obstruction is incomplete, and a channel within the fibrosis will persist. In such situations repeated injections must be performed to induce total obstruction. Otherwise recurrence is inevitable after a variable interval.

The formation of a thrombus is related to the endothelial lesion. The lesion induces adhesion and platelet aggregation, with activation of intrinsic pathways of coagulation. No risk of thrombotic embolization is present because the thrombus is firmly adherent to the vessel wall. However, if an excessively large thrombus forms and involves an exaggerated intravascular and extravascular inflammatory reaction, it may interfere with fibrosis, causing a high risk of recanalization. This mechanism is responsible for in situ recurrences associated with apparently perfect sclerotherapy. Effective compression after injections can prevent, or at least reduce, this phenomenon. Compression plays an essential role by limiting formation and extension of thrombosis and by facilitating endothelial fibrosis. Therefore the endothelial lesion induced by intravenous injection of a sclerosing agent must be as complete as possible. The resulting vascular necrosis must be sufficiently extensive to destroy the entire vessel wall without leaving significant thrombus.[3]

INDICATIONS AND CONTRAINDICATIONS

The indications for sclerotherapy of varicose veins may include any varicose veins not demonstrating reflux derived from the deep venous system. The principal indications recognized by major authors are as follows[3-6]:

1. Nonsaphenous varicose veins
   a. Varicose collaterals of normal saphenous veins
   b. Varicose veins supplied by:
      • One of several incompetent perforators
      • Cutaneous draining veins
   Examples are residual or new varicose veins after surgical treatment of saphenous veins.
2. Long or short saphenous varicose veins after isolated ligation/division of the saphenofemoral or saphenopopliteal junction
3. A more controversial indication for sclerotherapy involves incompetent long or short saphenous trunks for which surgery cannot be performed

for reasons such as patient refusal, surgical contraindication, or excessive separation from home.

Contraindications to sclerotherapy are related to either the patient or the sclerosing agent. Patient-related contraindications include concomitant deep venous thrombosis or superficial thrombophlebitis, postthrombotic syndrome when the venous dilatation acts as a collateral vessel, hypercoagulability, confinement to bed, pregnancy, and breast-feeding. Contraindications related to the sclerosing agent include (1) allergy to the agent itself, and (2) the sclerosant polidocanol in patients receiving disulfiram (Antabuse), since it contains 5% ethyl alcohol.

STRATEGY

Sclerotherapy of varicose veins must comply with certain basic principles for a satisfactory result for both patient and physician to be achieved.[2] These principles are easy to understand and are based on logical assumptions. Treatment must be performed from above in a downward direction and must proceed from the largest to the smallest vein; it must be complete (all-or-nothing rule) and must include short- and long-term follow-up.

Above-to-Downward Approach

The origin of varicose vein reflux is derived from the proximal part of the varicose vein, that is, at its upper extremity when the patient is standing. When the reflux is interrupted at this level, distal pressure is decreased, leading to a marked reduction in the caliber of distal varicose veins and thus facilitating sclerosis. This is the principle behind the therapeutic combination of ligation/division of the saphenofemoral junction and sclerotherapy of the distal long saphenous vein. When this approach is used, the sclerosing injections also must be started as proximally as possible, with the distal portion being finished over the course of subsequent sessions. If this principle is not followed, in situ recurrence is inevitable. Reflux will penetrate through the fibrotic wall of the varicose vein, leading to recanalization and recurrence.

Therefore before treatment is begun, it is essential to make sure that the obvious varicose vein is not actually supplied by a more proximal unseen varicose vein. Verification can be obtained by means of either a manual compression test or Doppler study (Figure 13-1). If this above-to-downward direction principle is not followed, a large patch of telangiectatic matting, venulectasias, or a new varicose vein parallel to the original one may develop at the injection site (worse yet, a combination of all three may occur).

Largest-to-Smallest-Vein Approach

In general, sclerotherapy of varicose veins is done by starting with the largest-diameter veins and finishing with the smallest ones. Schematically, the incompetent perforating vessels must be sclerosed first, followed by large varicose

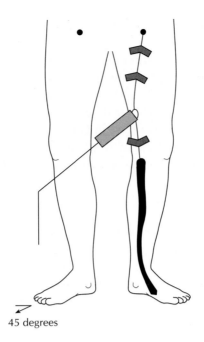

45 degrees

FIGURE 13-1. Palpation-percussion demonstrates varicose veins in leg but not in thigh. Doppler studies identify the origin of reflux: a perforator in adductor (Hunter's) canal.

veins, then smaller varicose veins, and finally venulectasias and telangiectasias.[3,7] Treatment of telangiectasias or small varicose veins before sclerosis of the varicose veins supplying these small vessels is associated with risk of treatment failure, early recurrence, or excessive inflammation.

Complete Approach

To obtain a good long-term result, the entire varicose vein must be sclerosed. Like surgical excision, such sclerosis ensures total disappearance of the varicose cluster without any portions of the varicose vein left intact for possible recurrence.

Follow-up

Regular follow-up, at least once a year, is essential. Such follow-up allows for treatment of new varicosities or those in evolution.

MATERIALS
Office Equipment

For examination of the patient in the standing position, a stable phlebologic stool with a solid base is essential. The examination table must be large and stable, with adjustable height, and it must be equipped with multiple planes that allow raising or lowering of the patient's body, trunk, or limbs. The physician should be seated on a stool (on casters) with adjustable height. Good lighting must be ensured, ideally with several light sources to avoid shadows.

Syringes

Disposable 2 to 5 ml plastic syringes graduated in 0.1 ml or 0.2 ml increments are the most widely used type. The tip of the syringe may be either central or eccentric, depending on the physician's preference. Glass syringes may be used, but they are less practical and require fastidious cleaning.

Needles

Long beveled needles are used: *usually* 0.4 to 20 mm (or 27-gauge, 3/4 inch), 0.45 to 16 mm (or 26-gauge, 5/8 inch), 0.5 to 16 mm (or 25-gauge, 5/8 inch); *occasionally* 0.6 to 25 mm (or 23-gauge, 1 inch); *more rarely* 0.7 to 40 mm (or 22-gauge, 1½ inch), 0.8 to 40 mm (or 21-gauge, 1½ inch). Certain specialists use butterfly needles, whereas others use short or long catheters. With small varicose veins or veins that are difficult to puncture in the supine position, the varicose vein is punctured while the patient is standing and the sclerosing agent is injected while the patient is lying down.

Sclerosing Agent

Numerous sclerosing agents are available on the market, although the choices vary from one country to another (Table 13-1). Each product has certain advantages and disadvantages, and the choice is based on personal experience. The best sclerosing agent is the one that the practitioner knows best.[8,9] Sclerosing agents can be classified according to the mechanism of action by which they induce the endothelial lesion.

Compression Material

Compression is an integral part of the technique required for sclerosing injection. Stockings and/or bandages may be used.[10] Elastic stockings must exert a pressure of approximately 30 mm Hg at the ankle (e.g., Sigvaris 503). If edema is present, the patient should systematically wear the stockings for 8 days before each injection session. This practice makes the varicose veins more accessible to palpation and therefore easier to inject.

Bandages should be nonelastic rather than elastic.[11] Nonelastic bandages are used to obtain maximum impact on the varicose dilatation. The bandage should not be applied too tightly.[12] In this way the varicose veins, emptied at the time of injection while the patient was in a supine position, are maintained flat by this semirigid bandage. When an adhesive bandage (e.g., Elastoplast or Micropore,

TABLE 13-1. Most widely used sclerosing agents

Active Ingredient	Trade Names	Supply	Maximum Dose per Session	Drug Companies
Chromated glycerin	Scleremo (France)	5 ml ampules	France: 10 ml	Laboratoire Bouteille 7 Rue des Belges 87100 Limoges, France
				Omega 11177 Rue Hamon Montreal, Canada H3M3A2
Polidocanol	Aetoxisclerol (France) Aethoxysklerol (Germany) Sclerovein (Switzerland) Etoxisclerol (Spain)	2 ml ampules (0.5%, 2%, and 3%)	France: 4 ml (0.5%), 2 ml (2% and 3%)	Dexo S.A. 31 Rue d'Arras 92000 Nanterre, France
				Globopharm AQ P.O. Box 1187 8700 Kusnacht, Switzerland
				Kreussler & Co. D 6200 Wiesbaden-Biebrich, Germany
Sodium tetradecyl sulfate	Thrombovar (France) Sotradecol (U.S.A.) Thromboject (Canada) STD (Great Britain)	2 ml ampules (1% and 3%)	France, U.S.A., and Canada: 10 ml (3%) Great Britain: 4 ml (3%)	Promedica 41 Rue C. Pelletan 92305 Levallois-Perret, France
				Elkins-Sinn, Inc. 2 Esterbrook Lane P.O. Box 5483 Cherry Hill, NJ 08034, U.S.A.
				STD Pharmaceutical Fields Yard, Plough Lane Hereford, England HR4 0EL
Dextrose/ sodium chloride	Sclerodex (Canada)	10 ml ampules	10 ml	Omega 11177 Rue Hamon Montreal, Canada H3M3A2

8 cm wide) is used, it remains firmly in place. If an elastic bandage is used, segmental compression is obtained by means of four or five turns without tightening. The main problem with this type of bandage is keeping it in place. An elastic stocking is worn by the patient after application of this segmental compression.

Protection Against Contamination

Gloves must be worn. Needles must not be reused; they must be collected in a special container for sharp instruments. Containers and contaminated wastes must be treated in accordance with local regulations. Glasses must be worn to protect the eyes from possible projection of blood.[13]

Emergency Kit

The equipment required to treat any immediate consequences of problems caused by sclerosing injections must be at hand. This equipment is discussed further in Chapter 16.

TECHNIQUE

Sclerotherapy should be a harmless therapeutic modality. Varicose veins are not a sufficiently serious condition to justify taking the slightest risk. At each session the practitioner must be well prepared, act effectively, and inform the patient wisely.

The pretreatment visit must include clinical examination; ideally, the examination is combined with a Doppler ultrasound study, which offers greater sensitivity.[14,15] Based on the examination findings, a precise map of the varicose lesions is drawn. The origin of the various refluxes, vein morphology, presence of branches or perforating vessels, and varicose vein diameter should be indicated in the patient's medical record.[16]

In preparation for a sclerotherapy session, a clinical history must be recorded and a search for allergic reactions must be done. The latter may require suspension of injections or use of another agent. Injection sites, carefully identified by palpation and percussion, are marked by two parallel lines on either side of the varicose vein. The clinical measurement of diameter is recorded beside these two parallel lines so that the dose of the sclerosing agent can be calculated in relation to the size of the varicose vein.

The patient remains supine because this is the most comfortable position that helps to reduce excessive venous pressure so that the sclerosing agent can be injected into an empty varicose vein.[17] Complete emptying ensures optimal contact between the sclerosing agent and the wall of the varicose vein. The practitioner must assume a stable and comfortable position and needs good illumination of the operating field. Varicose veins are located again because the patient's new position may have modified previous markings by several millimeters.

Puncture, aspiration, and injection are theoretically simple procedures. Puncture must never be performed blindly. It always must be performed on a clearly identified and, better still, palpable varicose vein. The axis of the vessel is indicated by the two parallel lines, with the angle of entry between 30 and 45 degrees. The skin puncture should be swift. Perforation of the vein wall sometimes can be detected easily.

Occasionally, when the varicose vein is small or when it is situated in a dangerous zone such as the popliteal fossa, the puncture is performed with a butterfly needle while the patient is standing.[18] The injection is administered several seconds later with the patient lying down. An inclining table can be very useful in this situation.

Negative pressure within the plastic syringe can be produced by withdrawing the piston so that, as the bevel of the needle crosses the wall of the vessel, blood is aspirated into the syringe by suction, immediately indicating the correct position of the needle. Users of glass syringes think that the piston slides sufficiently easily in the chamber of the syringe that it will rise on its own when in contact with arterial blood. One recommendation has been to insert the needle, not attached to the syringe, into the injection site.[19] The color and pressure of the blood coming from the needle are used to confirm correct intravenous position.

The injection must not be performed precipitously. It must be painless, and the patient must be asked to describe what he/she feels.[20] The injection should be slowed or even stopped in the event of pain.

Selective compression of the puncture site during injection with the index finger of the free hand keeps the varicose vein flat (distention of the wall can be painful), ensures good contact between the sclerosing agent and the endothelium, and confirms nonextravasation of the sclerosing agent injected.

Treatment Session Report

All the information concerning the injection session is recorded in the patient's medical record, including the side and sites of injection, the diameter of the varicose vein at these sites, the sclerosing agent used (with concentration and volume injected specified), and the results obtained. This information must be clearly presented and understandable to all members of the health care team. The following format for a treatment session report serves as a guide for the practitioner in subsequent treatment sessions:

Right	1	2	3	etc.
Diameter				mm
1% STS				ml
Results				

Compression

Compression is an integral part of treatment, just as it is after surgery.[3,21] Injection without compression is generally followed by intravaricose thrombosis associated with an inflammatory reaction and hematoma. Digital compression over the puncture site during or after injection, reinforced by segmental compression, constitutes the best way of preventing thrombosis and generally obviates the need for thrombectomy.

Pigmentation and matting are the principal aesthetic complications. They usually appear alone, but occasionally they are present together. Pigmentation and matting are generally secondary to an intense inflammatory reaction, usually related to lack of control of the sclerosing process by means of a compressive bandage. Therefore a compressive bandage always must be applied, and the patient must be convinced to keep the bandage on for several days to avoid subsequent aesthetic complaints.

Sclerosing Agent and Starting Dose

Sclerotherapy of varicose veins usually gives excellent results, particularly in the hands of an experienced practitioner. Nevertheless, the choice of sclerosing agent and the dose to be injected remain a delicate problem. The most appropriate sclerosing agent should be selected after its advantages and disadvantages have been considered in relation to the patient's clinical context and the lesions to be treated.

The choice of dose is more difficult since it is impossible to predict the effects of a given dose on a particular type of varicose vein. A number of factors are probably involved: age, sex, body weight, elasticity of the cutaneous tissue, skin fragility, skin color, and type of varicose vein (its age, tortuosity or straight appearance, and diameter). For these reasons a standard dose does not exist. However, there is a close relationship between the diameter of the varicose vein and the dose.[22] It is referred to as the "minus one" technique. It can be used to calculate the ideal starting dose for all nonsaphenous varicose veins, with 1% sodium tetradecyl sulfate (STS) used as the sclerosing agent.

The ideal starting dose is the quantity of sclerosing agent sufficient to obtain a good result by the first injection without inducing any harmful effects. It is calculated as follows:

$$\text{Ideal starting dose (ml 1\% STS)} = \frac{\text{Diameter of varicose vein (mm)} - 1}{10}$$

where ideal dose is one that ensures maximum efficacy (resolution or painless cord) with a minimum of side effects (little or no painful induration, pigmentation, or additional telangiectasias) (Table 13-2). The starting dose is the dose injected for the first time into one point of a varicose vein. The dose of sclerosing

TABLE 13-2. Relationship between clinical diameter of nonsaphenous varicose veins and ideal starting dose

Diameter of Varicose Veins (mm)*	Ideal Starting Dose (ml 1% STS)
3	0.2
4	0.3
5	0.4
6	0.5
7	0.6
8	0.7

STS, Sodium tetradecyl sulfate.
*Diameter as measured at injection site with patient standing.

agent corresponds to the volume (ml) injected multiplied by its concentration. If the initial concentration used is 1%, the dose corresponds to the volume injected. The diameter (mm) of the varicose vein is determined at the injection site by palpation (caliber rule) or by ultrasonography with the patient standing.

In practice, when this "minus one" technique is used with injections every 5 cm, and when principles of dual, segmental, and global compression of the limb are used, the results are excellent in approximately 70% of cases, ineffective in about 20%, and excessive in slightly less than 10%. This technique is easy to use because the diameter is often relatively constant along the varicose vein and rarely exceeds 8 mm. This diameter-dose relationship has been used by other authors with other sclerosing agents.[23]

The therapeutic approach at subsequent sessions is guided by evaluation of the results obtained with the first injections. The system of scoring the results (Table 13-3) has been used in the various statistical studies mentioned here. It is easy to use, can be adapted for computer processing, and effectively completes the treatment session report. This score can be used to complete the fourth line of the treatment session report (see sample report, p. 232). Thus, at a single glance, this report describes the initial session, tells what was done, and notes the results obtained. When no reaction is observed at the injection site (result scored as 0), the volume injected is increased by 0.1 ml. When the diameter is reduced by one half (result scored as 1) and the entire length of the vein remains patent, the same volume of sclerosing agent is reinjected. When sclerosis of part of the vein occurs, the "minus one" technique is pursued. In the case of total resolution of a cord (scores 2 and 3, respectively), the "minus one" technique is applied to the other varicose veins.

In the case of an excessive reaction, such as a cord with inflammatory reaction lasting more than 1 week, a cord with pigmentation, or a cord with telangi-

TABLE 13-3. Scoring of results of sclerotherapy at injection site

Score	Effect Obtained
0	No result
1	Reduction in diameter by one half
2	Total resolution
3	Cord
4	Cord and inflammatory reaction >8 days
5	Cord and pigmentation
6	Cord and development of telangiectasias

ectasias (scores 4, 5, and 6, respectively), the initial dose was excessive and should be decreased by one half for other varicose veins. Rigorous application of compression is essential in such a situation. With intense inflammatory reactions, local anti-inflammatory treatment should be applied. If the thrombus is not reabsorbed after 30 days, thrombectomy must be performed by incising the indurated zone with a large-caliber needle (21 gauge) or a No. 11 scalpel blade and pressing on the edges of the varicose vein. In most cases evacuation of the thrombus will prevent pigmentation of the zone.

Timing of Treatment Sessions

Treatment sessions must not occur too frequently because complete response to treatment can occur as late as 2 to 3 weeks after injections. Therefore an interval of at least 1 month should be allowed between each session for each varicose vein. If other varicose veins need treatment, particularly on the opposite leg, treatment sessions can be scheduled more frequently.

Patient preference concerning frequency of sessions and number of injections also should be considered. It is important to listen and clearly define the patient's reasons for consulting the physician so that the technique can be adapted to achieve the defined objectives.

Injection of Saphenous Veins After Ligation

When the long (greater) saphenous vein (LSV) and short (lesser) saphenous vein (SSV) do not require stripping, simple ligation of the saphenofemoral and saphenopopliteal junctions can be performed. This ligation is generally followed by a reduction in the diameter of the tributary veins. Sclerotherapy should be performed according to the rules defined in the following discussion. Initial doses injected into a palpable saphenous vein correspond to twice the "minus one" technique (e.g., 6 mm dilatation requires a dose of 1 ml of 1% STS). The "minus one" technique then is applied to the remaining tributaries.

Treatment of Saphenous Veins
With Sclerotherapy Alone

Treatment of long and short saphenous veins by sclerotherapy alone is controversial and does not appear to be indicated as first-line treatment.[6,24] Sclerosis of the junction regions, where blood flow and reflux are maximal, is difficult to achieve. Even when sclerosis is obtained, recanalization is usually inevitable because of underlying reflux. Therefore surgical treatment with ligation/division of the junctions, with or without stripping of distal varicose veins, appears to be the treatment of choice.

However, sclerotherapy of the LSV and SSV sometimes can be performed with a satisfactory success rate, particularly in the case of long-standing varicose veins. These veins are generally sufficiently large to be palpable over their entire length and therefore are easy to inject, which allows complete treatment to be done from above in a downward direction. Sclerotherapy of the LSV has a greater chance of success when the vein is sinusoid with dilatations at different levels and in male patients. In such cases compression is applied with stockings or superimposed nonadhesive bandages.

Additional indications for sclerotherapy of the SSV include improvement in functional testing after application of a 20 mm Hg elastic stocking and only minor reflux into the deep venous system. Because of the large number of anatomic variants in the popliteal fossa, a complete venous Doppler ultrasound study must be performed systematically. The sclerosing agent of choice is STS at a concentration of 3% for the LSV and 2% for the SSV. The modalities of compression are identical to those used for nonsaphenous varicose veins.

LONG-TERM RESULTS

Patients should be seen at least once a year after treatment. Follow-up should consist of a clinical examination and Doppler studies (whenever possible, combined with duplex to avoid missing a residual patent lumen within the sclerosis). This approach is designed to evaluate the efficacy of previous treatments and to demonstrate the appearance of varicose veins in previously untreated territories. Complementary treatment then can be instituted as a means of limiting disease progression.

Most authors agree that correctly performed sclerotherapy gives very satisfactory results in the majority of cases.[4,25] This view is supported by certain statistical studies.[8] Other authors monitor the intensity of sclerosis obtained and its subsequent course by ultrasound.[26,27] However, there is no easy way of differentiating among residual varicose veins, recurrent varicose veins, and natural progression of the disease. No method of quantification of varicose disease has been established. These points remain limiting factors for demonstrating the efficacy of any treatments.

A topographic and quantitative assessment of the lesions should be performed before any treatment is repeated, and this assessment should be performed at regular intervals.[28] Topographic differences between subsequent examinations allow for in situ recurrent varicose veins to be distinguished from new varicose veins. Quantitative differences allow for a quantitative assessment of the rate of disease progression.

OTHER METHODS
Ultrasound-Guided Sclerotherapy

Duplex ultrasound has become the gold standard for the diagnosis and evaluation of venous disease of the lower limbs.[29] It allows precise assessment of venous function and provides anatomic mapping.

Duplex ultrasound can be used to optimize sclerotherapy[30,31] when it is difficult, or even dangerous, to perform according to the usual clinical guidelines (palpation and direct vision). The ultrasound examination permits visualization of the vein to be injected and then allows guidance of the needle and control of the injection of sclerosing agent.[32,33]

Advantages. This method improves safety through visualization of the varicose vein to be treated, the zone of injection, and injection of the product. It therefore limits the risks of intra-arterial and/or extravascular injection. It also improves efficacy by visualizing spasm induced by the injection (indicator of efficacy).[34] Finally, it allows selective compression of the treated vein to ensure impregnation of all of the venous endothelium by the sclerosing agent and to increase the contact time.[2]

Indications. General indications for ultrasound-guided sclerotherapy are the same as those described previously. Specifically, ultrasound guidance is used for deep varicose veins (in obese patients), nonpalpable incompetent perforators, residual channels resulting from incomplete efficacy of previous sclerotherapy, LSV or SSV when sclerotherapy is indicated, and tributaries of the upper third of the LSV or SSV.

Materials and technique. The ultrasound apparatus and transducer must allow visualization of superficial planes and therefore must have a high frequency (7.5 MHz or more). This equipment should be light and easy to use and should be covered with a disposable membrane to avoid contamination. The use of sterile ultrasound gel is also recommended.

Continuous-Wave Doppler–Guided Injections

The usual method of injection of sclerosing agents is based simply on clinical recognition and visualization of the varicose vein.

The purpose of the technique named Doppler sclerotherapy[35] is to allow more accurate sclerotherapy in situations where varicose veins are not palpable in the supine position but are palpable during standing.

Technique. This technique consists of injecting the sclerosing agent by means of an uncomplicated continuous-wave Doppler, a syringe, and a needle, according to a method consisting of four well-defined steps ensuring avoidance of arterial

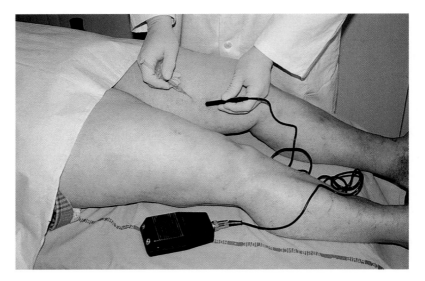

FIGURE 13-2. Doppler-guided injection.

vessels and constant appreciation of the varicose vein to be treated, even during the injection. It requires no assistants and allows the treating physician's gaze to remain at the injection site while listening for very specific Doppler sounds of aspiration and injection (Figure 13-2).

Indications and limitations. The principle indication is the treatment of varicose veins that are palpable while the patient is standing but impalpable in the supine position. In addition, varicose veins in the groin region, the lower third of the thigh, and those along the axis of the small saphenous vein may be treated with this technique. In these situations it is a more accessible, faster, and economical technique, although it does not replace duplex ultrasound–guided injections. The needle must be of sufficient caliber to be echogenic, and its length should be adapted to the depth of the varicose veins. We generally use a 0.7 to 40 mm (22-gauge, 1½ inch) or 0.8 to 40 mm (21-gauge, 1½ inch) needle.

To improve the efficacy and especially the safety of the technique, it is recommended to use a needle guide[36] or a catheter.[37] The sclerosing agent and dose are selected as already described.

The varicose vein to be injected is first located with the patient standing. The zone is then identified in semidarkness with the patient lying down. Ultrasound visualization of the vein to be injected is performed on transverse or longitudinal sections. The injection is performed, and progression of the needle is followed on the screen. Visualization of the tip of the needle in the form of a highly echogenic bright point in the middle of the venous lumen confirms correct positioning of the needle (Figure 13-3). The operator must control the syringe visually. Gentle traction on the piston must induce reflux of venous blood. The injection can be performed and is visualized in the form of echogenic interfaces with turbulence within the blood. The absence of any localized parietal deformity of the injected

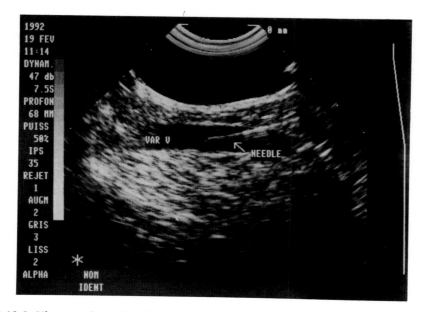

FIGURE 13-3. Ultrasound visualization of needle correctly located in varicose vein to be injected.

vein, possibly reflecting intraparietal or extravascular injection, must be verified during the injection.

The injection is administered slowly (1 ml over approximately 5 seconds). The injected vein is compressed by the transducer. Subsequent injections are administered more and more distally. When all injections have been performed and complete spasm has been obtained, compression is applied.

Limitations. Ultrasound-guided sclerotherapy does not eliminate the risks related to the technique,[37] but it must be considered as an instrumental aid, essential to standard sclerotherapy in certain situations. The improved efficacy and safety provided by this technique can be achieved only when the operator is perfectly familiar with sclerotherapy techniques and their limitations.

Endoscopic Injection

Venous endoscopy allows visualization of the venous endothelium, the valves, and the tributaries. However, this technique is still under investigation, and endoscopic sclerotherapy is only a research technique at present.[38]

SPECIAL CASES
Pregnancy

In general, sclerotherapy is not indicated during pregnancy. The combination of diurnal compression with leg elevation at night halts disease progression during gestation.[39] During pregnancy, compression should exert 30 to 40 mm Hg and the foot of the patient's bed should be raised 10 to 12 cm. This dual approach should be continued at least until delivery. An assessment should be performed after pregnancy to determine the indications for curative treatment. Depending on the patient's desires, treatment can proceed, but plans for a future pregnancy should not alter the therapeutic approach.

Postthrombotic Syndrome

Sclerotherapy cannot be considered until the thrombosed deep vein has become recanalized and if the superficial dilatation is the site of constant blood flow, indicating a collateral vessel. This problem area can be detected by repeated noninvasive investigations. In fact, noninvasive venous investigation is imperative in such a situation to assess the respective importance of the superficial and deep veins. A clotting survey should be done to eliminate possible hypercoagulability.

■ ■ ■

A 56-year-old woman presented with a painful varicose vein of the right thigh. She had no history of deep venous thrombosis and had not undergone treatment. The diagnosis of nonsaphenous varicose veins was based on clinical examination and Doppler studies. The patient had a large varicose vein (9 mm in greatest diameter) on the anterolateral surface of the right lower extremity (Figure 13-4, A) with a clinically normal LSV; no

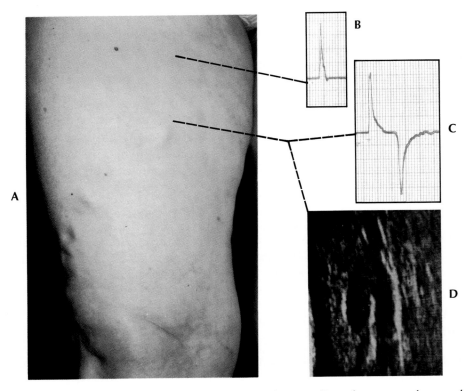

FIGURE 13-4. **A,** Nonsaphenous varicose vein. **B,** Doppler recording of competent long saphenous vein. **C,** Doppler recording of nonsaphenous varicose vein. **D,** Ultrasound examination.

reflux was present on the cough test. Manual compression of the saphenofemoral junction had no effect (the varicose vein filled at the same rate when the patient stood up). Doppler examination confirmed the integrity of the LSV; no reflux was present (Figure 13-4, *B*). However, marked reflux into the varicose vein was noted (Figure 13-4, *C*), and on ultrasound examination the dilatation measured 9 mm at its most proximal point (Figure 13-4, *D*). The remainder of the examination produced normal findings, with no other varicose veins, good patency and competence of the deep veins, and no arterial disease noted.

This patient's nonsaphenous varicose vein constituted a perfect indication for sclerotherapy. Treatment was commenced after the procedure was explained to the patient and after informed written consent had been obtained (Figure 13-5). Injection sites were marked, and the corresponding diameter was measured with the patient in a standing position (Figure 13-6, *A*).

PATIENT INFORMATION

Sclerotherapy of varicose veins is not devoid of risks. The technique consists of the injection of a sclerosing agent into your varicose veins. This agent acts by inducing irritation of the wall of the varicose vein. When a sufficient dose is injected, it causes complete obstruction of the varicose vein, leaving a more or less sensitive cord for several days. Your body will gradually resorb this cord, which finally disappears completely.

The objective of these injections is to eliminate your varicose veins, exactly as if they were removed surgically. In the same way as after surgery, compressive bandages are extremely important after the procedure. The aesthetic results obtained when these bandages are used are much more satisfactory and longer lasting.

You must comply with the following rules:
1. Lead a normal life during the hours following the injection. Specifically, do not rest but walk and go about your usual activities. Avoid prolonged sitting, such as in a car (stop every 20 minutes for a walk) or in a train (walk up and down the aisle).
2. Over the following 3 to 8 days, avoid excessive heat, shower rather than bathe, and do not cover your legs with heavy blankets. Avoid excessively violent sports.
3. Keep the bandages on for 8 days. If for any reason you must remove them, replace them within hours. If you need to wear an elastic stocking, continue to do so by putting it on over the bandage (without removing the bandage). When showering, protect your leg with a plastic bag.
4. Several minor events may occur in the treated regions, such as a sensitive cord or a hematoma. These are usual phenomena that are no cause for concern.

Do not hesitate to contact me by phone (or leave a message) if you have any questions or concerns.

Doctor _____

Patient _____

Telephone # _____

FAX # _____

Date _____

FIGURE 13-5. Patient information form for sclerotherapy.

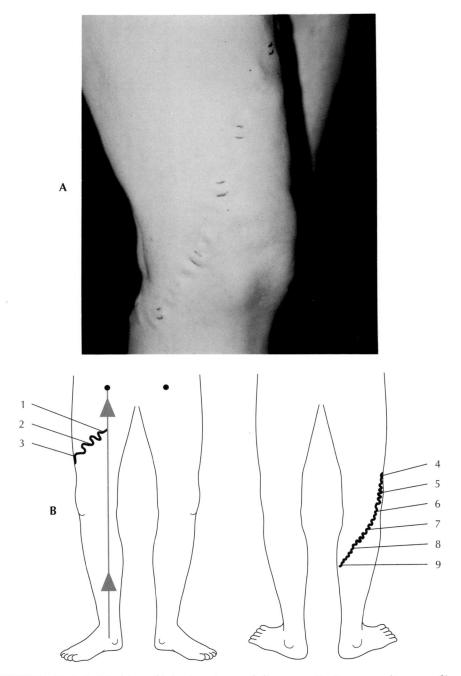

FIGURE 13-6. A, Marking of injection sites and diameters. B, Corresponding case file.

In this first session, the doses for injection were established according to the "minus one" technique. For the first three injection sites, which measured 9 mm, 6 mm, and 7 mm, the volumes of 1% STS were 0.8 ml, 0.5 ml, and 0.6 ml, respectively. A total of nine injections at intervals of 5 cm were done along this varicose vein (Figure 13-6, *B*). A nurse specialist applied the segmental compression (Figure 13-7, *A*); the bandage was

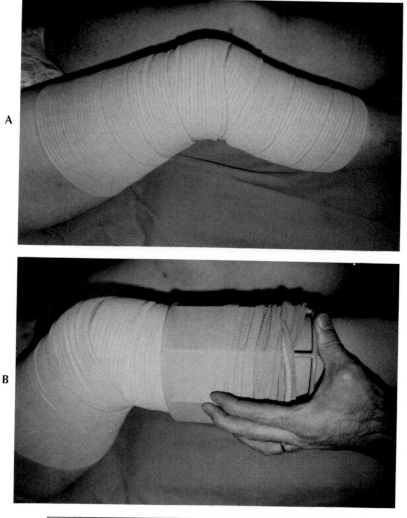

Right	1	2	3	4	
Diameter	9	6	7		mm
1% STS	0.8	0.5	0.6		ml
Results					

FIGURE 13-7. **A,** Application of segmental compression. **B,** Elastic stocking is put on with Sigvaris extensor. **C,** Establishment of treatment session report.

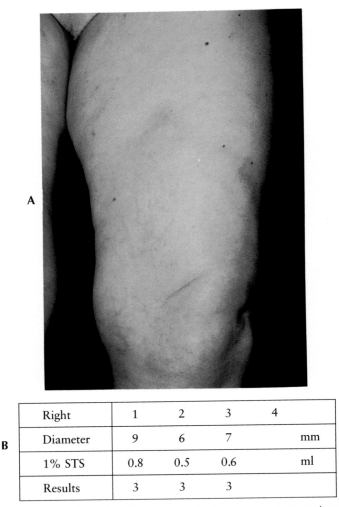

Right	1	2	3	4	
Diameter	9	6	7		mm
1% STS	0.8	0.5	0.6		ml
Results	3	3	3		

FIGURE 13-8. Clinical result (**A**) and transcription to treatment session report (**B**).

worn for 8 days. The elastic stocking was put on with an extensor (Figure 13-7, *B*). The treatment session report includes all pertinent data (Figure 13-7, *C*).

One month after treatment, the results were assessed (Figure 13-8, *A*) and scored to complete the treatment session report (Figure 13-8, *B*). In this case each injection site was scored as 3, corresponding to a cord. This single session was considered to be satisfactory, and the patient was scheduled for follow-up every 6 months for 2 years and annually thereafter.

CONCLUSION

Sclerotherapy remains a cornerstone in the treatment of superficial venous insufficiency. It occupies an important place among other available treatments.

Sclerotherapy always must comply with two essential imperatives: safety and efficacy. A rigorous approach must be taken in defining the indications and administering the treatment.

REFERENCES

1. MacLatchie JD. The Treatment of Varicose Veins by Intravenous Injection. New York: Macmillan, 1929.
2. Tournay R. La Sclérose des Varices, 4th ed. Paris: L'Expansion Scientifique Française, 1985.
3. Goldman MP. Sclerotherapy: Treatment of Varicose and Telangiectatic Leg Veins. St. Louis: Mosby, 1991.
4. Boivin P, Hutinel B. Indications de la sclérothérapie dans l'insuffisance veineuse superficielle des membres inférieurs. Sang Thrombose Vaisseaux 5:463-467, 1993.
5. deGroot WP. Practical phlebology. Sclerotherapy of large veins. J Dermatol Surg Oncol 17:589-595, 1991.
6. Perrin M. L'Insuffisance Veineuse Chronique des Membres Inférieurs. Paris: Medsi/McGraw-Hill, 1990.
7. Boivin P. Traitement des télangiectasis. Phlebologie 39:233-239, 1986.
8. Hutinel B. Phlébologie Esthétique. Paris: Arnette, 1990.
9. Sapin G, Parpex P. Choix du sclérosant. Phlebologie 38:183-185, 1985.
10. Stemmer R. The choice of compressive stocking. Phlebologie 35:107-116, 1982.
11. Stemmer R. Sclérose des varices et compression. Phlebologie 44:49-67, 1991.
12. Ducros R. Intérêt de la compression dans le traitement sclérosant. Phlebologie 27:205-207, 1974.
13. Guex JJ. Matériels utilisés en sclérothérapie. Phlebologie 44:49-67, 1991.
14. Fronek HS. Noninvasive examination of the venous system in the leg: Presclerotherapy evaluation. J Dermatol Surg Oncol 15:170-173, 1989.
15. Large J. Doppler testing as an important conservation measure in the treatment of varicose veins. Aust N Z J Surg 54:357-359, 1984.
16. Cornu-Thénard A, Boivin P, Parpex P. Essai d'une quantification clinique des varices pour l'épidémiologie, la thérapeutique et l'informatique. Phlebologie 39:661-676, 1986.
17. Wallois P. The condition necessary to achieve an effective sclerosant treatment. Phlebologie 35:337-344, 1982.
18. Raymond-Martimbeau P. Sclérothérapie de la saphène interne en position debout et en position assise. Etude comparative. Phlebologie 44:97-110, 1991.
19. Bernbach HR. Le traitement sclérosant selon SIGG. Phlebologie 44:31-36, 1991.
20. Fronek A. Injection compression sclerotherapy of varicose veins. In Ernst CB, Stanley JC, eds. Current Therapy in Vascular Surgery, 2nd ed. Philadelphia: BC Decker, 1991.
21. Sladen JG. Compression sclerotherapy: Preparation, technique, complications, and results. Am J Surg 146:228-232, 1983.
22. Cornu-Thénard A, de Vincenzi I, Valty J. Sclérothérapie des varices: Intérêt de la mesure clinique de leur diamètre avant les premières injections. In Davy A, Stemmer R, eds. Phlebologie '89. Montrouge: John Libbey Eurotext, 1989.
23. Sadick NS. Minimal sclerosant concentration of hypertonic saline and its relationship to vessel diameter. J Dermatol Surg Oncol 17:65-70, 1991.
24. Hobbs JT. Surgery and sclerotherapy in the treatment of varicose veins: A random trial. Arch Surg 109:793-796, 1974.
25. Eklöf B. Modern treatment of varicose veins. Br J Surg 75:297-298, 1988.
26. Schadeck M. Doppler and echotomography in sclerosis of the saphenous veins. Phlebology 2:221-240, 1987.
27. Bishop C, Fronek H, Fronek A, Dilley R, Bernstein E. Real-time color-duplex scanning after sclerotherapy of the greater saphenous vein. J Vasc Surg 14:505-510, 1991.

28. Cornu-Thénard A, de Vincenzi I, Maraval M. Evaluation of different systems for clinical quantification of varicose veins. J Dermatol Surg Oncol 17:345-348, 1991.
29. Kanter A, Thibault P. Saphenofemoral incompetence treated by ultrasound-guided sclerotherapy. Dermatol Surg 22:648-652, 1996.
30. Zummo M. Sclérose de la veina saphène interne sous écho-guidage: Etude prospective. Phlebologie 50:261-268, 1997.
31. Isaacs M, Forrestal M, Harp J, Gardener M. Sclérothérapie écho-guidée (UDS) des troncs saphéniens. Phlebologie 50:247-249, 1997.
32. Knight RM, Vin F, Zygmunt JA. Ultrasonic guidance of injections into the superficial venous system. In Davy A, Stemmer R, eds. Phlebologie '89. Montrouge: John Libbey Eurotext, 1989.
33. Miserey G, Reinharez D, Ecalard P. Sclérose sous échographie dans certaines zones à risques. Phlebologie 44:85-96, 1991.
34. Schadeck M. Echosclérose de la grande saphène. Phlebologie 50:189-195, 1997.
35. Cornu-Thénard A, DeCottreau H, Weiss RA. Sclerotherapy: Continuous wave Doppler-guided injections. Dermatol Surg 21:867-870, 1995.
36. Marley W. Utilisation d'un guide-aiguille pour les injections sous échographie. Phlebologie 49:473-476, 1996.
37. Grondin L, Young R, Wouters L. Sclérothérapie écho-guidée et sécurité: Comparaison des techniques. Phlebologie 50:241-245, 1997.
38. van Cleef JF, Desvaux P, Griton P, Cloarec M. Sclérose de la sàphene externe sous contrôle endoscopique. Phlebologie 44:131-136, 1991.
39. Boivin P, Hutinel B. Varices et grossesse. J Mal Vasc 12:218-221, 1987.

Chapter 14

Compression Sclerotherapy for Large Varicose Veins and Perforator Veins: Details of an Empty Vein Technique

Joseph G. Sladen and John D.S. Reid

In North America the traditional approach to treating large varicose veins and complicated venous disease has been surgical.[1-3] The recent addition of subfascial endoscopic ligation of perforators has made surgical treatment of perforators more appealing[4,5] (see Chapter 17). In the last decade sclerotherapy, with or without the use of compression, has gained popularity for treatment of small superficial veins and telangiectasias. Cosmetic appearance is usually the primary indication for this procedure, although some of these veins are symptomatic. Compression sclerotherapy for large veins was initially described by Sigg[6] in 1952 and was reported in the English literature by Fegan[7] in the 1960s. A random trial comparing surgery with compression sclerotherapy that was published by Hobbs[8] in 1974 demonstrated that compression sclerotherapy controlled perforators effectively.

We have practiced compression sclerotherapy using the "empty vein technique," described by all the authors noted in the preceding discussion, for the last 20 years. We have concentrated on patients with symptoms, large veins, and perforators.[9] It soon became obvious that thigh reflux was poorly controlled by compression sclerotherapy alone. Flush ligation of the saphenofemoral junction that involved taking all the branches was added. This approach led to improved results, particularly in the control of thigh varicosities.[10,11] Thigh stripping gives more definitive control in the thigh and is widely recommended.[12,13] Apart from stripping the occasional vein for smoldering superficial phlebitis, compression sclerotherapy is our primary below-knee treatment.

INITIAL EXAMINATION

An organized examination is directed specifically at the venous system. The findings are recorded on a specialized form (Figure 14-1). Initially the patient is asked to stand for 10 minutes. This standing loads the venous system and usually precipitates symptoms. Saphenofemoral incompetence often can be identified by a cough impulse in the upper saphenous vein, but use of a hand-held continuous-wave Doppler device is standard practice today.

Duplex ultrasound examination is useful in documenting more complicated disease. The upper saphenous vein is insonated approximately 8 cm below the inguinal ligament with the Doppler probe while pressure is applied and released

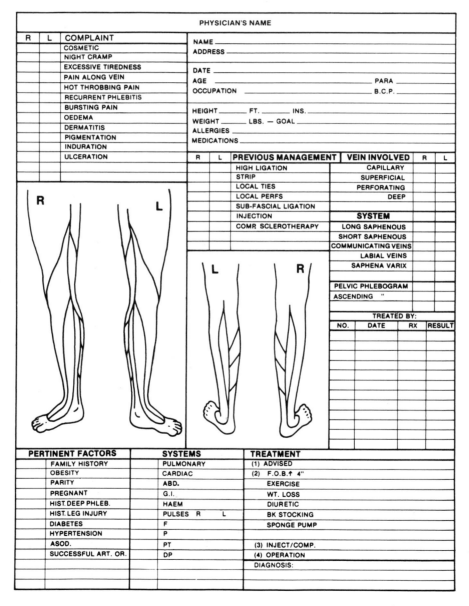

FIGURE 14-1. Form on which venous complaints, findings, and treatment are recorded. (Modified from Sir Patrick Dunn Hospital, Dublin, Ireland.)

over the saphenous vein in the lower thigh (Figure 14-2). Reflux of blood in the saphenous vein that occurs when the palpating hand is released indicates sapheno-femoral incompetence. This finding can be enhanced by a Valsalva maneuver performed by having the patient blow against the back of his/her hand while it is pressed against the mouth. The patient must not move during the Valsalva maneuver because Doppler sounds indicate blood passing the probe in either direction, and movement of the leg can produce a false-positive result. The short (lesser) saphenous vein is examined while the patient is standing, with notation of distention over its course in the middle posterior calf and particularly at the crow's foot configuration above the lateral malleolus. Along with palpation, the Doppler probe can be used to identify the course of the vein by manually tapping the short saphenous vein near its lower end. Doppler examination is more difficult in the popliteal fossa than in the groin because of the adjacent deep venous system, but it can be helpful in identifying reflux.

The varicose veins are then examined for control or entry points and for perforators. While the patient remains standing, the veins are manually stripped of blood. The examiner controls the vein with the fingers of one hand and uses the fingers of the other hand, moving proximally on the leg, to strip the blood from the vein. Sudden reappearance of blood filling the vein as the second examining

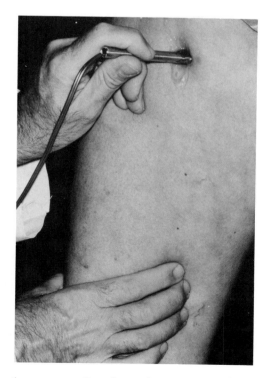

FIGURE 14-2. Use of continuous-wave Doppler probe to assess saphenofemoral reflux with release of pressure over long saphenous vein and use of Valsalva maneuver.

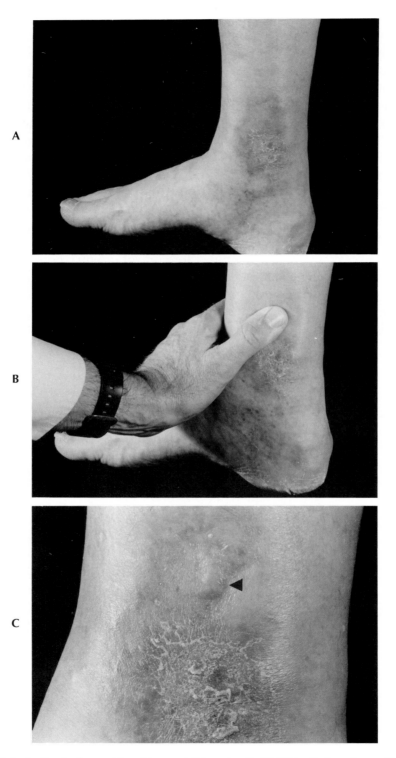

FIGURE 14-3. A, Stasis dermatitis with no visible vein. **B,** "Milking" the edema. **C,** Close-up of same area showing visible and easily palpable high-pressure vein *(arrowhead)* fed by Cockett perforator after "milking."

hand moves up the leg indicates a control point or an incompetent perforator. Pressure applied at a control point may control a nest of varicosities. The anatomic perforator sites on the medial side of the lower leg are examined by palpating with the thumb, searching for tenderness, and milking away edema with repetitive pressure (Figure 14-3).

Frequently a high-pressure vein that has not been obvious emerges from the surrounding edema when examination is done with this technique. Tender or warm areas are the most important injection sites for compression sclerotherapy. They reflect high-pressure veins and are usually venous "lakes" fed by perforators or control points. Differentiation between perforators and control points is not especially important clinically because both should be treated. Edema, dermatitis, induration, and pigmentation are noted. While in a supine position, the patient is then examined for pulses and ankle pressures, if indicated, to rule out arterial disease. We do not find that the standard Trendelenburg test adds any useful information. The patient's complaints and examination are recorded on the venous form during the examination.

PREPARATION OF PATIENT

The patient must understand the basic principles of venous disease for satisfactory management. Concepts of venous drainage, valves, and the calf pump need to be discussed. We stress control, not cure, of disease and spend time allaying fears of ulceration and amputation, which frequently concern the patient with venous disease. It is helpful to involve the office nurse in the discussion and to provide handouts that address many of the questions the patient may have later.

Pressure

As an integral part of treatment, all patients are fitted with a below-knee pressure-gradient stocking (30 to 40 mm Hg). Many patients state that they cannot tolerate a stocking, but a well-fitted stocking improves venous disease and symptoms. In fact, we often use the stocking as a "therapeutic trial" to help confirm the diagnosis of venous insufficiency. Although trained stocking fitters have improved significantly during the last 15 years, an experienced physician can often improve on a measured fit. A full range of stocking sizes kept in the office is recommended to the physician specializing in the treatment of venous disease. This supply allows the fitting of alternative stocking sizes and the stretching of the stocking by the physician to achieve a comfortable fit.

The patient is instructed in the use of the stocking at the first visit (Figure 14-4). The stocking is most easily applied by turning it inside out and then inverting the foot portion to the heel. The patient's foot is inserted into the stocking to the heel, and the remaining stocking is everted over the foot and up the leg. The stocking should slip off the thumbs during this part of the application rather than being stretched up the leg. There should be room for one or two fingers above the stocking in the popliteal fossa with the knee bent. Frequently the stocking needs to be loosened by vigorous stretching of its cuff and ankle before appli-

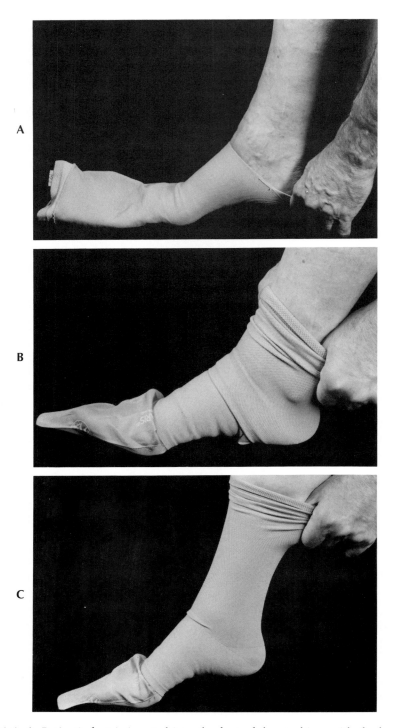

FIGURE 14-4. A, Patient's foot is inserted into the foot of the stocking, with the leg of the stocking inside out over the foot. **B,** Stocking is eased over the heel, one layer at a time without bunching. **C,** Tension is distributed by slipping the stocking off the thumbs to place the stocking on the leg, rather than by stretching it upward on the leg.

cation to prevent constriction of the calf and to allow it to pass over the heel easily. Patient compliance is important because the stocking is worn over the bandage after compression sclerotherapy and must be well tolerated.

Compression

If diffuse tenderness, induration, or ulceration is present on the medial lower calf, a "sponge pump" is added rather than increasing the pressure of the stocking (Figure 14-5). Initially very few patients can tolerate stockings with a pressure gradient of 40 to 50 mm Hg or greater. A sponge pump is made from soft ½-inch latex foam rubber, measuring approximately 8 × 20 cm. The pump is rounded and beveled so that the edges do not indent the tissue, and it can be modified to apply more pressure behind the medial malleolus. The sponge pump is placed on the medial perforator area over the pressure-gradient stocking and wrapped with approximately one half of a 4-inch tensor bandage. The bandage is applied tightly with crisscrossing wraps on the lower part of the sponge pump; as the bandage is applied upward, the pressure is reduced by spreading the wraps and easing the pressure.

Activity

The patient is directed to walk 2 miles a day to ensure adequate deep venous outflow. If the patient has difficulty tolerating the stocking or the sponge pump, we do not proceed with high ligation or compression sclerotherapy but persist in conservative management. Patients who are unable to walk because of arthritic or cardiac problems are taught to exercise their calf against resistance. An air-mattress foot pump works well for this purpose.

If the patient is comfortable for a few days with the pressure-gradient stocking and sponge pump, if indicated, we proceed with treatment.

THIGH REFLUX

Although thigh reflux is not the primary focus of this chapter, effective treatment of thigh reflux (saphenofemoral thigh perforators and short saphenous vein) is mandatory in the treatment of complicated venous insufficiency.

Burnand et al.[14] have shown that an incompetent long saphenous vein may contribute more than 50% of the increase in ambulatory venous pressure at the ankle seen in venous disease, even in the presence of incompetent perforators. Approximately 60% of patients who present with large varicosities but have not had a previous saphenofemoral ligation have saphenofemoral reflux. Moderate reflux is compatible with excellent initial results of compression sclerotherapy; however, these results are not lasting, particularly when thigh varicosities are present. Ignored or recurrent saphenofemoral reflux is probably the most common cause of poor result from compression sclerotherapy and often leads the patient to seek other treatment.

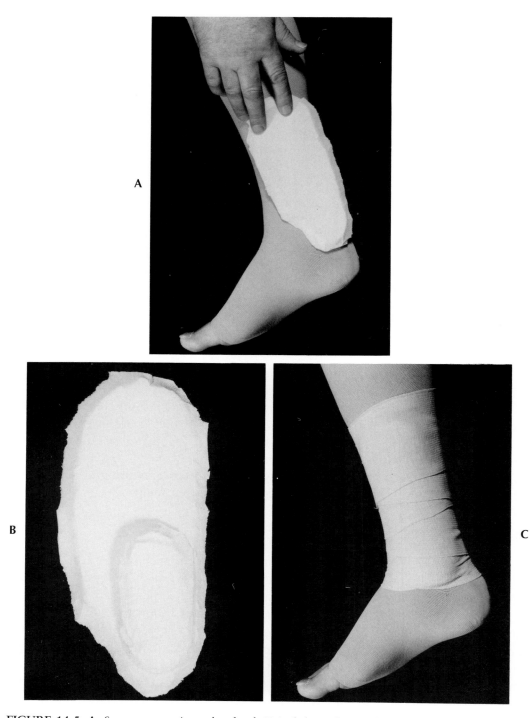

FIGURE 14-5. A, Sponge pump is made of soft ½-inch latex foam rubber sculpted to fit the area. **B,** Additional piece of latex foam can be used to apply more pressure behind the medial malleolus if there is an ulcer in that area. **C,** Four-inch elasticized bandage is applied tightly on the lower part of the sponge, easing the pressure above.

Surgery is the treatment of choice for saphenofemoral and thigh reflux. The most definitive approach is ligation and thigh stripping[12,13,15] with careful attention to the groin tributaries[16] (see Chapter 17). The option of saving the saphenous vein in the thigh but treating saphenous varices locally at the time of flush ligation has been our choice because patients usually are not concerned about a few residual veins. If the varix is large, it is ligated proximally during the operation. After surgery a 3 ml syringe is filled with 3% sodium tetradecyl sulfate (STS), which is used to inject the thigh varicosities while the patient is supine or sitting. Up to six sites are each injected with 0.5 ml of STS from the syringe. An abdominal pad, folded in thirds, is placed over the varix and wrapped with a 6-inch tensor bandage to apply pressure. The thigh is wrapped in a random crisscrossing fashion, with an early wrap made high, near the groin, to reduce the chance of slippage. The wrap is extended distally to meet the pressure-gradient stocking so that the bandage is contiguous with the stocking. Half of an abdominal dressing pad may be placed behind the knee to prevent the bandage from piling. The patient is advised to rewrap the thigh when the bandage loosens or slips. This operation can be done easily with the patient under local anesthesia. Most patients are ready to return to work 3 or 4 days after surgery, and a follow-up office visit is scheduled within 7 to 10 days.

Compression Sclerotherapy

Approximately half of our patients have no significant saphenofemoral reflux or have had previous venous ligation or stripping (done by other practitioners) and require only compression sclerotherapy. It is important that the patient understand the basic principles of venous disease and learn to master the use of the pressure-gradient stocking. Therefore compression sclerotherapy is not performed at the initial visit.

Materials. An injection tray that includes prefilled syringes, precut ½-inch tape in 8 cm lengths, cotton fluffs, crepe bandages, sponge, adhesive elastic bandage (Elastoplast), scissors, and porous plastic tape (Micropore) is essential if the procedure is to be accomplished expediently (Figure 14-6). Syringes are prefilled with 0.5 ml of either 1% or 3% concentrations of STS.* A 3% concentration is used for the large high-pressure veins, and a 1% concentration is used for the smaller veins. The different concentrations are clearly coded on the syringes with tape. We prefer 3 ml syringes with 25-gauge needles because of better tactile feedback during injection. A standing stool is provided for the patient so that the physician can sit in a comfortable position while injecting. Applying a layer of carpeting under each end of an examining table allows it to slide over a smooth floor so it can be moved to the patient easily when it is time for the patient to lie down.

---

*EDITOR'S NOTE: Wyeth-Ayerst Laboratories (Philadelphia), the manufacturer of STS, does not advise allowing STS to remain in contact with the rubber stopper of a syringe for longer than a few hours because of degradation of the rubber (personal communication, 1992).

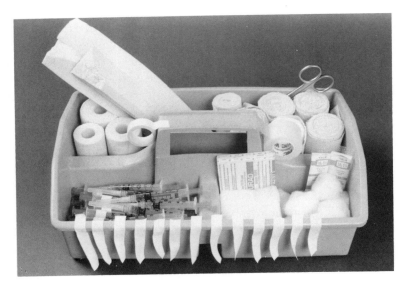

FIGURE 14-6. An organized tray expedites compression sclerotherapy.

Technique. The technical steps in compression sclerotherapy can be summarized in the following way:

1. Have the patient stand for 10 minutes.
2. Make multiple oblique punctures, noting a flash of blood in the syringe.
3. Elevate the patient's leg.
4. Inject the sclerosant and trap it with cotton fluffs.
5. Hold the cotton fluffs in place with a crepe bandage while applying moderate pressure.
6. Apply a latex sponge to the course of the vein.
7. Wrap the leg with a crepe bandage in a random crisscrossing fashion.
8. Apply Elastoplast to stabilize the crepe bandage.
9. Cover the bandage with an old nylon stocking.
10. Add compression through the use of a below-knee pressure-gradient stocking (30 to 40 mm Hg) and a 6-inch elasticized bandage or tube for the knee or thigh.

The preceding steps are illustrated in Figure 14-7.

The patient should stand for 10 minutes to load the veins. This loading facilitates needle placement within the vein lumen. Some patients are prone to vasovagal syncope and may be treated while sitting if the veins are large enough to palpate. The needle is introduced into the vein obliquely so that there is good tissue friction on the needle. A flash of blood into the hub of the needle indicates that the needle is in the vein lumen. Care is taken not to puncture the main saphenous trunk but rather the venous lake over the perforator or control point branches, if possible. The syringe is then secured to the leg with ½-inch tape.

When all the sites have been punctured, the patient lies supine on the examining table and the leg is elevated (with the foot resting on the physician's shoul-

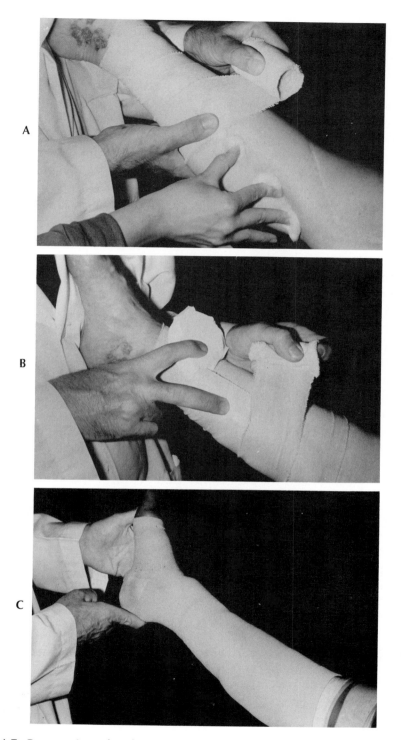

FIGURE 14-7. Compression sclerotherapy for large veins. **A,** After injection, sclerosant is trapped with cotton fluffs and compressed with a bandage. **B,** Precut latex sponge is applied to the course of the vein. **C,** Prefitted pressure-gradient stocking is worn over the bandage.

der) to empty the veins. The sclerosant is then injected slowly; it is trapped by digital pressure applied over cotton fluffs placed approximately 5 cm proximal to the injection site; the pressure is worked upward on the leg when possible. Assistance from the nurse is necessary at this stage. If the sclerosant extravasates, it burns severely, like a bee sting. The patient is warned of this possibility, and the injection is stopped if there is a suggestion of extravasation. Infiltration of 1% lidocaine solution controls the pain and may reduce the incidence of injection ulceration (see Chapter 16).

The needles are left in place, and the wrapping is begun in a distal to proximal direction, with syringes and needles removed as they are encountered. Leakage from the needle hole is controlled by applying a cotton fluff over the area of the vein pierced by the needle, which is slightly proximal to the skin puncture site. If there are many injection sites on the leg, it is easier to inject and wrap the lower half of the leg and then proceed with the upper half. We use a crepe bandage rather than an elasticized bandage because the former makes it much easier to control the amount of pressure applied. The wrap is first applied above, then over the infection site, if possible. Precut wedged and tapered 1-inch latex sponge rubber is applied along the course of the vein, which can be seen by the outline of the cotton fluffs through the crepe bandage. The sponge is held in place with a second and third layer of random wrapping. The wrap must be applied smoothly, and the second and third layers are applied in a random fashion to support the whole wrapped area equally. The wrap should be applied firmly but not tightly.[17]

In a lean leg tension must be reduced slightly over the anterior border of the tibia or the area padded with cotton batten; otherwise, the bandage may cause blisters or pressure symptoms such as burning pain. In wrapping a large leg it is useful to compress the sponge with the thumb as the leg is wrapped to produce more pressure locally over the course of the vein. Elastoplast is used at the top and bottom of the bandage to stabilize it. Contact with the skin is avoided to minimize the potential for skin reaction. Bandages are covered with an old nylon stocking that is used both day and night to protect the bandage. The crepe bandage loosens over the course of a day or so but serves to keep the sponge in place over the injected veins. During the day the 30 to 40 mm Hg pressure-gradient stocking is applied over the nylon stocking and slides on quite easily. Injection sites and areas of suspected extravasation are recorded on the vein chart.

ADVICE

The patient is advised to take three or four walks daily, totaling approximately 2 miles, and to apply extra pressure with a sanitary napkin or similar pad over any area of tenderness. Patients who are unable to walk are advised to use an air-mattress foot pump to exercise 10 minutes four times a day. The foot is always cyanotic and congested when dependent, but the congestion is controlled by the pressure-gradient stocking and activity. We encourage the patient to wear the stocking the first night and alternate nights for the first week. Analgesic or anti-inflammatory medication is not prescribed, but the patient is advised to walk if

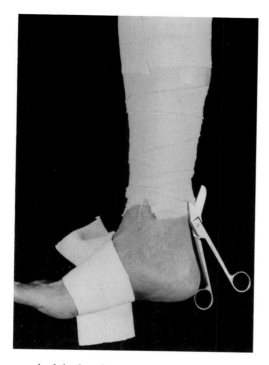

FIGURE 14-8. Without removal of the bandage, tension on the bandage can be eased by the patient by removing the lower Elastoplast and cutting the lower third of successive wraps at the 12, 4, and 8 o'clock positions, as required.

the limb feels congested. It may be necessary to get up once during the first night and take a short walk if the leg is uncomfortable.

If the foot swells to the point that wearing a shoe is uncomfortable or if the lower edge of the bandage digs into the leg, the patient should reduce the tension of the bandage, particularly at its lower end. This reduction is accomplished by cutting the lower edge of the bandage in successive layers at the 12, 4, and 8 o'clock positions, with the cut made approximately one third of the width of the bandage (Figure 14-8). The Elastoplast is then reapplied to produce a neat bandage with tapered pressure. The bandage is removed by the patient in 3 weeks (if large high-pressure veins were treated) or in 10 days (if smaller low-pressure veins were treated). The pressure-gradient stocking is reapplied and should be used at all times that the leg is dependent. A handout is supplied to guide the patient through this period. The patient is examined in follow-up 3 or 4 days after the bandage is removed.

FOLLOW-UP

Residual veins are injected if necessary, and local areas of phlebitis are aspirated (see discussion of complications). These veins are usually low pressure, so unless a perforator is reinjected, 10 days of compression bandaging is usually adequate. All patients should continue to wear the pressure-gradient stocking for at least 3 weeks after the bandage is removed. Extra pressure is applied with a pad placed under the stocking over any tender area. Unless there is a great deal of standing or kneeling involved in the patient's occupation, there should be no interruption in work schedule.

We try to minimize the number of sessions. For example, we complete treatment of the thigh at the time of surgery for saphenofemoral reflux because bandages are more easily tolerated if the thigh and calf are not wrapped at the same time. Varicosities of the foot are also more easily managed alone after treatment of the calf. Approximately 75% of the patients are treated in one session; 20%, in two sessions; and 5% in three sessions. An average of six or seven sites are injected at the first session; two or three are done thereafter.

When treatment is completed, the patient is advised to "listen to the leg." If the leg feels better with the stocking, this situation reflects residual venous insufficiency and the use of a pressure-gradient stocking is encouraged. In such cases the stocking should always accompany the patient on trips and should be worn for prolonged sitting or standing, particularly during air travel. The word "control" (rather than "cure") is reiterated, and a review appointment is suggested in 3 to 5 years.

DIFFICULT PRESENTATIONS

Exact anatomic diagnosis is important, particularly if venous disease is to be treated surgically. Venous duplex ultrasound is the most useful examination when the anatomy of reflux is unclear. Varicograms give a useful road map of venous drainage but do not demonstrate reflux.[18] Venograms are rarely indicated in the investigation of chronic venous disease.

Gross saphenofemoral reflux after flush ligation or stripping is best treated by reoperation, with careful reexploration of the origin of the saphenous vein from the femoral vein. Minor recurrence in this area can be treated by injection. Thigh perforators are sometimes difficult to treat with compression sclerotherapy. Local ligation and compression sclerotherapy, or thigh stripping, should be considered. Veins that drain directly from the pelvis posteriorly or laterally are best treated by ligation at their control point before injection because it is too difficult to apply effective compression in this area. Short saphenous vein incompetence is rare in the absence of long saphenous vein incompetence, but it is a significant cause of calf pain and should be considered in symptomatic venous disease. Varicograms are very helpful in delineating popliteal venous anatomy.[19] Recurrent veins found in the popliteal fossa after short saphenous ligation demand an anatomic diagnosis before retreatment. The only episode of deep phlebitis after compression sclerotherapy in our experience followed injection of recurrent varicosities in this area.

Large veins in the foot can hemorrhage and may be tender; they are often disfiguring. With a few modifications, the results of compression sclerotherapy are very good. Bandages that incorporate the ankle may cause blisters and sometimes ulceration over the Achilles tendon because of pressure and friction. It is always necessary to protect this area when treating veins of the foot. Friction on the Achilles tendon can be reduced by covering the area with Telfa or Tegaderm. Smaller cotton fluffs are used on the foot, supplemented with a piece of ½-inch foam, custom fitted and beveled to cover the injection sites. This method reduces the bulk so that a shoe can be worn.

COMPLICATIONS

Small areas of local phlebitis occur in approximately 20% of injected limbs, particularly in the thigh and upper calf, where it is more difficult to sustain compression. If the area is more than 3 mm in diameter, the tarlike thrombus can be expressed easily by opening the skin with a No. 11 scalpel blade, or it can be aspirated with an 18-gauge needle up to 6 weeks after injection. Removal of the thrombus results in immediate relief of pain and tenderness and reduces subsequent pigmentation in the area. The area should be compressed for 3 days to avoid recurrence of phlebitis. We express or aspirate thrombi in 12% of injected limbs. Noticeable pigmentation is present in 10% of patients at 3 months, but usually the appearance is quite acceptable at the end of a year. Oriental and East Indian patients have a greater tendency toward permanent pigmentation and should be advised of this fact.

More generalized superficial phlebitis, usually located in the thigh above the injected area, occurs in 5% to 10% of limbs. This condition is treated with early application of pressure by using a sanitary napkin or folded abdominal dressing pad placed longitudinally over the area of tenderness and wrapped with a tensor bandage to give comfortable support. We use a 6-inch elasticized bandage or elasticized tube in the thigh and a 4-inch bandage in the calf for this purpose. In our treatment of several thousand limbs, there have been no occurrences of embolization and no cases requiring high ligation.

Ulceration occurs in 3% of limbs after compression sclerotherapy of large veins. Three causes should be considered: (1) extravasation (injection ulcer, Figure 14-9); (2) pressure necrosis; and (3) local hypersensitivity. Reducing the concentration of the sclerosant from 3% to 0.5% or 1% decreases the incidence of injection ulcer but in our experience has not been as effective in controlling large high-pressure varicosities. Injection ulcers may be more than 2 cm in diameter and tend to occur in the lower half of the calf. The large ones may take 3 or 4 months to heal as the fat and capillary bed are necrosed as well as the skin. Fortunately, such ulcers are not painful and are easily managed by placing a dry or occlusive dressing under a pressure-gradient stocking. We advise excising the large ulcers early because this practice shortens the healing time and results in a very acceptable scar. Patients with large symptomatic veins accept this complication much more easily than those with asymptomatic small reticular veins or telangiectasias for whom the cosmetic result is important. This matter should be considered in choosing the sclerosant and its concentration.

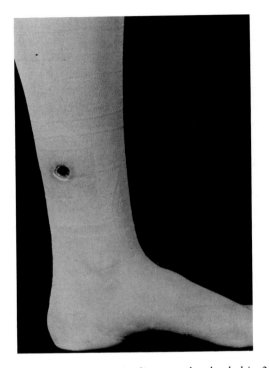

FIGURE 14-9. Injection ulcer measuring 1 cm in diameter that healed in 3 months and left a small scar. Excision would have expedited healing.

Ulceration also can be caused by pressure from cotton fluffs that are too thick and firm, particularly if they are placed over the anterior subcutaneous surface of the tibia. Such ulcers tend to heal more quickly than injection ulcers, and they do not have the characteristic depth of injection ulcers. This problem can be reduced by thinning the cotton fluffs and avoiding the injection sites over the surface of the tibia. Occasionally, we have seen one or even two small ulcers at injection sites in patients who have had no apparent or undue pressure but usually have had previous courses of sclerotherapy. Such ulcers may represent local hypersensitivity to the small amount of sclerosant that leaks from the vein when the needle is removed. Frothing the sclerosant may reduce this leakage. We have seen a few cases of saphenous neuritis, one of which was permanent but localized. This complication is minimized by keeping the puncture site away from the saphenous vein and nerve.

MANAGEMENT OF INDURATION AND ULCERATION

Compression sclerotherapy is particularly applicable to the treatment of severe symptomatic disease and venous ulceration (CEAP clinical class 3-6).[20] The aim is to isolate the pressure in the deep calf pump from the surface by obliterating the venous connecting veins and perforators. Injections should be made through normal, or at least noninfected, subcutaneous tissue and rarely adjacent to an ulcerated area.

The patient is seen and examined as described. Characteristically, venous ulcers are not painful and are only slightly tender. If the ulcer is painful, there is either a significant infective component or it is a combined ulcer, associated with occlusive disease or hypertension. Ulcers on the lateral aspect of the leg are more suggestive of this condition. Hospitalization is rarely necessary. Most patients can be managed as outpatients with application of 3 × 3–inch cotton gauze to the ulcer. The gauze is backed with a portion of abdominal padding to absorb moisture and is held in place with a nylon stocking. A pressure-gradient stocking is applied over the nylon and then wrapped with a sponge pump for additional pressure. This dressing is changed in the morning and evening. Patients are carefully taught that pressure heals. They are instructed to walk 2 miles daily and to resume their normal activities as much as possible. It usually takes two or three follow-up office visits for the physician to be certain that the patient is using the sponge pump effectively. The sponge must be sculpted to fill the concave area behind the medial malleolus, and it may be necessary to add another layer of sponge to heal an ulcer in this area (see Figure 14-5, B). When the ulcer is clean and relatively dry, Telfa is substituted for gauze and the need for the abdominal pad is soon eliminated. Patient compliance with this treatment is high. Tenderness and induration subside quickly; the patient is fully mobile and can easily monitor the progress of healing.

In an unpublished study of our experience, 100 stasis ulcers, ranging from 0.5 to 8 cm in minimum diameter, were treated in this manner. It took 1 to 2 months for ulcers approximately 1 cm in diameter to heal. Larger ulcers healed at a rate of approximately 1 cm per month (8 months for an 8 cm ulcer). Most stasis ulcers remain healed with continued use of a sponge pump or conversion to a higher-grade compression stocking.[21] Such ulcers are usually associated with obvious venous insufficiency and incompetent perforators. We treat patients with this type of ulcer with compression sclerotherapy because it gives them more freedom in long-term management. All these patients are instructed to use a compression stocking with a pressure gradient of 30 to 40 mm Hg permanently and to return temporarily to the sponge pump if the tenderness or induration recurs. The recurrence rate for stasis ulcer was less than 5% at 4 years after compression sclerotherapy, confirming the work of others.[22] Recurrent ulcer, even after fasciotomy, is often related to a recurrent perforator and responds to repeat compression sclerotherapy.

SUMMARY

Venous disease is effectively managed through surgical control of thigh reflux and compression sclerotherapy for perforating veins and major control points. Most of the long saphenous vein can be preserved when desirable, and treatment can be repeated easily when necessary. Compression sclerotherapy for large veins is not surgery-free. It is also not a cure and rarely produces a "Hollywood leg." Patients with edema, dermatosclerosis, or ulceration (CEAP clinical class 3-6) are ideal candidates for compression sclerotherapy if perforators are present. This method is particularly applicable to patients who are elderly, obese, or at high risk for other reasons. Compression sclerotherapy, with its attendant bandaging, is well accepted by patients in North America and is an extremely useful tool in the management of venous disease.

REFERENCES

1. Homans J. The operative treatment of varicose veins and ulcers. Surg Gynecol Obstet 22:143-158, 1916.
2. Linton RR. The postthrombotic ulceration of the lower extremity: Its etiology and surgical treatment. Surgery 138:415, 1953.
3. DePalma RG. Surgical therapy for venous stasis ulcer. Surgery 76:910, 1975.
4. Bergan JJ, Murray J, Greason K. Subfascial endoscopic perforator vein surgery (SEPS): A preliminary report. Ann Vasc Surg 10:211-219, 1996.
5. Gloviczki P, Bergan JJ, Menawat SS, Hobson RW, et al. Safety, feasibility, and early efficacy of subfascial endoscopic perforator surgery: A preliminary report from the North American Registry. J Vasc Surg 25(1):94-105, 1997.
6. Sigg K. The treatment of varicosities and accompanying complications. Angiology 3:355-379, 1952.
7. Fegan WB. Continuous compression technique of injecting varicose veins. Lancet 2:109, 1963.
8. Hobbs JI. Surgery and sclerotherapy in the treatment of varicose veins. A random trial. Arch Surg 109:793-796, 1974.
9. Sladen JG. Compression sclerotherapy: Preparation, technique, complications and results. Am J Surg 146:228-232, 1983.
10. McCaffery J. An approach to the treatment of varicose veins. Med J Aust 1:1379, 1969.
11. Sladen JG. Flush ligation and compression sclerotherapy in control of venous disease. Am J Surg 152:535-538, 1986.
12. McMullin GM, Coleridge-Smith PD, Scurr JH. Objective assessment of ligation without stripping the long saphenous vein. Br J Surg 78:1139-1142, 1991.
13. Neglén P. Treatment of varicosities of saphenous origin: Comparison of ligation, selective excision, and sclerotherapy. In Bergan JJ, Goldman MP, eds. Varicose Veins and Telangiectasias: Diagnosis and Treatment. St. Louis: Quality Medical Publishing, 1993.
14. Burnand JC, O'Donnell TF, Thomas ML, Browse NL. The relative importance of incompetent communicating veins in the production of varicose veins and venous ulcers. Surgery 82:9-14, 1977.
15. Darke SG. Recurrent varicose veins. In Goldman MP, Bergan JJ, eds. Ambulatory Treatment of Venous Disease. St. Louis: Mosby, 1996.
16. Hobbs JT. Operations for varicose veins. Rob and Smith's operative surgery. In De Weese JA, ed. Vascular Surgery, 4th ed. St. Louis: Mosby/London: Butterworth, 1985, p 278.
17. Gunderson J. Bandaging of the lower leg. Phlebology 7:50-53, 1992.
18. Thomas ML, Bowles JN. Incompetent perforating veins: Comparison of varicography and ascending phlebography. Radiology 154:619-623, 1985.
19. Hobbs JT. Perioperative venography to ensure accurate sapheno-popliteal vein ligation. BMJ 2:1578-1580, 1980.
20. Porter JM, Moneta GL and International Consensus Committee. Reporting standards in venous disease: An update. J Vasc Surg 21(4):635-645, 1995.
21. Moneta GL, Porter JM. Varicose veins and venous ulceration: Rationale for conservative treatment. In Bergan JJ, Goldman MP, eds. Varicose Veins and Telangiectasias: Diagnosis and Treatment. St. Louis: Quality Medical Publishing, 1993.
22. Henry MEF, Fegan WG, Pegum JM. Five-year survey of the treatment of varicose ulcers. BMJ 2:493-494, 1971.

Chapter 15

Role of Sclerotherapy in Greater Saphenous Vein Incompetence

Pauline Raymond-Martimbeau

As one of the two major vessels that comprise the superficial venous system, the greater (long) saphenous vein (GSV) is particularly vulnerable to incompetence, a disorder characterized by venous reflux and dilatation. Although traditionally managed surgically, GSV incompetence also may be treated by means of sclerotherapy, a nonsurgical approach in which injection of a chemical agent into the diseased vessel induces a sterile inflammatory reaction that results in fibrosis or sclerosis, thereby permanently obliterating the vein. Ideally, the vessel is reduced in diameter and reabsorbed. The technique, which is painless and nonscarring, is performed on an outpatient basis.

This chapter gives a brief review of the history of sclerotherapy and offers guidelines for preoperative evaluation and patient selection in the treatment of GSV incompetence. Sclerotherapeutic technique is described, and a discussion of postoperative management, evaluation, and potential complications is presented.

HISTORICAL OVERVIEW

Sclerotherapy of the GSV is believed to have been introduced in 1905 by Tavel, who injected a 5% phenic acid solution into the GSV of a patient after surgical ligation. During the first quarter of the twentieth century, sclerotherapy was practiced mainly in Europe, sometimes in combination with surgical ligation. Unfortunately, sclerosants remained relatively toxic and often produced undesirable side effects. In 1928 brief trials of sclerotherapy were undertaken in the United States, primarily at the Mayo Clinic, but the results were disappointing, and physicians in the United States continued to favor surgery.

Modern sclerotherapy is based on progress made during the past 50 years. A key factor was the advent of improved chemical agents, including less toxic powerful sclerosants such as iodine sodium iodide and sodium tetradecyl sulfate. Several schools of thought evolved, each with its own technique. In the 1950s Fegan[1] and his followers recommended that the injection sequence progress from bottom to top, beginning with the most distal incompetent perforating vein. Because this technique relies heavily on postoperative bandaging and compressive therapy, it is known as compression sclerotherapy. In contrast, the French school, led by Tournay, progressively expanded the concept that treatment should begin at the highest point of reflux and proceed downward. This top-to-bottom arrangement followed the logical sequence of surgical treatment. Initially, injection was performed at the junction itself, but the danger of accidentally puncturing the deep venous or arterial systems was soon recognized. Safety was increased by moving the injection site several centimeters below the saphenofemoral junction (SFJ). Digital compression of the SFJ during injection, as proposed by Chatard[2] and studied by Cloutier,[3,4] was also an important advance.

During the past 20 years sclerotherapy has become a more exact discipline, and the results of experienced sclerotherapists now compare favorably with those of surgeons. In light of the current widespread trend toward noninvasive technology and minimally invasive techniques, sclerotherapy can be expected to gain increased popularity.

ANATOMY

On the basis of location and function, the vessels of the lower limb are divided into three main groups: (1) high-pressure deep veins, which are responsible for 90% of venous return; (2) low-pressure superficial veins, which drain blood from the skin and serve as a reservoir for blood storage; and (3) perforating veins, which link the deep and the superficial systems. In each of these groups one-way flow is normally maintained by a series of bicuspid valves that direct the blood upward and inward. When one of these valves malfunctions, venous reflux and hypertension eventually result in varicosities. This disorder primarily affects the superficial veins because, unlike the deep vessels, they have little external support.

The two major superficial veins are the GSV, which drains much of the lower limb, and the short saphenous vein (SSV), which drains mainly the calf region. The GSV arises from the internal marginal vein in the foot, courses anteriorly toward the medial malleolus, traverses the medial portion of the tibia, following its posteromedial border, and passes behind the condyle of the femur. It then crosses the sartorius and adductor longus muscles before entering the common femoral vein at Scarpa's triangle to form the SFJ (Figure 15-1). This junction is usually crescent-shaped. Blood flow through the SFJ is regulated by a constant valve, called the ostial valve, which is particularly vulnerable to malfunction (Figure 15-2). When the ostial valve is incompetent, the resulting venous reflux causes distention of the distal truncal vein; in turn, the valves of that vein become incompetent, leading to varicosity.

In a recent study of duplex ultrasonographic assessment, I found that (1) the GSV terminates in the common femoral vein at Scarpa's triangle in 91.4% of cases; (2) the SFJ is crescent-shaped in 76.2% of cases; and (3) the sapheno-

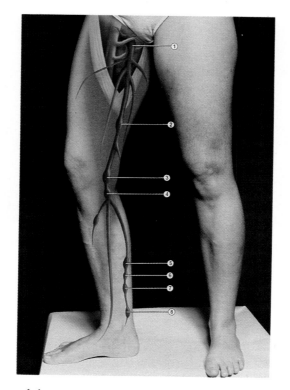

FIGURE 15-1. Anatomy of the greater saphenous vein. *1*, Saphenofemoral junction; *2*, hunterian perforator group; *3*, geniculate perforator group; *4*, Boyd perforator group; *5*, 24 cm perforating vein; *6*, Cockett III (18.5 cm); *7*, Cockett II (13.5 cm); *8*, Cockett I (6-7 cm).

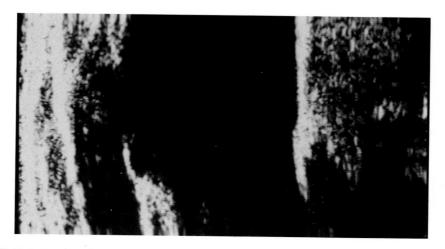

FIGURE 15-2. Duplex ultrasonographic longitudinal section shows the saphenofemoral junction as crescent-shaped. Note the presence of the ostial valve. (From Raymond-Martimbeau P, ed. Phlebologia Houston '91. Dallas: PRM Editions, 1991.)

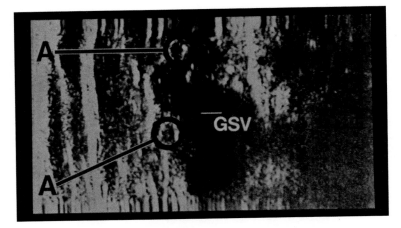

FIGURE 15-3. Duplex ultrasonographic transverse section of the greater saphenous vein *(GSV)* and the pudendal arteries *(A)*.

femoral valve can be visualized in 82.4% of cases.[5] The GSV has a single continuous trunk in 84.3% of cases, a double trunk in 12.2%, and a triple trunk in 3.5%. Two groups of tributaries, the upper and lower tributaries, enter the proximal segment of the GSV. The major upper tributaries, which enter the GSV near the fossa ovalis, are the superficial circumflex iliac vein, the superficial epigastric vein, and the external pudendal vein. The most important lower tributaries, which enter the GSV in the thigh, are the anterior accessory (anterior crural) saphenous vein and the posterior accessory (posterior crural) saphenous vein (also known as the Cruveilhier vein). Both groups of tributaries have a variable termination. Failure to recognize variations can lead to relapses after sclerotherapy or surgery. My study showed that the upper tributaries and the proximal segment of the GSV have a common termination in the common femoral vein in 8.4% of cases. The upper tributaries terminate in the GSV near the junction in 45.1% of cases and directly in the common femoral vein in 1.9% of cases. In the remaining cases the upper tributaries cannot be visualized. The termination site of the lower tributaries varies from the midaspect of the thigh to Scarpa's triangle. The Giacomini vein, an anastomotic vein that links the SSV and the GSV, enters the trunk of the GSV at variable levels, ranging from near the SFJ to the knee. If the Giacomini vein enters near the SFJ, and if it is incompetent and left untreated, it can contribute to the recurrence of GSV incompetence.

In the upper third of the leg, the main trunk is joined by the anterior arch branch and the posterior arch branch (Leonardo's vein). Arteries that lie near the GSV include the external pudendal arteries at the SFJ level (Figure 15-3) and the posterior tibial artery at the distal end of the GSV. The external pudendal arteries exhibit considerable variability in their topography.

> **TYPES OF GREATER SAPHENOUS VEIN INVOLVEMENT***
>
> SFJ only
> SFJ + tributaries
> SFJ + saphenous trunk
> SFJ + saphenous trunk + single perforating vein
> SFJ + saphenous trunk + multiple perforating veins
> Attendant perforating vein: single or multiple
> Postoperative neovascularization of GSV at SFJ
> Mixed form: SSV terminating in GSV
> Giacomini vein anastomosing SSV with GSV
>
>
> *SFJ,* Saphenofemoral junction; *GSV,* greater saphenous vein; *SSV,* short saphenous vein.
> *At any of these levels, a stasis ulcer may be present.

CLASSIFICATION

Incompetence of the GSV can originate at one or more levels (see box), at which a stasis ulcer may also be present (Figure 15-4). In my practice 64% of patients who present with GSV incompetence have reflux at the SFJ (Figures 15-5 through 15-7). In such cases control of incompetence at this level is a prerequisite for the treatment of more distal varicosities.

Alternatively, the SFJ may be functional, in which case GSV incompetence originates from valvular malfunction at any of the following levels: (1) the tributaries (Figure 15-8), (2) the GSV trunk, (3) one or more perforating veins (Figure 15-9), (4) the SSV, or (5) an anastomotic vein (Figure 15-10). Therefore GSV incompetence denotes a wide spectrum of disease, the development of which is progressive; such disease ranges from a localized telangiectasia (Figure 15-11) or varicosity (Figure 15-12) in early cases to involvement of the entire vessel in advanced cases.

SYMPTOM COMPLEX

Incompetence of the GSV generally evolves through three stages, each of which is characterized by a different main symptom. Early mild disease is often the most painful stage because it is associated with mild venous dilatation and minimal changes in the venous wall. In more advanced disease the patient usually complains of limb heaviness rather than pain. In complicated disease the overall venous return is impaired, and manifestations such as edema and cutaneous discoloration may be present. Patients report tiredness, tingling of the limb, and generalized malaise. At this stage pain may be totally absent.

Text continued on p. 274.

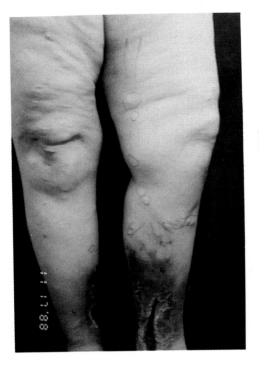

FIGURE 15-4. Bilateral saphenofemoral junction incompetence with the presence of a bilateral stasis ulcer.

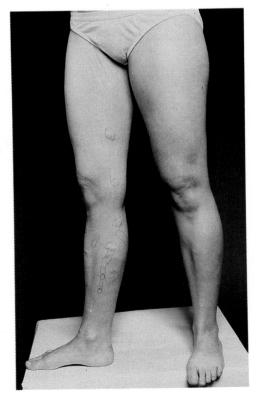

FIGURE 15-5. Saphenofemoral junction incompetence. (From Raymond-Martimbeau P, ed. Phlebologia Houston '91. Dallas: PRM Editions, 1991.)

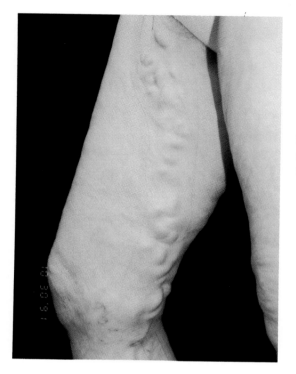

FIGURE 15-6. Saphenofemoral junction incompetence. In this case the junction is laterally located.

FIGURE 15-7. Saphenofemoral junction incompetence. Note the location of the tortuous venous dilatations in the territory of the short saphenous vein.

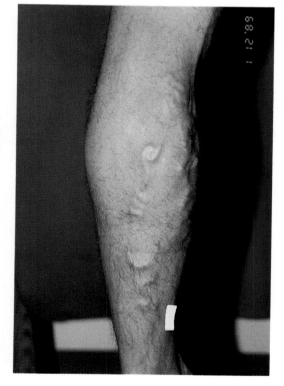

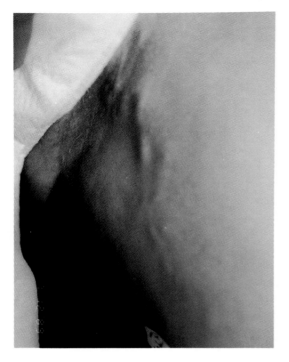

FIGURE 15-8. Incompetence of an upper tributary of the greater saphenous vein.

FIGURE 15-9. Perforating vein incompetence.

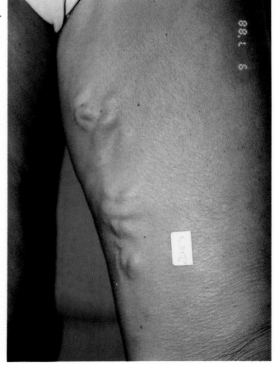

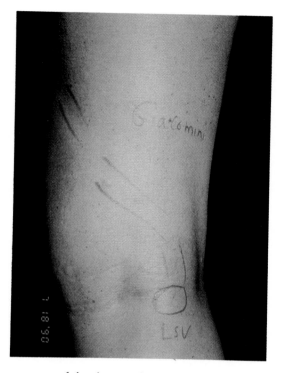

FIGURE 15-10. Incompetence of the short saphenous vein and anastomotic Giacomini vein.

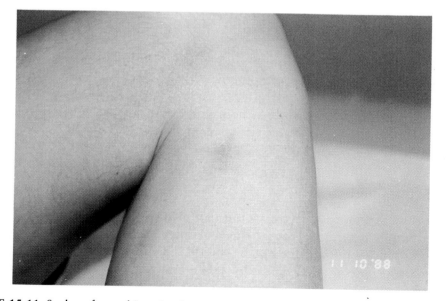

FIGURE 15-11. Saphenofemoral junction incompetence. In this case only a telangiectasia in the upper portion of the calf is visible.

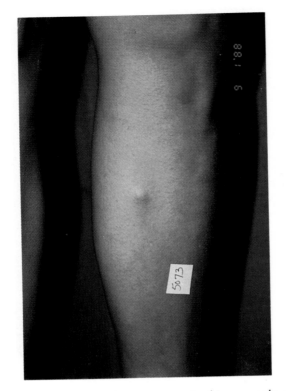

FIGURE 15-12. Saphenofemoral junction incompetence. In this case only an isolated dilatation in the midportion of the leg is visible.

PREOPERATIVE EVALUATION

Clinical examination and duplex ultrasonography are the twin cornerstones of preoperative evaluation for sclerotherapy of GSV incompetence. Although clinical assessment can yield abundant information concerning the origin and extent of disease, noninvasive studies are necessary for elucidating the topologic and morphologic aspects of the superficial veins and for ruling out disease of the deep venous system.

Clinical Examination

In each case the first step is a thorough medical and surgical history, including information regarding the patient's lifestyle, professional activities, medications, and drug allergies. Information should include whether or not the patient has ever had deep venous thrombosis. If the patient is a woman, the number of pregnancies (if any) should be noted. The type of venous symptoms should be reported so that the stage of incompetence can be ascertained. Specifying when and under what circumstances the symptoms were first noted is also important.

For the physical examination, the patient should stand on a support high

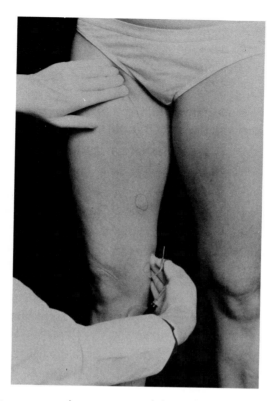

FIGURE 15-13. Schwartz maneuver in assessment of the saphenofemoral junction with the patient standing.

enough to allow the seated physician to inspect the limbs at eye level (for this purpose, I use a specially made stepped cube that measures 50 cm in height). First, the physician should determine whether the varicosities are caused by GSV or SSV incompetence or by a mixed form of incompetence. The answer is not always obvious. For evaluation of GSV incompetence, the leg should be abducted and rotated externally. The examiner should inspect the lower abdomen and the front and back of the thigh and leg. If the vein is dilated anterior to the medial malleolus, this finding can signify distention of the entire GSV trunk. The main points of reflux are identified by means of inspection, palpation, and percussion (Schwartz maneuver) (Figure 15-13). In the Schwartz maneuver pressure is applied at a downstream site to diagnose a deficiency in upstream flow; to assess SFJ competence, percussion should be applied over the point where the GSV passes posterior to the condyle of the femur, and a finger should be placed in Scarpa's triangle to detect retrograde blood flow. The patient also can be asked to cough or perform a Valsalva maneuver while the phlebologist holds a finger on the SFJ to detect a thrill and evaluate the presence of reflux. The points of reflux located with the Schwartz maneuver can always be verified clinically with the Trendelenburg maneuver and Doppler ultrasound to confirm the highest point of incompetence. Photoplethysmography may be used to assess vein function before sclero-therapy.

The SFJ also should be examined with the patient in the sitting position with the leg abducted, rotated externally, and hanging with the knee flexed. Particular care is necessary in the case of obese patients, who are relatively difficult to examine. The position described here may be useful for such patients because it facilitates exposure of Scarpa's triangle (Figure 15-14).

Duplex Scanning

Although Doppler ultrasound examination may be sufficient for evaluating uncomplicated sites of incompetence, this technique alone is inadequate for assessing an intricate SFJ or perforating veins with an indirect trajectory. Therefore duplex scanning is performed with a high-resolution, real-time, gray-scale B-mode imager equipped with a 4, 8, or 10 MHz transducer and coupled with an integrated 5 MHz pulsed Doppler probe. With the patient in reverse Trendelenburg position, the GSV and its tributaries are scanned distally and are evaluated transversely and longitudinally as necessary. Important variables include luminal and parietal diameter, venous compressibility, echogenicity, direction of blood flow,

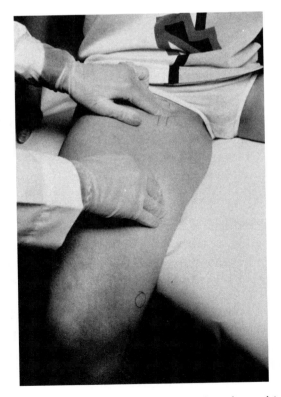

FIGURE 15-14. Schwartz maneuver in assessment of the saphenofemoral junction with the patient sitting.

and valve-leaflet motion and coaptation, particularly at the SFJ and perforator sites.

Failure to recognize variations in the termination of the upper and lower tributaries of the GSV and in the anastomotic veins to the SSV may be an important cause of relapse after sclerotherapy. The ability to pinpoint topographic and morphologic irregularities at the SFJ greatly enhances operative success. In addition, the external pudendal arteries, the common femoral vein, and the common femoral artery (all of which are subject to wide anatomic variations) must be identified to avoid puncture during sclerotherapy. Duplex scanning also has the advantage of supplying information about the perivenous tissues and extrinsic obstructing lesions.

Color-Flow Doppler Imaging

Because duplex ultrasonography is not always totally accurate, color-flow Doppler imaging and/or magnetic resonance imaging may be necessary in specific cases for clarifying equivocal findings. This method also uses duplex technology, but the Doppler signals appear as colored pixels on the B-mode scan. The color changes from red to blue, depending on whether blood is flowing toward, or away from, the transducer.

Intravenous Ultrasonography

In some cases intravenous ultrasonography with a 20 or 25 MHz transducer may be helpful to obtain even more precise data concerning the architecture of the venous wall and preoperative and postoperative venous changes (Figure 15-15).

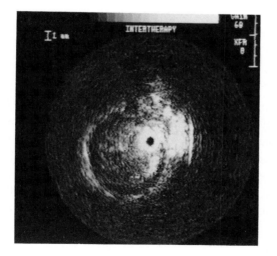

FIGURE 15-15. Intravascular ultrasonographic cross-sectional image from a segment of the greater saphenous vein after injection of iodine sodium iodide. Note the presence of intimal thickening and intimal destruction at the 12 o'clock position.

Intravenous ultrasonography yields exceptionally detailed two-dimensional, cross-sectional images of intraluminal and intramural architecture.[6,7] This approach relies on a disposable, flexible 5.1 Fr catheter containing a high-resolution 20 or 25 MHz ultrasound transducer. The catheter is introduced through either an 18-gauge needle or an introducer/dilator set with a side-arm. Conventional echographic guidance may be used to position the catheter properly within the target vein. Unlike fiberoptic venoscopy, intravenous echography can be performed in the presence of flowing blood. Because of its unique viewpoint, intravenous echography can reveal clinically important information that may be missed by extravascular methods.

Echo-Enhanced Contrast Agents

By augmenting the intensity of echographic signals, echo-enhanced contrast agents are increasing the success of ultrasonographic studies. Most of these agents contain galactose microparticles or sonicated albumin. One of the most widely used products is SHU 508 (Levovist; Schering AG, Berlin, Germany), a galactose/palmitic acid–based microbubble preparation. More than 99% of this agent's bubbles are <8 μm in diameter, and more than 50% are <2 μm in diameter.[8] The microbubbles cause a dose-dependent increase in the backscatter of ultrasound, producing harmonic echoes at twice the frequency of the transmitted signal and eliminating interference from tissue signals. The resulting B-mode or color-flow Doppler images are remarkably clutter-free.

By offering improved echographic resolution of both large and small vessels, echo-enhanced agents can image portions of veins that would otherwise not be visualizable. Because these agents increase the reflectivity of blood, they are unusually sensitive to blood flow and are able to detect low-velocity flow missed by other methods. Echoenhancement is extremely accurate at identifying points of reflux, clarifying intricate venous pathways, and detecting volume changes in nearby tissues.

PATIENT SELECTION
Indications

Sclerotherapy of the GSV is indicated for eradicating incompetent veins, which, if left untreated, can cause a series of progressively severe effects, including edema, dermatitis, and eventual ulceration (see Figure 15-4). Any patient with GSV incompetence is eligible for treatment, regardless of the patient's age or degree of reflux, unless contraindications are present. No incompetent vein should be excluded because it is deemed too large; in my experience sclerotherapy has proved successful for veins ranging from 3.5 mm to >20 mm.

Contraindications

Sclerotherapy is inappropriate for bedridden patients or others who cannot follow the necessary postoperative exercise regimen. The technique is also inappropriate for patients with infectious disease, acute septic reactions (e.g., cellulitis, abscess, and adenitis), severe arterial occlusive disease, a history of thrombophlebitis and deep venous thrombosis, pregnant women, nursing mothers, women less than 3 months postpartum, patients with severe systemic disease (including malignancy), and those with coagulopathies (protein C and protein S deficiency). Although patients with previous thrombophlebitis and previous deep venous thrombosis are not absolutely excluded, sclerotherapy should not be considered until the signs and symptoms of the disease have abated. In patients with postphlebitic varices sclerotherapy should be postponed until at least 6 months after the phlebitic reaction has stabilized. Allergic individuals require special consideration. Patients taking disulfiram (Antabuse) should not be treated with a sclerosant that contains alcohol; nor should persons with a history of tuberculosis or hyperthyroidism be treated with a sclerosant that contains iodine.[9]

SCLEROTHERAPY TECHNIQUE

Once the preoperative workup has confirmed the need for sclerotherapy, treatment may be initiated with or without ultrasonographic monitoring. Success depends on following a rational treatment plan.[10] Treatment consists of injecting a chemical irritant capable of traumatizing the endothelium. The goals are as follows: (1) to produce a sterile, inflammatory intimal reaction (Figure 15-16) that induces a thrombotic reaction, permitting the resulting thrombus to adhere to the venous wall; and (2) to induce a fibrotic reaction that permanently destroys the vein. In this manner the vein is transformed into a hard fibrotic cord through which blood can no longer circulate. This cord is then reabsorbed.

If the inflammatory reaction is excessive and affects all the layers of the tunica and surrounding tissue, the resulting thrombus may not be adherent and ascending recanalization may ensue. This chemical phlebitis may extend proximally to the point of injection, inducing widespread cutaneous hyperpigmentation (Figure 15-17).

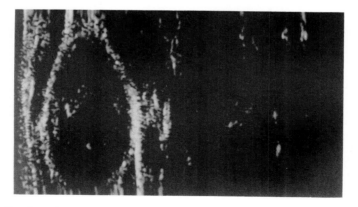

FIGURE 15-16. Duplex ultrasonographic transverse section of the incompetent greater saphenous vein shows intimal thickening.

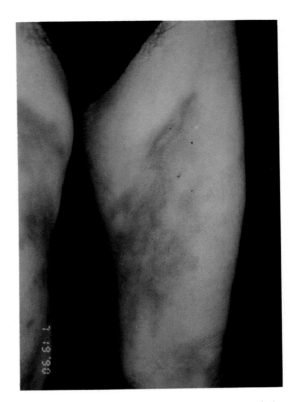

FIGURE 15-17. Permanent skin hyperpigmentation after injection of the greater saphenous vein with sodium tetradecyl sulfate.

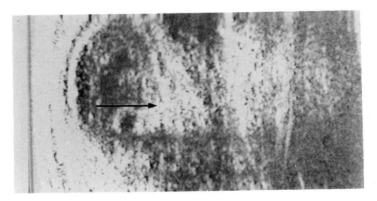

FIGURE 15-18. Duplex ultrasonographic transverse section of the greater saphenous vein after sclerotherapy. Note also the presence of incompressible adherent heterogeneous material *(arrow)* within the lumen and thickening of the intima. Note also the presence of arteries in the top portion of the vessel.

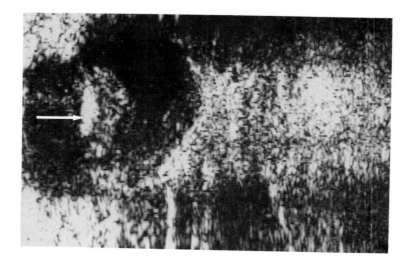

FIGURE 15-19. Duplex ultrasonographic transverse section of the greater saphenous vein shows an inappropriate sclerosing reaction: minimal intimal thickening, partial adherence of thrombus *(arrow)*, inflammatory reaction involving the surrounding tissue, and echogenic blood flow.

The stages that characterize a permanent ideal sclerosing reaction (Figure 15-18) and those that indicate a failed or inappropriate sclerosing reaction (Figure 15-19) are presented in the boxes on p. 282.

Successful sclerotherapy depends on three main factors. In order of importance they are (1) site of injection, (2) type of sclerosing agent (major rather than minor), and (3) dosage.

Failure results from injecting at a location distal to the point of reflux, attempting to treat GSV incompetence with a minor sclerosing agent, and/or giving too strong a dose of a major sclerosing agent.

Site of Injection

The injection sequence always proceeds from top to bottom, starting at the highest point of reflux and proceeding to the next highest point until the entire GSV has been sclerosed. If the highest site of incompetence is the SFJ, the junction should be treated first because complete eradication of the proximal portion of the GSV is necessary to abolish venous reflux. To prevent accidental penetration of the deep venous or arterial systems, the injection should be done several centimeters below the SFJ rather than at the junction itself (Figure 15-20). The injection sequence proceeds methodically toward the most distal incompetent perforating vein, the dosage being proportionally decreased as the site of injection progresses downward.

An exception is made for stasis ulcers and ruptured varices. When these conditions are present, the first step is to inject either at the closest point of reflux or

---

STAGES OF PERMANENT IDEAL SCLEROSING REACTION

1. Endothelial trauma
2. Endothelial thickening
3. Thrombus formation
4. Thrombus adherence to site of endothelial thickening
5. Endothelial destruction
6. Reduction of venous diameter
7. Fibrous reaction, which should stop at limits of deep venous system
8. Reabsorption of vein

STAGES OF FAILED OR INAPPROPRIATE SCLEROSING REACTION

1. Minimal endothelial trauma + premature thrombus formation
2. Adventitial thickening
3. Enlargement of venous diameter
4. Inflammatory reaction involving surrounding tissue
5. Cutaneous hyperpigmentation
6. Recanalization
7. Neovascularization (telangiectasias or reticular veins)

---

into a venous dilatation near the ulcer or ruptured varices to accelerate the healing process. In these cases proper postoperative bandaging is mandatory. The second step is to inject the highest point of reflux at a later date.

Sclerosing Agent

Sclerosing agents are classified as major, intermediate, or minor according to their strength. It is extremely important that a major sclerosing agent be selected for the treatment of GSV incompetence. Only two such agents are appropriate: iodine sodium iodide (ISI) and sodium tetradecyl sulfate (STS) (see box on p. 284). The others are either too toxic or too weak.

It might be erroneously assumed that the use of a weaker sclerosant would provide an extra margin of safety. If administered in this setting, however, a minor agent would be swept away by the bloodstream before the desired local endothelial reaction could occur. The result would be distal sclerosis characterized by a nonadherent thrombus, which could lead to deep venous thrombosis. Use of

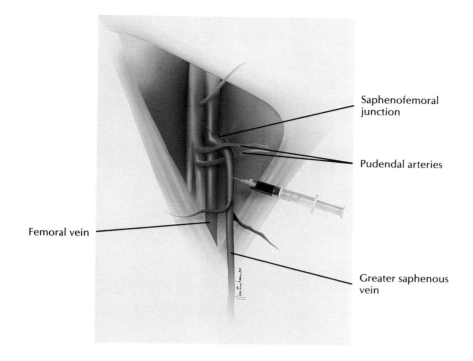

Saphenofemoral
junction

Pudendal arteries

Femoral vein

Greater saphenous
vein

FIGURE 15-20. Injection of the sclerosing agent is done below the saphenofemoral junction and away from the external pudendal arteries. (From Raymond-Martimbeau P, ed. Phlebologia Houston '91. Dallas: PRM Editions, 1991.)

a major sclerosant is crucial in order to produce an immediate local inflammatory reaction.

ISI is a chemical irritant that has both a strong sclerosing action and a low diffusing power. Because it is lighter than blood, it is not readily swept away from the injection site. It also has the advantage of producing pain with extravascular or intra-arterial injection, thereby immediately alerting the practitioner to these complications.

STS is a detergent irritant that has a strong sclerosing action and a high diffusing power; because it is heavier than blood, it is easily swept away from the injection site. It produces slight pain with intra-arterial injection but does not cause pain with extravascular injection. Therefore sodium salicylate should be added to STS so that it will produce pain when injected extravascularly.

Dosage

The dosage depends primarily on the site of injection, not solely on the size of the vein. It is important to follow a strict protocol and not be influenced by a

MAJOR AGENTS USED WORLDWIDE FOR SCLEROSING GREATER SAPHENOUS VEIN

Iodine, Sodium or Potassium Iodide

France: Iodo-iodurée solution 1% to 3% (Meram Laboratory, Paris)
Switzerland: Variglobin* 2%, 4%, 8%, 12% (Globopharm SA, Zurich)
Canada: Sclerodine 6% (Omega Laboratories, Montreal, Quebec)
U.S.A.:   Iodine crystals USP, sodium iodide granules USP, and potassium iodide granules USP (Fisher Scientific Company, Fair Lawn, N.J.)

Sodium Tetradecyl Sulfate

France: Trombovar 1%, 3%, 5% (Promedica, France)
Canada: Thromboject 1%, 3% (Omega Laboratories, Montreal, Quebec)
U.S.A.:   Sotredecol 1%, 3% (Elkins-Sinn, Cherry Hill, N.J.)

*Variglobin 2%, 4%, 8%, 12% is equivalent to Sclerodine and Iodo-iodurée solution 1%, 2%, 4%, 6%.

large venous diameter. Ironically, it may take a larger dose to sclerose a small tubular GSV than a large GSV. The more endothelial damage, the easier it is to achieve sclerosis. If a large dose is injected into a large vein, the stages of sclerosing action may not occur methodically and the risk of deep venous thrombosis is increased. It is important to prepare the intima with a relatively low dose to ensure that satisfactory intimal thickening takes place before thrombus formation occurs.

For this treatment the physician may use either a commercial preparation of 1% to 6% ISI diluted with 0.9% sodium chloride or sterile water or a preparation of 1% to 5% STS. I do not consider volume to be the most important parameter. If the dose needs to be augmented to enhance the sclerosing power, it is better to increase the concentration, not the volume. The target is focused, and the action needs to be as local as possible; therefore increasing the volume may not greatly affect the sclerosing capability. If too large a volume of sclerosing agent is injected, the extra amount may be swept into the deep system or to distal incompetent points, where the reaction would be excessive.

SCLEROTHERAPY FOR SAPHENOFEMORAL JUNCTION INCOMPETENCE

If incompetence is isolated at the SFJ only and does not produce symptoms, the sclerotherapist should observe the progression of the disease and postpone treatment. If the incompetence produces signs and symptoms, the vein may be injected; however, care must be used because the injection must be given almost at the junction itself. As mentioned earlier, the danger of accidentally entering the ar-

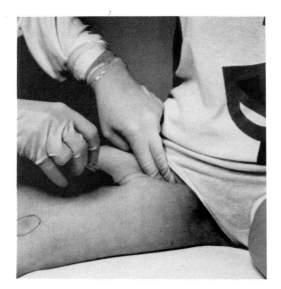

FIGURE 15-21. Injection of the incompetent saphenofemoral junction done with the patient sitting.

terial or deep venous system is great because the relationship between the common femoral vein and the common femoral artery is variable; moreover, the number and size of the pudendal arteries are variable (the inferior pudendal artery overlaps or crosses the arch of the GSV at, or close to, the SFJ). In cases in which the incompetence is isolated at the SFJ and the reflux is mild or nonexistent, the physician should start with a low dose (1 ml of 2% ISI or STS); if sclerosis does not occur, the concentration should then be increased sequentially (e.g., to 1 ml of a 3% solution or 1 ml of a 4% solution).

If incompetence involves more than the junction itself, treatment is performed with the patient either standing or sitting. I have found that the standing position is associated with more extensive occlusion and a greater reduction in venous caliber, as well as less postoperative inflammation and pigmentation.[11] Moreover, surprisingly fewer vagal reactions seem to occur when the patient is standing.

Different Positions for Injection

If the sitting position (Figure 15-21) is chosen, the sclerotherapist remains standing while the patient is seated on the examining table with his or her leg abducted, rotated externally, and hanging with the knee flexed. The patient's leg must be very relaxed. The injection is administered 5 to 9 cm below the SFJ with a disposable standard 25-gauge, ⅝-inch needle and a 3 ml disposable plastic syringe. Digital pressure is applied at the SFJ with the nondominant hand and is maintained for several minutes after the injection has been completed. Such pressure may be applied by an assistant (but never by the patient) in order to free the

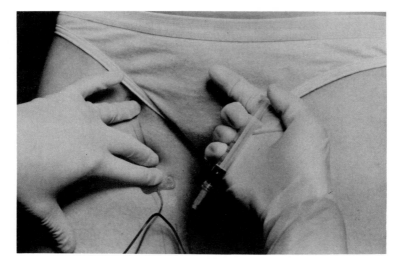

FIGURE 15-22. Injection of the incompetent saphenofemoral junction done with the patient standing. Digital pressure is applied at the junction with the annular finger of the nondominant hand. (From Raymond-Martimbeau P, ed. Phlebologia Houston '91. Dallas: PRM Editions, 1991.)

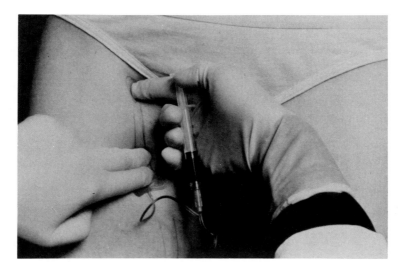

FIGURE 15-23. Injection of the incompetent saphenofemoral junction with the patient standing. With the index finger of the dominant hand, digital pressure is applied at the junction.

sclerotherapist's nondominant hand to secure the needle at the injection site and to ascertain its stability.

If the standing position (Figures 15-22 and 15-23) is preferred, the patient stands on a platform with the leg abducted and rotated externally and the knee unflexed. The patient should stand perfectly still, without bending, and should look straight ahead. The patient should not touch anything because doing so may cause movement during the puncture. To ensure stability of position, the patient should apply weight to the leg to be injected. The sclerotherapist should be seated, with his or her leg and elbow secured to prevent unwanted motion during injection. The sclerotherapist should not explain or discuss the technique at this point because doing so may increase the patient's apprehension and thereby increase the likelihood of a vasovagal reaction. The injection is administered 4 to 7 cm below the SFJ with a disposable 25-gauge, ¾-inch butterfly needle with 12 inches of tubing and a 3 ml plastic disposable syringe. Digital pressure is applied in two places: (1) at the junction with either the annular finger of the nondominant hand (see Figure 15-22) or the index finger of the dominant hand (see Figure 15-23) and (2) below the site of injection with the third finger of the nondominant hand to cause sequestration and empty the vein as much as possible, thereby allowing maximal endothelial contact with the sclerosing agent. Pressure at the junction is maintained throughout the injection and is continued for a few minutes afterward; the distal pressure is released as soon as the injection is completed.

Injection Technique

In either position, before injection the syringe should be examined for air, which reduces the degree of negative pressure and interferes with aspiration of blood. Once the depth and precise location of the injection site have been confirmed by means of a percussion maneuver or duplex ultrasound, alcohol is applied and the vein is punctured briskly. The needle is generally aimed toward the torso, in the direction of the SFJ. With the patient in the standing position, the butterfly needle permits better manipulation of the syringe, allows the syringe to be oriented with the plunger facing upward, and facilitates examination of aspirated blood. When the patient is standing, ISI is preferable to STS. Because STS is heavier than blood, it tends to diffuse distally, leaving the proximal segment of the GSV unchanged.

Aspiration of a small amount of venous blood confirms proper needle placement (unfortunately, the darkness of the iodine agent may be a disadvantage for the inexperienced sclerotherapist). The appearance of pulsatile or bright-red blood suggests that the needle has entered an artery and is an indication for immediate cessation. If the return of venous blood is not obvious, or if there is any doubt about the return, the injection should be stopped.

The injection involves three steps: (1) injecting half of the dose very slowly, (2) reaspirating the blood to confirm correct needle positioning, and (3) injecting the second half of the dose quickly to prevent spasm of the vessel, which will already be reacting to the sclerosant. The patient should be instructed to report any pain during injection because such pain can herald a serious complication. Applying digital pressure at the SFJ when injecting below the junction prevents the sclerosant from dispersing into the deep venous system and increases the local reaction.

Whichever position is used, as soon as the injection is finished, the patient should lie down while the sclerotherapist maintains digital pressure at the SFJ. The limb then is elevated to ensure optimal exposure of the SFJ to the sclerosing agent.

A selective noncircumferential compressive dressing is placed over the SFJ and should extend a few centimeters below the injection site; the dressing is left in place for 48 hours. A light compressive stocking may be applied. For daywear only, I use an 18 to 22 mm Hg pressure-gradient stocking for progressive stage II disease, since injecting the highest point of reflux should lower pressure distally. For progressive stage I or III disease, I use a class 1 or 2 stocking or an elastic bandage because the sclerosing reaction may be increased in these stages.

Injection Protocol

The injection protocols for ISI and STS are described in Tables 15-1 and 15-2, respectively. The protocol for ISI is similar to that reported and described by Cloutier.[3,4] Protocols for STS other than the one described here have been advocated by other authors.[12] Some experts have proposed an accelerated protocol in which the initial treatment comprises multiple injections of a major sclerosing agent into different sites of reflux.[9]

SEQUENTIAL SCLEROTHERAPY FOR OTHER AREAS OF INCOMPETENCE

After the highest point of reflux has been sclerosed flush with the common femoral vein, sclerotherapy of distal points can be started in a top-to-bottom sequential manner (Table 15-3). The injection is given at the site where the previous sclerosis stopped in the GSV. It is better to obtain a short but firm sclerosis than a long, weak one.

Perineal Veins or Tributaries

When left untreated, perineal vein and upper tributary incompetence (see Figure 15-8) often leads to recurrent GSV incompetence. These veins are "sclerosensible" and require 0.5 to 0.75 ml of 0.5% to 1% STS.

Saphenous Trunk at Thigh Level

If the next highest point of incompetence is the saphenous trunk in the upper or middle third of the thigh, 1 ml of 3% ISI or STS should be injected at the lim-

TABLE 15-1. Schedule and dosage of iodine sodium iodide (Sclerodine) injections for treating GSV incompetence secondary to SFJ malfunction*

Visit	Dosage	Site
1	2 ml at 3% concentration	Below SFJ
2	2 ml at 4% concentration	Below SFJ
3	2 ml at 6% concentration	Below SFJ
4	2 ml at 6% concentration 1 ml at 3% concentration	Below SFJ Midthigh level
5	2 ml at 6% concentration 1 ml at 3% concentration 1 ml at 2% concentration	Below SFJ Midthigh level Knee level

GSV, Greater saphenous vein; SFJ, saphenofemoral junction.
*Data from Raymond-Martimbeau P. Two different techniques for sclerosing the incompetent saphenofemoral junction: A comparative study. J Dermatol Surg Oncol 16:626-631, 1990.

TABLE 15-2. Schedule and dosage of sodium tetradecyl sulfate injections for treating GSV incompetence secondary to SFJ malfunction

Visit	Dosage	Site
1	2 ml at 2% concentration	Below SFJ
2	2 ml at 3% concentration	Below SFJ
3	2 ml at 4% concentration OR 2 ml at 3% concentration 1 ml at 3% concentration	Below SFJ Below SFJ Midthigh level
4	2 ml at 5% concentration OR 2 ml at 3% concentration 1 ml at 3% concentration 1 ml at 2% concentration	Below SFJ Below SFJ Midthigh level Knee level

GSV, Greater saphenous vein; SFJ, saphenofemoral junction.

TABLE 15-3. Top-to-bottom sequential sclerotherapy for points of incompetence other than SFJ: Initial treatment with iodine, sodium iodide, or sodium tetradecyl sulfate*

Location	Concentration (%)	Volume (ml)
Perineal veins and tributaries	0.5-1	0.5-0.75
Saphenous trunk		
Upper or midthigh	3	1
Lower thigh	2	1
Perforating veins		
Thigh	3	1
Knee	1-2	1
Upper leg	1-1.5	1
Lower leg	1	0.5

SFJ, Saphenofemoral junction.
*If the SFJ is competent or sclerosed, these sites should be treated in sequence.

its of sclerosis and permeability; if that point is in the lower third of the thigh, 1 ml of a 2% major sclerosing agent should be used.

Perforating Veins

If the highest point of incompetence is located in a GSV-related perforator, the injection sequence should proceed methodically toward the most proximal incompetent perforating vein, with the dosage being decreased proportionally as the site of injection progresses downward.

Van Limborg and Hage[13] detailed the topography of 142 perforating veins of the leg, including 49 in the foot, 44 in the lower leg, 13 at knee level, and 36 in the thigh. However, few such veins are constant. In the upper thigh a perforator sometimes is found that causes significant dilatation and reflux (see Figure 15-9). In the midthigh the Dodd or hunterian perforators (see Figure 15-1), at the site of Hunter's canal, range from six to eight in number; as the longest perforating veins, they are often indirect and may cause significant reflux. When these thigh-level perforators are incompetent, 1 ml of a 3% major sclerosing agent should be injected as initial treatment.

At knee level the geniculate group of perforating veins (Figure 15-24) causes a milder degree of reflux. Therefore a lower dosage is necessary for treatment at this site; 1 ml of 1% or 2% STS is normally sufficient for initiating sclerosis.

In the upper leg the Boyd group of perforating veins (see Figure 15-1) causes a moderate degree of reflux and requires 1 ml of 1.0% to 1.5% STS. In the lower leg the perforators of the Cockett group comprise three to four veins located on the posterior branch of the GSV (called Leonardo's vein), along a vertical line depicted by Linton (see Figure 15-1). When incompetent, these perforators are very

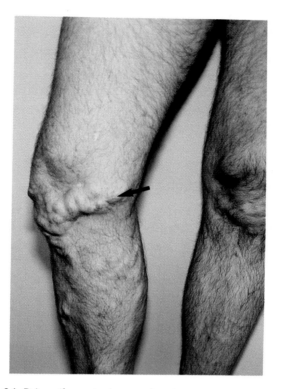

FIGURE 15-24. Primarily geniculate perforating vein incompetence *(arrow)*.

noxious to cutaneous structures and are frequently responsible for trophic problems and stasis ulcers. They are often involved in postphlebitic and posttraumatic varices, and the degree of reflux can be severe in these cases. Because these veins have a short trajectory and are located distally, they should be sclerosed with caution. Injection of 0.5 ml of a 1% major sclerosing agent should be sufficient for the initial treatment.

Occasionally, the highest point of incompetence is in small (0.5 to 2 mm) unexpected perforators not obvious on clinical or Doppler ultrasound examination. Such perforators must always be sought because they can be present all along the GSV pathway and can cause significant reflux, resulting in medium-sized distal varicosities. Eradication of these perforators is essential to ensure a successful outcome with a decreased risk of complications. Injection of 1 ml of 1.0% STS is needed to sclerose these small perforators.

I treat incompetent perforating veins by injecting the sclerosing agent into their trajectory at a 90-degree angle; small ones are injected with the patient in the standing position. This controversial approach depends on satisfactory duplex ultrasonographic monitoring and occasionally duplex guidance.

After sclerosing incompetent perforator sites, I routinely apply selective noncircumferential compressive dressings for 24 to 48 hours; this compression regimen is similar to that used after SFJ injection.

Mixed Incompetence

The termination point of the SSV varies considerably. When the SSV terminates in the GSV and becomes incompetent (Figure 15-25), eradication of the SSV is imperative to obtain permanent sclerosis of the GSV to prevent recurrence.

When an anastomotic vein (especially the Giacomini vein) (see Figure 15-10) is incompetent, eradication or permanent obliteration of this vein is essential to reduce the recurrence rate.

Postoperative Neovascularization

The highest point of incompetence may be located in vessels formed by neovascularization at the SFJ. Occlusion of these vessels is necessary to stop disease progression. These vessels are not easy to enter with a needle because they have a very thin, soft wall and do not normally cause a severe degree of reflux. Puncture should be brisk to allow intraluminal, rather than extravascular, injection. Normally, 1 ml of 1% to 3% STS is necessary. Preinjection duplex ultrasonographic monitoring is essential in these cases because vessels formed by neovascularization

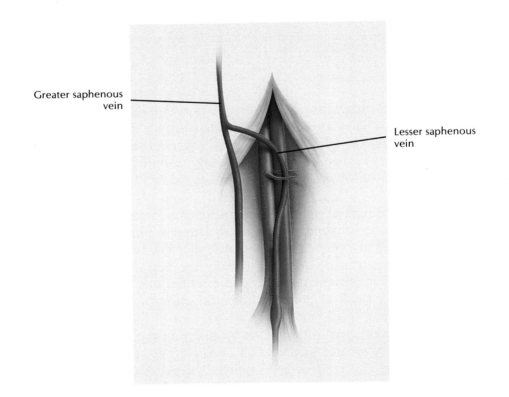

Greater saphenous vein

Lesser saphenous vein

FIGURE 15-25. Termination of the short saphenous vein in the greater saphenous vein. (From Raymond-Martimbeau P, ed. Phlebologia Houston '91. Dallas: PRM Editions, 1991.)

often have an anarchic presentation and are surrounded by small or medium-sized arteries.

When a major sclerosant is injected in top-to-bottom fashion, a minimal number of injections and therapeutic sessions is needed for permanent obliteration of the GSV and few adverse reactions occur. Injecting the sites of origin according to a proper technique and protocol is often sufficient to make tortuous distal visible varicosities disappear.

ECHO-GUIDED SCLEROTHERAPY

In selected cases echography may be used to guide the injection and assess the vein's immediate response[14-17] (Figure 15-26). Instead of being a new sclerotherapy technique, echo-guided sclerotherapy (EGS) is a treatment modality that increases the precision of sclerotherapeutic injection. It is especially valuable for the SFJ and the saphenopopliteal junction. This method is helpful for treating perforating veins, recurrent varicosities, and dilated veins associated with severe ulcerations. It can also facilitate the treatment of obese patients and those with previous varicose vein operations, in whom a sclerosant might otherwise be hard to administer.

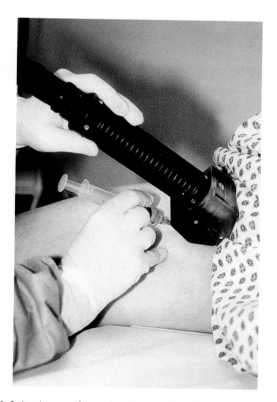

FIGURE 15-26. Injection performed with the aid of ultrasonographic equipment.

Echography may be performed with duplex ultrasonography, color-flow Doppler imaging, or intravenous ultrasonography. It may be instituted at the beginning of the procedure, to guide the physician to the target vein and monitor the injection. Alternatively, echography may be instituted after the vein is punctured, to confirm that the needle is in the correct place.

Shortly after a successful injection, echography should show spasm of the target vein, followed by blurring of the vessel as the sclerosing reaction progresses.[16] Ideally, the vein should undergo the stages listed in the box at the top of p. 282 rather than those listed in the box below it. On the duplex display an unsuccessful response is indicated by mobile echoes around or within the intraluminal material. Signs of an inadequate response include an enlarged luminal diameter, minimal parietal changes, partial venous compressibility, echogenic blood flow, a lumen partially filled with echogenic material, and increased echogenicity of the surrounding tissue.[18] These signs indicate that the treatment plan should be adjusted or that further injections are necessary.

The success of EGS may be increased with the use of echo-enhanced contrast agents. Echographic guidance may also be simplified by two new techniques that improve needle visualization. In one technique (SMART Needle; CardioVascular Dynamics, Inc., Irvine, Calif.), visualization is enhanced by a Doppler probe incorporated in the tip of the needle.[19] The probe is used to guide the needle toward the target vein or confirm proper positioning within the vessel. In the other ap-

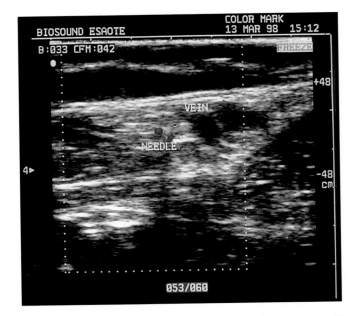

FIGURE 15-27. The ColorMark needle with duplex ultrasound equipment. (Courtesy EchoCath, Princeton, N.J.)

proach (The ColorMark System; EchoCath, Princeton, N.J.) (Figure 15-27), the needle's location is indicated by a colorful line generated by piezoelectrically induced flexural waves.[20]

By permitting direct visualization of the diseased vein, EGS prevents accidental extravascular, intra-arterial, or deep venous injection. Therefore the minimal effective dose of sclerosant can be given safely and accurately. Because EGS offers no benefit in easy cases, it is used only when the anatomy is so complex that the diseased vein(s) would otherwise be unapproachable. EGS is no substitute for proper sclerotherapeutic training, practice, and experience. Injecting a sclerosant with the aid of echography is a challenging process that should be undertaken only by experts in both sclerotherapy and echography. In a few extremely rare cases intra-arterial injection has occurred even with echographic guidance.[21] When used appropriately by a skilled sclerotherapist, however, EGS is a useful injection modality. Because it enhances the safety and efficacy of sclerotherapy in difficult or high-risk cases, it makes such therapy available to many patients who might otherwise need varicose vein surgery.

POSTOPERATIVE MANAGEMENT
Compression Therapy

One of the most widely held tenets of sclerotherapy is that treatment of a large vein such as the GSV can occur only if the vessel remains compressed for several weeks postoperatively so that the lumen is reduced as much as possible. Some experts recommend that the compressive bandage remain in place for 3 weeks, after which the patient returns to the physician for follow-up examination and rebandaging.[22] During this period the bandage should not be loosened or removed. Moreover, the patient should avoid any activities that might promote venous distention (i.e., hot baths, saunas, or exercises involving increased abdominal pressure).

I do not routinely use this regimen for the following reason: if the treatment is successful (i.e., the injection is performed at the highest point of reflux according to proper protocol, as described earlier, and closure of this point allows normalization of the distal pressure), the compromise of venous return caused by the use of strong compression might actually undermine the treatment. Therefore I use compression therapy discriminatingly, prescribing light elastic support in most cases and strong compression for patients in whom the degree of immediate operative success is uncertain (i.e., those who have pain during the immediate [<5 minutes] postinjection period).

Ambulation

Postoperative ambulation is critical for preventing venous congestion. The patient should exercise after sclerotherapy. Walking, bicycling, and swimming are recommended, but high-impact activities are inadvisable.

COMPLICATIONS

Sclerotherapy of the GSV results in a minimum of complications, which may be classified as major or minor, depending on their severity.[23-25] Because these complications and their treatment are described elsewhere in this book, they will not be discussed here.

POSTOPERATIVE EVALUATION

Follow-up visits are mandatory to assess treatment results, and duplex ultrasonography is especially important to evaluate venous changes. Within several days of injection, the vein should have been converted into a thin, irregular cord. The goal of therapy is thorough fibrosis, evidenced by a markedly reduced luminal diameter, a thickened intima, and an incompressible lumen that contains a dense echogenic heterogeneous material.

Excessive thrombosis is the most frequent cause of recanalization after sclerotherapy. If postoperative scanning yields images of superficial thrombophlebitis (i.e., enlarged venous diameter, partial compressibility, and slight parietal changes, as well as intraluminal blood flow and only partial luminal filling with an echogenic material), the patient should be evaluated for proximal reflux and further treatment will be necessary. In such cases the type and dosage of sclerosant may need to be adjusted.

Recanalization and recurrence also can be caused by failure to recognize anatomic variants involving the SFJ or SSV termination. In some cases recurrence is the result of an incompetent parietal valve within the common femoral vein.

Experience has shown that certain patients (i.e., those with a light complexion, blond hair, and blue eyes) are more "sclerosable" than others and that some veins (i.e., superficial) are more amenable to sclerotherapy than others. Surprisingly, the likelihood of a successful outcome appears to be inversely related to the degree of preoperative venous dilatation. Small-diameter tubular veins with a relatively intact endothelium are more difficult to sclerose than large-diameter vessels with thin, diseased walls.

If occlusion has not been induced after the initial injection, the patient is treated according to the injection protocols described in Tables 15-1 and 15-2. Treatment sessions are spaced at intervals of between 7 and 21 days.

In some cases lack of control in recurrence is not the result of inadequate treatment but is related to an uncontrollable cause, such as heredity or persistent aggravating factors. When sclerotherapy alone fails to relieve GSV incompetence, the patient may benefit from surgery or a combined approach. Neither surgery nor sclerotherapy, however, can cure the underlying venous disease, which is progressive in character. Therefore follow-up visits are important to control further disease progression. When treatment has been completed, the patient is seen for clinical follow-up assessments at 3-, 6-, and 12-month intervals and yearly afterward.

DISCUSSION

Until recently, surgical ligation and stripping of the incompetent GSV has been the primary therapeutic approach. Because distal dilatations of the GSV may be tortuous and not easily accessible for stripping, multiple incisions are necessary. Potential complications include deep vein thrombosis and pulmonary embolization, arterial hemorrhage, and lymphatic disorders, as well as postoperative hematomas, paresthesias, infection, and scar formation. Occasionally the femoral artery or vein is erroneously ligated or stripped; arterial involvement of this type can necessitate amputation. Surgical relapses may be caused by incomplete crossectomy or inaccessibility of indirect multitruncal perforating veins.

As a safe, painless, and highly effective outpatient procedure, sclerotherapy is an attractive alternative to surgical treatment of varicose veins. Unfortunately, many physicians are skeptical about sclerotherapy. They may have heard of poor results obtained with early sclerosing agents or without the use of a strict protocol, or they may have tried sclerotherapy haphazardly in a few cases, with unimpressive results, and then blamed the method for their own lack of proficiency. Critics may not realize that, during the past two decades, sclerotherapy has been transformed into a less empirical, more exact science. This transformation has been the result of improved technique and increased understanding of the mechanism of action of sclerosing agents, as well as a more rigid adherence to sound protocols. Moreover, the advent of high-technology diagnostic modalities such as duplex scanning has permitted better patient selection and assessment of injection sites, as well as the detection of early recanalization. Evolving experience has shown that practitioners can lower the incidence of adverse effects and/or recurrence by modifying their protocols.

Reported clinical experience in thousands of cases indicates that sclerotherapy of the GSV is well tolerated and that the injection of a major sclerosing agent yields a successful outcome in 85% to 90% of cases.[4,11,26] The precise mechanism of various sclerosing agents has not yet been clarified, but these agents all disrupt vascular endothelium, by means of cellular dehydration, maceration of intracellular cement, or direct destruction. In a recent prospective study regarding the effects of sclerotherapy on blood coagulation, injection of various doses of ISI (Sclerodine) into 26 consecutive patients with lower-extremity varicosities produced no evidence of activation of blood coagulation.[27] With procedures performed under optimal biologic conditions, this study has helped allay the fear that sclerotherapy could promote systemic fibrin formation.

Most risks and iatrogenic complications of sclerotherapy can be prevented with proper preoperative assessment, intraoperative technique and protocol, and postoperative care: intra-arterial injection can be averted with preoperative duplex ultrasonography; cutaneous necrosis secondary to extravascular injection can be avoided with proper technique; phlebitis and residual pigmentation caused by overdosage can be minimized by following a sound protocol; and deep venous thrombosis resulting from incorrect dosage and/or site of injection can also be prevented with a suitable protocol.

From the patient's viewpoint, sclerotherapy is obviously the treatment of choice, and many patients simply refuse to undergo varicose vein surgery. In addition to being painless and nonscarring, sclerotherapy eliminates the need for hospitalization, general anesthesia, and intense postoperative care. The patient can return to work immediately after treatment, which has economic benefits. Furthermore, a sclerosant can be used to treat hard-to-reach vessels (e.g., perforating veins with intricate trajectories) that would be unapproachable by a scalpel. Nevertheless, surgery and sclerotherapy are not opposed to each other but are complementary therapeutic options that may be combined in selected cases.

Whichever method is used, early and late success rates are subject to many variables, including patient age, vein size, location (proximal vs. distal), and severity and complexity of the disease. Operator experience is also a crucial factor. Moreover, in discussing optimal treatments, experts tend to underestimate the complexity of the population at risk. Ultimately, the value of different therapeutic modalities can be assessed only on the basis of prospective randomized studies in which patients are stratified according to similar disease states.

In the treatment of GSV incompetence, sclerotherapy at the SFJ is a particularly challenging procedure that remains highly controversial and is practiced by only a small number of experts. In a 6-year follow-up study, I have shown that the success rate of this procedure approaches 90% for experienced physicians.[18] Injection of the SFJ requires not only extensive sclerotherapeutic skill but also an excellent background in duplex scanning technique. Physicians who lack these qualifications are ill advised to perform sclerotherapy at this site. Before attempting the procedure, practitioners should honestly assess their capabilities. They also must realistically assess the demands of their practices to determine whether the procedure can be performed frequently enough to attain the required skill.

CONCLUSION

Sclerotherapy can be viewed as a forerunner of the minimally invasive techniques that are currently revolutionizing surgical practice. In the management of GSV incompetence, injection of the SFJ is a valuable adjunct. The technique seems well tolerated by patients, and complications are minimal when a strict protocol is followed. If sclerotherapy fails, surgery or a combined therapeutic regimen is indicated.

REFERENCES

1. Fegan G. Varicose Veins. London: William Heinemann Medical Books, 1967.
2. Chatard H. Thérapeutique. In Bassi G, ed. Les Varices des Membres Inférieurs. Paris: Doin, 1967, p 353.
3. Cloutier G. La sclérose des crosses des saphènes internes et externes; nouvelle approche. Phlebologie 29:227-232, 1976.
4. Cloutier G. La sclérose des crosses des saphènes internes et externes avec compression. Résultats. Phlebologie 33:731-735, 1980.

5. Raymond-Martimbeau P. Duplex ultrasonography assessment of anatomical variations as a guide to sclerotherapy. In Raymond-Martimbeau P, ed. Phlebologia Houston '91. Dallas: PRM Editions, 1991, pp 48-55.
6. Raymond-Martimbeau P. Echographie endovasculaire. J Mal Vasc 17:123-126, 1992.
7. Raymond-Martimbeau P. Intravenous ultrasound in the management of varicose veins. In Negus D, et al., eds. Phlebology '95. Phlebology (Suppl) 1:326-329, 1995.
8. Goldberg BB, Liu JB, Burns PN, Merton DA, Forsberg F. Galactose-based intravenous sonographic contrast agent: Experimental studies. J Ultrasound Med 12:463-470, 1993.
9. Vin F, Schadeck M. La Maladie Veineuse Superficielle. Paris: Masson, 1991.
10. Wallois P. The conditions necessary to achieve an effective sclerosant treatment. Phlebologie 35:337-348, 1982.
11. Raymond-Martimbeau P. Two different techniques for sclerosing the incompetent saphenofemoral junction: A comparative study. J Dermatol Surg Oncol 16:626-631, 1990.
12. Schadeck M. Sclerotherapy of the great saphenous vein. In Raymond-Martimbeau P, ed. Phlebologia Houston '91. Dallas: PRM Editions, 1991, pp 245-249.
13. Van Limborg J, Hage RW. L'anatomie systémique des veines perforantes de la jambe, en particulier des veines de Cockett. Phlebologie 35:19-28, 1982.
14. Schadeck M. Ultrasound guided sclerotherapy. In Schadeck M, ed. Duplex and Phlebology. Napoli: Ed. Gnocchi, 1994, pp 115-128.
15. Kanter AH, Thibault PK. Ultrasound-directed sclerotherapy for junctional incompetence: Follow-up at two years [abstract]. Dermatol Surg 21:91, 1995.
16. Thibault PK, Lewis WA. Recurrent varicose veins. Part 2. Injection of incompetent perforating veins using ultrasound guidance. J Dermatol Surg Oncol 18:895-900, 1992.
17. Raymond-Martimbeau P. Echo-guided sclerotherapy. Phlebol Digest, Jan. 1997.
18. Raymond-Martimbeau P. The role of duplex ultrasound in the sclerotherapy of varicose veins. Phlebol Digest, 1994, pp 4-10.
19. Vucevic M, Tehan B, Gamlin F, Berridge JC, Boylan M. The SMART needle. A new Doppler ultrasound–guided vascular access needle. Anaesthesia 49:889-891, 1994.
20. Kurohiji T. Motion marking in colour Doppler ultrasound needle and catheter visualization. J Ultrasound Med 9:243-245, 1990.
21. Biegeleisen K, Neilsen RD, O'Shaughnessy A. Inadvertent intra-arterial injection complicating ordinary and ultrasound-guided sclerotherapy. J Dermatol Surg Oncol 19:953-958, 1993.
22. Browse NL, Burnand KG, Lea TM. Diseases of the Veins. London: Edward Arnold, 1988.
23. Raymond-Martimbeau P. Complications of sclerotherapy. In Raymond-Martimbeau P, ed. Phlebologia Houston '91. Dallas: PRM Editions, 1991, pp 269-274.
24. Goldman MP. Sclerotherapy: Treatment of Varicose and Telangiectatic Leg Veins. St. Louis: Mosby, 1995.
25. Bernard R. Emergency measures. In Raymond-Martimbeau P, ed. Phlebologia Houston '91. Dallas: PRM Editions, 1991, pp 286-287.
26. Cloutier G, Zummo M. La sclérose des crosses avec compression. Résultats à long terme. Phlebologie 39:145-148, 1986.
27. Raymond-Martimbeau P. Effects of sclerotherapy on blood coagulation: A prospective study [abstract]. J Dermatol Surg Oncol 17:91, 1991.

Chapter 16

Complications and Adverse Sequelae of Sclerotherapy*

Mitchel P. Goldman

As with any therapeutic technique, sclerotherapy carries with it a number of potential adverse sequelae and complications. Fairly common, and often self-limiting, side effects include cutaneous pigmentation, edema of the injected extremity, a flare of new telangiectasias, pain with injection of certain sclerosing solutions, localized urticaria over injected sites, blisters or folliculitis caused by postsclerosis compression, and recurrence of previously treated vessels. Relatively rare complications include localized cutaneous necrosis, systemic allergic reactions, thrombophlebitis of the injected vessel, arterial injection with resultant distal necrosis, and deep vein thrombosis (DVT), which may result in chronic venous insufficiency or pulmonary emboli and nerve damage. This chapter addresses the pathophysiology of these reactions, methods for reducing their incidence, and treatment of their occurrence.

ADVERSE SEQUELAE
Postsclerotherapy Hyperpigmentation

To some degree cutaneous pigmentation is a relatively common occurrence after sclerotherapy with any sclerosing solution. This complication has been reported in 11% to 80% of patients treated with sodium tetradecyl sulfate (STS).[1-3] One study found that a 0.1% concentration of STS produced an incidence of pigmentation in 11% of patients. The incidence of pigmentation with hypertonic saline (HS) has been reported to range from 10% to 30%.[3-7] Patients treated with polidocanol (POL) have a reported incidence of pigmentation from 6.7%[8,9] to 30%.[5,10] A 35% incidence has been reported in 7200 patients treated with POL,

*Adapted from Goldman MP. Sclerotherapy Treatment of Varicose and Telangiectatic Leg Veins. St. Louis: Mosby, 1995.

300

ethanolamine oleate (EO), or iodine-iodide solution.[11] An incidence of 15.7% has been reported for Sclerodex.[9] An incidence of 32% has been reported with use of Sclerodine.[9] A 2% incidence of hyperpigmentation was reported from one series of patients treated with POL, chromated glycerin (CG), and sodium salicylate (SAL).[12] Therefore the true incidence of hyperpigmentation is a result of many factors, including treatment technique, sclerosing solution, and the definition of pigmentation. It is my opinion that the definition of pigmentation should be any brown-black staining of the skin that occurs after sclerotherapy; persistent pigmentation refers to brown staining that is present after 1 year. As discussed later, it is my hypothesis that pigmentation develops through extravasation of red blood cells (RBCs) from damaged vessels with resulting inflammation, which contributes to ineffective digestion of hemosiderin. This process results in a hemosiderin tattoo.

When pigmentation occurs, it is usually temporary. Physicians report a 1% to 2% incidence of pigmentation persisting after 1 year.[12,13] Pigmentation is usually linear, along the course of the treated blood vessel. I use the term "ghost of the blood vessel" to explain to patients that it represents a resolving, not a functioning, vessel. However, in addition to linear lines of pigmentation, osmotic sclerosing solutions may produce punctate pigmentation at points of injection, which may be related to their mechanism of action through an osmotic gradient that produces maximal osmolality and resultant endothelial destruction at the injection site. In contrast, detergent-type sclerosing solutions destroy the treated vessel for a few centimeters along its length, producing a more linear golden-brown color (Figure 16-1).

Etiologic factors. The etiology of this pigmentation most likely results from a combination of postinflammatory hyperpigmentation (incontinence of melanin pigment) and hemosiderin deposition.[14-16] However, histologic examination has demonstrated that this pigmentation is caused only by hemosiderin staining of the dermis irrespective of the type of sclerosing solution used, pigmentation of the patient, or length of time after injection[17-20] (Figure 16-2). Defects in iron storage or transport mechanisms or both have also been found in a significant number of patients who developed postsclerotherapy pigmentation.[21]

Hemosiderin deposition predominantly occurs in the superficial dermis, although it may be present in periadnexal and middermal locations, particularly in the ankle area. This phenomenon probably occurs when RBCs extravasate into the dermis after the rupture of treated vessels.[22] Erythrocyte diapedesis may also occur after inflammation of the vessel and is commonly seen after thrombophlebitis. Perivascular inflammation is presumed to promote degranulation of perivascular mast cells. Released histamine leads to endothelial cell contraction, which results in widening of endothelial gaps through which extravasation of RBCs can occur.[23-27] Thus injecting a sclerosing solution both dilates the vessel directly through pressure generated by the syringe and indirectly through histamine-induced endothelial cell contraction.

Perivascular phagocytosis of RBCs occurs either by intact cells or in piecemeal manner after fragmentation by macrophages.[28,29] The intracellular frag-

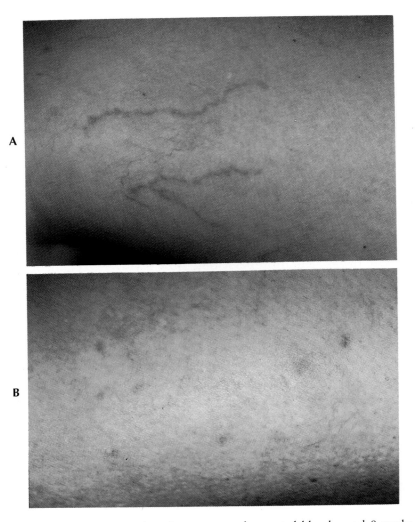

FIGURE 16-1. A, Linear pigmentation along course of a treated blood vessel 8 weeks after treatment with POL 0.5%. **B,** Punctate pigmentation 8 weeks after treatment with Sclerodex.

ments in the macrophage cytoplasm are further compartmentalized into hemoglobin-containing globules. They are referred to as *secondary liposomes.* Since hemosiderin is an indigestible residue of hemoglobin degradation, it may appear as aggregates up to 100 mm in diameter.[30] Hemosiderin has a variable concentration. Iron concentrations vary from 24% to 36%.[31] Iron hydroxide contained in hemosiderin occurs in different forms, with differing amounts of ferritin.[32] On unstained tissue iron hydroxide appears golden and is 30% iron by weight. Its elimination from the area may take years (if it ever occurs).

In addition to being insoluble, hemosiderin may directly affect cellular function. Histologic examination with x-ray fluorescence analysis of patients with varicose ulceration disclosed an elevation of mean iron levels in periulcerated

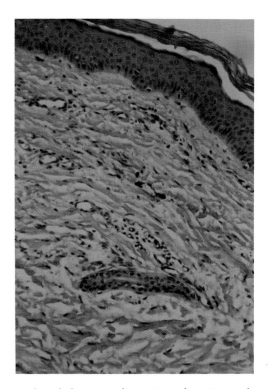

FIGURE 16-2. Section stained with hematoxylin-eosin; taken 6 months after injection with POL 0.75%. Note scattered foci of golden-brown pigment. (Original magnification ×50.) (From Goldman MP, Kaplan RP, Duffy DM. Postsclerotherapy hyperpigmentation: A histologic evaluation. J Dermatol Surg Oncol 13:547, 1987. Copyright © 1987 Elsevier Science Publishing Co., Inc. Reprinted with permission.)

skin.[33] The authors speculate that free radical formation resulting from local iron accumulation may cause melanocytic stimulation, thereby augmenting brown pigmentation. Indeed, several authors have demonstrated melanin incontinence in the presence of venous stasis, complicated by extravascular RBCs.[34-36] Whether melanocytic stimulation plays a role in the early appearance of postsclerotherapy pigmentation is unlikely, but it may contribute to the persistence of pigmentation in certain patients.

Regardless of the etiology of pigmentation, its incidence apparently is related to multiple factors, including (1) sclerosing solution type and concentration, (2) sclerotherapy technique, (3) gravitational and other intravascular pressures, (4) innate tendency toward cutaneous pigmentation (total body iron stores and/or altered iron transport and storage mechanisms, innate enhanced histamine release or hypersensitivity, and vessel fragility), (5) postsclerotherapy treatment (graduated compression), (6) vessel diameter, and (7) concomitant medication.

Solution type and concentration. The type and concentration of the sclerosing solution affect the degree of endothelial destruction. The extent of endothelial destruction with resulting inflammation and extravasation of RBCs is thought to influence the development of postsclerotherapy hyperpigmentation. The increased incidence of pigmentation with STS and HS, which produces a greater reaction than POL, confirms this hypothesis.[2,37-39] Sclerosing solutions reported to have the lowest incidence of postsclerotherapy pigmentation also produce minimal inflammation. These are CG[13,37,40-44] and SAL.[13,16]

A higher concentration of the same sclerosing solution also produces increased inflammation.[45] Thus the inflammatory response after treatment should be kept to a minimum, and sclerosing solutions and concentrations should be altered accordingly from treatment session to session.

Technique. Optimal technique consists of limiting pressure into damaged (sclerosed) veins to prevent extravasation of RBCs. To limit the degree of intravascular pressure, larger feeding varices, incompetent varices, and points of high pressure reflux should be treated first. A greater incidence of pigmentation occurs if vessels distal to the saphenofemoral junction (SFJ) are treated before successful closure of the junction with a decreased incidence of pigmentation when treatment is from proximal to distal (C. Guardi, personal correspondence, 1989).[46]

The degree of injection pressure is also important. Because telangiectasias and small venules are composed essentially of endothelial cells with a thin (if any) muscular coat and basement membrane, excessive intravascular pressure from injection may cause vessel rupture. In addition, endothelial pores and spaces between cells in the vascular wall will dilate in response to pressure, leading to extravasation of RBCs. It is therefore important to inject intravascularly with minimal pressure. Since injection pressure is inversely proportional to the square of the piston radius, using a syringe with a larger radius will result in less pressure.

The average piston radius is 8 mm for a 2 ml syringe and 5 mm for a 1 ml syringe. The calculated pressure with an implied force of 250 g is 180 mm Hg for a 2 ml syringe and more than 300 mm Hg for a 1 ml syringe.[47] This is one reason I recommend using a 2 to 3 ml syringe for sclerotherapy.

Gravitational and other intravascular pressures. Postsclerotherapy pigmentation appears most commonly in vessels treated below the knee,[16] but they can occur anywhere on the leg, probably as a result of a combination of increased capillary fragility and increased intravascular pressure by gravitational effects in this location.

Vessel diameter. It is commonly observed that telangiectasias that have the maximal incidence of pigmentation are those between 0.6 and 1.2 mm in diameter. Chatard[16] also has observed an increased incidence of pigmentation when blue venulectasias are treated as opposed to the treatment of red telangiectasias. The explanation for the latter observation is unknown but may be related to vessel diameter since blue telangiectasias are usually of larger diameter than red telangiectasias. An evaluation of 113 patients treated with sclerotherapy demonstrated rare pigmentation in vessels less than 1 mm in diameter.[48]

Predisposition to pigmentation. Certain individuals appear to be predisposed to the development of pigmentation. Pigmentation has been reported as more common and pronounced in patients with dark hair and "dark-toned" skin.[14] This effect is believed to be caused by an increased incidence of postinflammatory hyperpigmentation in patients with such coloring. However, Chatard[16] reported that pigmentation is unrelated to skin or hair color. I agree with Chatard's assessment.

Pigmentation resolves from a gradual resorption of ferritin particles from macrophage digestion. It is hypothesized that the patient's iron storage and transport mechanisms may influence the rate of clearance of dermal hemosiderin.[49] A preliminary study of 16 patients with age-matched controls disclosed that patients who developed pigmentation had higher serum ferritin levels. Serum ferritin levels correlate with total body iron stores.[50] To clarify the relationship between serum ferritin and postsclerotherapy pigmentation, a prospective study of 233 consecutive patients was done.[51] A linear relationship between the occurrence of pigmentation and pretreatment serum ferritin levels was found at each posttreatment assessment date. This finding supports the hypothesis that high total body iron stores increase the susceptibility toward hyperpigmentation. However, serum ferritin levels are not an absolute predictor for the development of hyperpigmentation. A patient with hemochromatosis having a serum ferritin level of 1200 ng/ml did not develop pigmentation after sclerotherapy of telangiectasias 0.6 mm in diameter with 0.2% STS.[52] The explanation may be that this patient's physician probably used outstanding technique to avoid extravasation of RBCs.

Therefore serum ferritin levels may be used to identify patients at risk for this complication. These patients may require special attention with meticulous microthrombectomy, and an increase in time and extent of posttreatment compression is advocated.

If histamine-induced endothelial contraction promotes extravasation of RBCs or hemosiderin, or both, histamine antagonists should prevent or limit its occurrence. The catecholamines norepinephrine and isoproterenol antagonize histamine-induced edema in canine brachial artery preparations.[53] Similarly, corticosteroids decrease the size of histamine-induced endothelial gap junctions.[54] Terbutaline also inhibits macromolecular leakage from postcapillary venules in hamster femoral veins.[55] Cimetidine blocks histamine-induced widening of endothelial gaps in rat femoral veins.[56] Therefore patients who develop postsclerotherapy pigmentation may be pretreated with one of these medications or a combination of them to block or limit histamine effects.

Vessel fragility may also result in an innate predisposition toward pigmentation. Capillary strength is related to both menstrual cycles and circulating estrogen.[57] Decreased capillary strength occurs 3 to 5 days before and 2 days after menses and during ovulation. Fragility has been found to improve with intravenous (IV) and oral (PO) administration of conjugated equine estrogen (Premarin) in postmenopausal women.

Patients taking minocycline may have an increased risk for developing postsclerotherapy pigmentation.[58,59] This propensity may be related to the inflammatory effects of sclerotherapy. Unlike the golden to deep-brown color characteristic of typical sclerotherapy-induced pigmentation, pigmentation resulting from minocycline is typically blue-gray. Minocycline produces pigmentation in a variety of organs and structures.[60,61] One form of minocycline pigmentation develops in depressed acne scars or at other sites of inflammation.[7,62-66] A second form of pigmentation has been described on ultraviolet light–exposed legs.[67] The pigment involved in minocycline hyperpigmentation is hemosiderin or some other iron-chelating compound.[65,67-70] It has been hypothesized that minocycline or a metabolite interferes with degradation of hemosiderin through lysosomal disruption, leading to macrophage death and deposition of pigment.[66] Therefore it may be prudent to withhold minocycline therapy in sclerotherapy patients. Further studies are needed to establish this direct relationship.

Postsclerotherapy coagula. Removal of postsclerotherapy coagula may decrease the incidence of pigmentation. Thrombi are thought to occur after sclerotherapy of all veins to some degree, regardless of size, because of the inability to occlude the vascular lumen completely with external pressure. The persistence of a small vascular lumen, even with maximal external pressure, has been predicted with experimental models of vein wall.[71] It has also been directly observed with fiberoptic varicography (H. Muntlak, personal communication, 1989).

Persistent thrombi are thought to produce a subacute "perivenulitis" that can persist for months.[72-74] The perivenulitis favors extravasation of RBCs through a damaged endothelium or by increasing the permeability of treated endothelium. In addition, intratissue fixation of hemosiderin may occur.[16] These possibilities provide a rationale for drainage of all foci of trapped blood 2 to 4 weeks after sclerotherapy. Sometimes blood can be released even 2 months after sclerotherapy.

Thrombi are best removed by gentle expression of the liquefied clot through a small incision made with a 21-gauge needle, No. 11 blade, or a lancet (Figure 16-3). A rocking action applied around the clot may aid in its expulsion. This action should be continued until all dark blood is removed. The art of this procedure is to find the right place to puncture, which is best perceived as a soft, fluctuating spot. If the thrombosis is located in the deep dermis, the area should be marked, and 1% lidocaine can be infiltrated around the area to facilitate a less painful removal. Compression pads and/or stockings are then worn an additional day or two to prevent further thrombosis formation and to aid in adherence of the opposing endothelial walls to establish effective endosclerosis.

Perchuk[75] raises the possibility of infection occurring from stab incisions. This danger was presumed to be caused by the presence of bacteria in varicose veins—a belief commonly held by physicians 40 to 50 years ago.[76,77] However, there have been no reports of infections occurring in patients treated with stab incisions into postsclerotherapy clots in the modern medical literature. This problem has not occurred in my practice, in which this procedure is used routinely.

Duration. Despite therapeutic attempts, pigmentation often lasts from 6 to 12 months.[19] Rarely, pigmentation may last more than 1 year. Georgiev[13] estimates that 1% of his patients have pigmentation lasting more than 1 year; Duffy[5] estimates that up to 10% of his patients do so. Izzo et al.[12] report a 2% incidence after 1 year. Persistent telangiectasias may be due to factors other than sclerotherapy itself. In certain patients pigmentation may be present over superficial vari-

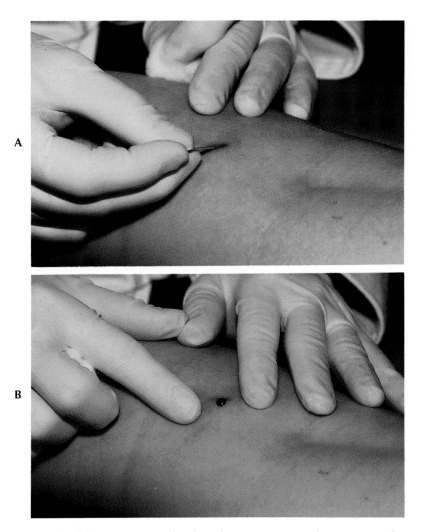

FIGURE 16-3. Method for evacuation of a thrombosis in a 1 mm–diameter reticular varicose vein 2 weeks after sclerotherapy. **A,** Small incision is made. **B,** Clot is expelled. (From Goldman MP. Sclerotherapy: Treatment of Varicose and Telangiectatic Leg Veins. St. Louis: Mosby, 1991, p 226. Reprinted with permission.)

cosities and telangiectasias before sclerotherapy is performed.[13,16] Hyperpigmentation as a result of "physiologic" diapedesis of RBCs through fragile vessels is common in patients with venous stasis or over varicose veins. Therefore preoperative documentation, including photographs, may be beneficial during follow-up patient visits.

Prevention. To prevent the development of pigmentation, sclerotherapy should produce limited endothelial necrosis, not total destruction with its resulting diapedesis of RBCs. This result may be achieved by using meticulous technique, avoiding excessive injection pressures, selecting the appropriate solution concentration, and treating areas of reflux venous return in a proximal-to-distal manner.

Thibault and Wlodarczyk[51] recommend that patients avoid taking all iron supplements during the course of treatment and for 1 month after treatment. This precaution presumably will decrease serum ferritin levels. Alternatively, the serum ferritin levels of patients may be assessed before sclerotherapy to determine if iron chelation therapy is warranted. The latter recommendation awaits further study.

Treatment. Treatment of pigmentation after its appearance is often unsuccessful. Because this pigmentation is primarily caused by hemosiderin deposition and not melanin incontinence, bleaching agents that affect melanocytic function are usually ineffective. Exfoliants (e.g., trichloroacetic acid [TCA]) may hasten the apparent resolution of this pigmentation by decreasing the overlying cutaneous pigmentation or promoting the exfoliation of hemosiderin, but they carry a risk of scarring, permanent hypopigmentation, and postinflammatory hyperpigmentation. However, some physicians have reported apparent success with this therapeutic modality.[12,78] The combination of 20% TCA with retinoic acid and hydroxyquinone has also been reported to result in total fading of pigmentation in 76% of patients whose pigmentation persisted from 6 months to 5 years.[12] The remaining patients had a reduction in their pigmentation. Treatments were given every 7 to 10 days from 4 to 12 weeks.

Chatard[16] has found that using light cryotherapy to exfoliate the epidermis and "evict the pigment" is helpful. I have not found cryotherapy useful in my practice.

Terezakis (personal communication, 1989) has found that the use of topical retinoic acid enhances resolution of the pigmentation. She speculates that retinoids enhance fibroblastic removal of hemosiderin. I have used topical tretinoin (Retin-A 0.1% cream) to treat patients who have pigmentation beyond 3 months. Although formal placebo control studies have not been completed, it appears that this therapy may be effective. It does not appear to have any adverse sequelae and has the advantage of bringing the patient into active therapy.

A seemingly logical form of treatment would be chelation of the subcutaneous iron deposition. Myers[79] reported the use of a 150 mg/ml ointment of disodium ethylenediamine tetraacetic acid (EDTA) in the treatment of 10 patients with pigmentation after sclerotherapy or vein stripping or with pigmentation in chronic postphlebitic legs. He reported a consistent reduction in the shade of the pigmentation in every patient treated. Unfortunately, this study was uncontrolled, and there have been no further reports of this form of treatment since its presentation in 1965. In my experience intradermal injections of deferoxamine in an attempt to cause chelation of the hemosiderin appear to be somewhat effective, but they are painful and expensive. The timing, concentration, and quantity of deferoxamine injections have not been systematically studied.

The topical iron chelator 2-furildioxome (FDO) has been found to provide a level of photoprotection.[80] However, the product manufacturer has no interest at present in providing this agent for clinical testing of postsclerotherapy pigmentation (personal correspondence, Proctor & Gamble, October 1994).

Graduated elastic compression with coadministration of the anabolic steroid stanozolol decreases pigmentation in patients with lipodermatosclerosis who also have varicose veins.[81] There was no change in skin pigmentation when patients used graduated compression stockings alone. Stanozolol may exert its effect through reduction in perivascular fibrin from fibrinolytic enhancement. In addition, compression alone improves lipodermatosclerotic skin changes, including hyperpigmentation (H. Partsch, personal communication, 1992). Although it seems reasonable to promote wearing graduated support stockings after treatment, further studies are needed before recommending systemic stanozolol therapy.

Finally, laser treatment has been efficacious in 45%[21] to 69%[49] of patients with pigmentation of 12 or 6 months' duration, respectively. Hemosiderin has an absorption spectrum that peaks at 410 to 415 nm, followed by a gradually sloping curve throughout the visible spectrum[82,83] (Figure 16-4). The copper vapor laser (CVL) at 511 nm in a continuous airbrush technique and the flashlamp-excited pulsed dye laser (FLPDL) at 510 nm should interact relatively specifically with the hemosiderin absorption spectrum. Competition from oxygenated hemoglobin (peak absorption at 577 nm) should be low. However, interaction with epidermal melanin, which has a higher absorption rate at these wavelengths, may be significant. These lasers are thought to result in physical fragmentation of pigment granules, which are later removed by phagocytosis. However, penetration of laser

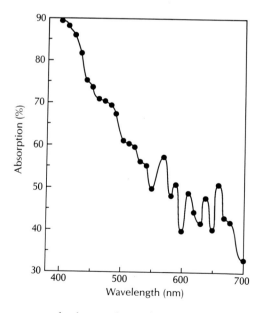

FIGURE 16-4. Absorption spectra for hemosiderin (freshly frozen, average of two determinations). (Redrawn from Wells CI, Wolken JJ. Biochemistry: Microspectrophotometry of haemosiderin granules. Nature 193:988, 1962.)

energy at 510 and 511 nm is limited to 1 mm below the granular layer. Since hemosiderin may occur up to 2.8 mm below the granular layer, nonthermal effects may result in clinical resolution. An inflammatory reaction from thermal and/or photoacoustic effects may stimulate hemosiderin absorption. Although CVL-treated pigmentation responded better than that treated with FLPDL therapy, thermal relaxation times used by the latter laser system should be more selective.

The Q-switched ruby laser (694 nm) may also be effective in removing recalcitrant pigmentation. Hemosiderin does have a peak at 694 nm, and the Q-switching impulse at 20 to 30 nsec is effective in removing tattoo granules. In addition, 694 nm is not absorbed to a significant extent by melanin or hemoglobin and thus has a relative specificity for hemosiderin. I have found this laser to be effective in a number of patients (Figure 16-5).

Weiss[84] has reported successful clearing in 10 patients with pigmentation persisting after 1 to 2 months with intense pulsed light (IPL) (Photoderm PL). He used the IPL at 30 to 40 J/cm^2 given in a single 4 msec pulse with a 590 nm cutoff filter. Significant lightening occurred in 6 of 10 patients.

The recommended treatment is "flashbulb therapy" or "chronotherapy." Since the majority of patients will have a resolution of pigmentation within 1 year,

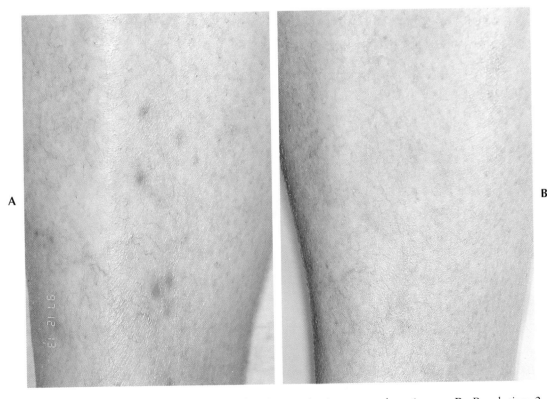

FIGURE 16-5. A, Pigmentation from sclerotherapy lasting more than 1 year. **B,** Resolution 2 months after the second of two treatments with the Q-switched ruby laser at 8.0 J/cm^2.

time and photographic documentation usually are very satisfactory for the understanding patient.

Temporary Swelling

Etiologic factors. Multiple factors are responsible for swelling of a treated area. These factors include changes in the pressure differential between the intravascular and perivascular space and changes in endothelial permeability. Edema is most common when varicose veins or telangiectasias below the ankle are treated. This relates both to the increase in gravitational intravascular pressure in this area and the relative sparsity of perivascular fascia at the ankle. Riddock[85] speculates that edema is caused by an unduly prolonged reflex spasm spreading to some of the subfascial (deep) veins.

The extent of edema appears to be related to the strength of the sclerosing solution. This result apparently correlates with the degree of perivascular inflammation produced by the sclerosing solution. The by-products of inflammation, including release of histamine and various mediators, increase endothelial permeability. In addition to the degree of inflammation induced by sclerotherapy itself, the innate sensitivity of a patient's perivascular mast cells (possibly related to their atopic or asthma history), concomitant medications that may promote or inhibit mast cell degranulation (e.g., corticosteroids, antihistamines, nonsteroidal anti-inflammatory agents), and previous exposure sensitivity to the sclerosing agent may all contribute to edema. Duffy[5] and Goldman[10] estimate the occurrence of pedal edema as 2% to 5%.

Edema may also occur if compression is not applied in a graduated manner. Edema may be produced when application of localized pressure on the thigh over an injected vein is attempted with the addition of a tape dressing over or under a graduated compression stocking. If patients are informed of the possibility of the production of a tourniquet effect by the extra compression, they can be advised to remove the dressing at the first sign of edema distal to the dressing.

Prevention and treatment. Two techniques may limit temporary swelling. First, limit perivascular inflammation, as previously described. Ankle edema occurs much less frequently if the quantity of sclerosing solution is limited to 1 ml per ankle.

One method that I have found helpful is topical application of a strong-potency corticosteroid. Application of pharmacologic agents either topically or systemically may be beneficial in patients with excessive postsclerotherapy edema. Methylprednisolone acts both to stabilize mast cell membranes, preventing histamine release, and to exert part of its anti-inflammatory action directly on the endothelial cell, rendering it less responsive to various mediators.[86] Ruscus extract inhibits macromolecular permeability, increasing the effect of histamine in the hamster cheek pouch model.[87] This effect is due to stabilization of endothelial pore size. Beta-receptor agonists such as terbutaline and theophylline counteract histamine-induced venular permeability. This effect also occurs with verapamil and glucocorticoids.[88]

A second method for limiting the degree of pedal or ankle edema is to apply a graduated pressure stocking routinely after injections in this area.[89]

Telangiectatic Matting

The new appearance of previously unnoticed fine red telangiectasias occurs in a number of patients after either sclerotherapy or surgical ligation of varicose veins and leg telangiectasias (Figure 16-6). This occurrence has been termed "flares" by Arenander and Lindhagen,[90] "distal angioplasia" by Terezakis,[91] and "telangiectatic matting" (TM) by Duffy.[5] The reported incidence varies from 5%[10] to 75%.[39,90] Two retrospective analyses of 2120 and 7200 patients with leg telangiectasias each reported a 16% incidence.[11,92] This incidence has been confirmed in a random sample of 113 female sclerotherapy patients.[38]

Reasons for the development of TM are multiple. Recovery from an ischemic injury, such as closing blood vessels with sclerotherapy, may produce a hypoxia-induced neovascularization. This response is probably a fundamental feedback response, acting to satisfy tissue needs for oxygenation. For example, this response is commonly seen in myocardial collateralization. It is interesting that the incidence is not higher. Therefore other innate factors must predispose to the development of TM.

The incidence of TM increased with increasing patient age in one report,[90] but this correlation was not seen in another report.[92] Although most authors do not comment on a sexual predisposition,[5] I have seen the development of TM in only one male patient with leg telangiectasias. Because of the small number of men seeking treatment, an accurate appraisal of the sexual incidence of TM cannot be stated.

TM may appear anywhere on the leg and almost never on the face, chest, and hands after sclerotherapy treatment. One detailed study found that most TM occurred on the medial ankle and the medial and lateral calves.[90] However, TM has also been reported to occur more frequently on the thighs.[93] Duffy has reported that 80% of his patients develop TM within 10 inches of the knees (personal communication, October 1994). Duffy postulates that relative ischemia occurs in this area from tissue hypoxia, which results from the thighs and knees pressing on each other during sleep when one lies on his or her side. Hypoxia has been found both in the retina as well as around compressive tumors to promote vascular endothelial growth.[94-96]

Etiologic factors. Postsclerosis TM was first described in the 1960s by Ouvry and Davy.[97] They observed that the incidence of matting was proportional to the degree of inflammation and thrombus formation. The etiology of TM is unknown, but it is believed to be related either to angiogenesis[5,98] or to a dilation of existing subclinical blood vessels by the promotion of collateral flow through arteriovenous anastomoses.[98,99] One or both of these mechanisms may occur.

Probable risk factors for the development of TM in patients with leg telangiectasias include obesity, use of estrogen-containing hormones, pregnancy, and a family history of telangiectatic veins. Excessive standing does not appear to influ-

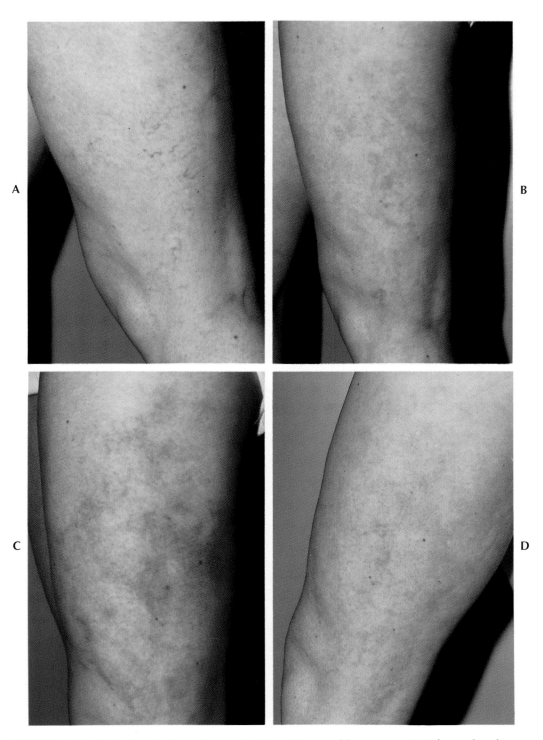

FIGURE 16-6. Typical telangiectatic matting in a 36-year-old woman. **A,** Before sclerotherapy treatment, telangiectasias are seen on left lateral thigh. **B,** Three months after treatment of reticular veins with POL 0.75%. **C,** Six weeks after treatment of telangiectatic veins with POL 0.5%. Note development of extensive matting. **D,** Six weeks later. Note complete resolution of matting without treatment.

ence the incidence of TM.[92] Excessive postsclerotherapy inflammation may also predispose toward development of TM.

Normally, the more than 1 trillion endothelial cells that line blood vessels have a turnover time of over 1000 days.[100] However, under appropriate conditions, the development of new vessels can occur in 2 to 3 days. Observations of mammalian systems have demonstrated the development of a vein from a capillary, an artery from a vein, a vein from an artery, or from any of these back to a capillary.[101,102] In coronary vessels increased numbers of arterioles and capillaries occur within 1 week after injury.[103]

Angiogenesis. Angiogenesis is a complex process in which capillary blood vessels grow in an ordered sequence of events. Angiogenic factors act either directly on the endothelium to stimulate locomotion and mitosis or indirectly by mobilization of host helper cells (mast cells and macrophages) with release of endothelial growth factors. When a new capillary sprout grows from the side of a venule, endothelial cells degrade basement membrane, migrate toward an angiogenic source, proliferate, form a lumen, join the tips of two sprouts to generate a capillary loop, and manufacture new basement membrane.[104] Obstruction of outflow from a vessel (which is the end result of successful sclerotherapy) is one of the most important factors contributing to angiogenesis.[105] Initiation of angiogenesis also follows disruption of endothelial continuity or intercellular contact. This contact results in endothelial cell sprouting and migration.[106]

In addition, endothelial damage leads to the release of heparin and other mast cell factors that both promote the dilation of existing blood vessels and stimulate angiogenesis.[107-110] Finally, neovascularization may be promoted by numerous other angiogenic factors, including but not limited to heparin-binding fibroblast growth factor (FGF),[13,111,112] tumor necrosis factor (TNF),[108,113,114] platelet-derived endothelial mitogen,[115] endothelial cell growth factor (ECGF),[116] and other macrophage-derived growth factors.[113,117,118] These factors and many others are released from perivascular mast cells.[119] FGF is released at cell death and is essential for the stimulation of angiogenesis and wound repair.[120,121] Thus sclerotherapy, through endothelial damage, promotes the release of endothelial angiogenic factors and perivascular mast cell angiogenic factors that provide multiple mechanisms for new blood vessel formation to occur. Indeed, it is remarkable that a greater incidence of postsclerosis TM does not occur.

Sclerotherapy-induced perivascular inflammation may also promote TM.[22] Inflammation may be considered a hypermetabolic state, with new vessel growth occurring as a result of increased metabolic demand.[122] In addition, mast cells are found in increased numbers in inflammatory states such as allergic contact dermatitis or delayed hypersensitivity reactions.[123] Since mast cell heparin is one factor responsible for capillary endothelial cell migration,[107] in an attempt to decrease angiogenic stimuli, one should try to limit the degree of inflammation as much as possible. This limitation is achieved by choosing an appropriate solution concentration for each type of vessel treated and limiting the quantity of solution to the amount that will not produce excessive endothelial damage. This method was confirmed by Weiss and Weiss,[38] who found that in a random sample of 113 sclerotherapy patients, 10 developed TM with injection of POL 1% into vessels less than 1 mm in diameter. When POL 0.5% was used for subsequent treatments in these patients, none developed further areas of TM. In a multicenter report of 16,804 legs, the use of low concentrations of POL was found to have an incidence of TM of 0.04%.[124] However, it is unclear how closely patients were followed up in this large prospective clinical trial.

Another group of investigators report TM in 12% of patients treated with Sclerodine 0.25%, 17% treated with Sclerodex, and 15% treated with 0.25% POL.[9] These agents should all be comparatively similar in their sclerosing power despite their different mechanism of action on endothelial cells. Interestingly, although their effectiveness in eliminating telangiectasias varied from 73% for POL to 44% for Sclerodine and Sclerodex, the incidence of TM was relatively similar.

As noted previously, assuming a role for the perivascular mast cell in the etiology of TM is intriguing. With aging, a 50% decrease in cutaneous mast cells occurs, associated with a 35% decrease in subepidermal venules.[48] Thus if TM develops predominantly from mast cell factors, its incidence should be decreased in the elderly. Such a decrease has not been noted in two studies.[90,92] Cutaneous mast cells usually occur perivascularly, with a distribution ranging from 7000/mm[5] to 20,000/mm.[5,125-128] These figures represent 0.2% to 0.7% of normal skin. In telangiectatic macules associated with mastocytosis, mast cells account for 3.5% (61.8 SEM) of cells, whereas telangiectasias not associated with mastocytosis have a mast cell volume of 0.4% (0.1 SEM).[129] An analysis of mast cell content in TM lesions is needed.

Estrogen may play a role in the development of TM. It appears that there may be an increased incidence of persistent TM among patients taking systemic estrogen preparations.[5,38,92] Weiss and Weiss[38] found a relative risk of 3.17 ($p < 0.003$) for development of TM while patients were receiving exogenous estrogen. The mechanism for promotion of TM by estrogen is speculative, but it may be secondary to its effect on modulating mast cell responses.[130]

Estrogen receptors have been found in a number of tumors, including angioma of the nose, soft tissue sarcoma, breast carcinoma, endometrial carcinoma, and unilateral nevoid telangiectasia syndrome. Estrogens also play a role in the development of vascular tissues. In vitro estrogen and estradiol have promoted endothelial cell migration and proliferation.[131] Spider angiomas develop during pregnancy and resolve after delivery.[32,132] Spider nevi also occur in patients with hepatic cirrhosis associated with elevated serum estradiol levels.[133] In addition, Davis and Duffy[92] have reported on the virtual disappearance of leg telangiectasias and TM in a 51-year-old woman with estrogen-receptor–positive breast carcinoma after initiation of antiestrogen therapy with tamoxifen citrate (Nolvadex). This result may be due to the inhibition of angiogenesis by tamoxifen.[134,135] However, Sadick and Niedt[136] could not demonstrate estrogen receptors in a number of biopsy specimens from leg telangiectasias. An evaluation of estrogen receptors in TM lesions is needed. Since estrogen receptors have been implicated in the promotion of angiogenesis,[137] it may be prudent, although premature, to withhold estrogen therapy during sclerotherapy treatment.

Prevention and treatment. Regardless of the etiology of TM, since patients come for treatment to have leg telangiectasias eliminated, it is disconcerting for the sclerotherapist to produce new areas of telangiectasia. Unfortunately, despite one's best efforts, TM will occur in a significant percentage of patients. Fortunately, TM usually resolves spontaneously over 3 to 12 months.[5,38] It has been estimated that 10% to 20% of patients will have permanent TM.[92,138]

Treatment modalities for TM are limited. Reinjection with hypertonic solutions may be helpful. Because of the extremely small diameter of these vessels, the use of a 33-gauge needle is helpful. Injection of any feeding reticular veins or venulectases is also helpful.

Various vascular specific lasers and IPL sources may be useful in treating these vessels.[139-143] In my practice at least 75% of patients who develop persistent TM can be improved or treated completely with laser or IPL treatment. Interestingly, individual TM lesions may respond better to one laser or IPL than another. Reasons for the variable response are speculative. The 532 nm long-pulse Nd:YAG laser set at the highest fluence and pulse durations available has been found to be most effective on the most recalcitrant lesions. However, persistent and rarely permanent hypopigmentation may occur. Unfortunately, even with all of these therapeutic modalities, TM may be resistant to treatment. These resistant TM lesions may have a feeding arteriolar network that prevents persistent vessel elimination.

In patients who demonstrate a propensity to develop TM, additives to the sclerosing solutions or topical agents may minimize this complication. Protamine blocks the ability of mast cells and heparin to stimulate migration of capillary endothelial cells.[144] It also prevents the neovascularization induced by an inflammatory agent when it is applied locally or given systemically.[145] Protamine has no effect on established capillaries that are not proliferating.[146] In addition, beta-cyclodextrin tetradeasulfate administered with cortexolone is a potent inhibitor of angiogenesis.[147] Thus the use of these additives with the sclerosing solution may limit the development of TM.

Systemic treatment before or during sclerotherapy may also be helpful in limiting TM. Through suppression of TNF synthesis, pentoxifylline (Trental) may minimize angiogenesis.[148,149] Inhibition of mast cell mediators with the cell wall–stabilizing medication Ketoprofen (Ketotifen) may also be useful for preventing TM, edema, and localized urticaria. Ketoprofen, a benzocycloheptathiophene derivative, has H_1 antihistaminic properties in addition to decreasing mast cell mediator release.[150,151] Ketoprofen may also exert its effect by depleting mediators in cutaneous mast cells and thus require multiple doses over a few days to have maximal effect.[152] Its clinical beneficial effect in patients with chronic idiopathic urticaria, cutaneous mastocytosis, and urticaria pigmentosa has been established.[152-156]

Pain

Since most patients who come for treatment of leg telangiectasias require multiple treatment sessions, each consisting of numerous injections, an attempt should be made to minimize the unpleasantness of the procedure.

Prevention. Certain areas are slightly more painful, especially the ankles, upper medial thighs, and medial knees. Two variables that can be adjusted to minimize pain are the type and size of the needle used for injection and the type of sclerosing solution used.

Type and size of needle. Using the smallest possible diameter needle for injection is the most obvious way to minimize injection pain. Another factor to consider is the shape of the needle bevel. Needles, even those of the same gauge, are shaped differently and may or may not be coated with a layer of silicone. Acutely tapered needles, especially when tribeveled, and those that are silicone coated usually are perceived by the patient as less painful in my experience.

Technique. With sclerosing solutions that are inherently painful to inject (e.g., hypertonic solutions), pain can be minimized with slow infusion.[3,5] Slow injection produces a slower distention of tissue and may minimize endothelial cell separation, which may decrease perivascular nerve stimulation.

Type of sclerosing solution. HSs are notorious for causing pain on injection. The cramping pain that may develop after correct IV injection usually occurs a few minutes after injection. Weiss and Weiss[3] report that 72% of their patients injected with HS 23.4% experience pain that lasts less than 5 minutes; 4.5% of patients have pain that lasts more than 5 minutes. This pain probably occurs at the time the HS reaches the nerve fibers of the adventitia, either through the wall of the vein or through the capillaries. Subsequently, because of stimulation of sympathetic perivenous nerve fibers, an active contraction of the muscle occurs that may also produce a cramping pain.[157] In addition, vascular spasm caused by direct effects of the HS itself may occur.

HSs also produce muscle cramping after injection. With the injection of 5 to 10 ml of Heparsal (20% HS plus heparin, 10 U/ml) per injection site into varicose veins, Chou et al.[158] noted that 16% of 310 patients could not tolerate the pain associated with the procedure. Duffy[5] estimates that 82% of his patients treated with HS note moderate cramping or aching. This effect can be limited somewhat by keeping the volumes injected to 0.1 ml or less per injection site and by massaging the area immediately after injection.

Adding lidocaine to the sclerosing solution may lessen muscle cramping and allow placement of additional injections into the same area with less pain.[5,6] However, the addition of lidocaine to an HS is associated with two problems. First, if the lidocaine is acidified (in a multidose bottle), it produces pain during the injection. Therefore nonacidified lidocaine (found in single-dose "cardiac" ampules) should be used as an additive. Second, the addition of lidocaine gives the sclerosing solution the potential to produce an allergic reaction.

Chromated glycerin solutions are also painful during injection and may produce mild muscle cramping if more than 1 ml of solution is injected into a single vein.[42]

Two relatively painless solutions are POL and STS. STS has the advantage of being painful only when it is injected into perivascular tissues, thereby providing a noticeable check on inadvertent perivascular injection. POL is painless with both intradermal and IV injection. Therefore one does not have the additional sign of pain to ensure accurate placement of the sclerosing solution. In a double-blind comparison of STS, HS, and POL, patients preferred injection with POL.[159] Although relatively painless to inject, STS does produce a dull ache a few minutes after injection. This ache resolves in a few minutes. POL does not produce post-treatment aching.

Despite optimal technique and the use of mild sclerosing agents, posttreatment soreness for 1 or 2 weeks after injection occurs in 20% of patients.[5] With the use of nonosmotic sclerosing solutions and graduated compression stockings worn after treatment, I have not seen soreness in most patients after treatment. If patients do complain of soreness, the cause usually is thrombosed and/or inflamed vessels.

Localized Urticaria

Localized urticaria occurs after injection of all sclerosing solutions (Figure 16-7). It is usually transient (lasting approximately 30 minutes) and is probably the result of endothelial irritation with release of perivascular mast cell histamine. Localized urticaria is not an allergic response since it occurs even after injection of 23.4% unadulterated HS.

Urticaria may occur as the earliest manifestation of perivascular inflammation, again through release of endothelial- or platelet-derived factors, which lead to perivascular mast cell degranulation.[160] (See previous discussion in sections on pigmentation and edema.)

Approximately 40% of patients studied by Norris et al.[39] described temporary itching after injections with POL regardless of drug dosage. Duffy[5] reports an almost 100% occurrence of urticaria with injection of either POL or HS-heparin-lidocaine solutions. The urtication is usually more intense when more concentrated solutions are used.[5,10] Urtication may also be more intense with repeat injection sessions, especially when POL or STS is used.

Treatment. In my experience localized urticaria and itching can be diminished by applying topical steroids immediately after injection and by limiting the injection quantity per injection site. This method is particularly helpful in patients who will wear a graduated support stocking after treatment. High-potency topical corticosteroids, such as clobetasol propionate, have been shown to rapidly decrease histamine-induced pruritus.[161] Therefore I recommend application of a nongreasy, fast-absorbing, high-potency corticosteroid to all treated areas after sclerotherapy. A secondary effect of the topical corticosteroid is vasoconstriction, which may also help with vessel resolution and minimize posttreatment thrombosis with its sequelae.

Tape Compression Blister

Tape compression blisters (Figure 16-8) occur when a tape dressing is applied to an area of tissue movement or to thin skin (e.g., in elderly patients). The blister usually appears as a flaccid, fluid-filled sac overlying normal-appearing skin. It is usually not associated with induration or erythema of the adjacent skin. Common sites of occurrence are the posterior calf, medial thigh, and popliteal fossa.

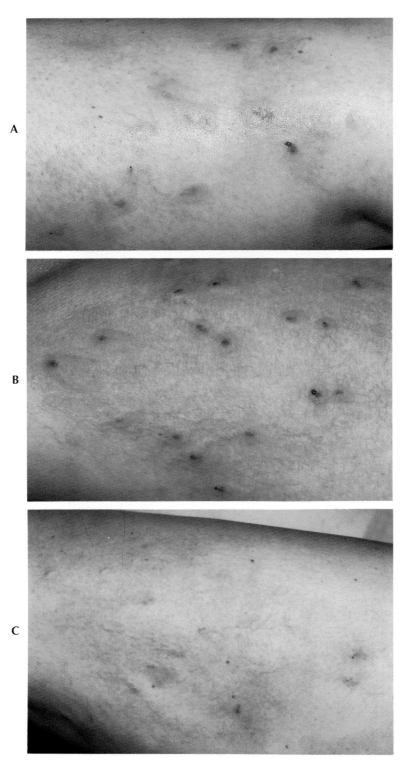

FIGURE 16-7. Urtication. **A,** Immediately after sclerotherapy with Sclerodex. **B,** Immediately after sclerotherapy with Scleremo. **C,** Immediately following sclerotherapy with POL 0.5%. Note relatively increased degree of edema and erythema as compared with urtication from Sclerodex and Scleremo.

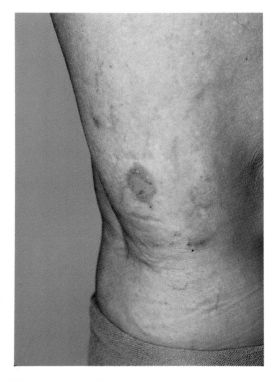

FIGURE 16-8. Superficial blister that developed 1 week after sclerotherapy treatment. Compression of treated area was produced with foam (sodium tetradecyl sulfate) pad overlaid with Microfoam tape and a 30 to 40 mm Hg graduated thigh-length compression stocking (shown pulled down below knee).

Blisters may occur with the use of any tape but appear more commonly when one uses Microfoam tape (3M Medical-Surgical Division, St. Paul, Minn.) as opposed to a hypoallergenic paper tape, such as Dermilite II (Johnson & Johnson, New Brunswick, N.J.), over foam pads or cottonballs, probably because of the greater adhesiveness of the Microfoam tape. In addition, Microfoam tape is usually placed over the foam dressing with a slight amount of tension, thus increasing the tension on either end of the tape. Blistering is also more common in the summer months, when the weather is hotter, and in elderly patients, who have thinner, more fragile skin.

The only problem with blistering is that it must be distinguished from early cutaneous necrosis, cutaneous infection, or an allergic reaction. Early cutaneous necrosis may appear as a superficial blister. In this situation the underlying and adjacent tissue is usually indurated and erythematous. Bullous impetigo can also have a similar physical appearance. In this condition the blister is usually overlying warm, erythematous skin. If not warned beforehand, patients may think that the blister is the result of an allergy to the sclerosing solution. A detailed explanation of the cause of the blister is usually required before treatment can continue.

Prevention. If compression pads are used under graduated stockings in a pa-

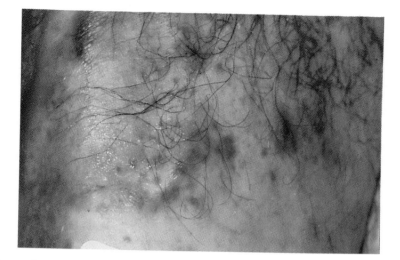

FIGURE 16-9. Folliculitis apparent 7 days after sclerotherapy. Compression of treated area was produced with foam (sodium tetradecyl sulfate) pads overlaid with Microfoam tape. (From Goldman MP. Sclerotherapy: Treatment of Varicose and Telangiectatic Leg Veins. St. Louis: Mosby, 1991, p 236. Reprinted with permission.)

tient susceptible to blistering, a Tubigrip tubular support bandage (Seton Products, Inc., Montgomeryville, Pa.) can be used over the pad to hold it in place while the stocking is being applied. Although somewhat costly, this dressing (similar to a net dressing used in burn patients) helps prevent blister formation. (It can also be used in patients with allergies to tape.)

Treatment. Resolution of the blister occurs within 1 or 2 weeks without any adverse sequelae. To aid healing and prevent infection of the denuded skin, the use of an occlusive hydroactive dressing such as Duoderm (ConvaTec, Princeton, N.J.) is helpful. Occlusive dressings may also help alleviate any pain associated with the blister.

Tape Compression Folliculitis

Occlusion of any hairy area can promote the development of folliculitis (Figure 16-9). If they do not have secondary alopecia associated with chronic venous insufficiency, men seeking treatment for varicose veins usually have hairy legs. If a tape dressing is placed over foam or cottonball pads under a graduated compression stocking, a follicular inflammation or infection may occur.

Folliculitis is more likely to occur in the summer months or when patients are active and perspire under the dressing.

Treatment. Treatment consists of removal of the occlusive dressing and application of topical treatment with an antibacterial soap such as chlorhexidine gluconate (Hibiclens Antimicrobial Skin Cleanser) or a topical antibiotic gel such as erythromycin 2% (Erygel Topical Gel) or clindamycin phosphate topical solution 1% (Cleocin T). The folliculitis usually resolves within a few days. Only rarely will use of systemic antibiotics be necessary.

Recurrence

Recurrence of sclerotherapy-treated vessels has been estimated to occur in 20% to nearly 100% of leg telangiectasias at 5-year follow-up.[162] Recanalization of initially thrombosed leg veins is procedure dependent. The larger the extent of intravascular thrombosis, the greater is the likelihood of recanalization of the thrombosis during vascular organization.[163,164] The recanalization of injected varices without subsequent compression or with inadequate compression is caused by clot contraction and the formation of sinuses that may become lined with endothelium, central clot liquefaction and the formation of vascular tunnels through the thrombosis, formation of vascular organization of the thrombosis and collateral vessel formation of the newly formed capillaries, and formation of peripheral sinuses filled with sludged blood[164,165] (Figure 16-10). Therefore the most important factor in preventing recurrence is the limiting of intravascular thrombosis.

Treatment. Tournay[166] was the first physician to stress the importance of postinjection removal of blood clots in 1938. The importance of draining these postsclerotherapy thrombi has since been emphasized by Sigg,[167] Pratt,[168] Hobbs,[169] and Orbach.[163]

With proper technique, recurrence of varicose veins only rarely occurs. A biopsy study of six patients with "recurrence" of previously treated veins demonstrated that the veins thought to have recurred were in reality new varicose veins.[170] When high recurrence rates are reported, the patients have usually been

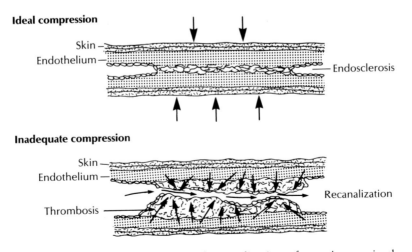

FIGURE 16-10. Diagrammatic representation of recanalization of a varicose vein through sclerotherapy-induced thrombosis. (Redrawn from Wenner L. Vasa 15:180, 1986. From Goldman MP. Sclerotherapy: Treatment of Varicose and Telangiectatic Leg Veins. St. Louis: Mosby, 1991, p 237. Reprinted with permission.)

treated with minimal compression.[163] For example, in one study of 310 patients, 83% required reinjection of a treated varicosity. These patients received only 48 hours of compression with elastic bandages.[158]

Unlike recanalization through a varicose vein cord, recanalization is not common through a sclerosed telangiectasia. Posttreatment histologic studies have demonstrated only fibrosis in an area treated with sclerotherapy.[4] One study of telangiectasias found a "recurrence rate" of 77%.[171] Examination of the telangiectasias present 1 year after treatment most likely indicated either untreated telangiectasias or new telangiectasias, not recurrent veins.

Stress-Related Symptoms

Vasovagal reflex. The vasovagal reflex is a common adverse sequela of any surgical or invasive procedure. It has been estimated to occur in 1% of patients during sclerotherapy[172] and is more frequent when the technique of Fegan or Sigg is used.[173] With the latter two techniques, 21- to 25-gauge needles are inserted while the patient is sitting or standing, and blood is allowed to flow freely from the punctured vein. Duffy,[5] who performs sclerotherapy with 30-gauge needles in reclining patients, estimates the incidence of vasovagal reactions as 0.001%. It is interesting that the percentage of men who experience this response far exceeds the percentage of women.

Vasovagal reactions have typical clinical findings. The usual symptoms include light-headedness, nausea, and sweating. The patient may also experience shortness of breath and palpitations. Syncope rarely occurs but usually provokes the most concern in the physician and staff. Vasovagal reactions are most often preceded by painful injection but may even occur from the patient's seeing the needle or smelling the sclerosing solution.

Prevention. The main concern in a vasovagal reaction is that the patient will fall and be injured. Therefore both the nurse and the physician should watch the patient closely for signs of restlessness and excessive perspiration. All patients should be warned to sit down if they become dizzy. When needle placement is performed on a standing patient, it is also helpful for the patient to hold onto an arm rail or other support. Vasovagal reactions are easily reversible when the patient assumes the supine or Trendelenburg position. Preventive measures consist of recommending that the patient eat a light meal before the appointment, affording good ventilation in the treatment room, and maintaining constant communication with the patient during the procedure.

The physician must recognize the vasovagal response in a patient and not assume that an anaphylactic reaction is occurring. If subcutaneous epinephrine is given in the mistaken belief that an anaphylactic reaction is occurring, the symptoms will become both exaggerated and obscured. This effect only further confuses the clinical situation and adds to the patient's apprehension about further treatment sessions.

Underlying medical disease. More serious stress-induced problems include exacerbation of certain underlying medical diseases. Patients with a history of asthma may experience wheezing, which can be treated with a bronchodilator such as metaproterenol sulfate (Alupent, Proventil) or over-the-counter epinephrine bitartrate in a metered-dose inhaler (Primatene).

Patients with cardiovascular disease may develop angina, which is treatable with sublingual nitroglycerin tablets. As discussed in detail later, POL is a negative inotropic agent that slows cardiac contractility in a dose-dependent manner. STS has also been reported to produce chest pain, but this effect is not cardiac in nature. In my practice one 65-year-old patient without a history of cardiac disease who was treated with STS developed acute chest pain on two separate occasions when using 0.5% STS, 2 to 4 ml. An electrocardiogram taken as soon as the patient began experiencing chest pain was normal, and sublingual nitroglycerin was ineffective in resolving the pain, which lasted approximately 5 minutes. Thus this effect may be an idiosyncratic reaction.

Urticaria is easily treated with an oral antihistamine but may be a sign of systemic allergy. Therefore the use of the sclerosing agent in future treatment sessions should be carefully evaluated. The incidence of urticaria with various sclerosing agents is detailed later. Throughout more than 15 years, urticaria has occurred in only one of my patients treated with STS. It lasted less than 1 hour and resolved with oral diphenhydramine. Subsequent treatment with POL was unremarkable.

It is intriguing that urticaria and periorbital edema have occurred even with injection of unadulterated HS solution (D.M. Duffy, personal communication, 1989). This effect may be related to histamine release from irritated perivascular mast cells. Finally, the triggering of frequent migraine headaches has also occurred after sclerotherapy.[5]

Localized hirsutism. Localized hypertrichosis developing after sclerotherapy with the use of multiple sclerosing agents has been described. The etiology is believed to be the result of an improved cutaneous oxygen content, which stimulates increased hair growth, or of a long-standing low-grade inflammatory reaction that increases vascularity. In support of this phenomenon, patients with chronic venous insufficiency have been reported to develop localized hair growth after surgical treatment.[174]

Hair growth at the site of injection has been described in three patients treated with STS.[175] All patients were given injections of 1 to 6 ml of STS over 5 to 10 sessions. Localized hair growth developed 4 to 7 months after the last injection. The site of hair growth was related to the area of skin most damaged by venous incompetence. Weissberg[176] has also reported on the development of localized hirsutism in 1 of 62 patients treated with STS. The hair growth occurred at the site of injection 1 month after treatment. It lasted 4 months and then subsided. Sclerotherapy with polyiodinated iodine has also been associated with hypertrichosis at the injection site in three cases.[170] Two cases of hirsutism were also noted after sclerotherapy with POL.[177] Therefore the sclerosing solution itself is not the cause; the action that the solution exerts on either the surrounding microcirculation or inflammation produces this rare effect. Although there have been a few case reports of hirsutism, this effect must be very rare because I have yet to see it in more than 15 years of an active practice in venous disease.

COMPLICATIONS
Cutaneous Necrosis

Etiology. Cutaneous necrosis may occur with the injection of any sclerosing agent, even under ideal circumstances, and does not necessarily represent physician error. Fortunately, its occurrence is both rare and usually of limited sequelae. Its cause may be the result of (1) extravasation of a sclerosing solution into the perivascular tissues, (2) injection into a dermal arteriole or an arteriole feeding into a telangiectatic or varicose vein, (3) a reactive vasospasm of the vessel, or (4) excessive cutaneous pressure created by compression techniques.

Extravasation. Extravasation of caustic sclerosing solutions may directly destroy tissue. The extent of tissue injury is directly related to both the concentration of the sclerosing solution as well as the quantity extravasated. Different sclerosing solutions have a greater or lesser ability to destroy tissue. Since the final clinical appearance of the skin may not be apparent for several days, therapeutic intervention must be undertaken as soon as possible in all cases.

Clinically, one sees bright erythema in the skin overlying the extravasated solution (Figure 16-11). With certain extravasation injuries, the formation of epidermal blistering may occur; however, it does not predict a partial-thickness injury but may precede eventual full-thickness necrosis.[178]

During injection of an abnormal vein or telangiectasia, even the most adept physician may inadvertently inject a small quantity of sclerosing solution into the perivascular tissue (Figure 16-12). A tiny amount of sclerosing solution may be left in the tissue when the needle is withdrawn, and sclerosing solution may leak

FIGURE 16-11. Porcelain-white cutaneous reaction immediately after injection with POL 0.25%. This area healed within 4 weeks without any complications. (From Goldman MP. Sclerotherapy: Treatment of Varicose and Telangiectatic Leg Veins. St. Louis: Mosby, 1991, p 244. Reprinted with permission.)

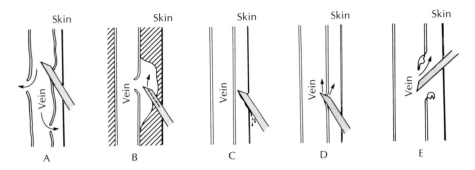

FIGURE 16-12. Mechanisms for extravasation of sclerosing solution. **A,** Through multiple needle puncture holes. **B,** From injection of solution after slight withdrawal of needle. **C,** Along needle shaft. **D,** From injection with needle bevel both in and out of vein. **E,** Through excessive destruction of vein wall. (Redrawn from Biegeleisen HI. Varicose Veins, Related Diseases, and Sclerotherapy: A Guide for Practitioners. Montreal: Eden Press, 1984. From Goldman MP. Sclerotherapy: Treatment of Varicose and Telangiectatic Leg Veins. St. Louis: Mosby, 1991, p 241. Reprinted with permission.)

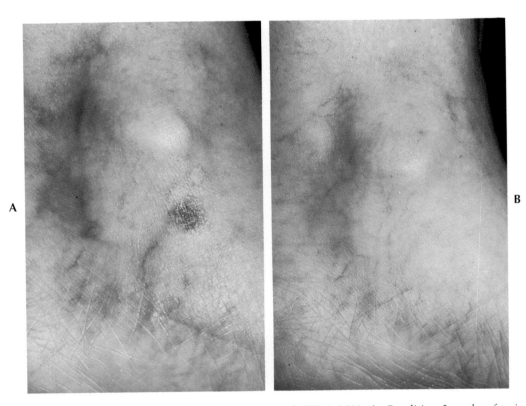

FIGURE 16-13. Cutaneous necrosis after injection with STS 0.25%. **A,** Condition 3 weeks after injection. **B,** Complete resolution of necrosis after 20 months.

out of the injected vessel, which has been traumatized by multiple or through-and-through needle punctures. Rarely, the injection of a strong sclerosing solution into a fragile vessel may lead to endothelial necrosis and rupture, producing a "blowout" of the vessel and perivascular extravasation of sclerosing solution (Figure 16-13). Therefore injection technique is an important but not foolproof factor in avoiding this complication, even under optimal circumstances.

Sclerosing solutions vary in the degree of cellular necrosis they produce. If minimal tissue necrosis is caused by a sclerosing agent, it may even be suitable for perivascular injection in the treatment of telangiectatic mats, whose vessels cannot be cannulated, even with a 33-gauge needle.

Hyperosmotic agents with an osmolality greater than that of serum (281 to 289 mOsm/L) can cause tissue damage as a result of osmotic factors. Epidermal necrosis has even occurred from extravasation of solutions containing 10% dextrose.[179] HS 23.4% is a caustic sclerosing agent, as demonstrated in intradermal injection experiments. Clinically, small punctate spots of superficial epidermal damage occur at points of injection, especially when a small bleb of the solution escapes from the vein. However, subcutaneous injection of up to 1 ml of HS 23.4% (by mistake) instead of lidocaine into the neck or cheek has been reported to result in no adverse sequelae.[180] In this situation cutaneous necrosis was most likely avoided by rapid physiologic dilution of HS. Alternatively, dermal tissue may be more resistant to the caustic effects of HSs. However, the increasing frequency of cutaneous necrosis occurring after extravasation of inadvertent subcutaneous injection of HS has moved the Department of Health and Human Services and the product manufacturer (American Regent Laboratories, Inc., Shirley, N.Y.) to recommend that storage of HS be done only in pharmacies where all dilutions would be performed before dispensing. This approach would eliminate the possibility of an iatrogenic medication error outside the pharmacy (Mary Helenek, American Regent Laboratories, Inc., written communication, May 1990). It is recommended that HS be stored in a location separate from other injectable solutions to avoid this potential complication.

Experimentally, POL apparently is minimally toxic to subcutaneous tissue. Duffy[181] has reported injecting 0.5 ml of a 3% solution of POL directly into his own skin without the development of an ulceration. Although some physicians advocate the use of intradermal POL 0.5% to treat tiny telangiectatic leg veins,[182,183] POL in sufficient concentration will cause cutaneous necrosis. Solutions of POL greater than 1% may produce superficial necrosis with intradermal injection.[182] Unfortunately, this occurred in my practice with the mistaken injection of 0.1 ml POL 5% solution into a leg telangiectasia of 0.2 mm in diameter. This injection resulted in extensive overlying cutaneous necrosis that took 8 weeks to heal. Therefore POL is not without the risk of cutaneous necrosis if a strong enough concentration is injected.

Although STS is more toxic to tissue than POL with extravasation, concentrations above 0.25% are usually necessary to produce ulceration. Banning[184] has reported on 5 of 4860 consecutive patients who developed ulcerations after tel-

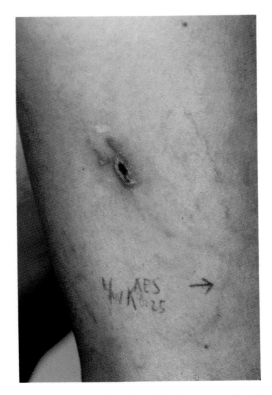

FIGURE 16-14. Cutaneous necrosis 6 weeks after sclerotherapy with POL 0.25%. Note that 2 ml of solution was injected into a feeder vein *(arrow)* approximately 10 cm distal to necrotic area.

angiectasias were injected with STS 0.1%. However, this result probably represents injection into an arteriole.

Glycerin or CG solutions have not been reported to produce cutaneous necrosis with extravasation. Duffy (personal communication, 1992) has shown that injection of "full strength" CG will not produce cutaneous necrosis when it is injected into the middle dermis. Histologic examination of his patient showed no evidence of dermal or epidermal damage.

Even when sclerotherapy is performed with expert technique and the safest sclerosing solutions and concentrations are used, cutaneous ulceration may occur (Figure 16-14). Therefore it appears that extravasation of caustic sclerosing solutions alone is not totally responsible for this complication.

Arteriolar injection. De Faria and Moraes[185] have observed that 1 in 26 leg telangiectasias is associated with a dermal arteriole. I think that inadvertent injection into or near this communication is the most common cause of cutaneous ulcerations.

POL has been injected intradermally to effect sclerosis of TM in my practice without the development of cutaneous ulceration, even with the injection of 0.5 ml of a 0.75% solution. However, I have noted the development of ulcera-

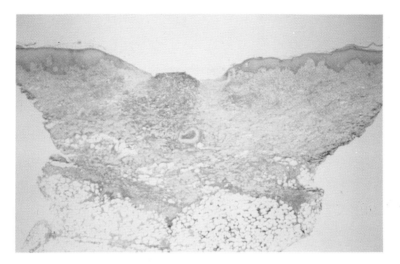

FIGURE 16-15. Low-power magnification view showing arterial ulceration and focal inflammation extending into subcutaneous fat. A thrombosed vessel, most likely an artery, is present directly under area of necrosis (hematoxylin-eosin ×25). (From Goldman MP. Sclerotherapy: Treatment of Varicose and Telangiectatic Leg Veins. St. Louis: Mosby, 1991, p 243. Reprinted with permission.)

tions of 3 to 6 mm in diameter in approximately 0.0001% of injections with POL 0.5%. Five consecutive ulcerations that appeared over the course of 12 months were excised. In these patients each cutaneous ulceration developed as a result of the occlusion of the feeding dermal arteriole. This occlusion produced a classic wedge-shaped arterial ulceration (Figure 16-15). At 2 years the Australian Polidocanol Open Clinical Trial reported 43 ulcers on 32 legs after sclerotherapy treatment of varicose and telangiectatic leg veins on 12,544 legs for an incidence of 0.23%.[186] Therefore it appears that this complication may be unavoidable to some extent.

Vasospasm. Rarely after injection of the sclerosing solution, an immediate porcelain-white appearance to the skin is noted at the site of injection (Figure 16-16). A hemorrhagic bulla usually forms over this area within 2 to 48 hours (Figure 16-17) and progresses to an ulcer.[73] This cutaneous reaction might represent an arterial spasm.

Vasospastic reactions of arteries occur in predisposed individuals for unknown reasons.[187-189] Such reactions may occur even with puncture of the artery without injection of sclerosing solution.[189] Thus small vessels, when irritated in susceptible patients, may spasm.

In an attempt to reverse the spasm, vigorous massage when the white macule appears has sometimes averted ulceration. However, prevention of the ulceration with massage alone is not always successful. Massaging in a 2% nitroglycerin ointment is more likely to prevent the development of ulcerations in this setting.

The major systemic action of nitrates is a direct reduction in venous smooth muscle tone.[190] Nitrates also relieve spasm of angiographically normal and dis-

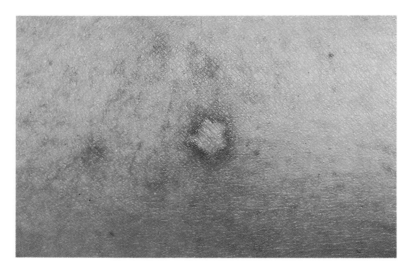

FIGURE 16-16. Porcelain-white cutaneous reaction immediately after injection with POL 0.5% in upper lateral thigh. Frank cutaneous ulceration later developed in this area. (From Goldman MP. Sclerotherapy: Treatment of Varicose and Telangiectatic Leg Veins. St. Louis: Mosby, 1991, p 245. Reprinted with permission.)

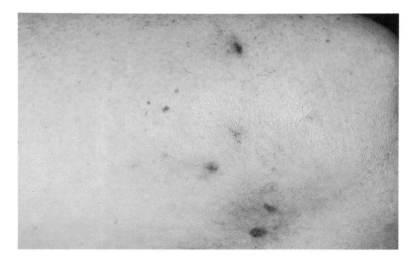

FIGURE 16-17. Hemorrhagic bulla, a macular reaction 1 week after injection with POL 0.5%. This area healed without any complications. (From Goldman MP. Sclerotherapy: Treatment of Varicose and Telangiectatic Leg Veins. St. Louis: Mosby, 1991, p 244. Reprinted with permission.)

eased arteries.[191] Topical nitroglycerin ointment has been reported as beneficial in treating both dopamine extravasation and vasoconstriction necrosis.[192,193] Although more experience from other investigators needs to be reported, it seems prudent to use this technique.

Arterial spasm may also explain the development of cutaneous ulceration upstream from the injection site (see Figure 16-14). In the latter case 2 ml of POL 0.25% was injected into a feeding reticular vein, as shown by the arrow. That was the only injection given to the patient in that sclerotherapy session.

Lymphatic injection. Injection into a lymphatic vessel may also lead to cutaneous necrosis. Histologic studies have disclosed evidence of lymphovenous anastomoses in humans.[194] It is possible that injection into such an anastomosis could result in necrosis of the associated lymphatic vessel and infiltration of the sclerosing solution extravascularly. If the sclerosing solution is caustic to extravascular tissues, the result may be tissue necrosis.

Excessive compression. Excessive compression of the skin overlying the treated vein may produce tissue anoxia with the development of localized cutaneous ulceration. Subcutaneous tissue flow in the leg is decreased when cutaneous pressure exceeds 20 mm Hg.[195] In addition, external pressure >30 mm Hg reduces muscle blood flow in some patients.[196] Therefore excessive compression may produce tissue ischemia. However, both of these studies used indirect measurements of subcutaneous tissue flow and calf muscle blood flow and thus must be viewed with caution. A more physiologic method for measuring the effect of compression on blood flow was recently performed through determination of femoral blood flow.[197] The authors demonstrated that, in the recumbent patient, static, graduated external compression of approximately 20 mm Hg at the ankle (reduced to approximately 10 mm Hg in the upper thigh) produces an increase in femoral flow of up to 75%. However, if calf pressures exceed 30 mm Hg when the patient is recumbent, a progressive fall in subcutaneous tissue flow and deep venous velocity occurs. Therefore it is recommended that patients not wear a graduated compression stocking of >30 to 40 mm Hg when lying down for prolonged periods of time.

One method for applying compression to treated veins that could be varied with patient position is that of using a double layer of graduated compression stockings. This approach would ensure that maximal pressure over the vein is maintained while the patient is ambulatory. When the patient is recumbent, the outer stocking is removed, thereby decreasing the cutaneous pressure to 20 to 30 mm Hg at the ankle, which should prevent a reduction in cutaneous and subcutaneous blood flow. Another method, described in Chapter 14, is to use foam or rolled cotton wool directly over the treated varicose vein, which increases the pressure under the foam by over 50%.

Prevention. If extravasation of sclerosing solution occurs, the solution must be diluted as soon as possible. HSs should be diluted with copious amounts of normal saline solution. At least 10 times the volume of extravasated solution should be injected to limit osmotic damage.

Detergent sclerosing solutions of adequate strength may also be toxic to tissues. Dilution is again of paramount importance. Dilution with hyaluronidase in normal saline solution limits the extent and prevents the development of cutaneous necrosis from 3% STS.[198] Hyaluronidase (Wydase, lyophilized, 150 USP U/ml) enzymatically breaks down connective tissue hyaluronic acid. This action is hypothesized to disrupt the normal interstitial fluid barrier to allow rapid diffusion of solution through tissues, thereby increasing the effective absorption.[199,200] This beneficial effect has been demonstrated in limiting IV extravasation injuries from 10% dextrose, calcium and potassium salts, contrast media, sodium bicarbonate, aminophylline, hyperalimentation solution, and doxorubicin.[199,201-204] In addition to its enhanced dilutional ability, hyaluronidase may have an independent cellular preservation function.

Hyaluronidase injection improves skin flap survival[205] and reduces myocardial infarction.[206] These effects have been postulated to occur through enhanced nutritive flow. Enhanced healing with resolution of painful induration was observed when 250 U of hyaluronidase was injected in an area where neoarsphenamine and mapharsen were extravasated subcutaneously.[207] Finally, hyaluronidase promotes wound repair in fetal skin, contributing to scarless repair of wounds by as yet unclear mechanisms.[208] In summary, accelerated dilution, cellular stabilization, and wound repair properties of hyaluronidase appear useful in preventing cutaneous necrosis from inadvertent sclerosing solution extravasation.

Side effects from hyaluronidase use are rare and generally of the urticarial type.[209,210] Because of its limited stability, hyaluronidase should be reconstituted with 0.9% sodium chloride solution immediately before use. The ideal concentration and quantity to inject after extravasation has been reported to be 75 U in a volume of 3 ml. Higher doses did not appear to improve clinical outcome after intradermal infiltration of 0.25 ml of 23.4% HS.[211] For maximal effectiveness, I recommend injecting the diluted solution into multiple sites around the extravasated area. Studies have demonstrated that hyaluronidase solution must be injected within 60 minutes of extravasation to be effective.[212]

Treatment. Whatever the cause of the ulceration, it must be dealt with when it occurs. Fortunately, ulcerations, when they do occur, are usually fairly small, averaging 4 mm in diameter in my practice. At this size primary healing usually leaves an acceptable scar (see Figure 16-13). In addition to various topical agents directly applied to the ulcer, elevation of the affected extremity and systemic pentoxifylline may be helpful in minimizing the ulcer size. In a series of 26 extravasation sloughs, less tissue damage occurred when limbs were elevated.[213]

Pentoxifylline may decrease tissue injury of ischemia-reperfusion by inhibiting the production of platelet-activating factor during reperfusion.[214] Pentoxifylline should improve microcirculatory dysfunction observed during reperfusion of ischemic tissues. Pentoxifylline causes increased deformability of red blood cells and lowers blood viscosity.[215-217] The optimal dosage appears to be 25 mg/kg for protective effects in experimental studies in the canine gracilis muscle model. However, the dosage that produces maximal protective effects in humans is unknown.

Bodian,[93] who uses 23.4% HS, notes that ulceration usually takes 3½ months to heal, even when judicious wound care is given. He advocates treatment with a daily application of 20% benzoyl peroxide powder (Vanoxide Acne Lotion) under moist dressings cut to fit snugly over the ulcer. However, benzoyl peroxide is cytotoxic for newly growing epidermis. Therefore its use cannot be recommended. I have found that the use of occlusive or hydrocolloid dressings results in an apparent decrease in wound healing time. Occlusive dressings do not speed healing of full-thickness ulcers until granulation tissue has formed. Hydrocolloid gel dressings enhance debridement of wounds, possibly through their pectin-gelatin base. Nongelatin, nonpectin hydrocolloid dressings act only to stimulate fibrinolysis. Thus its enhanced efficacy may be related to wound debridement, which should always be used either medically or surgically to promote granulation tissue formation.

More important, the use of occlusive dressings decreases the pain associated with an open ulcer. Dressings must be changed every 3 to 4 days, and necrotic tissue should be sharply debrided every week or two as needed to promote granulation tissue. However, because an ulcer may take 4 to 6 weeks to heal completely even under ideal conditions, if possible, excision and closure of these lesions are recommended at the earliest possible time. This approach affords the patient the fastest healing and an acceptable scar.

Systemic Allergic Reaction or Toxicity

Systemic reactions caused by sclerotherapy treatment occur very rarely.

Minor reactions. Minor reactions such as urticaria are easily treated with an oral antihistamine such as diphenhydramine (Benadryl), 25 to 50 mg PO, or hydroxyzine (Atarax), 10 to 25 mg PO. Rarely, the addition of corticosteroids is needed if the reaction does not subside readily. A short course of prednisone, 40 to 60 mg per day for 1 week, in conjunction with systemic antihistamine administered every 6 to 8 hours is helpful. Since suppression of the adrenal axis is not a problem with this short course, a tapering schedule is not necessary.

Because of the possibility of angioedema or bronchospasm, each patient with evidence of an allergic reaction should be examined for stridor and wheezing through auscultation over the neck and chest while the patient breathes normally. Supine and sitting blood pressure and pulse should be checked to rule out orthostatic changes, hypotension, or tachycardia, which might result from the vasodilation that precedes anaphylactic shock.

Minor degrees of angioedema can be treated with oral antihistamines; however, if stridor is present, an intramuscular (IM) injection of diphenhydramine and IV corticosteroids should be administered, and a laryngoscope and endotracheal tube should be available.

Bronchospasm is estimated to occur after sclerotherapy in 0.001% of patients.[5] It usually responds to the addition of an inhaled bronchodilator or IV aminophylline, 6 mg/kg over 20 minutes, or to the antihistamine-corticosteroid regimen already noted.

Wheezing has been reported to occur in up to 5% of patients treated with HS (M. Coverman, personal communication, 1991). Coverman notes wheezing that resolves spontaneously, occurring 15 minutes after the completion of sclerotherapy. He has found that if treatment sessions are performed with the patient sitting at a 45-degree angle, wheezing can be aborted. This wheezing is probably not an allergic reaction but an irritant phenomenon produced on the airways. Alternatively, it may be related to rapid infusion of histamine from perivascular mast cell degranulation with damage from the hyperosmotic solution.

Major reactions. Four types of potentially serious systemic reactions specific to the type of sclerosing agent have been noted: anaphylaxis, pulmonary toxicity, cardiac toxicity, and renal toxicity. These reactions are discussed both in general and separately for each sclerosing solution.

Anaphylaxis is a systemic hypersensitivity response caused by exposure or, more commonly, reexposure to a sensitizing substance. Anaphylaxis is usually an immunoglobulin E (IgE)–mediated, mast cell–activated reaction that occurs most often within minutes of antigen exposure. Other classes of immunoglobulin, such as IgG, may also produce anaphylaxis.[218] Since the risk of anaphylaxis increases with repeated exposures to the antigen, one should always be prepared for this reaction in every patient.[219]

The principal manifestations of anaphylaxis occur in areas where mast cell concentrations are highest: skin, lungs, and gastrointestinal tract. Histamine release is responsible for the clinical manifestations of this reaction. Although urticaria and abdominal pain are common, the three principal manifestations of anaphylaxis are airway edema, bronchospasm, and vascular collapse. Urticaria alone does not constitute anaphylaxis and should not be treated as such because of the potential side effects of treatment with epinephrine, especially in older patients.

The signs and symptoms of anaphylaxis initially may be subtle and often include anxiety, itching, sneezing, coughing, urticaria, and angioedema. Wheezing may be accompanied by hoarseness of the voice and vomiting. Shortly after these presenting signs, breathing becomes more difficult, and the patient usually collapses from cardiovascular failure resulting from systemic vasodilation. One helpful clue toward distinguishing between anaphylaxis and a vasovagal reaction is heart rate. Sinus tachycardia is almost always present in a patient with anaphylaxis, whereas bradycardia or cardiac rhythm disturbances are commonplace in vasovagal reactions.

The recommended treatment is to give epinephrine, 0.2 to 0.5 ml 1:1000 subcutaneously (SC). This dose can be repeated three to four times at 5- to 15-minute intervals to maintain a systolic blood pressure above 90 to 100 mm Hg. This administration should be followed by establishment of an IV line of 0.9% sodium chloride solution. Diphenhydramine hydrochloride, 50 mg, is given next along with cimetidine, 300 mg; both the IV solution and oxygen are given at 4 to 6 L/min. An endotracheal tube or tracheotomy is necessary for laryngeal obstruction. For asthma or wheezing, IV theophylline, 4 to 6 mg/kg, is infused over 15 minutes. At this point it is appropriate to transfer the patient to the hospital.

Methylprednisolone sodium succinate, 60 mg, is given intravenously and repeated every 6 hours for four doses. Corticosteroids are not an emergency medication since their effect appears only after 1 to 3 hours. They are given to prevent the recurrence of symptoms 3 to 8 hours after the initial event. The patient should be hospitalized overnight for observation.

Allergic reactions to sclerosing agents

Sodium morrhuate. Although touted by the manufacturer as "the natural sclerosing agent," sodium morrhuate (SM) causes a variety of allergic reactions, ranging from mild erythema with pruritus[220-222] to generalized urticaria[222-224] to gastrointestinal disturbances with abdominal pain and diarrhea[220,221] to anaphylaxis. It has been estimated that "unfavorable reactions" in the treatment of varicose leg veins occur in 3% of patients.[225] The incidence of allergic reactions in the treatment of esophageal varices ranges from 11% to 48%.[226] The reason for the high number of allergic reactions associated with SM may be related to the inability to remove all the fish proteins that are present in this product. In fact, 20.8% of the fatty acid composition of the solution is unknown.[227]

Many cases of anaphylaxis have occurred within a few minutes after the drug was injected or more commonly when therapy was reinstituted after a few weeks.[222,228-230] Most of these cases occurred before 1950. Rarely, anaphylaxis has resulted in fatalities,[224,225,231] many of which have not been reported in the medical literature.[220]

While under anesthesia, one patient developed bronchospasm when being given the twelfth injection of SM. This patient responded readily to antihistamine and epinephrine. Subsequently the patient was treated with STS without an adverse reaction.[232]

Pleural effusions with pulmonary edema and acute respiratory failure appearing as adult respiratory distress syndrome (ARDS) are common with esophageal injection.[227] It has been estimated that pleural effusions occur in 46% of patients with an esophageal injection.[233] With injection into esophageal varices, the sclerosing solution rapidly enters the pulmonary circulation, causing increased permeability of the pulmonary microvasculature.[227] There have been no reports of pleural effusions with injection into varicose veins of the legs.

Prolonged dysrhythmia requiring placement of a permanent pacemaker has been reported in two cases.[234] This complication has been attributed to a direct cardiotoxic effect of SM.

Ethanolamine oleate. EO (Ethamolin) is a synthetic mixture of ethanolamine and oleic acid with an empirical formula of $C_{20}H_{41}NO_3$. The minimal lethal IV dose in rabbits is 130 mg/kg.[223] The oleic acid component is responsible for the inflammatory action. Oleic acid may also activate coagulation in vitro by release of tissue factor and Hageman factor. Biegeleisen[235] observed no toxic effects in 500 injections. EO is thought to have a decreased risk of allergic reactions compared with SM or STS.[236] However, pulmonary toxicity and allergic reactions have been associated with EO.

Pleural effusion, edema, and infiltration and pneumonitis have been demonstrated in human trials with the injection of esophageal varices. Pleural effusion or infiltration has been estimated by the product manufacturer to occur in 2.1% of patients and pneumonia in 1.2% of patients. One study of 75 patients treated for esophageal varices disclosed abnormal chest x-ray films showing infiltration or effusion in 45 patients, an incidence of 60%.[237] These conditions usually resolve spontaneously within 48 hours.

Anaphylactic shock has been reported by the product manufacturer after injection in three cases (product information [1989] from Glaxo Pharmaceuticals, Research Triangle Park, N.C.). Another case of a nearly fatal anaphylactic reaction during the fourth treatment of varicose leg veins with 1 ml of solution has also been reported.[238] In one additional case a fatal reaction occurred in a man with a known allergic disposition (product information [1989] from Glaxo Pharmaceuticals, Research Triangle Park, N.C.). Another episode of a fatal anaphylactic reaction occurred in a woman having her third series of injections[220]; this episode represented one reaction in 200 patients from that author's practice. Generalized urticaria occurred in approximately 1 in 400 patients; this symptom responded rapidly to an antihistamine.[239]

Acute renal failure with spontaneous recovery occurred after injection of 15 to 20 ml of EO in two women (Clin-alert correspondence, 1992). A hemolytic reaction occurred in 5 patients in a series of more than 900 patients, with injection of more than 12 ml of 0.5% EO per patient per treatment session.[239] The patients were described as "feeling generally unwell and shivery, with aching in the loins and passage of red-brown urine. All rapidly recovered with bed rest and were perfectly normal the next day." Injections of less than 12 ml per treatment session have not resulted in this reaction.

Transient chest pain has also been reported in 13 of 23 patients treated for esophageal varices.[240] However, pyrexia and substernal chest pain are considered common sequelae of injection of esophageal varices with any sclerosing agent.[236]

EO has also been tested for carcinogenic activity in the albino rat by intradermal injection without induction of tumors.[241]

Sodium tetradecyl sulfate. A synthetic detergent developed in the 1940s, STS has been used throughout the world as a sclerosing solution. A comprehensive review of the medical literature (in multiple specialties and languages) until 1987 disclosed a total of 47 cases of nonfatal allergic reactions in a review of 14,404 treated patients. This review included six case reports.[242] A separate review of treatment in 187 patients with 2249 injections disclosed no evidence of allergic or systemic reactions.[243] An additional report of 5341 injections given to an unknown number of patients found "no unfavorable reaction."[244] Fegan[245] reviewed his experience with STS in 16,000 patients. He reported 15 cases of "serum sickness, with hot stinging pain in the skin, and an erythematous rash developing 30 to 90 minutes after injection." These patients subsequently underwent additional uneventful treatment with STS after premedication with antihistamines. Ten additional patients developed "mild anaphylaxis" that required treatment with an injection of epinephrine. If one were to combine only those reviews of more than 1000 patients, the incidence of nonfatal allergic reactions would be approximately 0.3%.[6,239,246-248]

The product manufacturer notes two fatalities associated with the use of STS, both from the sclerotherapy procedure itself and not specifically related to STS. One fatality occurred in a patient who was receiving an antiovulatory agent. Another death (fatal pulmonary embolism) was reported in a 36-year-old woman who was not taking oral contraceptives. Four deaths attributed to anaphylactoid reactions were reported to the Committee on Safety of Medicines for the United Kingdom between 1963 and 1988, with 22 nonfatal allergic reactions such as urticaria noted over the same period.[249]

A fatality has been reported after a test dose of 0.5 ml of STS 0.5% was given to a 64-year-old woman.[250] An autopsy performed by the Hennipin County, Minnesota, coroner's office revealed no obvious cause of death. Subsequently, mast cell tryptase studies were performed on blood collected approximately 1 hour after the reaction while the patient was receiving life support. A normal tryptase level is less than 5 ng/ml; in experimental anaphylactic reactions induced in the laboratory, levels up to 80 ng/ml have been seen. In this patient the levels were extremely high at 6000 ng/ml, suggesting that an anaphylactoid reaction had caused her death. Unfortunately, tryptase levels are experimental at this time, and it is unclear how such a high level could be obtained. Therefore it is also unclear whether fatal anaphylaxis is a significant possibility with STS.

Since all reported cases of allergic reactions are of the IgE-mediated immediate hypersensitivity type, it is recommended that patients remain in or near the physician's office for 30 minutes after sclerotherapy when STS is used. However, patients may also develop allergic reactions hours or days after the procedure.[248,251] For example, urticaria occurred 8 hours after treatment in one patient[251] and 2 weeks after treatment in two other patients.[248] Therefore patients should be warned about the possibility of allergic reactions and how to obtain care if a reaction should occur.

In a review of 2300 patients treated over 16 years, four cases of allergic reactions were reported (0.17% incidence).[252] Reactions in this study were described as periorbital swelling in one patient and urticaria in three. All reactions were easily treated with oral antihistamines. It is of interest that with STS French phlebologists advocate a 3-days-before and 3-days-after treatment course with an antihistamine. P. Flurie noted no episodes of allergic reactions in 500 patients treated in this manner.[253]

Between August 1985 and January 1990, a total of 37 reports of adverse reactions to STS were reported to the Drug Experience Monitoring Program of the Food and Drug Administration (FDA). These included five cases of suspected anaphylaxis and two cases of asthma induced by injection. One of the cases of anaphylaxis resulted in the death previously discussed. After a detailed review of this information, it is unclear to me whether anaphylaxis indeed occurred in every reported case.

The reports of the Clinical Drug Safety Surveillance Group of Wyeth-Ayerst Laboratories are compiled from voluntary reporting to the manufacturer and/or the FDA. The following are summaries of those reports. The January to July 1991 report disclosed one episode of erythema multiforme; one episode of ARDS; one episode of fever, lymphadenopathy, and rash; and three episodes of abdominal pain, nausea, vomiting, and diarrhea. The case report of erythema multiforme was reported in a woman after her thirteenth sclerotherapy treatment.[254] The patient developed pruritus the morning after the last injection, with the development of a generalized eruption beginning on the legs 4 days later. This reaction was followed by fever the next day. A rapidly tapering course of oral prednisone was given, and complete resolution of the rash occurred in 2 weeks.

From September 1991 to November 1992, there were five reports of urticaria and one episode of ARDS. From December 1992 to September 1993, there was only one case of a maculopapular rash. In short, anaphylaxis has been reported with rare fatal reactions.[255] From September 1993 through October 1994, there was one case of angioedema, and one patient developed generalized weakness after receiving 10 ml of 3% STS. From November 1994 through January 1996, there was one case of anaphylaxis. These reactions, which were voluntarily reported to Wyeth-Ayerst, occurred with approximately 500,000 2 ml ampules of 1% and 3% STS being sold yearly within the United States. Thus the incidence of adverse reactions is rare. In 1997 there was one report of a febrile reaction, one of vasculitis, and one of elevated fever function enzymes. (All information regarding adverse reactions from Sotradecol was provided by Paul Minicozzi, Ph.D., of Wyeth-Ayerst at yearly correspondence.)

A similar low incidence with adverse reactions was reported by STD Pharmaceuticals, a manufacturer of STS (correspondence from Robert Gardiner, Hereford, England, March 15, 1995, and the Adverse Drug Reaction Information Tracking Product Analysis from the Medicines Control Agency of Great Britain). The adverse drug reactions reported in Great Britain between 1963 and 1993 included one nonspecific allergic reaction, two cases of anaphylactic shock, six cases of GI disorder, two cases of bronchospasm, four patients with a nonspecific cutaneous eruption, and two patients who developed urticaria. This summary occurred over 30 years, during which time an estimated 7,200,000 ml of STS 1% and 3% was sold in the United Kingdom.

The most common systemic reaction consists of transient low-grade fever and chills lasting up to 24 hours after treatment. This reaction has also been noted in one of my patients. Of note is that three patients with allergic systemic reactions to monoethanolamine oleate had no evidence of allergy to STS.[256]

An interesting dilemma develops with patients who have a history of allergy to sulfa medication. STS contains a sulfate; therefore one can assume that such patients would be at increased risk for an allergic reaction. However, a review of all reported cases of allergic reactions to STS has not disclosed an independent allergic history to sulfa-containing medications (correspondence from Tom Udicious, R.Ph., Wyeth-Ayerst Laboratories, November 1993). I have treated many patients with a history of sulfa allergy with STS without adverse sequelae. This experience is also shared by Drs. Robert and Margaret Weiss (personal communication, 1998).

With any sclerosing solution, reactions can occur that are not allergic in nature but represent the effect of the sclerosing solution on the vascular system. One such reaction is hemolysis, which occurs through lysis of red blood cells present in the treated vein. A hemolytic reaction occurred in 5 patients in a series of more than 900 patients who were injected with more than 8 ml of STS 3%.[239] Similar to reactions that occurred with EO, patients were described as "feeling generally unwell and shivery, with aching in the loins and passage of red-brown urine. All rapidly recovered with bed rest and were perfectly normal the next day." Injections of <8 ml per treatment session did not result in this reaction. Intravascular hemolysis was also reported to the FDA after injection of STS into a hepatic artery feeding a hepatic tumor.

Although the lethal dose in humans or higher animals has never been reported, the IV median lethal dose (LD_{50}) in mice is 90 mg/kg.[257] The lethal volume after IV injection in the rat is approximately four to six times as high for STS as for POL in equivalent concentrations.[185] In my practice it is not uncommon for patients to be treated with up to 30 ml of 0.5% STS. In my practice there has not been an adverse reaction from this dose level of STS.

Polidocanol. Allergic reactions to POL are also rare and have been reported in only four patients in a review of the world's literature up to 1987, with an estimated incidence of 0.01%.[242] Amblard[258] reported no allergic reactions in more than 250 patients, including no allergic reactions in two patients who were intolerant to STS. Hoffer[183] reported no allergic reactions in more than 19,000 cases. In addition, patients who are allergic to STS or iodine have no allergic manifestations to injections of POL.[258-260] However, since 1987 rare allergic reactions have been reported, including a case of nonfatal anaphylactic shock to 1 ml of POL 2% injected into a varicose vein during the fourth treatment session.[252,261-263] Also, Ouvry et al.[264] reported on a patient who developed generalized urticaria with cough and dyspnea after receiving 2 ml of POL 2%; the condition resolved in 30 minutes with IV corticosteroid therapy.

Since the previous review, additional cases of allergic reaction have been reported. Guex[47] reported seven cases of minor general urticaria in nearly 11,000 patients treated over 12 years. The allergic reaction of these patients cleared completely in 1 to 2 days with antihistamine and topical corticosteroid therapy, with one patient requiring systemic corticosteroids. Kreussler GmbH, the product manufacturer in Germany, has documented 35 cases of suspected sensitivity from 1987 to 1993 (personal correspondence, January 1994). Of these reports, most were either vasovagal events or unproven allergic reactions. Nine patients were given repeat challenges with POL, with only three demonstrating an allergic reaction (urticaria or erythematous dermatitis). One patient died of anaphylactic shock 5 minutes after injection with 1 ml of POL despite maximal intervention. In 1994 Kreussler reported on two patients with urticaria. In 1995 two additional patients were reported as having urticaria; two, bronchospasm; and one, angioedema. In 1996 there were four reports of patients with urticaria, two with anaphylactoid reactions, one with angioedema, one with pruritus, and one with contact allergy. Therefore POL is *not* free from allergy, and, as with *all* sclerosing solutions, physicians must be prepared to evaluate and treat patients who develop an allergic reaction to the sclerosing solution.

A detailed account of three serious cases of anaphylaxis was reported from the Netherlands.[265] The affected patients developed anaphylaxis within 15 minutes after injection of POL. Two of them were receiving the drug for the first time. One patient was successfully resuscitated after cardiac arrest. She was a 70-year-old woman with a complicated medical history of two heart operations, two cerebrovascular accidents, and hyperthyroidism. She was receiving multiple medications, including digoxin, carbimazol, captopril, furosemide, mebeverine, and acenocoumarol. She had been treated with POL four previous times without complications. The second patient showed signs of ARDS after being treated with epinephrine and systemic methylprednisolone for "shock." The third patient developed urticaria, dyspnea, paresthesia, headache, and chest pain with electrocardiographic (ECG) findings of cardiac ischemia. No further studies were performed on these patients.

At 2 years the Australian Polidocanol Open Clinical Trial, with more than 8000 treated patients, reported nine local urticarial reactions and three generalized reactions, with two patients developing a rash, for a frequency of approximately 0.2%. There were no cases of anaphylaxis.[186] After an additional 8804 patients were evaluated, an additional three patients developed urticaria again without any additional significant adverse sequelae.[124] A 5-year experience in 500 patients treated with POL 3% reported five cases of allergic reaction (1% incidence). One patient had nonfatal anaphylactic shock, with the other patients experiencing urticaria.[266]

Two of 689 sequential patients were reported as developing an immediate type of hypersensitivity reaction with systemic pruritus and urticaria.[267] This number represented an incidence of 0.3% in their patient population and of 0.91% for the "true" population. These two reactions occurred without prior exposure to POL as a sclerosing agent. Since POL is used as an emulsifying agent in preprocessed foods, prior exposure may have occurred from ingestion of such foods. Both patients responded well to either a single dose of diphenhydramine, 50 mg PO, or 0.3 ml of epinephrine SC plus 50 mg diphenhydramine IM.

Jaquier and Loretan[182] believe that the decrease in antigenicity is the result of the absence of a benzene nucleus and a paramine group and the presence of a lone free alcohol group. Dexo SA Pharmaceuticals, the product manufacturer in France, recommends that this substance not be used in patients with an allergic diathesis (e.g., asthma) (product description of hydroxypolyethoxydodecane [May 1985] received with correspondence from Dexo SA Pharmaceuticals, France). Thus allergic reactions to POL are similar to those reported with STS.

An interesting adverse effect may be noticed in patients in whom a near-maximal dosage of POL is used. These patients report paresthesia or tingling of the tongue or a strange sensation in taste that resolves within 5 minutes. This effect has been reported to Kreussler five times from 1986 to 1993 (correspondence, January 1994) and also has been noted in my practice. This sensation may be explained by particular effects of the anesthetic properties of POL. Other unusual reactions reported to Kreussler (correspondence, January 1994) include rare episodes of short convulsive coughing, acute pressure sensation in the chest, acute difficulty with breathing, and one case of stabbing chest pain without demonstrable ECG changes or myoglobin-band creatine phosphokinase fluctuations.

Like EO and SM, POL has demonstrated a dose-dependent cardiac toxicity when injected into esophageal varices. POL has a negative inotropic effect and reduces atrioventricular and intraventricular conduction. Animal studies demonstrate a reversible, dose-dependent decrease in myocardial contractility, blood pressure, and pulse rate and a prolongation of the PQ interval.[268] This effect may explain the cause of heart failure in three elderly patients with severe liver failure who were given massive quantities of POL during esophageal sclerotherapy (760 mg in a 74-year-old woman; 600 mg in a 70-year-old woman; 750 mg in a 76-year-old woman).[269,270]

The LD_{50} of POL in rabbits at 2 hours is 0.2 g/kg, which is three to six times greater than the LD_{50} for procaine hydrochloride.[271] The LD_{50} in mice is 110 mg/kg.[272] The systemic toxicity level is similar to that of lidocaine and procaine.[273]

Finally, the teratogenicity of POL was evaluated by Fournier[274] in rabbits and rats. The pregnant animals received from 2.7 to 4.5 mg/kg/day and did not demonstrate a significant increase in the number of abnormal fetuses.[275] One severe malformation was seen in a rat pup, out of 530 normal pups (0.08%), whose mother received 4.5 mg/kg/day. This dosage is greatly in excess of the recommended doses of POL in humans. Kreussler has reported animal experiments that disclose a placental barrier to POL. However, no formal studies in pregnant women have been reported. Sigg[276] has reported treating 3600 pregnant women with 34,000 injections without fetal injury or abortion.

Chromated glycerin. CG 72% (Scleremo) is a sclerosing solution with a very low incidence of side effects (product information [1987]).[17,71,277] Hypersensitivity is a very rare complication.[278,279] Contact sensitivity to chromium occurs in approximately 5% of the population.[280] IV potassium dichromate leads to complete desensitization in chromium-sensitized guinea pigs. This effect occurs because chromium needs to bind to skin proteins to become an effective antigen.[281] This action may be related to the necessity for epidermal Langerhans' cells to produce an allergic response, whereas T-lymphocyte accessory cooperation is not optimal with IV injection and its resulting endothelial necrosis. Thus it is more common for the sclerotherapist to develop an allergic contact dermatitis to CG than for the patient to develop an allergic reaction to IV use of CG. Indeed, Ouvry has developed an allergic contact dermatitis from CG injected without the use of protective gloves (personal communication, 1995).

Ramalet et al.[282] have reported on seven patients who developed an allergic reaction to CG. One patient had a vasculitis, and six patients had an eczematous reaction. All allergic patients demonstrated a sensitivity to topically applied chrome.

Hematuria accompanied by urethral colic can occur transiently after injection of large doses of CG. Ocular manifestations, including blurred vision and a partial visual field loss, with resolution in less than 2 hours, have been reported by a single author.[283]

Recently an additional case of transient hypertension and visual disturbance was reported to have occurred after the injection of 12 ml of 50% CG into spider and "feeder" leg veins in a fourth treatment session. These symptoms occurred 2½ hours after treatment and lasted over a 3-hour period without treatment. These effects may have represented a retinal spasm or an ophthalmic migraine.[284]

Polyiodide iodine. Polyiodide iodine (Varigloban, Variglobin, Sclerodine 6) is a stabilized water solution of iodide ions, sodium iodine, and benzyl alcohol. Sigg et al.[285] reported on their experience in more than 400,000 injections with Variglobin. Paravenous injections readily produced tissue necrosis. In 1975 Sigg and Zelikovski[286] reported an incidence of 0.13 per 1000 allergic cutaneous reactions. No systemic allergic reactions were observed. Obvious contraindications to the use of Variglobin are hyperthyroidism and allergies to iodine and benzyl alcohol.

Iodine solutions may also produce bronchiomucosal lesions if they are used in high concentration. Therefore Wenner[287] recommends that a maximum of 5 ml of 12% solution be used in a single sclerosing session.

Sodium salicylate. In a literature review Saliject (Omega Laboratories, Montreal, Canada) has not been reported to cause allergic reactions. Dr. Beverly Kemsley has reported that 1 of 6000 patients developed an anaphylactic reaction following the use of Saliject. Thirty patients developed localized erythema and urticaria, which responded to the oral antihistamine terfenadine 120 mg (personal communication, 1996).

Hypertonic saline. Alone, HS solution shows no evidence of allergenicity or toxicity. Complications that may arise from its specific use include hypertension that may be exacerbated in predisposed patients when an excessive sodium load is given, sudden hypernatremia, central nervous system disorders, extensive hemolysis, and cortical necrosis of the kidneys (Mary Helenek, written correspondence, American Regent Laboratories, Inc., May 1990). These complications among others have led one manufacturer (American Regent Laboratories) to add to its label the warning "FOR IV OR SC USE AFTER DILUTION" in bold red type.

As discussed previously, hematuria can occur with any sclerosing agent. Dodd[288] has reported painless hematuria in five patients injected with HS. Sometimes blood appears in the urine after one to two acts of micturition and at additional times throughout the day. There are usually no other ill effects, and the hematuria resolves spontaneously. Hematuria probably occurs because of hemolysis of RBCs during sclerotherapy.

Coverman (personal communication, 1989) described two patients injected with up to 6 ml of HS 23.4% who developed "peculiar visual symptoms in just one eye." This effect was described as either blurred vision or an aura. There were no other symptoms, and each incidence passed quickly and spontaneously. Coverman speculates that this symptom may have been caused by the addition of lidocaine to the HS solution.

Heparin in hypertonic saline. Although unadulterated HS solutions in concentrations from 15% to 30% are used for the treatment of varicose and telangiectatic leg veins, adding heparin to the solution to prevent the theoretic risk of embolization associated with sclerotherapy has been advocated.[18] Although the necessity for heparin was discounted in a well-controlled 800-patient randomized study,[20] Foley's solution, Heparsal, consisting of HS 20% with heparin, 100 U/ml, and procaine 1%, is commonly used in the treatment of telangiectatic leg veins. Therefore the risk of adverse reactions to heparin should be mentioned.

Commercial preparations of heparin consist of straight-chain anionic polysaccharides of variable molecular weight (usually 7000 to 40,000). Heparin prepared from different tissues also appears to vary: more protamine is required to neutralize a unit of beef lung heparin than porcine mucosal heparin. Plasma lipolytic activity, antifactor Xa activity, and activated partial thromboplastin time ratios are significantly different.[289]

Fever, urticaria, and anaphylaxis occur occasionally after administration of heparin.[289-293] Necrosis has been reported in patients receiving subcutaneous heparin.[285,294-297] Necrosis usually occurred 3 to 10 days after multiple subcutaneous injections. Pruritus, local tenderness, and burning sensations associated with large indurated, erythematous plaques were also reported to occur in six patients 10 to 20 days after beginning prophylactic doses of heparin.[298] Thus there is a measurable risk of toxicity to heparin.

Although heparin is not a totally benign substance, there have been no reports by those who use Heparsal of any adverse reactions that could be attributed to the heparin component.[5,18,20,158] The lack of side effects has been reported in one series of 310 patients when volumes of 10 to 20 ml have been injected into varicose veins.[158] In the recommended doses, heparin in Heparsal may be without significant side effects, but one must be aware of the potential dangers associated with its use.

Lidocaine in hypertonic saline. Alderman[6] and Duffy[5] advocate the addition of lidocaine (to achieve a 0.4% final concentration) to minimize patient discomfort during injection of HS. This addition means that this sclerosing mixture can be potentially allergenic. Although the most common causes of previous allergic reaction to lidocaine in a patient are psychogenic or vasovagal reactions,[299] allergic reactions may occur. In one report 28 patients who had a variety of adverse reactions to lidocaine, including skin reaction, loss of consciousness, and vagal symptoms, were evaluated with skin testing and were found not to be allergic to lidocaine. Nineteen of these patients were subsequently treated with lidocaine without an adverse reaction.[300]

The amide class of anesthetics has a very low risk of allergic reaction.[301-306] Allergy is most likely caused by the methylparabens or sodium metabisulfite used as a preservative in the anesthetic solutions.[301,302,307-309] To keep the allergic risk as low as possible, single-dose vials of lidocaine without preservatives should be used.

Despite the low risk of allergenicity to lidocaine, there have been a few true allergic reactions, including anaphylaxis, reported.[310-317] Thus HS, when adulterated with lidocaine, may place the patient at risk for allergic reactions.

Superficial Thrombophlebitis

Before the advent of modern-day sclerotherapy, which uses graduated compression to limit thrombosis, thrombophlebitis—both superficial and deep—occurred in a significant number of sclerotherapy patients.[318] In fact, it was commonly thought that the incidence of phlebitis was so common a sequela of sclerotherapy that there was doubt whether this form of therapy was legitimate.[319] With the use of compression and the realization that many adverse effects resulted from thrombus formation in treated veins, the incidence of thrombophlebitis has greatly decreased.

There are many innate conditions that may predispose patients to the development of thrombophlebitis through hypercoagulopathy syndromes (see the section on pulmonary embolism and deep venous thrombosis on p. 351). In addition, the persistence of significant reflux into a vein that has been treated can also lead to phlebitis. Fegan[320] states that this complication occurs more commonly if perforator veins in the region of treatment are undiagnosed and not treated.

Etiology. Superficial thrombophlebitis appears 1 to 3 weeks after injection as a tender erythematous induration over the injected vein (Figure 16-18). Duffy[5] estimates that it occurs in 0.5% of his patients who have primarily small vessel varicose veins and telangiectasias. Mantse[248] reported an incidence of 1% in the treatment of varicose (nontelangiectatic) veins despite the use of a tensor bandage for 6 weeks. This author notes that the patients who developed superficial thrombophlebitis found that the bandage was too tight and reapplied it too loosely at

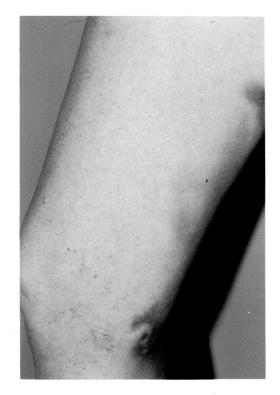

FIGURE 16-18. Superficial thrombophlebitis developed in this patient 14 days after sclerotherapy with STS 0.5%. Note ecchymosis from compression padding and graduated support stocking, worn for only 1 week on upper medial/posterior thigh.

home. In my experience this complication occurs to some degree in approximately 0.01% of patients. Most patients have minimal phlebitis and require no treatment. Rarely, in symptomatic patients treatment with compression and anti-inflammatory agents is given (0.001% of patients totaling more than 10,000 separate injections).

Prevention and treatment. The decreased incidence of superficial thrombophlebitis in my practice may be the result of the greater degree and length of compression used in treating all injected veins. Indeed, the cause of thrombophlebitis is related in part to treatment technique. An inadequate degree or length of compression results in excessive intravascular thrombosis. Sigg[321] notes that perivenous inflammation is observed only at those parts of the limb not covered by a compression dressing. Thus, to avoid this complication, one should prevent or minimize the development of postsclerosis thrombosis by using compression pads and hosiery over the entire leg and not just over the treated veins.

However, even when appropriate compression is used, thrombosis and perivascular inflammation may occur. Ascending phlebitis in the lesser saphenous vein (LSV) or its long tributaries that starts at the upper edge of the compression stocking is relatively common. Here the sclerosing action continues up the abnormal vessel (even beyond what apparently is the extent of the abnormality). It is thought that the sclerosing solution destroys damaged endothelium to a greater extent than it does normal endothelium (product description of hydroxypolyethoxydodecane received with correspondence, May 1985). Therefore the placement of a foam pad extending above the compression stocking or bandage to create a gradual transition of pressure from compressed to noncompressed vein may provide a safety margin. Also, it may prevent damage to the vein by the otherwise abrupt cutoff of the pressure stocking.

Thrombophlebitis is not a complication to be taken lightly. If untreated, the inflammation and clot may spread through perforating veins to the deep venous system. This extension may lead to valvular damage and possible pulmonary embolic events.[322-326] A study on a group of 145 patients with superficial thrombophlebitis found that 23% of affected limbs had proximal extent into the SFJ.[327]

Treatment. In addition to adequate compression, drainage of thrombi after liquefaction (approximately 2 weeks after sclerotherapy) will hasten resolution of the otherwise slow, painful resorption process.[321] Adequate compression and frequent ambulation should be maintained until the pain and inflammation resolve. Aspirin or other nonsteroidal anti-inflammatory agents may be helpful in limiting both the inflammation and the pain.

In patients with extensive involvement of leg varices, anticoagulation therapy should be used. This approach is particularly important if there is proximal involvement of the SFJ. In addition to propagation of the thrombus through the SFJ, from 11% to 40% of patients with subclavian vein thrombosis (SVT) at the SFJ have evidence of concurrent DVT.[328,329] In these patients anticoagulation for 6 months achieved resolution of the DVT/SVT while preventing pulmonary embolism. This success occurred despite duplex scanning evidence of progression of SVT to DVT in 2 of 20 patients.[328] Of interest is the fact that the incidence of coincidental DVT with SVT occurred more commonly in patients without varicose veins (60% vs. 20%). Thus other innate factors place the patient with SVT at additional risk for DVT.

Arterial Injection

The most feared complication in sclerotherapy is inadvertent injection into an artery. Fortunately, this complication is very rare.[330-332] Five examples of this complication had been reported to the Medical Defense Union in Great Britain by 1985.[333] Cockett[334] has reported 18 cases, including those reported to the two medical protection societies in the United Kingdom over a 10-year period. However, Cockett believes that even this number is too low because many cases occur that never reach the courts or the medical literature. Biegeleisen et al.[335] have reported seven cases in their practice history of more than 10 years. Forty cases over 17 years have been reported from France.[336]

Arterial injection of a sclerosing solution causes the development of an embolus. This result has been experimentally confirmed in the canine femoral artery.[337] These experiments demonstrate little effect on the artery itself with injection. Spasm does not occur. The sclerosing solution acts to denature blood and endothelial cells in smaller arteries, producing a sludge embolus that obstructs the microcirculation[338] (Figure 16-19). Stagnant blood flow, secondary thrombosis, and necrosis soon follow.

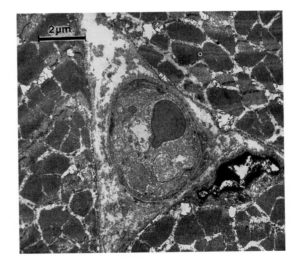

FIGURE 16-19. Terminal arteriole from the adductor musculature of the rat hind limb 60 minutes after injection of 4% Variglobin into the iliac artery. Lumen contains a large amount of cellular debris. Transmission electron micrograph, primary magnification ×3800; for final enlargement, see scale. (From Staubesand J, Seydewitz V. Ultrastructural changes following perivascular and intra-arterial injection of sclerosing agents: An experimental contribution to the problem of iatrogenic damage. Phlebologie 20:1, 1991.)

Occlusion of small arteries may lead to the development of a compartmental syndrome. Intracompartmental pressures of 30 mm Hg or more in humans usually produce neural deficits characterized by pain during stretching of the muscles involved, paresthesia, and then paresis and anesthesia in the sensory distribution of the nerve that courses through the affected compartment. The end result is paralysis.[251] Muscle necrosis then leads to leg atrophy. Sensory deficit in the first web space (deep peroneal nerve) implicates anterior compartmental syndrome. Sensory deficit on the dorsum of the foot (superficial peroneal nerve) implicates the lateral compartment. The superficial posterior compartment is indicated by sensory deficit of the sural nerve distribution (lateral foot). Deep compartmental syndrome is likely if the sole of the foot is affected (posterior tibial nerve).

Unless large arteries are blocked, peripheral pulses will be intact, and capillary filling is easily identified since the compartmental pressure must be greater than 80 mm Hg to occlude large-artery flow.[339] This situation may lull the physician into a false sense of security, and the underlying compartmental syndrome may not be recognized. Intracompartmental pressures between 30 and 40 mm Hg that last for 6 to 12 hours can cause irreversible damage to the nervous tissue because of impairment of microcirculation.[251] Magnetic resonance imaging (MRI) examination of the affected limb has been able to distinguish muscle destruction (Figure 16-20).

Etiology. The most common location for arterial injection to occur is the posterior or medial malleolar region, particularly when an effort is made to inject the internal ankle perforator vein, specifically in the posterior tibial artery.[320,332,334,340] The patient will usually, but not always, note immediate pain.

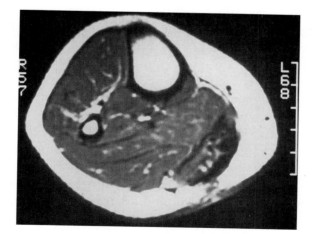

FIGURE 16-20. Magnetic resonance image of the medial calf a few weeks after inadvertent intra-arterial injection has produced muscular weakness and pain. Note atrophy of the gastrocnemius muscles with significant edema within fascial compartments. (Courtesy Professor Jean Natali, Paris. From Goldman MP. Sclerotherapy: Treatment of Varicose and Telangiectatic Leg Veins. St. Louis: Mosby, 1995. Reprinted with permission.)

The pain slowly propagates down into the foot and outer toes over the following 2 to 6 hours. During this time arterial pedal pulses are palpable. Ten to 12 hours later the four outer toes are white, with the sole of the foot becoming painful. Cutaneous blanching of the injected area usually occurs in an arterial pattern associated with a loss of pulse and progressive cyanosis of the injected area.

Natali and Farman[341] have noted 40 cases of arterial injection in their 20-year experience and review of the French medicolegal system. They found that injection of the short saphenous vein was the most common preceding event. Seven patients required amputations, including 2 above the knee and 5 below the knee, 6 peripheral amputations of one or more toes, and 27 abnormalities of the triceps and/or sural muscles. Muscle abnormalities consist of infarction with subsequent fibrosis and retraction of the affected area with or without limb atrophy.

Another area in which the artery and veins are in close proximity is the junction of the femoral and superficial saphenous veins. A review of one sclerotherapy practice over 20 years disclosed two cases of accidental arterial injection in this area, requiring thigh amputations.[342] A similar experience was noted by Biegeleisen et al.,[335] who reported seven cases of arterial injection during attempts to inject the greater or lesser saphenous vein at the groin or popliteal area, even done under color-flow ultrasound control. In this location the external pudendal artery bifurcates and may surround the LSV shortly after the location of its connection with the femoral vein. In addition, the junction of the LSV with the popliteal vein has been demonstrated to have a tortuous and variably located satellite arteriole.[343] Because these collateral arteries vary anatomically in these locations, duplex scanning may be useful before sclerosing of these vessels; however, this aid does not guarantee absolute safety.

With the onset of duplex-assisted sclerotherapy, small arteries in superficial and deep aspects of the thigh and calf have been inadvertently injected (Figure 16-21). As described previously, the usual sequelae are both loss of tissue (cutaneous and subcutaneous) and nerve damage, which may result in muscle atrophy and/or necrosis. For sclerosing these very tricky areas, color-flow duplex scanning and the use of open needles are recommended. A physician should be present at all times to give immediate treatment if needed.

Prevention and treatment. Arterial injection in sclerotherapy is a true emergency. The extent of cutaneous necrosis usually is related to the amount of solution injected. Therapeutic efforts to treat this complication are usually unsatisfactory but should be attempted.[332] Because the occurrence of arterial injection is extremely rare, I recommend that an emergency flowsheet be readily accessible (see box on p. 350). Hobbs (personal communication, 1991) recommends that, on realization of arterial injection, blood and sclerosing solution be aspirated back into the syringe to empty the needle of solution. In addition, aspiration of the injected artery as rapidly and completely as possible, if performed immediately, may help remove the injected sclerosing solution. The needle should not be withdrawn, but the syringe should be replaced with one containing 10,000 U of heparin, which should be injected slowly into the artery. Unfortunately, this maneuver is

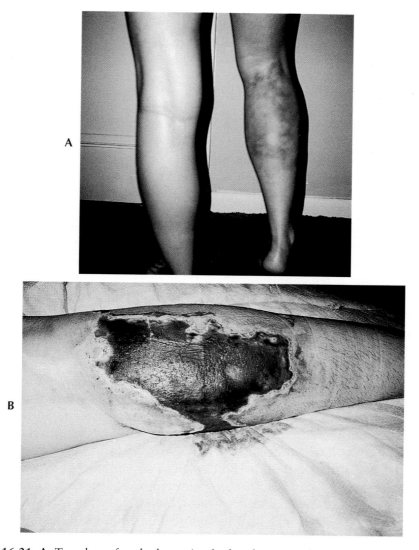

FIGURE 16-21. A, Two days after duplex-assisted sclerotherapy with STS 1.0% into the gastrocnemial area to treat cutaneous telangiectasia. Note mottled skin. **B,** Three weeks later a well-circumscribed necrotic area is apparent. (From Goldman MP. Sclerotherapy: Treatment of Varicose and Telangiectatic Leg Veins. St. Louis: Mosby, 1995. Reprinted with permission.)

ARTERIAL INJECTION TREATMENT

- Arterial and periarterial infiltration with procaine 1% (inactivates STS)
- Cooling of injected area with ice packs
- Immediate heparinization (continues 6 days or longer)
- Intravenous dextran 10%, 500 mg/day × 3 days
- Consider direct thrombolytic therapy with streptokinase
- Oral prazosin, hydralazine, or nifedipine × 30 days

difficult to accomplish since the patient is usually in considerable pain and may find it difficult to hold still (J. Hobbs, personal communication, 1991).

Some patients who experience arterial injection have no complaints of pain and only demonstrate a mild, sharply demarcated erythema that becomes dusky and cyanotic after a few hours.[335]

More practical treatments include periarterial infiltration with procaine 3%, 1 ml, which will form a complex with STS and render it inactive.[320,340] The foot should be cooled with ice packs to minimize tissue anoxia. Immediate heparinization (continued for 6 days) and administration of IV dextran 10%, 500 ml per dose, for 3 days is recommended. Use of IV streptokinase also may be considered if there are no contraindications for its use. Finally, use of oral prazosin, hydralazine, or nifedipine for 30 days should be considered. Cockett[334] has found that treatment that is delayed for more than 1 hour has no effect in limiting damage to the foot.

Use of intravenous heparin followed by subcutaneous heparin has been found to avert skin necrosis.[335] It was observed that warfarin (Coumadin) did not appear as effective as subcutaneous heparin in these patients. The protective effect of heparin may be unrelated to its anticoagulant activity.[344] Postischemic endothelial cell dysfunction was prevented with heparin perfusion in the rat hind limb model.[345] Heparin infusion at 0.5 U/ml resulted in endothelial-dependent vasodilation. Serum levels <0.5 U/ml (the average serum heparin level in a patient undergoing therapeutic anticoagulation) were less effective. It is postulated that direct interactions of heparin with the endothelium, inducing maintenance of a strong luminal charge, may produce beneficial membrane-stabilizing effects. Heparin may also modulate TNF activity, contributing to this effect.[346] In addition, a favorable resolution of arterial injection occurred in one patient with injection of tissue-type plasminogen activator (t-PA).[347] In this patient promazine was injected into an artery. The use of heparin, axillary plexus blockade, and IV sodium nitroprusside were not successful. Brachial artery injection of t-PA (Actilyse, 50 mg over 8 hours) resulted in therapeutic efficacy. Thus local fibrinolytic therapy should be considered if conservative treatments prove ineffective.

Given the known relationship of injection site to the development of this problem, one must consider the necessity for injecting vessels in the vicinity of the medial malleolus. The *British Medical Journal* has published an interesting report of a legal case brought against a physician for performing such an injection, which resulted in a transmetatarsal amputation.[330] The case was found in favor of the physician after several renowned sclerotherapists stated that if the patient would benefit from the injection, it should be attempted since the risks are infrequent and the benefits are significant.

Prevention of this dreaded complication is best accomplished by visualization of the blood emanating from the needle. If the blood is pulsatile and continues to flow after the leg is horizontal, injection should not be attempted at this site. Mantse[248] advises that when the medial malleolar area is treated, placement of the sclerosing needle should be performed while the patient is standing so the varix is bulged and the distance between the artery and the vein is increased.

Theoretically, visualization of arteries and veins with duplex-assisted sclerotherapy should negate this risk. Indeed, newer color-flow duplex imagery allows visualization of minute arteries and veins. However, a number of arterial ulcerations have occurred with this technique, even when posterior calf, gastrocnemius, and SFJ varicose veins were injected. Thus no technique is completely free from this complication.

Pulmonary Embolism and Deep Venous Thrombosis

Pulmonary embolism (PE) and DVT occur very rarely after sclerotherapy. The literature contains many case reports but does not permit an exact estimate of the incidence of postsclerotherapy DVT or PE. A recent review by Feied[348] summarizes the major reports and risk factors for DVT.

The diagnosis of DVT is often clinically difficult, with up to 50% of cases going unnoticed. The most common clinical finding is mild enlargement of the calf or thigh. Embolization of a thrombus occurs in more than 50% of patients[349] and is not diagnosed in up to 70% of cases,[350] with a mortality rate approaching 35% without treatment.[351] Both the use of preventive measures and maintaining clinical suspicion are important in preventing this complication. The clinical diagnosis of DVT is accurate only 50% of the time as compared to the use of fibrinogen scanning.[352] Venous Doppler examination has a 30% to 96% accuracy, depending on the experience of the investigator.[353-355] Likewise, impedance phlebography has a 40% accuracy.[355] Thus the reported incidence of DVT postsclerotherapy treatment may be greatly underestimated.

In the 1930s and 1940s PE after sclerotherapy of varicose veins occurred in 0.14% of patients at most.[356,357] In a series of 45,000 injections given to 7500 patients, only one episode of PE was reported.[358] In 1928 Sicard reported 325,000 injections without a pulmonary infarction.[359] Linser and Vohwinkel[360] reported four cases of PE after 75,000 injections, and only one case was fatal. More recently, with the onset of compression techniques in combination with sclerotherapy, this complication has become even less common. Sigg[361] has reported PE occurring only once with 42,000 injections. A French vascular surgeon who treats approximately 75 sclerotherapy patients a week, amounting to 25,000 yearly injections, reported only one case of PE in 20 years.[331] Fegan[245] reported that he has never seen conclusive evidence of DVT after injection treatment of 16,000 patients in his clinic. The 2-year Australian Polidocanol Trial reported one case of major DVT and two cases of minor DVT that occurred after injection of 4 ml of 0.5% POL, 4 ml of 0.5% POL, and 0.5 ml of 1% POL, respectively, in 12,544 injected legs, for an incidence of approximately 0.02%.[186] In a review of 28 cases of PE after sclerotherapy, most cases occurred in patients at bed rest. PE occurred 1 to 21 days after the treatment session. The incidence of PE in this series was estimated as 1 per 10,000 patients.[362]

To evaluate the true incidence more accurately, 13 patients undergoing compression sclerotherapy with Fegan's technique were studied with continuous-screening ascending venography. Not more than 1 ml of 3% STS was injected, with the total amount not exceeding 5 ml. Patients were seen at follow-up 1 week later for comparison venography. Patients did not develop radiographic evidence for DVT.[363]

An additional study using impedance plethysmography and Doppler ultrasonic examination was performed before and after sclerotherapy treatment by the classic Fegan technique in 67 legs.[364] This study confirmed that there were no alterations in deep venous blood flow at 1 and 2 weeks after injection treatment. This finding confirmed the clinical experience that sclerotherapy performed with the Fegan technique is highly unlikely to be complicated by the development of DVT. Venographic evaluation of the injection of 0.5 to 1 ml of sclerosing solution in 15 patients with incompetent perforator veins failed to demonstrate extension of radiocontrast media into the deep venous system.[363]

An additional reason why sclerotherapy treatment does not usually result in DVT may be related to platelet inhibition by sclerosing solutions.[365] One study found that platelet aggregation, the first step in thrombogenesis, is inhibited by the concentrations of sclerosing solution that usually occur in the deep venous system after sclerotherapy of superficial varicosities.[366,367]

Emboli without pulmonary involvement. Reversible ischemic neurologic defects after sclerotherapy have been reported.[368] In one case a 41-year-old woman was injected with 2 ml of 3% POL and 1 ml of 1% POL into varicose leg veins. One hour later the patient developed paresthesia in the right half of the body with loss of visual field in the right upper quadrant. The neurologic signs and symptoms resolved within 2 days. There was no evidence of DVT, and coagulation factors were all normal except for a transient elevation of antithrombin-III immediately after sclerotherapy that resolved within 5 days. Unfortunately, the patient was not evaluated for a patent foramen ovale, which is the probable etiologic event for this temporary cerebral vascular accident.

An additional patient sustained an immediate hemiparesis that lasted for 24 hours after injection of a left leg varix with a hypertonic solution.[369] In this patient an open atrial septal defect was demonstrated on ultrasound. However, thrombosis was not detected in either the varicose or deep veins of the leg or in the cerebral circulation.

Since 20% to 30% of unselected patients can be found to have a patent foramen ovale with present-day ultrasound techniques,[370] this complication may occur more often than reported. Thus any patient who complains or manifests neurologic symptoms should be carefully evaluated for both leg and cerebral thrombosis as well as a patent foramen ovale. Consideration should be given to anticoagulation therapy in these patients.

Cause. The cause of DVT, with or without PE, after sclerotherapy is unclear. The three major factors responsible for DVT were first elucidated more than 100 years ago by Virchow[371]: (1) endothelial damage; (2) vascular stasis; and (3) changes in coagulability. Sclerotherapy treatment always produces the first two causes in the triad, with coagulability changes related to the unique properties of sclerosing solutions in addition to the predisposing factors of the patient. Chemical endophlebitis produced by sclerotherapy should anchor the thrombus to the site of injection. Histologic examination of treated varicose veins has demonstrated that firm thrombosis occurs only on the damaged endothelium. Nonadherent thrombosis occurs on normal endothelium.[372] Therefore the most logical explanation for the development of emboli is damage to the deep venous system by migration of sclerosing solution or a partly attached thrombosis from treated superficial veins into deep veins. These effects may occur as a result of either injection of excessive volumes of sclerosing solution or physical inactivity after injection.[373]

An additional possibility concerns injection of tributary perforator veins, which may directly communicate with the deep venous system. In this situation inadequate compression or injection of even 0.5 ml of sclerosing solution may force nonadherent thrombi into the deep circulation with muscle contraction. Ascending venography and digital subtraction phlebography in women with leg telangiectasias found that 0.7 ml of contrast medium injected into telangiectatic branches spread into the saphenous system in 8 of 15 patients.[374] Two of the eight patients had telangiectasia as the only clinically perceptible abnormality. Therefore it is possible that up to 13% of patients with telangiectatic veins are at risk for the spread of sclerosing solution directly into the deep venous system. This possibility further emphasizes the importance of limiting injection volumes.

Amount of injection per site. The circulation and direction of blood flow in varicose veins have been determined radiographically as stagnant or reversed (away from the heart) so that the chemically induced thrombus is forced distally toward the smaller branching veins.[375] However, cinematographic studies documented that a small amount of sclerosing solution entered the deep circulation after injection of 0.5 to 1 ml of solution into a superficial varicosity during 7 of 15 injections in nine subjects[376] (Figures 16-22 and 16-23). No adverse effects were noted in these patients treated with POL 2%. The lack of adverse effects was probably related to rapid compression and ambulation of treated individuals and the resulting rapid dilution of the sclerosing agent within the deep venous system.

Although studies demonstrating the rarity of DVT after sclerotherapy are reassuring, DVT and embolic episodes usually occur 4 to 28 days after the sclerotherapy treatment session.[356] Therefore longer follow-up is necessary. In addition, nearly 40% of patients with DVT have asymptomatic PE.[377]

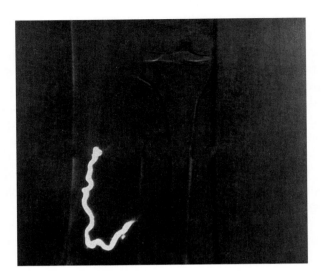

FIGURE 16-22. Injected contrast media, 1.5 ml, shown 9½ seconds after injection into a varicose vein with the patient standing. (From Goldman MP. Sclerotherapy: Treatment of Varicose and Telangiectatic Leg Veins. St. Louis: Mosby, 1995. Reprinted with permission.)

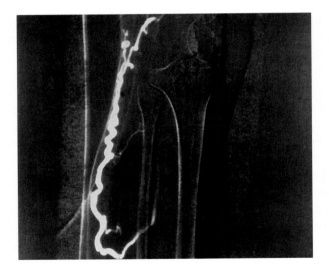

FIGURE 16-23. Injected contrast media, 1.5 ml, shown 9½ seconds after injection into a varicose vein with the patient supine. (From Goldman MP. Sclerotherapy: Treatment of Varicose and Telangiectatic Leg Veins. St. Louis: Mosby, 1995. Reprinted with permission.)

DVT and PE have been reported to occur with injection of large quantities of sclerosing solution (12 ml) in a single site.[378] Two separate case reports of this complication, occurring with injection of <0.5 ml of POL 1% in two patients in each report, have been published.[186,379] In both reports the injected veins involved leg telangiectasias. In addition, the injection of 0.5 to 1 ml of sclerosing solution above the midthigh resulted in a presumed thrombus at the SFJ with associated pulmonary emboli.[239] These effects prompted Reid and Rothine[239] to recommend that injections not be given above the midthigh. Thus the quantity of sclerosing solution per injection site must be limited to ensure that the agent will remain within the superficial system, and blood flow in the deep venous system must be rapidly stimulated after sclerotherapy with compression and muscle movement.

Finally, sclerotherapy of pedal veins may be hazardous since the lack of valves or the reversal of valves allows inward flow from superficial to deep veins.[380] These factors may produce DVT. Therefore, when treatment is necessary, phlebectomy may be preferable to sclerotherapy.

Inappropriate compression. The inappropriate tourniquet effect of an excessively tight wrap on the thigh is a rare cause for the development of DVT.[381] Occlusion of deep venous flow results in popliteal vein thrombosis, which can be resolved with conservative treatment. The adverse effects of nongraduated compression emphasize the importance of using properly fitted graduated support stockings in sclerotherapy treatment.

Hypercoagulable states. A number of primary and secondary hypercoagulable states exist that can be ruled out through the use of an appropriate patient history and a review of systems in the presclerotherapy treatment evaluation. The prevalence of inherited thrombotic syndromes in the general population is 1 in 2500 to 5000 but increases to 4% in patients with a history of thrombosis.[382] In addition, a history of DVT raises the likelihood of new postoperative venous thrombosis from 26% to 68%, whereas a history of both DVT and PE gives an almost 100% incidence of thrombosis.[352] Thus sclerotherapy should be undertaken cautiously in patients with previous DVT. Further detail on all hypercoagulable states is beyond the scope of this chapter. Only the most common states are discussed here. The reader is referred to multiple review articles on this important subject.[348,382,383,384]

Oral contraceptive agents and estrogen replacement therapy. The mechanism for thromboembolic disease in women who use oral contraceptives is multifactorial. Both estrogens and progestogens have been implicated in promoting thrombosis despite low-dose therapy.[385-387] All studies have indicated that the increased risk occurs only while the preparations are actually in use and perhaps for 1 week or so after discontinuation.[388,389] Total correction of the potentially hemostatic changes that occur during oral contraceptive therapy requires 4 weeks of abstinence.[390]

The highest rates of thromboembolism occur with the use of higher levels of estrogen[385-388,391]; some studies show an elevenfold increase.[389,392] Nevertheless, the risk of postoperative PE still appears to be increased in women who use oral contraceptive agents with minimal amounts of estrogen.[393] Interestingly, a detailed review of the statistical methodologies of these studies did *not* prove a *definite* risk.[394] The following is a brief review on this topic.

The incidence of DVT after use of oral contraceptive agents varies on the type and concentration of estrogen. In addition, there is at least a 200-fold difference in potency between the native estrogens—estrone, estradiol, and ethinyl estradiol—and the estrogens found in oral contraceptive agents.[395] Women undergoing hormone replacement therapy with 0.625 mg of conjugated equine estrogens and 2.5 mg of medroxyprogesterone have a risk of DVT that is 2 to 3.6 times higher than that of nonusers.[396]

It has been estimated that oral contraceptives are responsible for one case of superficial or deep vein thrombosis per 500 women users per year.[397] This estimate of hypercoagulability may be low because an examination of plasma fibrinogen chromatography demonstrated a 27% incidence of silent thrombotic lesions in 154 new contraceptive users of either mestranol, 100 mg, or ethinyl estradiol, 50 mg.[398] Oral contraceptive users as a group have numerous alterations in their coagulation system that promote a hypercoagulable state. These changes include hyperaggregable platelets, decreased endothelial fibrinolysis,[399] decreased negative surface charge on vessel walls and blood cells,[400] elevated levels of procoagulants, reduced RBC filterability,[401] increased blood viscosity secondary to elevated RBC volume,[402] and decreased levels of antithrombin III.[403-405] Any of these factors, alone or in combination, may predominate in women taking oral contraceptives. The extent of this derangement in the hemostatic system determines whether thrombosis will occur. When endothelial damage through sclerotherapy is initiated in this population, an increased incidence of thrombosis may result.

The most important factors preventing clot propagation are antithrombin III and vascular stores of t-PA.[403,406-408] Antithrombin III levels have been demonstrated as 20% lower in some women taking oral contraceptive agents[406] or undergoing estrogen replacement therapy.[409] Of women using oral contraceptive agents who have thromboembolic events, 90% have a twenty-five–fold decrease in releasable t-PA[403,406,407]; 51.6% have an abnormally low plasminogen activator content in the vein walls.[408] Therefore a certain subgroup of women taking oral contraceptives is at particular risk for thromboembolic disease.

In addition, increased distensibility of peripheral veins may occur with use of systemic estrogens and progestins.[410,411] This change may promote valvular dysfunction and a relative stasis in blood flow to add to the hypercoagulable state. Since it is practically impossible (and also impractical) at this time to determine which women are at risk, it seems prudent to recommend that patients consider discontinuing this medication before sclerotherapy treatment.

An alternative for women who cannot discontinue oral estrogen replacement therapy is the use of transdermally administered 17-beta-estradiol. Since estrogen is delivered directly into the peripheral circulation, the "first-pass effect" of liver metabolism is eliminated. This method decreases hepatic estrogen levels with subsequent minimization of estrogen-induced alteration of coagulation proteins. Thus the use of transdermal estrogen is recommended in patients at risk for thromboembolism since alterations in blood clotting factors have not been demonstrated during such treatment.[412]

Tamoxifen. For multiple reasons, including prevention of breast cancer in high-risk populations, adjunctive treatment of breast cancer, and possibly treatment and/or prevention of osteoporosis, tamoxifen is not an uncommon medication for patients who are scheduled for sclerotherapy, surgical treatment, or both. An unusual and poorly understood complication of tamoxifen use is the development of thrombophlebitis and DVT. This complication occurs in up to 1% of treated patients.[413,414] Results from evaluation of various coagulation parameters and factors, including sex hormone–binding globulin, antithrombin III fibrinogen level, platelet count, protein C, and fibrinopeptide A, have been normal.[414-418] Until more is known about this theoretical predisposing factor to thrombosis, note should be taken of patients receiving tamoxifen.

Pregnancy. As early as 1579, it was common medical practice not to tamper with varicose veins during pregnancy.[419] However, some physicians advocate removal of varicose veins to prevent postpartum venous thrombosis.[420] These authors report a distinct lack of complications to both mother and infant with this practice, even though treatment spanned the first and eighth months of gestation. However, in addition to the possible effects on the fetus through passage of sclerosing solution through the placental barrier, there is a potential for stimulating placental thrombosis.

Endothelial cell damage (presumably caused by sclerotherapy) releases t-PA to promote coagulability on the already formed clot, which invariably occurs in the immediate postsclerotherapy period.[421] In addition, coexistent hypercoagulability may promote excessive (uncontrolled) thrombosis. The hypercoagulable state in the immediate antepartum period is largely responsible for the development of superficial thrombophlebitis and DVT in 0.15% and 0.04% of this patient population, respectively.[422] Even more important is the immediate postpartum period during which the incidence of superficial thrombophlebitis and DVT is 1.18% and 0.15%, respectively.[422] DVT developed by the second postpartum day in 50% of patients. This development may be due to the rapid decrease in coagulation factors at delivery, which normalizes in most patients on the third day.[423] However, other factors must also play a role since an additional 21% of the patients developed DVT 2 to 3 weeks postpartum. Interestingly, two thirds of the patients who developed postpartum DVT had varicose veins. The age of the mother was also linked to venous thrombosis, with the rate changing from approximately 1 in 1000 in women younger than 25 years to 1 in 1200 in women over 35.[391]

During pregnancy an increase in most procoagulant factors and a reduction in fibrinolytic activity occur. Plasma fibrinogen levels gradually increase after the third month of pregnancy to double those of the nonpregnant state. In the second half of pregnancy, factors VII, X, VIII, and IX are also elevated.[424] Decreased fibrinolytic activity probably is related to a decrease in circulating plasminogen activator.[425] In addition, a 68% reduction in protein S levels has been measured during pregnancy and in the postpartum period.[426] Protein S levels do not return to normal until 12 weeks postpartum. These changes are necessary to prevent hemorrhage during placental separation. Thus, in addition to avoiding the potential adverse effects on the fetus, sclerotherapy should not be performed near term but should be postponed until coagulability returns to normal at 6 weeks postpartum.

Inherited factor deficiency. Another subgroup of patients is also at increased risk for DVT. Protein C and protein S are two vitamin K–dependent proteins that are important anticoagulant factors that prevent thrombosis. Protein S is a cofactor for activated protein C (APC) on factor Va. It has been estimated that the prevalence of heterozygous protein C deficiency is 1 in 300 to 1 in 60 healthy adults in the United States.[427] More than 95% of these subjects are asymptomatic and without a history of thrombotic disease. However, these deficiencies may predispose these individuals to the development of DVT. Seventy-five percent of patients homozygous for protein S deficiency will develop venous thrombosis before age 35.[428]

It has been speculated that damaged endothelium in combination with this deficiency may be necessary for symptomatic thrombosis to occur.[429] In otherwise healthy patients under age 45 who are referred for evaluation of venous thrombosis, the prevalence of deficiencies of antithrombin III, protein C, and protein S is approximately 5% each.[430] A resistance to APC is at least 10 times more common than any known genetic defect for venous thrombosis and has been found in approximately one third of patients referred for evaluation of DVT.[431,432] Precipitating factors for thrombosis, such as pregnancy and the use of oral contraceptives, were present in 60% of these patients. Therefore patients who exhibit excessive thrombosis with sclerotherapy and patients with a family history of thrombotic disease should be screened for deficiencies of protein C and protein S before treatment.

There is also a heterozygous mutation having an incidence of 2% to 5% for APC.[433] This mutation results in an eight- to tenfold increased incidence of venous thromboembolism.

A rare cause of acquired protein S deficiency occurs from a transient circulating autoantibody. An 11-year-old boy with varicella was described as having this transient abnormal immune response, which resulted in severe thromboembolic disease.[434] With chickenpox, endothelitis that may disrupt normal production of protein S occurs.[435] In this patient thrombosis was resistant to heparin therapy, and it was postulated that infusions of protein S would have been therapeutic. Although this type of immune response is an extremely rare cause of DVT, withholding sclerotherapy treatment in febrile patients, especially those with varicella, Rocky Mountain spotted fever, and vasculitis, is recommended.

Antithrombin III deficiency occurs in 1 in 2000 to 1 in 5000 people in the general population.[436,437] Acquired antithrombin III deficiency may occur during liver disease and may result from the use of oral contraceptives, as previously discussed.

Defects in the fibrinolytic system, specifically plasminogen, occur in up to

10% of the normal population.[438] When they occur alone, there is little risk of thrombosis. Abnormal plasminogen levels may also predispose to thrombosis.

Lupus-like anticoagulants are present in 16% to 33% of patients with lupus erythematosus, but they are also associated with a variety of autoimmune disorders.[439-441] From 30% to 50% of patients with lupus-like anticoagulants develop thrombosis.[441-443]

Finally, if a patient develops thrombophlebitis or DVT after sclerotherapy and a workup for hypercoagulability is normal, consideration must be given to search for an occult malignancy. I have had one patient develop thrombophlebitis of superficial reticular veins (despite adequate compression) who was found to have an occult breast carcinoma on further examination.

Prevention. Because of the potentially lethal nature of excessive thrombosis, all attempts should be made to minimize its occurrence. The quantity of sclerosing solution should be limited to 0.5 to 1 ml per injection site to prevent leakage of the solution into the deep venous system.[340] Other techniques that minimize damage to the deep venous system include rapid compression of the injected vein with a 30 to 40 mm Hg pressure stocking, followed by immediate ambulation or calf movement of the injected extremity and frequent ambulation thereafter to promote rapid dilution of the solution from the injected area. Full dorsiflexion of the ankle empties all deep leg veins, including muscular and soleal sinuses.[444] Using these recommendations, Fegan[445] reported no cases of DVT or pulmonary emboli in 13,352 patients when the sclerosing solution quantity was limited to 0.5 ml and rapid compression was used.

The critical period for thrombus formation in sclerotherapy-treated vessels is approximately 9 hours after treatment. Therefore compression stockings or bandages are of most benefit during the night after sclerotherapy treatment and during other periods of relative vascular stasis, when an intravascular thrombus may be being formed.

Foley[446] advocates the addition of heparin, 100 U/ml, to HS to prevent the theoretical possibility of embolization associated with "microthrombus formation" in sclerotherapy. However, in a well-controlled randomized study of 800 patients treated with and without heparin in the sclerosing solution, no evidence for embolization and no difference in the incidence of thrombophlebitis or microthrombosis requiring puncture evacuation were found.[447]

Consideration must be given to treating elderly patients because they have a reportedly increased risk for DVT.[218,448-450] It is hypothesized that the major cause for this increased risk is the relative pooling of blood in the soleal venous sinuses, which occurs from decreased calf muscle pump infusion.[451] In the elderly population it may be best to perform small treatments, with calf pumping done manually immediately after injection.

Venous stasis is the most likely mechanism for DVT after sclerotherapy. This condition can occur from a tourniquet effect caused by an improperly bandaged extremity or immobilization of a treated limb. At least one case of fatal PE after sclerotherapy has been attributed to improper bandaging coupled with a prolonged car ride immediately after treatment.[452] If a patient becomes ill or injured after sclerotherapy, he or she must avoid immobilization. In this scenario it is strongly recommended that consideration be given to heparin prophylactic anti-coagulation therapy until ambulation is restored.[348]

Treatment. DVT has many sequelae and is also a potentially life-threatening complication. The most serious manifestation of DVT is the development of PE, which can be life-threatening. Late sequelae of DVT are common and frequently symptomatic. A study of 86 patients who developed DVT found that 70 of the patients were symptomatic 5 to 10 years later.[453] Typical symptoms were evening pain, edema, restless legs, and pigmentation. Up to 50% of the patients judged their symptoms to be severe 10 years after the DVT. Simple leg elevation improved symptoms in only 56% of patients. There was no difference between calf DVT and proximal DVT. Thus DVT treatment must be rapid and decisive.

PE usually occurs during the first 5 to 7 days of thrombus formation.[454] After effective anticoagulation with IV heparin has been achieved, oral anticoagulation therapy with warfarin and other inhibitors of vitamin K metabolism should be initiated. Alternatively, the patient may continue receiving subcutaneous heparin. IV heparin should be continued for 3 to 5 days after initiation of warfarin to prevent an early reduction in anticoagulant protein C and protein S function before procoagulant activity is affected. It is recommended that patients receive at least 3 months of oral anticoagulation therapy to decrease the risk of recurrent DVT to less than 4%.[455] However, additional studies on patients with reversible causes to DVT show that they need only be treated for 6 weeks.[456,457]

Peripheral infusions of lytic agents may be superior to anticoagulation therapy for rapidly reducing a clot, which should reduce late symptoms and the risk of recurrent thrombosis.[458] If peripheral systemic lytic therapy is ineffective, direct infusion of lytic agents into the thrombus may be useful.[459] To prevent recurrence, thrombolytic therapy should be followed by the use of antiplatelet agents such as aspirin, or warfarin, or both. A more complete discussion of the various lytic agents is beyond the scope of this chapter.

Nerve Damage

Because of their proximity to veins, the saphenous and sural nerves may be injected with solution during sclerotherapy. Injection into a nerve is reported as very painful and, if continued, may cause anesthesia and sometimes a permanent interruption of nerve function.[173] Five episodes of injection into a nerve were reported from France over 18 years.[335] Various degrees of nerve paralysis or paresis occurred.

One patient with a large vascular malformation was treated with sclerotherapy into vessels overlying the lateral aspect of the knee. During the third injection of sodium morrhuate, a foot drop developed, which lasted 3 months, followed by full recovery. The authors postulate that the venous anomaly involved the perineal nerve and the inflammatory edema/reaction resulted in neuropraxis.[232]

Occasionally a patient complains of an area of paresthesia in the treated leg. This effect is probably caused by perivascular inflammation extending from the sclerosed vein to adjacent superficial nerves. Steps to limit inflammation, including therapy with nonsteroidal anti-inflammatory medications and high-potency topical steroids, may hasten resolution of this minor annoyance. However, this complication may take 3 to 6 months to resolve.[245]

Air Embolism

When air-block[460,461] or foam techniques are used to inject sclerosing solutions, the theoretical possibility of air embolism is raised. The danger would be that if enough air entered the heart at one time, it might lead to vascular collapse. In addition, if air enters a cerebral vascular artery, a cerebral vascular infarction may occur. More likely, transient ischemic symptoms might occur with this injection technique.

Introduction of air in small amounts into the venous system does not lead to clinical air embolism.[460,461] It appears that small amounts of air are absorbed into the bloodstream before the blood enters the pulmonic circulation. It has been estimated that it would be necessary to put 480 ml of air into the venous system within 20 to 30 seconds to cause death in a person weighing 60 kg.[462] This occurrence has never been reported in the medical literature and has not been noted in a series of 297 cases with the air-block technique.[460]

Scintillating Scotomata

Although this effect has not been reported in the literature, many physicians have told me of patients who develop temporary blindness or unusual visual disturbances after sclerotherapy. These physical findings most likely suggest ischemia of the calcarine cortex, which may occur through either embolism of ophthalmic arteries via the internal carotid artery or a vasospastic event. Arterial embolism appears unlikely unless the patient has a patent foramen ovale because venous injection and possible embolic events terminate in the pulmonary system. Monocular retinal migraine may occur in patients with a migraine diathesis. In such a case the patient's history is helpful and the outcome is usually benign. It is recommended that a complete ophthalmologic examination be obtained to rule out other more serious and treatable causative factors.

Membranous Fat Necrosis

A single patient with multiple tender, erythematous subcutaneous nodules noted after sclerotherapy with HS solution has recently been reported.[463] This rare dermatologic effect is secondary to subcutaneous inflammation with alteration and necrosis of adipose tissue. The etiologic complex may also be secondary to trauma, thromboangiitis obliterans, arteriosclerosis, or scleroderma. It is essen-

TABLE 16-1. Summary of complications associated with use of sclerosing agents

Agent	Active Ingredient	Allergic Reaction	Necrosis	Pain
Sodium morrhuate*	Fatty acids in cod liver oil	Occasional	Frequent‡	Moderate
Sotradecol*	Sodium tetradecyl sulfate	Rare	Occasional‡	Mild
Ethamolin*	Ethanolamine oleate	Occasional	Rare‡	Mild
Polidocanol†	Hydroxypolyethoxy-dodecane	Very rare	Very rare‡	None
Hypertonic saline	10%-30% Saline	None	Occasional‡	Moderate
Sclerodex†	10% Saline and 5% dextrose	Very rare	Rare	Mild
Scleremo†	1.11% Chromated glycerin	Very rare	Very rare	Moderate
Variglobin†	Iodide sodium iodine	Very rare	Frequent‡	Moderate

*Approved for use by the Food and Drug Administration.
†Not approved for use in the United States.
‡Concentration-dependent, especially with extravasation.

tially a diagnosis of exclusion made at biopsy. In the reported patient, extravasation of HS solution or vessel rupture with subsequent exposure of HS to subcutaneous tissues was the probable causative event.

SUMMARY

Sclerotherapy of varicose and telangiectatic leg veins may be associated with a number of complications and adverse sequelae, which may occur despite optimal treatment. Some adverse sequelae are preventable to a limited degree, but, given a large enough number of procedures, such sequelae will occur in any practice. Complications also are avoidable to some extent. As with any procedure, however, sclerotherapy has inherent risks. Thus each patient should be evaluated and cautioned accordingly before treatment is initiated. A summary of the common complications that can occur with routinely used sclerosing agents is presented in Table 16-1.

REFERENCES

1. Tretbar LL. Spider angiomata: Treatment with sclerosant injections. J Kans Med Soc 79:198, 1978.
2. Tournay PR. Traitement sclérosant des très fines varicosités intra ou sous-dermiques. Soc Fran Phlebol 19:235, 1966.

3. Weiss R, Weiss M. Resolution of pain associated with varicose and telangiectatic leg veins after compression sclerotherapy. J Dermatol Surg Oncol 16:333, 1990.

4. Bodian EL. Techniques of sclerotherapy for sunburst venous blemishes. J Dermatol Surg Oncol 11:696, 1985.

5. Duffy DM. Small vessel sclerotherapy: An overview. In Callen JP, et al., eds. Advances in Dermatology, vol 3. Chicago: Year Book Medical Publishers, 1988.

6. Alderman DB. Surgery and sclerotherapy in the treatment of varicose veins. Conn Med 39:467, 1975.

7. White SW, Besanceney C. Systemic pigmentation from tetracycline and minocycline therapy. Arch Dermatol 119:1, 1983.

8. Cacciatore E. Experience of sclerotherapy with Aethoxysklerol. Minn Cardioangiol 27:255, 1979.

9. Gawrychowski J, Lazar-Czyzewska B, Romanski A. A comparative study of three sclerosing agents in the treatment of telangiectasias. Phlebology (Suppl) 1:530, 1995.

10. Goldman P. Sclerotherapy of superficial venules and telangiectasias of the lower extremities. Dermatol Clin 5:369, 1987.

11. Avramovic A, Avramovic M. Complications of sclerotherapy: A statistical study. In Raymond-Martimbeau P, Prescott R, Zummo M, eds. Phlebologie '92. Paris: John Libbey Eurotext, 1992.

12. Izzo M, et al. Postsclerotherapy hyperpigmentation: Incidence, clinical features and therapy. Phlebology (Suppl) 1:550, 1995.

13. Georgiev M. Postsclerotherapy hyperpigmentations: A one-year follow-up. J Dermatol Surg Oncol 16:608, 1990.

14. Biegeleisen HI, Biegeleisen RM. The current status of sclerotherapy for varicose veins. Clin Med 83:24, 1976.

15. Chrisman BB. Treatment of venous ectasias with hypertonic saline. Hawaii Med J 41:406, 1982.

16. Chatard H. Discussion de la question de J-C Allart: Pigmentations post-sclérotherapiques. Phlebologie 29:211, 1976.

17. Shields JL, Jansen GT. Therapy for superficial telangiectasias of the lower extremities. J Dermatol Surg Oncol 8:857, 1982.

18. Barner FR, Holzegel K, Voigt K. Über Hyperpigmentation nach Krampfaderverödung. Phlebol u Proktol 6:54, 1977.

19. Goldman MP, Kaplan RP, Duffy DM. Postsclerotherapy hyperpigmentation: A histologic evaluation. J Dermatol Surg Oncol 13:547, 1987.

20. Cuttell PJ, Fox JA. The etiology and treatment of varicose pigmentation. Phlebologie 35:387, 1982.

21. Goldman MP. Postsclerotherapy hyperpigmentation: Treatment with a flashlamp-excited pulsed dye laser. J Dermatol Surg Oncol 18:417, 1992.

22. Goldman MP, et al. Sclerosing agents in the treatment of telangiectasia: Comparison of the clinical and histologic effects of intravascular polidocanol, sodium tetradecyl sulfate, and hypertonic saline in the dorsal rabbit ear vein model. Arch Dermatol 123:1196, 1987.

23. Grega GJ, Svensjo E, Haddy FJ. Macromolecular permeability of the microvascular membrane: Physiological and pharmacological regulation. Microcirculation 1:325, 1981-1982.

24. Majno G, Palade GE, Schoefl GI. Studies on inflammation: The site of action of histamine and serotonin along the vascular tree—A topographic study. J Biophysiol Biochem Cytol 11:607, 1961.

25. Bjork J, Smedegard G. The microvasculature of the hamster cheek pouch as a model for studying acute immune-complex–induced inflammatory reactions. Int Arch Allergy Appl Immunol 74:178, 1984.

26. Fox J, Galey F, Wayland H. Action of histamine on the mesenteric microvasculature. Microvasc Res 19:108, 1980.

27. Simionescu N, Simionescu M, Palade G. Open junctions in the endothelium of the postcapillary venules of the diaphragm. J Cell Biol 79:27, 1978.

28. Bessis M. Living Blood Cells and Their Ultrastructure. Berlin: Springer-Verlag, 1973.

29. Leu HJ, et al. Veränderungen der transendothelialen Permeabilität als Ursache des Ödems bei der chronisch-venösen Insuffizienz. Med Welt 31:781, 1980.

30. Bessis M, Lessin LS, Beutler E. Morphology of the erythron. In Williams WJ, et al., eds. Hematology, 3rd ed. New York: McGraw-Hill, 1983.

31. Ludewig S. Hemosiderin. Isolation from horse spleen and characterization. Proc Soc Exp Biol Med 95:514, 1957.

32. Richter GW. The nature of storage iron in idiopathic hemochromatosis and in hemosiderosis. J Exp Med 112:551, 1960.

33. Ackerman Z, et al. Overload of iron in the skin of patients with varicose ulcers. Arch Dermatol 124:1376, 1988.

34. Chatarel H, Dufour H. Note sur la nature mixture, hématique et mélanique, des pigmentations en phlébologie. Phlebologie 36:303, 1983.

35. Merlen JF, Coget J, Sarteel AM. Pigmentation et stase veineuse. Phlebologie 36:307, 1983.

36. Klüken N, Zabel M. La pigmentation est-elle un signe caractéristique de l'insuffisance veineuse chronique? Phlebologie 36:315, 1983.

37. Cloutier G, Sansoucy H. Le traitement des varices des membres inférieurs par les injections sclérosantes. L'Union Médicale du Canada 104:1854, 1975.

38. Weiss RA, Weiss MA. Incidence of side effects in the treatment of telangiectasias by compression sclerotherapy: Hypertonic saline vs polidocanol. J Dermatol Surg Oncol 16:800, 1990.

39. Norris MJ, Carlin MC, Ratz JL. Treatment of essential telangiectasia: Effects of increasing concentrations of polidocanol. J Am Acad Dermatol 20:643, 1989.

40. Hutinel B. Esthétique dans les scléroses de varices et traitement des varicosités. La Vie Med 20:1739, 1978.

41. Nebot F. Quelques points techniques sur le traitement des varicosités et des telangiectasies. Phlebologie 21:133, 1968.

42. Landart J. Traitement médical des varices des membres inférieurs. La Rev du Pract 26:2491, 1976.

43. Tournay R. La Sclérose des Varices. Paris: Expansion Scientifique Française, 1980.

44. Lucchi M, Bilancini S. Sclerotherapy of telangiectasia [English abstract]. Minerva Angiol 15:31, 1990.

45. Georgiev M. Postsclerotherapy hyperpigmentation: Chromated glycerin as a screen for patients at risk (a retrospective study). J Dermatol Surg Oncol 19:649, 1993.

46. Marley W. Low-dose Sotradecol for small vessel sclerotherapy. Newsletter North Am Soc Phlebol 3:3, 1989.

47. Guex J-J. Indications for the sclerosing agent polidocanol. J Dermatol Surg Oncol 19:959, 1993.

48. Gilchrest BA, Stoff JS, Soter NA. Chronologic aging alters the response to ultraviolet-induced inflammation in human skin. J Invest Dermatol 79:11, 1982.

49. Thibault P, Wlodarczyk J. Postsclerotherapy hyperpigmentation: The role of serum iron levels and the effectiveness of treatment with the copper vapor laser. J Dermatol Surg Oncol 18:47, 1992.

50. Pippard MJ, Hoffbrand AV. Iron. In Hoffbrand AV, Lewis SM, eds. Postgraduate Haematology. Oxford: Heinemann Medical Books, 1989.

51. Thibault P, Wlodarczyk J. Correlation of serum ferritin levels and postsclerotherapy pigmentation: Prospective study. J Dermatol Surg Oncol 20:684, 1994.

52. Scott C, Seiger E. Postsclerotherapy pigmentation: Is serum ferritin level an accurate indicator? Dermatol Surg 23:281, 1997.

53. Marciniak DL, et al. Antagonism of histamine edema formation by catecholamines. Am J Physiol 234:H180, 1978.

54. Svensjo E. Pharmacological modulation of venular permeability with some antiinflammatory drugs. Return circulation and norepinephrine: An update. Paris: John Libbey Eurotext, 1991.

55. Svensjo E, Persson CGA, Rutili G. Inhibition of bradykinin-induced macromolecular leakage from post-capillary venules by a B_2-adrenoreceptor stimulant, terbutaline. Acta Physiol Scand 101:504, 1977.

56. Heltianu C, Simionescu M, Simionescu N. Histamine receptors of the microvascular endothelium revealed in situ with a histamine-ferritin conjugate: Characteristic high-affinity binding sites in venules. J Cell Biol 93:357, 1982.

57. Clemetson CAB, Blair L, Brown AB. Capillary strength and the menstrual cycle. Ann N Y Acad Sci 93:277, 1962.

58. Jacoby WD. Comment 21. Schoch Lett 41:2, 1991.

59. Leffell DJ. Minocycline hydrochloride hyperpigmentation complicating treatment of venous ectasia of the extremities. J Am Acad Dermatol 24:501, 1991.

60. Poliak SC, et al. Minocycline-associated tooth discoloration in young adults. JAMA 254:2930, 1985.

61. Billano RA, Ward WQ, Little WP. Minocycline and black thyroid [letter]. JAMA 249:1887, 1983.

62. Dwyer CM, et al. Skin pigmentation due to minocycline treatment of facial dermatoses. Br J Dermatol 129:158, 1993.

63. Fenske NA, Millns JL, Greer KE. Minocycline-induced pigmentation at sites of cutaneous inflammation. JAMA 244:1103, 1980.

64. Eedy DJ, Burrows D. Minocycline-induced pigmentation occurring in two sisters. Clin Exp Dermatol 16:55, 1991.

65. Basler RSW, Kohnen PW. Localized hemosiderosis as a sequela of acne. Arch Dermatol 114:1695, 1978.

66. Basler RSW. Minocycline therapy for acne [letter]. Arch Dermatol 115:1391, 1979.

67. Ridgway HA, et al. Hyperpigmentation associated with oral minocycline. Br J Dermatol 107:95, 1982.

68. Sato S, et al. Ultrastructural and x-ray microanalysis observations of minocycline-related hyperpigmentation of the skin. J Invest Dermatol 77:264, 1981.

69. Gordon G, Sparano BM, Iatropoulos MJ. Hyperpigmentation of the skin associated with minocycline therapy. Arch Dermatol 121:618, 1985.

70. Okada N, et al. Skin pigmentation associated with minocycline therapy. Br J Dermatol 124:247, 1989.

71. Moreno AH, et al. Mechanics of distention of dog veins and other thin-walled tubular structures. Circ Res 27:1069, 1970.

72. Wenner L. Sind endovarikose hamitische Ansammlungen eine Normalerscheinung bei Sklerotherapie? Vasa 10:174, 1981.

73. Leu HJ, Wenner A, Spycher MA. Erythrocyte diapedesis in venous stasis syndrome. Vasa 10:17, 1981.

74. Orbach EJ. Hazards of sclerotherapy of varicose veins—Their prevention and treatment of complications. Vasa 8:170, 1979.

75. Perchuk E. Injection therapy of varicose veins: A method of obliterating huge varicosities with small doses of sclerosing agent. Angiology 25:393, 1974.

76. De Takats G. Problems in the treatment of varicose veins. Am J Surg 18:26, 1932.

77. Biegeleisen HI. Sclerotherapy: Clinical significance. Clin Med Surg 47:140, 1940.

78. Bernier EC, Escher E. Treatment of postsclerotherapy hyperpigmentation with trichloroacetic acid, a mild and effective procedure. In Proceedings of the Second Annual International Congress of the North American Society of Phlebology. New Orleans, La., Feb. 25, 1989.

79. Myers HL. Topical chelation therapy for varicose pigmentation. Angiology 17:66, 1966.

80. Bissett DL, Oelrich M, Hannon DP. Evaluation of a topical iron chelator in animals and in human beings: Short-term photoprotection by 2-furildioxome. J Am Acad Dermatol 31:572, 1994.

81. Burnand K, et al. Venous lipodermatosclerosis: Treatment by fibrinolytic enhancement and elastic compression. BMJ 280:7, 1980.

82. Shoden A, Sturgeon P. Hemosiderin: I. A physio-chemical study. Acta Haematol (Basel) 23: 376, 1960.

83. Wells CI, Wolken JJ. Biochemistry: Microspectrophotometry of haemosiderin granules. Nature 193:977, 1962.

84. Weiss RA. Intense pulsed light (Photoderm PL) treatment of postsclerotherapy hyperpigmentation: Preliminary report. Presented at the Annual Meeting of the North American Society of Phlebology. Washington, D.C., Nov. 1996.

85. Riddock J. Treatment of varicose veins. BMJ 2:671, 1947.

86. Bjork J, et al. Methylprednisolone acts at the endothelial cell level reducing inflammatory responses. Acta Physiol Scand 123:221, 1985.

87. Bouskela E, Cyrino FZ, Marcelon G. Inhibitory effect of the Ruscus extract and the flavanoid hesperidine methylchalcone on increased microvascular permeability induced by various agents in the hamster cheek pouch. J Cardiovasc Pharmacol 22:225-230, 1993.

88. Svensjo E, Grega GJ. Evidence for endothelial cell–mediated regulation of macromolecular permeability by postcapillary venules. Fed Proc 45:89, 1986.

89. Goldman MP, et al. Compression in the treatment of leg telangiectasia. J Dermatol Surg Oncol 16:322, 1990.

90. Arenander E, Lindhagen A. The evolution of varicose veins studied in a material of initially unilateral varices. Vasa 7:180, 1978.

91. Terezakis N. Sclerotherapy treatment of leg veins. Presented at the summer session of the American Academy of Dermatology. San Diego, Calif., June 17, 1989.

92. Davis LT, Duffy DM. Determination of incidence and risk factors for post-sclerotherapy telangiectatic matting of the lower extremity: A retrospective analysis. J Dermatol Surg Oncol 16:327, 1990.

93. Bodian EL. Sclerotherapy. Semin Dermatol 6:238, 1987.

94. Miller JW, et al. Vascular endothelial growth factor/vascular permeability factor is temporally and spatially correlated with ocular angiogenesis in a primate model. Am J Pathol 145:574, 1994.

95. Aiello LP, et al. Vascular endothelial growth factor in ocular fluid of patients with diabetic retinopathy and other retinal disorders. N Engl J Med 331:1480, 1994.

96. Shweiki D, et al. Vascular endothelial growth factor induced by hypoxia may mediate hypoxia-initiated angiogenesis. Nature 359:843, 1992.

97. Ouvry P, Davy A. Le traitement sclérosant des telangiectasies des membres inférieurs. Phlebologie 35:349, 1982.

98. Merlen JF. Telangiectasies rouges, telangiectasies bleues. Phlebologie 23:167, 1970.

99. Biegeleisen K. Primary lower extremity telangiectasias, relationship of size to color. Angiology 38:760, 1987.

100. Denekamp J. Angiogenesis, neovascular proliferation and vascular pathophysiology as targets for cancer therapy. Br J Radiol 66:181, 1993.

101. Clark ER, Clark EL. Observations on living performed blood vessels as seen in a transparent chamber inserted into the rabbit's ear. Am J Anat 49:441, 1932.

102. Clark ER, Clark EL. Microscopic observations on the extracellular cells of living mammalian blood vessels. Am J Anat 66:1, 1940.

103. Yanagisawa-Miwa A, et al. Salvage of infarcted myocardium by angiogenic action of basic fibroblast growth factor. Science 257:1401, 1992.

104. Shing Y, et al. Angiogenesis is stimulated by tumor-derived endothelial cell growth factor. J Cell Biochem 29:275, 1985.

105. Ashton N. Corneal vascularization. In Duke-Elder S, Perkins ES, eds. The Transparency of the Cornea. Oxford: Blackwell Scientific Publications, 1960.

106. Haudenschild CC. Growth control of endothelial cells in atherogenesis and tumor angiogenesis. In Altura BM, ed. Advances in Microcirculation, vol 9. Basel: Karger, 1980.

107. Folkman J, Klagsbrun M. Angiogenic factors. Science 235:442, 1987.

108. Frater-Schroder M, et al. Tumor necrosis factor type alpha, a potent inhibitor of endothelial cell growth in vitro, is angiogenic in vivo. Proc Natl Acad Sci U S A 84:5277, 1987.
109. Fujita M, et al. Improvement of treadmill capacity and collateral circulation as a result of exercise with heparin pretreatment in patients with effort angina. Circulation 77:1022, 1988.
110. Ryan TJ. Factors influencing the growth of vascular endothelium in the skin. Br J Dermatol 82(Suppl 5):99, 1970.
111. Baffour R, et al. Enhanced angiogenesis and growth of collaterals by in vivo administration of recombinant basic fibroblast growth factor in a rabbit model of acute lower limb ischemia: Dose-response effect of basic fibroblast growth factor. J Vasc Surg 16:181, 1992.
112. Lindner V, et al. Role of basic fibroblast growth factor in vascular lesion formation. Circ Res 68:106, 1991.
113. Leibovitch SJ, et al. Macrophage-induced angiogenesis is mediated by tumor necrosis factor-alpha. Nature 329:630, 1987.
114. Piquet PF, Grau GE, Vassalli P. Subcutaneous perfusion of tumor necrosis factor induces local proliferation of fibroblasts, capillaries, and epidermal cells, or massive tumor necrosis. Am J Pathol 136:103, 1990.
115. Miyazono K, et al. Purification and properties of an endothelial cell growth factor from human platelets. J Biol Chem 262:4098, 1987.
116. Shing Y, Folkman J, Haudenschild C. Angiogenesis is stimulated by tumor-derived endothelial cell growth factor. J Cell Biochem 29:275, 1985.
117. Sporn MB, et al. Transforming growth factor beta: Biologic function and chemical structure. Science 233:532, 1987.
118. Martin BM, et al. Stimulation of nonlymphoid mesenchymal cell proliferation by a macrophage-derived growth factor. J Immunol 126:1510, 1981.
119. Rothe MJ, Nowak M, Kerdel FA. The mast cell in health and disease. J Am Acad Dermatol 23:615, 1990.
120. Flaumenhaft R, et al. Role of extracellular matrix in the action of basic fibroblast growth factor: Matrix as a source of growth factor for long-term stimulation of plasminogen activator production and DNA synthesis. J Cell Physiol 140:75, 1989.
121. Vlodavsky I, et al. Endothelial cell–derived basic fibroblast growth factor: Synthesis and deposition into subendothelial extracellular matrix. Proc Natl Acad Sci U S A 84:2292, 1987.
122. Barnhill RL, Wolf JE Jr. Angiogenesis and the skin. J Am Acad Dermatol 16:1226, 1987.
123. Dvorak AM, Mihm MC Jr, Dvorak HF. Morphology of delayed-type hypersensitivity reactions in man. II. Ultrastructural alterations affecting the microvasculature and the tissue mast cells. Lab Invest 34:179, 1976.
124. Conrad P, Malouf GM, Stacey MC. The Australian polidocanol (Aethoxysklerol) study: Results at 2 years. Dermatol Surg 21:334, 1995.
125. Enerback L. Mast cells in rat gastrointestinal mucosa. I. Effects of fixation. Acta Pathol Microbiol Scand 66:289, 1966.
126. Mikhail GR, Miller-Milinska A. Mast cell population in human skin. J Invest Dermatol 43:249, 1964.
127. Hellstrom B, Holmgren HJ. Numerical distribution of mast cells in human skin and heart. Acta Anat (Basel) 10:81, 1950.
128. Eady RAJ, et al. Mast cell population density, blood vessel density, and histamine content in normal human skin. Br J Dermatol 100:623, 1979.
129. Kasper CS, Freeman RG, Tharp MD. Diagnosis of mastocytosis subsets using a morphometric point counting technique. Arch Dermatol 127:1017, 1987.
130. Schiff M, Burn HF. The effect of intravenous estrogens on ground substance. Arch Otolaryngol 73:43, 1961.
131. Kleinman HK, et al. Role of estrogens in inflammation and angiogenesis. Presented at the Joint Meeting of the Wound Healing Society and European Tissue Repair Society. Amsterdam, Aug. 23, 1993.

132. Bean WB. The vascular spider in pregnancy. In Bean WB, ed. Vascular Spiders and Related Lesions of the Skin. Springfield, Ill.: Charles C Thomas, 1958.

133. Pirovino M, et al. Cutaneous spider nevi in liver cirrhosis: Capillary microscopical and hormonal investigation. Klin Wochenschr 66:298, 1988.

134. Gagliardi A, Collins DC. Inhibition of angiogenesis by antiestrogens. Cancer Res 53:533, 1993.

135. Haran EF, et al. Tamoxifen enhances cell death in implanted MCF7 breast cancer by inhibiting endothelial growth. Cancer Res 54:5511, 1994.

136. Sadick NS, Niedt GW. A study of estrogen and progesterone receptors in spider telangiectasias of the lower extremities. J Dermatol Surg Oncol 16:620, 1990.

137. Saski GH, Pang CY, Wittcliff JL. Pathogenesis and treatment of infant skin strawberry hemangiomas: Clinical and in vitro studies of normal effects. Plast Reconstr Surg 73:359, 1984.

138. Puisseau-Lupo ML. Sclerotherapy—A review of results and complications in 200 patients. J Dermatol Surg Oncol 15:214, 1989.

139. Goldman MP, Fitzpatrick RE. Pulsed-dye laser treatment of leg telangiectasia: With and without simultaneous sclerotherapy. J Dermatol Surg Oncol 16:338, 1990.

140. Goldman MP, Eckhouse S. Photothermal sclerosis of leg veins. Dermatol Surg 22:323, 1996.

141. Goldman MP. Treatment of benign vascular lesions with the Photoderm VL high-intensity pulsed light source. Adv Dermatol 13:503, 1998.

142. Adrian RM. Treatment of leg telangiectasias using a long-pulse frequency-doubled neodymium:YAG laser at 532 nm. Dermatol Surg 24:19, 1998.

143. Perez B, et al. Progressive ascending telangiectasia treated with the 585 nm flashlamp-pumped pulsed dye laser. Lasers Surg Med 21:413, 1997.

144. Azizkhan RG, et al. Mast cell heparin stimulates migration of capillary endothelial cells in vitro. J Exp Med 152:931, 1980.

145. Rakusan K, Turek Z. Protamine inhibits capillary formation in growing rat hearts. Circ Res 57:393, 1985.

146. Taylor S, Folkman J. Protamine is an inhibitor of angiogenesis. Nature 297:307, 1982.

147. Folkman J, et al. Control of angiogenesis with synthetic heparin substitutes. Science 243:1490, 1989.

148. Zabel P, Schade FU, Schlaak M. Pentoxifylline—An inhibitor of the synthesis of tumor necrosis factor alpha. Ammun Infekt (Germany) 20:80, 1992.

149. Wang P, et al. Mechanism of the beneficial effects of pentoxifylline on hepatocellular function after trauma hemorrhage and resuscitation. Surgery 112:451, 1992.

150. Martin U, Roemer D. Ketotifen: A histamine release inhibitor. Monogr Allergy 12:145, 1977.

151. Mansfield LE, et al. Inhibition of dermographia, histamine, and dextromethorphan skin tests by ketotifen. A possible effect on cutaneous response to mediators. Ann Allergy 63:201, 1989.

152. Huston DP, et al. Prevention of mast cell degranulation by Ketotifen in patients with physical urticarias. Ann Intern Med 104:507, 1986.

153. Kuokkanen K. Comparison of a new antihistamine HC 20-511 (Ketotifen) with cyproheptadine (Periactin) in chronic urticaria. Acta Allergica 32:316, 1977.

154. Saihan EM. Ketotifen and terbutaline in chronic urticaria. Br J Dermatol 104:205, 1981.

155. Shear NH, MacLeod SM. Diffuse cutaneous mastocytosis (DCM): Treatment with Ketotifen and cimetidine. Clin Invest Med 6(Suppl):36, 1983.

156. Czarnetzki BM. A double-blind cross-over study of the effect of Ketotifen in urticaria pigmentosa. Dermatologica 166:44, 1983.

157. De Takats G, Quint H. The injection treatment of varicose veins. Surg Gynecol Obstet 50:545, 1930.

158. Chou F-F, et al. The treatment of leg varicose veins with hypertonic saline–heparin injections. J Formos Med Assoc 83:206, 1984.

159. Carlin MC, Ratz JL. Treatment of telangiectasia: Comparison of sclerosing agents. J Dermatol Surg Oncol 13:1181, 1987.

160. Natbony SF, et al. Histologic studies of chronic idiopathic urticaria. J Allergy Clin Immunol 71:177, 1983.

161. Yosipovitch G, et al. High-potency topical corticosteroid rapidly decreases histamine-induced itch but not thermal sensation and pain in human being. J Am Acad Dermatol 35:118, 1996.

162. Alderman DB. Therapy for essential cutaneous telangiectasias. Postgrad Med 61:91, 1977.

163. Orbach EJ. The importance of removal of postinjection coagula during the course of sclerotherapy of varicose veins. Vasa 3:475, 1974.

164. Orbach EJ. A new approach to the sclerotherapy of varicose veins. Angiology 1:302, 1950.

165. Fegan WG. Varicose veins—Compression sclerotherapy [sound film]. Produced by Pharmaceutical Research Limited, 6-7 Broad St., Hereford HR4 9AE, England.

166. Tournay R. Collections hématiques intra ou extra-veineuses dans les phlebites superficielles ou après injections sclérosantes de varices a quel moment la thrombectomie? Soc Fran Phlebol 19:339, 1966.

167. Sigg K. Varizenverödung am hochgelgerten Bein. Deutsches Arzteblatt—Ärztliche Mitteilungen. 69. Jahrgang, Heft 14, S. 809-818. 6. April 1972, Postverlagsort Köln.

168. Pratt D. The technique of injection and compression. Stoke Mandeville Hospital Symposium: The treatment of varicose veins by injection and compression. Hereford, England, Oct. 15, 1971.

169. Hobbs JT. The management of recurrent and residual veins. Stoke Mandeville Hospital Symposium: The treatment of varicose veins by injection and compression. Oct. 15, 1971.

170. Holzegel VK. Über Krampfaderverödungen. Dermatol Wochenschr 153:137, 1967.

171. Lucchi M, Bilancini S, Tucci S. Sclerotherapy for telangiectasias of the leg: Results of a 5-year follow-up. Phlebology 11:73, 1996.

172. Winstone N. The treatment of varicose veins by injection and compression. In Proceedings of the Stoke Mandeville Symposium. Hereford, England, Pharmaceutical Research STD Ltd., 1992.

173. Browse NL, Burnard KG, Thomas ML. Diseases of the Veins: Pathology, Diagnosis, and Treatment. London: Edward Arnold, 1988.

174. Schraibman IG. Localized hirsuties. Postgrad Med J 43:545, 1967.

175. Marks G. Localized hirsuties following compression sclerotherapy with sodium tetradecyl sulphate. Br J Surg 61:127, 1974.

176. Weissberg D. Treatment of varicose veins by compression sclerotherapy. Surg Gynecol Obstet 151:353, 1980.

177. Strejcek J. Localised hypertrichosis after sclerotherapy performed with Aethoxysklerol. First observation. Scripta Phlebologica 2:41, 1994.

178. Upton J, Mulliken JB, Murray JE. Major extravasation injuries. Am J Surg 137:489, 1979.

179. Yosowitz P, et al. Peripheral intravenous infiltration necrosis. Ann Surg 182:553, 1975.

180. Eaglstein W. Inadvertent intracutaneous injection with hypertonic saline (23.4%) in two patients without complications. J Dermatol Surg Oncol 16:878, 1990.

181. Duffy DM. Setting up a vein treatment center—Incorporating sclerotherapy into the dermatologic practice. Semin Dermatol 12:150, 1993.

182. Jaquier JJ, Loretan RM. Clinical trials of a new sclerosing agent, Aethoxysklerol. Soc Fr Phlebol 22:383, 1969.

183. Hoffer AE. Aethoxysklerol (Kreussler) in the treatment of varices. Minn Cardioangiol 20:601, 1972.

184. Banning LL. Presentation at the Eighth Annual Meeting of the North American Society of Phlebology. Ft. Lauderdale, Fla., Feb. 28, 1995.

185. de Faria JL, Moraes IN. Histopathology of the telangiectasias associated with varicose veins. Dermatologia 127:321, 1963.

186. Conrad P, Malouf GM. The Australian Polidocanol (Aethoxysklerol) Open Clinical Trial results at two years. Presented at the Annual Meeting of the North American Society of Phlebology, Maui, Hawaii, Feb. 21, 1984.

187. Bassi G. In Santler R, Lindemayer H, Bolliger A, eds. Grenzen und Gefahren in der Phlebologie und Proktologie (Tischgespräch 1). Erg Angiol. Stuttgart: Schattauer, 1978, p 19.

188. Leun W, Langmaack BH. Die Grenzen und Gefahren der Varizenverödung. Dtsch Med Wochenschr 80:257, 1955.

189. Buri P, Brunner U. Die versehentliche Injektion von Verödungsmitteln in die Arteria tibialis posterior. In Brunner U, ed. Die Knoechelregion. Aktuelle Probleme in der Angiologie. Berne: Huber, 1980, p 40.

190. Dinkler JA, Cohen BE. Reversal of dopamine extravasation injury with topical nitroglycerin ointment. J Plast Reconstr Surg 84:811, 1989.

191. AMA Drug Evaluation, 6th ed. Chicago: American Medical Association, 1986.

192. Franks AG. Topical glyceryl trinitrate as adjunctive treatment in Raynaud's disease. Lancet 1:76, 1982.

193. Ross M. Dopamine-induced localized cutaneous vasoconstriction and piloerection. Arch Dermatol 127:586, 1991.

194. Chavez CM. The clinical significance of lymphatico-venous anastomoses. Vasc Dis 5:35, 1968.

195. Chant ADB. The effects of posture, exercise, and bandage pressure on the clearance of 24Na from the subcutaneous tissues of the foot. Br J Surg 59:552, 1972.

196. Campion EC, Hoffman DC, Jepson RP. The effects of external pneumatic splint pressure on muscle blood flow. Aust N Z J Surg 38:154, 1968.

197. Lawrence D, Kakkar V. Graduated, static, external compression of the lower limb: A physiological assessment. Br J Surg 67:119, 1980.

198. Zimmet SE. The prevention of cutaneous necrosis following extravasation of hypertonic saline and sodium tetradecyl sulfate. J Dermatol Surg Oncol 19:641, 1993.

199. Senk KE. Management of intravenous extravasation. Infusion 5:77, 1981.

200. Dorr RT, Alberts DS. Vinca alkaloid skin toxicity: Antidote and drug disposition studies in the mouse. J Natl Cancer Inst 74:113, 1985.

201. Laurie SWS, et al. Intravenous extravasation injuries: The effectiveness of hyaluronidase in their treatment. Ann Plast Surg 13:191, 1984.

202. Zenk KE, Dungy CL, Greene GR. Nafcillin extravasation injury: Use of hyaluronidase as an antidote. Am J Dis Child 135:1113, 1981.

203. Razka WV, et al. The use of hyaluronidase in the treatment of intravenous extravasation injuries. J Perinatol 10:146, 1990.

204. Dorr RT, Alberts DS. Pharmacologic antidotes to experimental doxorubicin skin toxicity: A suggested role for beta-adrenergic compounds. Cancer Treat Rev 65:1001, 1981.

205. Grossman JA, et al. The effects of hyaluronidase and DMSO on experimental flap survival. Ann Plast Surg 11:222, 1983.

206. Campbell CA, Przyklenk K, Kloner RA. Infarct size reduction: A review of the clinical trials. J Clin Pharmacol 26:317, 1986.

207. Haire RD. Use of Alidase in prevention of painful arm in accidental perivascular injection of neoarsphenamine and mapharsen. Rocky Mt Med J 600, 1950.

208. Lorenz HP, Adzick NS. Scarless skin wound repair in the fetus. West J Med 159:350, 1993.

209. Britton RC, Habif DV. Clinical uses of hyaluronidase. A current review. Surgery 33:917, 1953.

210. Schwartzman J. Hyaluronidase: A review of its therapeutic use in pediatrics. J Pediatr 39:491, 1951.

211. Zimmet SE. Hyaluronidase in the prevention of sclerotherapy-induced extravasation necrosis: A dose response study. Dermatol Surg 22:73, 1996.

212. Heckler FR, McCraw JB. Calcium-related cutaneous necrosis. Plast Surg 27:553, 1976.

213. Brown AS, Hoelzer DJ, Piercy SA. Skin necrosis from extravasation of intravenous fluids in children. Plast Reconstr Surg 64:145, 1979.

214. Adams JG Jr, et al. Effect of pentoxifylline on tissue injury and platelet-activating factor production during ischemia-reperfusion injury. J Vasc Surg 21:742, 1995.

215. Ehrly AM. The effect of pentoxifylline on the flow properties of human blood. Curr Med Res Opin 5:608, 1978.

216. Kobaladze SG, Schonia GS. Pentoxifylline and some physiochemical aspects of hemorrheology in patients with ischemic heart disease. Curr Med Res Opin 6(Suppl 4):5, 1979.

217. Weithmann KU. The influence of pentoxifylline on interactions between blood vessel wall and platelets. IRCS Med Sci 8:293, 1980.

218. Beall GN, Casaburi R, Singer A. Anaphylaxis—Everyone's problem (Specialty Conference). West J Med 144:329, 1986.

219. Wasserman SI. Anaphylaxis. In Middleton E, Reed CE, Ellis EF, eds. Allergy: Principles and Practice, 2nd ed. St. Louis: Mosby, 1983.

220. Shelley J. Allergic manifestations with injection treatment of varicose veins: Death following injection of monoethanolamine oleate. JAMA 112:1792, 1939.

221. Schmier AA. Clinical comparison of sclerosing solutions in injection treatment of varicose veins. Am J Surg 36:389, 1937.

222. Zimmerman LM. Allergic-like reactions from sodium morrhuate in obliteration of varicose veins. JAMA 102:1216, 1934.

223. Meyer NE. Monoethanolamine oleate: A new chemical for obliteration of varicose veins. Am J Surg 40:628, 1938.

224. Lewis KM. Anaphylaxis due to sodium morrhuate. JAMA 107:1298, 1936.

225. Dick ET. The treatment of varicose veins. N Z Med J 65:310, 1966.

226. Sarin SK, Kumar A. Sclerosants for variceal sclerotherapy: A critical appraisal. Am J Gastroenterol 85:641, 1990.

227. Monroe P, et al. Acute respiratory failure after sodium morrhuate esophageal sclerotherapy. Gastroenterology 85:693, 1983.

228. Dale ML. Reaction due to injection of sodium morrhuate. JAMA 108:718, 1937.

229. Ritchie A. The treatment of varicose veins during pregnancy. Edinburgh Med J 40:157, 1933.

230. Probstein JG. Major complications of intravenous therapy of varicose veins. J Missouri Med Assoc 33:349, 1936.

231. Dodd H, Oldham JB. Surgical treatment of varicose veins. Lancet 1:8, 1940.

232. de Lorimier AA. Sclerotherapy for venous malformations. J Pediatr Surg 30:188, 1995.

233. Kilby A, et al. Abnormal chest roentgenograms following endoscopic injection sclerosis of esophageal varices. Hepatology 2:709, 1982.

234. Perakos PG, Cirbus JJ, Camara S. Persistent bradyarrhythmia after sclerotherapy for esophageal varices. South Med J 77:531, 1984.

235. Biegeleisen HI. Fatty acid solutions for the injection treatment of varicose veins: Evaluation of four new solutions. Ann Surg 105:610, 1937.

236. Hedberg SE, Fowler DL, Ryan LR. Injection sclerotherapy of esophageal varices using ethanolamine oleate: A pilot study. Am J Surg 143:426, 1982.

237. Hughes RW Jr, et al. Endoscopic variceal sclerosis: A one-year experience. Gastrointest Endosc 28:62, 1982.

238. Foote RR. Severe reaction to monoethanolamine oleate. Lancet 2:390-391, 1942.

239. Reid RG, Rothine NG. Treatment of varicose veins by compression sclerotherapy. Br J Surg 55:889, 1968.

240. Harris OD, Dickey JD, Stephenson PM. Simple endoscopic injection sclerotherapy of esophageal varices. Aust N Z J Med 12:131, 1982.

241. Shubik P, Hartwell JL. Survey of compounds which have been tested for carcinogenic activity. Washington, D.C.: US Department of Health, Education, and Welfare, Public Health Service, 1969.

242. Goldman MP, Bennett RG. Treatment of telangiectasia: A review. J Am Acad Dermatol 17:167, 1987.

243. Steinberg MH. Evaluation of Sotradecol in sclerotherapy of varicose veins. Angiology 6:519, 1955.

244. Nabatoff RA. Recent trends in the diagnosis and treatment of varicose veins. Surg Gynecol Obstet 90:521, 1950.

245. Fegan G. Varicose Veins: Compression Sclerotherapy. Oxford: Heinemann Medical, 1967.

246. Wallois P. Incidents et accidents au cours du traitement sclérosant des varices et leur prévention. Phlebologie 24:217, 1971.

247. Mantse L. A mild sclerosing agent for telangiectasias. J Dermatol Surg Oncol 11:855, 1985.

248. Mantse L. The treatment of varicose veins with compression sclerotherapy: Technique, contra-indications, complications. Am J Cosmetic Surg 3:47, 1986.

249. Tibbs DJ. Treatment of superficial vein incompetence. Part 2. Compression sclerotherapy. In Tibbs DJ, ed. Varicose Veins and Related Disorders. Oxford: Butterworth-Heinemann, 1992.

250. Clinical Case 1. Presented at the Third Annual Meeting of the North American Society of Phlebology. Phoenix, Ariz., Feb. 21, 1990.

251. Mubarak SJ, et al. Acute compartment syndromes: Diagnosis and treatment with the aid of the wick catheter. J Bone Joint Surg 60A:1091, 178.

252. Fronek H, Fronek A, Saltzbarg G. Allergic reactions to Sotradecol. J Dermatol Surg Oncol 15:684, 1989.

253. Passas H. One case of tetradecyl-sodium sulfate allergy with general symptoms. Soc Fran Phlebol 25:19, 1972.

254. Shick LA, Laing K. Possible allergic reaction to agent used in sclerotherapy. Clin Cases Dermatol 4:2, 1992.

255. Schneider W. Contribution à l'historique du traitement sclérosant des varices et à son étude anatomo-pathologique. Soc Fran Phlebol 18:117, 1965.

256. Dingwall JA, Lin W, Lyon JA. The use of sodium tetradecyl sulfate in the sclerosing treatments of varicose veins. Surgery 23:599, 1948.

257. Reiner L. The activity of anionic surface active compounds in producing vascular obliteration. Proc Soc Exp Biol Med 62:49, 1946.

258. Amblard P. Our experience with Aethoxysklerol. Phlebologie 30:213, 1977.

259. Hartel S. Complications and side effects of sclerotherapy. Zarztl Furtbild (Jena) 78:331, 1984.

260. Heberova V. Treatment of telangiectasias of the lower extremities by sclerotization: Results and evaluation. Cesk Dermatol 51:232, 1976.

261. Eichenberger H. Results of phlebosclerosation with hydroxypolyethoxydodecane. Zentralbl Phlebol 8:181, 1969.

262. Jacobesen BH. Aethoxysklerol: A new sclerosing agent for varicose veins. Ugeskr Laeger 136:532, 1974.

263. Feuerstein W. Anaphylactic reaction to hydroxypolyaethoxydodecon. Vasa 2:292, 1973.

264. Ouvry P, Chandet A, Guillerot E. First impressions of Aethoxysklerol. Phlebologie 31:75, 1978.

265. Stricker BHC, et al. Anafylaxie na gebruik van polidocanol. Ned Tijdschr Geneeskd 135:240, 1990.

266. Tombari G, et al. Sclerotherapy of varices: Complications and their treatment. In Raymond-Martimbeau P, Prescott R, Zummo M, eds. Phebologie '92. Paris: John Libbey Eurotext, 1992.

267. Feied CF, Jackson JJ. Allergic reactions to polidocanol for vein sclerosis: Two case reports. J Dermatol Surg Oncol 20:466, 1994.

268. Thies E, Lange V, Iven H. Cardiac effects of polidocanol, a sclerotherapeutic drug—Experimental evaluations. Chir Forum 192:313, 1982.

269. Imperiali G, et al. Heart failure as a side effect of polidocanol given for esophageal variceal sclerosis. Endoscopy 18:207, 1986.

270. Paterlini A, et al. Heart failure and endoscopic sclerotherapy of variceal bleeding. Lancet 2:1241, 1984.

271. Siems KJ, Soehring K. Die Ausschaltung sensibler Nerven duren peridurale und paravertebrale Injektion von Alkylpolyathylenoxydathern bei Meerschweinchen. Arzneimittelforschung 2:109, 1952.

272. Soehring K, et al. Beiträge zur Pharmakologie der Alkylpolyathylenoxyd-derivate. I. Untersuchungen über die acute und subchronische Toxizität bei verschiedenen Tierarten. Arch Int Pharmacodyn Ther 87:301, 1951.

273. Soehring K, Frahm M. Studies on the pharmacology of alkylpolyethyleneoxide derivatives. Arzneimittelforschung 5:655, 1955.

274. Fournier PE. Expertise tératologique du produit Aethoxysklerol. 1970 (unpublished).

275. Forschungsbericht Chem Fabrik Kreussler & Co. Untersuchung zur Placentagängigkeit von 14C-Polidocanol an Ratten I und II. Battelle Institut. Marz und Juli 1986 (unpublished).

276. Sigg K. Varizen, Ulcus cruris und Thrombose. S 107-18, 4.Aufl. Berlin: Springer-Verlag, 1976.

277. Nguyen VB. Sclérotherapie des varices des membres inférieurs: Étude de 522 cas. Le Saguency Med 23:134, 1976.

278. Ouvry P, Arlaud R. Le traitement sclérosant des telangiectasies des membres inférieurs. Phlebologie 32:365, 1979.

279. Ouvry P, Davy A. Le traitement sclérosant des telangiectasies des membres inférieurs. Phlebologie 35:349, 1982.

280. Jager H, Pelloni E. Tests epicutanes aux bichromates, positifs dans l'eczéma au ciment. Dermatologica 100:207, 1950.

281. Polak L, Turk JL, Frey JR. Studies on contact hypersensitivity to chromium compounds. Prog Allergy 17:145, 1973.

282. Ramalet AA, Ruffieux C, Poffet D. Complications après sclérose à la glycérine chromée. Phlebologie 48:337, 1995.

283. Wallois P. Incidents et accidents de la sclérose. In Tournay R, ed. La Sclérose des Varices, 4th ed. Paris: Expansion Scientifique Française, 1985.

284. Zimmet SE. Letter to the editor. J Dermatol Surg Oncol 16:1063, 1990.

285. Sigg K, Horodegen K, Bernbach H. Varizen-Sklerosierung: Welches ist das wir Usamste Mittel? Dtsch Arzteblatt 34/35:2294, 1986.

286. Sigg K, Zelikovski A. Kann die Sklerosierungotherapie der Varizen ohne Operation in jedem Fallwirksam sein? Phlebol Proktol 4:42, 1975.

287. Wenner L. Anwendung einer mit Athylalkahol modifizierten Polijodidjonenlosung bei sklerose-resistenten Varizen. Vasa 12:190, 1983.

288. Dodd H. The operation for varicose veins. BMJ 2:510, 1945.

289. Anticoagulants. In Bennett R, ed. AMA Drug Evaluations, 5th ed. Chicago: American Medical Association, 1983.

290. Zinn WJ. Side reactions of heparin in clinical practice. Am Cardiol 14:36, 1964.

291. Gervin AS. Complications of heparin therapy. Surg Gynecol Obstet 140:789, 1975.

292. White PW, Sadd JR, Nensel RE. Thrombotic complications of heparin therapy, including six cases of heparin-induced skin necrosis. Ann Surg 190:595, 1979.

293. Dukes MNG, ed. Meyler's Side Effects of Drugs: An Encyclopaedia of Adverse Reactions and Interactions, 9th ed. Amsterdam: Excerpta Medica, 1980.

294. O'Toole RD. Heparin: Adverse reaction. Ann Intern Med 79:759, 1973.

295. Hume M, Smith-Petersen M, Fremont-Smith P. Sensitivity to intrafat heparin. Lancet 1:261, 1974.

296. Hall JC, McConahay D, Gibson D. Heparin necrosis: An anticoagulation syndrome. JAMA 244:1831, 1980.

297. Shelley WB, Ayen JJ. Heparin necrosis: An anticoagulant-induced cutaneous infarct. J Am Acad Dermatol 7:674, 1982.

298. Tuneu A, Moreno A, de Moragas JM. Cutaneous reactions secondary to heparin injections. J Am Acad Dermatol 12:1072, 1985.

299. DeShago RD, Nelson HS. An approach to the patient with a history of local anesthesia hypersensitivity: Experience with 90 patients. J Allergy Clin Immunol 63:387, 1979.

300. Wasserfallen J-B, Frei PC. Long-term evaluation of usefulness of skin and incremental challenge tests in patients with history of adverse reaction to local anesthetics. Allergy 50:162, 1995.

301. de Jong RH. Local Anesthetics, 2nd ed. Springfield, Ill.: Charles C Thomas, 1977.

302. Swanson JG. Assessment of allergy to local anesthetic. Ann Emerg Med 12:316, 1983.

303. de Jong RH. Toxic effects of local anesthetics. JAMA 239:1166, 1978.

304. Incaudo G, et al. Administration of local anesthesia to patients with a history of adverse reaction. J Allergy Clin Immunol 61:339, 1978.

305. Thomas RM. Local anesthetic agents and regional anesthesia of the face. J Assoc Military Dermatol 8:28, 1982.

306. Fregert S, Tegner E, Thelin I. Contact allergy to lidocaine. Contact Dermatitis 5:185, 1979.

307. Covino BG, Vassallo HG. Local Anesthetics: Mechanisms of Action and Clinical Use. New York: Grune & Stratton, 1976.

308. Eriksson E. Illustrated Handbook of Local Anesthesia, 2nd ed. Philadelphia: WB Saunders, 1980.

309. Baker JD, Blackmon BB. Local anesthesia. Clin Plast Surg 12:25, 1985.

310. Kennedy KS, Cave RH. Anaphylactic reaction to lidocaine. Arch Otolaryngol Head Neck Surg 112:671, 1986.

311. Promisloff RA, Dupont D. Death from ARDS and cardiovascular collapse following lidocaine administration. Chest 83:585, 1983.

312. Aldrete JA. Sensitivity to lidocaine. Anesth Intensive Care 7:73, 1979.

313. Gill C, Michaelides PL. Dental drugs and anaphylactic reactions: Report of a case. Oral Surg 50:30, 1980.

314. Chin TM, Fellner MJ. Allergic hypersensitivity to lidocaine hydrochloride. Int J Dermatol 19:147, 1980.

315. Ravindranathan N. Allergic reaction to lidocaine: A case report. Br Dent J 111:101, 1975.

316. Lehner T. Lidocaine hypersensitivity. Lancet 1:1245, 1971.

317. Fischer MM, Pennington JC. Allergy to local anaesthesia. Br J Anaesth 54:893, 1982.

318. Garber N. A criticism of present-day methods in the treatment of varicose veins. S Afr Med J 21:338, 1947.

319. Ogilvie WH. Some applications of the surgical lessons of war to civil practice. BMJ 1:619, 1945.

320. Fegan WG. The complications of compression sclerotherapy. Practitioner 207:797, 1971.

321. Sigg K. The treatment of varicosities and accompanying complications. Angiology 3:355, 1952.

322. Plate G, et al. Deep vein thrombosis, pulmonary embolism and acute surgery in thrombophlebitis of the long saphenous vein. Acta Chir Scand 151:241, 1985.

323. Gjores JE. Surgical therapy of ascending thrombophlebitis in the saphenous system. Angiology 13:241, 1962.

324. Bergqvist D, Lindblad B. A 30-year survey of pulmonary embolism verified at autopsy: An analysis of 1274 surgical patients. Br J Surg 72:105, 1985.

325. Bergqvist D, Jaroszewski H. Deep vein thrombosis in patients with superficial thrombophlebitis of the leg. BMJ 292:658, 1986.

326. Galloway JMD, Karmody AM, Mavor GE. Thrombophlebitis of the long saphenous vein complicated by pulmonary embolism. Br J Surg 56:360, 1969.

327. Bendick PJ, et al. Clinical significance of superficial thrombophlebitis. J Vasc Technol 19:57, 1995.

328. Sacer E, et al. Preliminary results of a nonoperative approach to saphenofemoral junction thrombophlebitis. J Vasc Surg 22:616, 1995.

329. Chengelis DL, et al. Progression of superficial venous thrombosis to deep vein thrombosis. J Vasc Surg 24:745, 1996.

330. From our legal correspondent: Hazards of compression sclerotherapy. BMJ 3:714, 1975.

331. Goldstein M. Les complications de la sclérotherapie. Phlebologie 32:221, 1979.

332. Oesch A, Stirnemann P, Mahler F. Das akute Ischämiesyndrom des Fusses nach Varizenverödung. Schweiz Med Wochenschr 114:1155, 1984.

333. MacGowan WAL. Sclerotherapy: Prevention of accidents. A review. J Roy Soc Med 78:136, 1985.

334. Cockett FB. Arterial complications during surgery and sclerotherapy of varicose veins. Phlebology 1:3, 1986.

335. Biegeleisen K, Neilsen RD, O'Shaughnessy A. Inadvertent intra-arterial injection complicating ordinary and ultrasound-guided sclerotherapy. J Dermatol Surg Oncol 19:953, 1993.

336. Natali J, Maraval M, Carrance F. Recent statistics on complications of sclerotherapy. Presented at the Annual Meeting of the North American Society of Phlebology. Maui, Hawaii, Feb. 21, 1994.

337. MacGowan WAL, et al. The local effects of intra-arterial injections of sodium tetradecyl sulphate (STD) 3%. Br J Surg 59:101, 1972.

338. Staubesand J, Seydewitz V. Ultrastructural changes following perivascular and intra-arterial injection of sclerosing agents: An experimental contribution to the problem of iatrogenic damage. Phlebologie 20:1, 1991.

339. Matsen FA, et al. A model compartmental syndrome in man with particular reference to the quantification of nerve function. J Bone Joint Surg 59A:648, 1977.

340. Orbach J. A new look at sclerotherapy. Folia Angiologia 25:181, 1977.

341. Natali J, Farman T. Implications medico-legales au cours du traitement sclérosant des varices. J Mal Vasc 21:227, 1996.

342. Benhamou AC, Natali J. Les accidents des traitements sclérosant et chirurgical des varices des membres inférieurs: A propos de 90 cas. Phlebologie 34:41, 1981.

343. Somer-Leroy R de, Wang A, Ouvry P. Echographie du creux poplité recherche d'une artériole petite saphène avant sclérotherapie. Phlebologie 44:69, 1991.

344. Sternbergh WC, Sobel M, Makhoul RG. Heparinoids with low anticoagulant potency attenuate postischemic endothelial cell dysfunction. J Vasc Surg 21:477, 1995.

345. Sternbergh WC III, Makhoul RG, Adelman B. Heparin prevents postischemic endothelial cell dysfunction by a mechanism independent of its anticoagulant activity. J Vasc Surg 17:318, 1993.

346. Lantz M, et al. On the binding of tumor necrosis factor (TNF) to heparin and the release in vivo of the TNF-binding protein I by heparin. J Clin Invest 88:2026, 1991.

347. Bounumeaux H, et al. Severe ischemia of the hand following intra-arterial promazine injection: Effects of vasodilatation, anticoagulation, and local thrombolysis with tissue type plasminogen activator. Vasa 19:68, 1990.

348. Feied CF. Deep vein thrombosis: The risks of sclerotherapy in hypercoagulable states. Semin Dermatol 12:135, 1993.

349. Kistner RL. Incidence of pulmonary embolism in the course of thrombophlebitis of the lower extremities. Am J Surg 124:169, 1972.

350. Coon WW. Venous thromboembolism—Prevalence: Risk factors and prevention. Clin Chest Med 5:391, 1984.

351. Dalen JE, Alpert JS. Natural history of pulmonary embolism. Prog Cardiovasc Dis 17:259, 1975.

352. Kakkar VV, et al. Deep vein thrombosis of the leg: Is there a high-risk group? Am J Surg 120:527, 1970.

353. Evans DS, Cockett FB. Diagnosis of deep-vein thrombosis with ultrasonic Doppler technique. Br J Med 28:802, 1969.

354. Milne RM, et al. Postoperative deep venous thrombosis. A comparison of diagnostic techniques. Lancet 2:445, 1971.

355. Burrow M, Goldson H. Postoperative venous thrombosis. Evaluation of five methods of treatment. Am J Surg 141:245, 1981.

356. Smith L, Johnson MA. Incidence of pulmonary embolism after venous sclerosing therapy. Minn Med 31:270, 1948.

357. Natali J, Marmasse J. Enquête sur le traitement chirurgical des varices. Phlebologie 15:232, 1962.

358. Barber THT. Modern treatment of varicose veins. BMJ 1:219, 1930.

359. Kern MM, Angle LW. The chemical obliteration of varicose veins: A clinical and experimental study. JAMA 93:595, 1929.

360. Linser P, Vohwinkel H. Moderne Therapie der Varizen, Hämorrhoiden und Varicocele. Stuttgart: Ferdinand Enke, 1942.

361. Sigg K. Zur Behandlung der Varicen der Phlebitis und ihrer Komplikationen. Hautarzt 1-2:443, 1950.

362. Marmasse J. Enquête sur les embolies pulmonaires au cours du traitement sclérosant. Phlebologie 22:255-257, 1969.

363. Stevenson IM, Seddon JA, Parry EW. The occurrence of deep venous thrombosis following compression sclerotherapy. Angiology 27:311, 1976.

364. Williams RA, Wilson SE. Sclerosant treatment of varicose veins and deep vein thrombosis. Arch Surg 119:1283, 1984.

365. Van Der Molen HR. Le risque de thrombose profonde lors des injections intra-variqueuses pourquoi est-il quasi inexistant? Phlebologie 42:137, 1989.

366. Cepelak V. Effect of sclerosing agents on platelet aggregation. Folia Angiologia 30-31:363, 1982.

367. Zelikowski A, et al. Compression sclerotherapy of varicose veins. A few observations and some practical suggestions. Folia Angiologia 26:61, 1978.

368. Van del Plas JPL, et al. Reversible ischemic neurological deficit after sclerotherapy of varicose veins. Lancet 343:428, 1994.

369. Dral E, et al. Sclérose de varices des membres inférieurs responsable d'un accident ischemique cérébral. La Presse Médicale 23:182, 1994.

370. Lechat P, et al. Prevalence of patent foramen ovale in patients with stroke. N Engl J Med 318:1148, 1988.

371. Virchow R. Cellular Pathology as Based on Physiological and Pathological Histology. London: Churchill Livingstone, 1860.

372. Schneider W, Fischer H. Fixierung und bindegewebige Organisation artifizieller Thromben bei der Varizenverödung. Dtsch Med Wochenschr 89:2410, 1964.

373. Atlas LN. Hazards connected with the treatment of varicose veins. Surg Gynecol Obstet 77:136, 1943.

374. Bohler-Sommeregger K, et al. Do telangiectases communicate with the deep venous system? J Dermatol Surg Oncol 18:403, 1992.

375. McPheeters HO, Rice CO. Varicose veins—The circulation and direction of venous flow. Surg Gynecol Obstet 49:29, 1929.

376. Muller JHA, Petter O, Kostler H. Kinematographische Untersuchungen bei der Varizenverödungstherapie. Z Arztl Fortbild (Jena) 78:345, 1984.

377. Moser KM, et al. Frequent asymptomatic pulmonary embolism in patients with deep venous thrombosis. JAMA 271:223, 1994.

378. D'Addato M. Gangrene of a limb with complete thrombosis of the venous system. J Cardiovasc Surg 7:434, 1966.

379. Goor W, Leu HJ, Mahler F. Thrombosen in tiefen Venen und in Arterien nach Varizensklerosierung. Vasa 16:124, 1987.

380. Askar O, Abullah S. The veins of the foot. J Cardiovasc Surg 16:53, 1975.

381. Tretbar LL, Pattisson PH. Injection-compression treatment of varicose veins. Am J Surg 120:539, 1970.

382. Thomas JH. Pathogenesis, diagnosis and treatment of thrombosis. Am J Surg 160:547, 1990.

383. Samlaska CP, James WD. Superficial thrombophlebitis. II. Secondary hypercoagulable states. J Am Acad Dermatol 23:1, 1990.

384. Schafer AI. The hypercoagulable states. Ann Intern Med 102:814, 1985.

385. Kaplan NM. Cardiovascular complications of oral contraceptives. Ann Rev Med 29:31, 1978.

386. Durand JL, Bressler R. Clinical pharmacology of the steroidal oral contraceptives. Adv Intern Med 24:97, 1979.

387. Stooley PD, et al. Thrombosis with low-estrogen oral contraceptives. Am J Epidemiol 102:197, 1975.

388. Vessey M, et al. Oral contraceptives and venous thromboembolism: Findings in a large prospective study. Br J Med 292:526, 1986.

389. Helmrich SP, et al. Venous thromboembolism in relation to oral contraceptive use. Obstet Gynecol 69:91, 1987.

390. Robison GE, et al. Changes in haemostasis after stopping the combined contraceptive pill: Implications for major surgery. BMJ 302:269, 1991.

391. Seigel DG. Pregnancy, the puerperium and the steroid contraceptive. Milbank Mem Fund Q 50(Suppl 2):15, 1972.

392. Boston collaborative drug surveillance program: Oral contraceptives and venous thromboembolic disease, surgically confirmed gallbladder disease, and breast tumours. Lancet 1:1439, 1973.

393. Quinn DA, et al. A prospective investigation of pulmonary embolism in women and men. JAMA 29:1689, 1992.

394. Realini JP, Goldzieher JW. Oral contraceptives and cardiovascular disease: A critique of the epidemiologic studies. Am J Obstet Gynecol 152:729, 1985.

395. Mashchak CA, et al. Comparison of pharmacodynamic properties of various estrogen formulations. Am J Obstet Gynecol 144:511, 1982.

396. Grady D, Hulley SB, Furberg C. Venous thromboembolic events associated with hormone replacement therapy. JAMA 278:477, 1997.

397. Stadel BV. Oral contraceptives and cardiovascular disease. N Engl J Med 305:612, 1981.

398. Alkjaersig N, Fletcher A, Burstein R. Association between oral contraceptive use and thromboembolism: A new approach to its investigation based on plasma fibrinogen chromatography. Am J Obstet Gynecol 122:199, 1975.

399. Siegbahn A, Ruusuvaara L. Age dependence of blood fibrinolytic components and the effects of low-dose oral contraceptives on coagulation and fibrinolysis in teenagers. Thromb Haemost 60:301, 1988.

400. Srinivasan S, et al. The alteration of surface charge characteristics of the vascular system by oral contraceptive steroids. Contraception 9:291, 1974.

401. Oski FA, Lubin B, Buchert ED. Reduced red cell filterability with oral contraceptive agents. Ann Intern Med 77:417, 1972.

402. Aronson HB, Magora F, Schenker JG. Effect of oral contraceptives on blood viscosity. Am J Obstet Gynecol 110:997, 1971.

403. Dreyer NA, Pizzo SV. Blood coagulation and idiopathic thromboembolism among fertile women. Contraception 22:123, 1980.

404. Sagar S, et al. Oral contraceptives, antithrombin-III activity, and postoperative deep-vein thrombosis. Lancet 1:509, 1976.

405. von Kaulla E, von Kaulla KN. Oral contraceptives and low antithrombin-III activity. Lancet 1:36, 1970.

406. Pizzo SV. Venous thrombosis. In Koepke JA, ed. Laboratory Hematology, vol 2. New York: Churchill Livingstone, 1984.

407. Miller KE, Pizzo SV. Venous and arterial thromboembolic disease in women using oral contraceptives. Am J Obstet Gynecol 144:824, 1982.

408. Astedt B, et al. Thrombosis and oral contraceptives: Possible predisposition. BMJ 4:631, 1973.

409. Judd HL, et al. Estrogen replacement therapy: Indications and complications. Ann Intern Med 98:195, 1983.

410. Goodrich SM, Wood JE. Peripheral venous distensibility and velocity of venous blood flow during pregnancy or during oral contraceptive therapy. Am J Obstet Gynecol 90:740, 1964.

411. McCaldeb TA. The inhibitory action of oestradiol-17-B and progesterone on venous smooth muscle. Br J Pharmacol 53:183, 1975.

412. Alkjaersig N, et al. Blood coagulation in postmenopausal women given estrogen treatment: Comparison of transdermal and oral administration. J Lab Clin Med 111:224, 1988.

413. Lipton A, Harvey HA, Hamilton RW. Venous thrombosis as a side effect of tamoxifen treatment. Cancer Treat Rev 68:887, 1984.

414. Fisher B, et al. A randomized clinical trial evaluating tamoxifen in the treatment of patients with node-negative breast cancer who have estrogen-receptor-positive tumors. N Engl J Med 320:479, 1989.

415. Jordan VC, Fritz NF, Tormey DC. Long-term adjuvant therapy with tamoxifen: Effects on sex hormone binding globulin and antithrombin III. Cancer Res 47:4517, 1987.

416. Love RR, Surawicz TS, Williams EC. Antithrombin III level, fibrinogen level, and platelet count changes with adjuvant tamoxifen therapy. Arch Intern Med 152:317, 1992.

417. Auger MJ, Mackie MJ. Effects of tamoxifen on blood coagulation. Cancer 61:1316, 1988.

418. Bertelli G, et al. Adjuvant tamoxifen in primary breast cancer: Influence on plasma lipids and antithrombin III levels. Breast Cancer Res Treat 12:307, 1988.

419. Paré A. Cited by Ritchie A. Edinburgh Med J 157, 1933.

420. Hamilton HG, Pittam RF, Higgins RS. Active therapy of varicose veins in pregnancy. South Med J 42:608, 1949.

421. Finley BE. Acute coagulopathy in pregnancy. Med Clin North Am 73:723, 1989.

422. Aaro LA, Johnson TR, Juergens JL. Acute deep venous thrombosis associated with pregnancy. Obstet Gynecol 28:553, 1966.

423. Beller FK. Thromboembolic disease in pregnancy. In Anderson A, ed. Thromboembolic Disorders. New York: Harper & Row, 1968.

424. Bonnar J. Hemostatic function and coagulopathy during pregnancy. Obstet Gynecol Annu 7: 195, 1978.

425. Bonnar J, McNicol GP, Douglas AS. Fibrinolytic enzyme system and pregnancy. BMJ 3:387, 1969.

426. Comp PC, et al. Functional and immunologic protein levels are decreased during pregnancy. Blood 68:881, 1986.

427. Miletich J, Sherman L, Broze G Jr. Absence of thrombosis in patients with heterozygous protein C deficiency. N Engl J Med 317:991, 1987.

428. Engesser L, et al. Hereditary protein S deficiency: Clinical manifestations. Ann Intern Med 106:677, 1987.

429. Rick ME. Protein C and protein S: Vitamin K–dependent inhibitors of blood coagulation. JAMA 263:701, 1990.

430. Bauer KA. Pathobiology of the hypercoagulable state: Clinical features, laboratory evaluation, and management. In Hoffman R, et al., eds. Hematology: Basic Principles and Clinical Practice. New York: Churchill Livingstone, 1991.

431. Svensson PJ, Dahlback B. Resistance to activated protein C as a basis for venous thrombosis. N Engl J Med 330:517, 1994.

432. Peus D, Heit JA, Pittelkow MR. Activated protein C resistance caused by factor V gene mutation: Common coagulation defect in chronic venous leg ulcers? J Am Acad Dermatol 36:616, 1997.

433. Nichols WI. Activated protein C resistance and thrombosis. Mayo Clin Proc 71:897, 1996.

434. D'Angelo A, et al. Brief report: Autoimmune protein S deficiency in a boy with severe thromboembolic disease. N Engl J Med 328:1753, 1993.

435. Fair DS, Marlar RA, Levin EG. Human endothelial cells synthesize protein S. Blood 67:1168, 1986.

436. Collen D, et al. Metabolism of antithrombin III (heparin cofactor) in man: Effects of venous thrombosis and of heparin administration. Eur J Clin Invest 7:27, 1977.

437. Odegaard OR, Abildgaard U. Antithrombin III: Critical review of assay methods. Significance of variations in health and disease. Haemostasis 7:127, 1978.

438. Towne JB. Hypercoagulable states and unexplained vascular graft thrombosis. In Bernhard VM, Towne JB, eds. Complications in Vascular Surgery. St. Louis: Quality Medical Publishing, 1991.

439. Espinoza LR, Hartmann RC. Significance of the lupus anticoagulant. Am J Haematol 22:331, 1986.

440. Tabechnik-Schor NF, Lipton SA. Association of lupus-like anticoagulant and nonvasculitic cerebral infarction. Arch Neurol 43:851, 1986.

441. Shi W, et al. Prevalence of lupus anticoagulant and anticardiolipin antibodies in a healthy population. Aust N Z J Med 20:231, 1990.

442. Mueh JR, Herbst KD, Rapaport SI. Thrombosis in patients with the lupus anticoagulant. Ann Intern Med 92:156, 1980.

443. Elias M, Eldor A. Thromboembolism in patients with the "lupus" type circulating anticoagulant. Arch Intern Med 144:510, 1984.

444. Kiely PE. A phlebographic study of the soleal sinuses. Angiology 24:230, 1973.

445. Fegan WG. Continuous compression technique of injecting varicose veins. Lancet 2:109, 1963.

446. Foley WT. The eradication of venous blemishes. Cutis 15:665, 1975.

447. Sadick N. Treatment of varicose and telangiectatic leg veins with hypertonic saline: A comparative study of heparin and saline. J Dermatol Surg Oncol 16:24, 1990.

448. Crandon AJ, et al. Postoperative deep vein thrombosis: Identifying high-risk patients. BMJ 281:343, 1980.

449. Sue-Ling HM, et al. Pre-operative identification of patients at high risk of deep vein thrombosis after major abdominal surgery. Lancet 1:1173, 1986.

450. Coon WW. Epidemiology of venous thromboembolism. Ann Surg 186:149, 1977.

451. Schina MJ Jr, et al. Influence of age on venous physiologic parameters. J Vasc Surg 18:749, 1993.

452. McMaster P, Everett WG. Fatal pulmonary embolism following compression sclerotherapy for varicose veins. Postgrad Med J 49:517, 1973.

453. Saarinen J, et al. Late sequelae of acute deep venous thrombosis: Evaluation five and ten years after. Phlebology 10:106, 1995.

454. Matzdorff AC, Green D. Deep vein thrombosis and pulmonary embolism: Prevention, diagnosis and treatment. Geriatrics 47:48, 1992.

455. Hull R, et al. Warfarin sodium versus low-dose heparin in the long-term treatment of venous thrombosis. N Engl J Med 301:855, 1979.

456. Hirsh J. The optimal duration of anticoagulant therapy for venous thrombosis. N Engl J Med 332:1710, 1995.

457. Schulman S, et al. A comparison of six weeks with six months of oral anticoagulant therapy after a first episode of venous thromboembolism. N Engl J Med 332:1661, 1995.

458. Arneson H, Hoseth A. Streptokinase or heparin in the treatment of deep vein thrombosis. Follow-up results of a prospective study. Acta Med Scand 211:65, 1982.

459. Schulman S, Lockner D. Local venous infusion of streptokinase in DVT. Thromb Res 34:213, 1984.

460. Orbach EJ. Sclerotherapy of varicose veins: Utilization of intravenous air block. Am J Surg 66:362, 1944.

461. Orbach EJ. Clinical evaluation of a new technique in the sclerotherapy of varicose veins. J Int Coll Surg 11:396, 1948.

462. Richardson HF, Coles BC, Hall GE. Experimental air embolism. Can Med J 36:584, 1937.

463. Yen D, Robison DL, Tschen J. Multiple tender, erythematous subcutaneous nodules on the lower extremities. Arch Dermatol 129:1331, 1993.

PART FOUR

Complex Problems
Involving Varicose Veins

Chapter 17

Chronic Venous Insufficiency and Its Surgical Care

John J. Bergan

Venous dysfunction has occupied the attention of many great minds. These include Ambroise Paré, John Hunter, Friedrich Trendelenburg, and John Homans. Homans is of particular importance because he tied the development of severe sequelae of venous dysfunction to prior deep venous thrombosis.[1] Therefore the condition of brawny induration, lipodermatosclerosis, medial and lateral ankle hyperpigmentation in gaiter areas, and characteristic "punched-out" ulceration has been referred to as the postphlebitic or postthrombotic state.

Gradually, it has become known that the disability produced by those conditions and the advanced skin changes are not dependent on a prior episode of deep venous thrombosis.[2] This new knowledge has important therapeutic implications. If the advanced condition of venous stasis is referred to as chronic venous insufficiency or, even better, chronic venous dysfunction, it is implied that correction can be obtained through surgical or pharmacologic manipulation. If the term "postphlebitic state" is used, the implication is that there is very little that can be done for the patient or his limb.[3] Amplification and elucidation of the details of this distinction are the subject of this chapter.

CUTANEOUS STIGMATA OF VENOUS DYSFUNCTION

Although elevated distal venous pressure has been linked to venous ulceration, more recent observations relative to lower extremity white blood cell trapping in situations of venous hypertension are more informative.[4] Such white cell trapping is found to be excessive in limbs with lipodermatosclerosis.[5] If leukocytes are activated when they are trapped, it would be expected that proteolytic enzymes would be released and free radical activity would be observed. Such a phenomenon would be the fundamental common pathophysiologic pathway that explains tissue damage in myocardial ischemia, stroke, shock, and other conditions.[6] Leukocyte trapping and subsequent release would also produce a reperfusion phenomenon, the effects of which in limbs, mesentery, and myocardium have already been shown to be due to white cell trapping and activation.[7]

Studies have shown that the predominant infiltrating cells in limbs with lipodermatosclerosis are T lymphocytes and macrophages.[8] However, it is uncertain whether this accumulation of macrophages and T cells is the cause of chronic venous insufficiency or an effect of it. An inflammatory response to tissue damage from any cause would lead to similar findings.

DIAGNOSTIC EVALUATION IN VENOUS DYSFUNCTION

Physical examination reveals the evidence of venous varicosities and, in many instances, of axial reflux through saphenous trunks. Visual examination can be supplemented by noting a downward-going impulse on coughing. Tapping the venous column of blood also demonstrates pressure transmission through the static column to incompetent distal veins.

Also, historically important tests such as the Perthes' test for deep venous occlusion[9] and the Brodie-Trendelenburg tests of axial reflux are heavily quoted.[10,11] These tests have been replaced by in-office use of the continuous-wave hand-held Doppler instrument supplemented by duplex evaluation.[12,13] The hand-held Doppler device can confirm an impression of saphenous reflux, and this finding, in turn, dictates the operative procedure to be performed in a given patient. Through imaging of the superficial and deep veins, duplex ultrasound technology more precisely defines which veins are refluxing. The duplex examination is commonly done with the patient supine, but this position results in an erroneous evaluation of reflux. When the patient is in the supine position, even when there is no flow, the valves remain open. Valve closure requires a reversal of flow with a pressure gradient that is higher proximally than distally.[14] Thus the duplex examination should be done with the patient standing or in the markedly trunk-elevated position.

TECHNIQUE OF EXAMINATION

Gloviczki and his colleagues have provided a succinct description of the patient examination in the *Atlas of Endoscopic Perforator Vein Surgery.* During examination the patient stands in a 60- to 80-degree near-upright position on a tilted examination table with the extremity to be examined abducted and externally rotated and the weight borne by the opposite extremity. A pneumatic cuff connected to an automatic inflator is placed on the calf. The examination is performed with a 5 or 7 MHz linear-array transducer.

To ascertain valvular incompetence, venous flow must be augmented and prolonged retrograde flow must be confirmed during the relaxation phase. Incompetence is confirmed if the duration of retrograde flow exceeds 1 second. Competence of proximal valves can be evaluated using the Valsalva maneuver, but with this technique normal deep vein valves do not close at all levels. Flow can also be augmented manually by compressing the calf or the thigh of the patient distal to the probe. However, an automatic pneumatic cuff placed on the calf is the best technique available and therefore its use is recommended. Compression with the pneumatic cuff is standardized and more reproducible and eliminates variability related to limb size and to the sonographer's technique. With automatic insufflators a cuff pressure of 100 mm Hg can be reached within 0.3 seconds.

The examination begins at the groin with identification of the saphenofemoral junction in the longitudinal plane. A sample volume is then placed in the common femoral vein 2 to 3 cm superior to the saphenofemoral junction. The patient is instructed to perform the Valsalva maneuver, or the flow is augmented by using a pneumatic cuff connected to the automatic inflator. Color duplex images and the Doppler spectrum in the compression and relaxation phases are recorded. Reflux at the common femoral vein level may be a normal variant.

The examination is repeated by placing the sample volume in the greater saphenous vein 2 to 3 cm inferior to the saphenofemoral junction. Competence of the greater saphenous vein is evaluated in the same way as with the common femoral vein. The examination continues caudally with longitudinal imaging of the greater saphenous vein at the level of the midfemur and knee. At midthigh the hunterian and Dodd perforators can be imaged and their valvular competence can be evaluated. The examination is continued, and the patency and competence of the middle and lower superficial femoral vein and the popliteal vein are studied. Valvular incompetence of the tibial veins and the lesser saphenous vein can also be evaluated in a similar manner, although these vessels are not routinely studied in all patients. At each of these venous segments, Doppler sampling is performed as the calf is compressed, augmenting cephalad flow, and then released.

DUPLEX IMAGING OF CALF PERFORATOR VEINS

The medial aspect of the leg is surveyed routinely from the knee to the malleolus. The examination begins near the paired posterior tibial veins at the level of the medial malleolus. B-mode imaging is used to survey the fascia and to identify perforators connecting the posterior arch vein, the greater saphenous vein, or one of its tributaries with posterior tibial veins (Figure 17-1). A spectral tracing within the perforator is obtained during and following augmentation of venous flow above or below the sample site through manual compression. Color duplex scanning is most helpful to confirm bidirectional flow, even in smaller perforators, because color changes indicate reversal of flow. At the site of the perforators the skin is marked with a permanent marker. An X represents incompetence and an O means that the vein is competent and the duration of retrograde flow is less than 0.3 second. In patients with lateral ankle ulcers the examination is continued to identify incompetent lateral calf perforators.

As the two ultrasound modes of direct evaluation of venous function have emerged, other earlier indirect testing methods have been discarded. Although these tests may have utility in specific situations, their clinical importance has been displaced in the evaluation of venous insufficiency (Table 17-1). These methods include photoplethysmography (PPG), light reflection rheography (LRR),

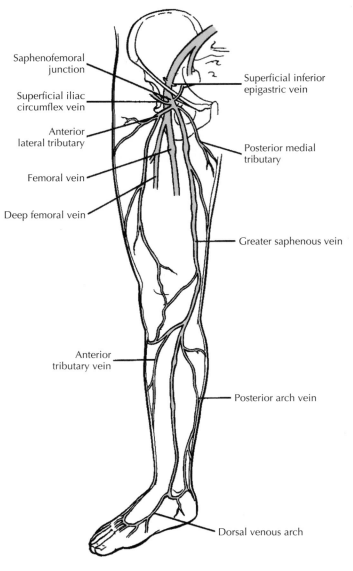

FIGURE 17-1. Duplex scanning examination of the vertical leg must encompass the anatomic landmarks shown here. If saphenofemoral reflux is not present, the saphenous vein may be refluxing throughout its length because of contributions from the major tributaries, which are illustrated. Reflux should be noted at the saphenofemoral and saphenopopliteal junctions and from the perforating veins shown in the medial leg. Perforating veins should be identified and measured from the heel pad or the floor so that they can be accurately identified during surgical maneuvers.

mercury strain-gauge plethysmography (MSG), and newer, but still unproven, air plethysmography (APG).

In deciding on therapy for a limb with chronic venous insufficiency, it is important to know which pathologic process—obstruction or reflux—is dominant. Although reflux is easily detected by physical examination and the hand-held

TABLE 17-1. Methods of assessing venous stasis

Testing Modality	Detects Chronic Obstruction	Detects Reflux	Useful Physiologically	Useful Clinically
Dynamic venous pressure	No	Yes	Yes	No
Photoplethysmography (PPG)	No	Yes	Yes/no	Yes
Light reflection rheography (LLR)	No	Yes	Yes/no	Yes
Air plethysmography (APG)	Yes	Yes	Yes	No
Phlebography, ascending	Yes	No	No	Yes
Phlebography, descending	Yes	Yes	No	Yes
MR phlebography	Yes	No	No	Yes
Continuous-wave Doppler	Yes	Yes	No	Yes
Duplex, supine position	Yes	No	No	No
Duplex, standing position	No	Yes	Yes/no	Yes

Doppler device and confirmed by duplex scanning techniques, functional obstruction is much more difficult to assess. Further, it is important to know whether reflux or obstruction or both of these is present in each major vein segment. The PPG, LLR, MSG, and APG instruments do not provide this information. Only imaging techniques can identify the anatomic location of obstructions. Physiologic venous obstruction is more difficult to ascertain, and no single method emerges that is entirely reliable. At present, imaging techniques include magnetic resonance phlebography, which is totally patient acceptable; radiologic contrast phlebography, which provides anatomic information as well as physiologic venous pressure changes before and after limb exercise; and duplex evaluation, which can identify obstruction. When a surgical decision is made toward reconstruction of major veins by valvoplasty or bypass, phlebography is mandatory. This radiography must be done in both the ascending and descending modes before surgical therapy.[15]

OPTIONS FOR TREATMENT

Physical examination, including history taking and supplemented by noninvasive evaluation, will determine the need for therapy. Options in therapy include a conservative nonoperative approach that employs various techniques of compression therapy, a minimally invasive approach to ablation of abnormally functioning vein segments as achieved by sclerotherapy, and a maximally invasive approach involving removal of malfunctioning veins, perforating vein interruption, and even valvoplasty. Improved understanding of cellular mechanisms in venous disease will make a pharmacologic approach to therapy possible in the future.

Conservative treatment of chronic venous insufficiency always precedes consideration of intervention. Such conservative treatment relies on limb compression to counteract the effects of venous hypertension.[16] This compression is achieved by various forms of gradient elastic support that do not affect intravascular pressure as much as it does interstitial tissue. In order of ascending pressure effects, external compression can be applied as support stockings, gradient elastic supports, long-stretch and short-stretch elastic bandages, gelatin cast boots (Unna boot), and a most recent addition, the semirigid Velcro support (CircAid appliance).

Patients with class 2 or 3 venous insufficiency may derive benefit from simple over-the-counter support stockings.[17] Those with class 4 venous insufficiency will require ankle pressures in the range of 20 to 30 mm Hg, and those with class 5 or 6 venous insufficiency with present or healed ulcerations will require 40 mm Hg ankle pressure. Treatment of stasis ulceration, complicated sepsis, and cellulitis demands more aggressive therapy. This treatment includes bedrest, leg elevation, antibiotics, and surgical wound care.[18] Organism-specific antibiotics tailored to bacteria cultured from the ulcer bed may be used, but tetracycline is thought to have a nonspecific effect on the cytokine activation phenomenon.

Specific drug therapy for venous insufficiency is not available in the United States. However, methylxanthines have a certain attraction. These agents improve red cell deformability and, more important, white cell deformability. They inhibit alterations in the microvasculature induced by interleukin 2 (IL-2). Placebo-controlled trials have suggested a more rapid rate of healing and more complete healing in a shorter time in drug-treated individuals compared to controls given placebo.[19]

In a multi-institutional cooperative study, pentoxifylline, 400 mg, administered three times a day orally was compared to placebo.[20] Complete healing of the ulcers occurred in 28 of 30 limbs in which the patients received the active agent. This result was compared to that of 12 of 42 limbs in patients treated with placebo ($p < 0.01$).

Following ulcer healing, ulcer recurrence is the rule rather than the exception, although Porter's group[18] has reported an exceptional recurrence rate of only 29% at 5 years.

OPERATIVE INTERVENTION

While conservative therapy is being pursued or ulcer healing is being achieved, appropriate diagnostic studies should reveal patterns of venous reflux or segments of venous occlusion so that specific therapy can be prescribed for the individual limb being examined (see box on p. 389). As mentioned earlier, imaging techniques must be used to detect obstruction because maximum venous outflow studies may prove inaccurate because of profuse collateralization. Imaging by duplex scanning will suffice for detection of reflux if the examination is carried out with the individual standing. Such noninvasive imaging may prove to be the only testing necessary beyond the continuous-wave hand-held Doppler instrument if superficial venous ablation is contemplated. If direct venous reconstruction by by-

OPTIONS FOR TREATMENT OF VENOUS STASIS

Compression, support
Unna boot, CircAid
Proximal ligation (with sclerotherapy, phlebectomy)
Proximal stripping (with phlebectomy)
Perforator interruption (superficial, subfascial, subfascial endoscopic)
Valvoplasty (open, external, external and angioscope-assisted)
Bypass of obstruction

pass or valvoplasty techniques is planned, ascending and descending phlebography will be required.

Superficial reflux may be the only abnormality uncovered by diagnostic testing. This is almost always true with simple varicose veins and telangiectasias, but it is also a surprising fact that in advanced chronic venous stasis, superficial reflux may be the only abnormality that will be found.[21] Obviously, correction of this pathophysiologic condition will be an important step toward permanent relief of the chronic venous dysfunction and its cutaneous effects. Using duplex ultrasound technology, Hanrahan et al.[22] found that in 95 extremities with current venous ulceration, 16.8% had only superficial incompetence; another 19% showed superficial incompetence combined with perforator incompetence. Similarly, in a study of 118 limbs, the Middlesex group[23] found that "in just over half of the patients with venous ulceration, the disease was confined to the superficial venous system."

In our own study of 58 limbs with class 3 venous insufficiency, 10 patients (17%) exhibited only superficial reflux, and superficial reflux was a major contributor to the chronic venous dysfunction in another 17 limbs. Our own study of limbs after greater saphenous vein stripping in which superficial femoral and popliteal venous incompetence was present has revealed correction of the deep reflux by superficial venous stripping in a vast majority of limbs.[24]

TREATMENT OF SUPERFICIAL REFLUX

Principles of inversion stripping of the saphenous vein from above to downward are quite simple (Figure 17-2). The upper groin incision is made above the inguinal skin crease. A heavy ligature is used to fix the upper end of the saphenous vein to the intraluminal stripper, which is removed through a wound exiting in a transverse skin line in the medial aspect of the popliteal fossa. In practice the ligature is used to draw into the saphenous tunnel a 10 cm gauze strip that has been soaked in lidocaine 0.5% with added adrenaline (1:1000). If the saphenous vein should be torn during downward stripping, the gauze pack will pick up the torn segment and deliver it into the distal incision. Important middle and distal

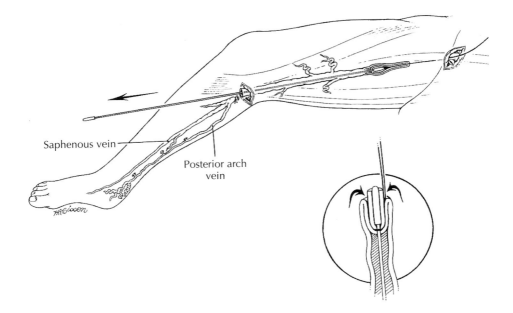

FIGURE 17-2. Groin incision exposes the saphenofemoral junction and the tributaries to the saphenous vein. This incision is placed 1 cm above the inguinal skin crease. The inset shows the technique of inversion of the saphenous vein, but the hemostatic pack is not shown. The same ligature that ties the saphenous vein to the stripper can be used to lead the hemostatic pack into the saphenous vein. This portion of the pack is removed through the distal incision, but the remaining pack acts like a tamponade leading from the disrupted vein's tributary to the saphenous vein. (From Bergan JJ. Ambulatory surgery of varicose veins. In Goldman MP, Bergan JJ. Ambulatory Treatment of Venous Disease: An Illustrative Guide. St. Louis: Mosby, 1995, p 150. Reprinted with permission.)

thigh perforating veins are detached. These maintain the patency of the saphenous vein if only proximal ligation is performed without stripping. The distal incision can be used to remove anterior tributary varicosities or the upper portion of the posterior arch vein and the important anteromedial calf Boyd perforating vein. The location of Cockett perforating veins and their relationship to the posterior arch vein must be noted.

Dealing with perforating veins has been a major concern since the early 1940s. Today, while the exact etiology of venous ulceration is incompletely understood, there is no doubt that chronic venous ulceration is related to venous hypertension. This hypertension in turn is related to venous reflux and, less commonly, to obstruction. Elevated ambulatory venous pressure leads to perimalleolar leukocyte trapping and activation with degradation of surrounding soft tissue. The transmission of high venous pressure toward the skin is facilitated by incompetent perforating calf veins. Failed valves in these veins permit venous blood to flow from the deep to the relatively unsupported superficial venous system. This fact explains the importance of perforator vein interruption to eliminate the pathologic outflow of venous blood toward the skin.

Until the mid-1980s, a number of investigators reported the efficacy of subfascial perforating vein interruption performed through a long, full-leg midcalf or stocking seam incision (Linton operation). For some time this procedure was the most popular operation for very severe chronic venous ulceration, and it led to permanent healing of venous ulcers in 57% to 98% of patients. Yet in recent years there has been little interest in performing the Linton procedure because of associated delayed wound healing, skin necrosis, and wound infections.

SUBFASCIAL ENDOSCOPIC PERFORATOR VEIN SURGERY

We became aware of subfascial endoscopic perforator vein surgery (SEPS) as reports of this procedure emerged after 1985. The appeal of performing this therapeutic procedure without the morbidity of an open operation led us to begin to develop endoscopic perforator vein surgery after 1993. Only patients with open ulcer, healed ulcer, or severe lipodermatosclerosis (stages 6, 5, 4) have been treated. Sixty-seven limbs have been treated by our group in San Diego. Two thirds had open ulcerations, and all patients had been studied by duplex ultrasonography, with phlebography being performed only in the earliest experience. Only 30% had evidence of prior deep venous thrombosis.

The operative procedure was accomplished through a 20 mm midcalf incision with a thigh tourniquet applied to an Esmarch-exsanguinated limb. Approximately 20 cm above the medial malleolus an endoscope was inserted through a fasciotomy incision. Subfascial space was developed with blunt finger dissection and was enlarged with a pendulum motion of the inserted scope. The leg was examined endoscopically distally and then proximally, with particular attention paid to searching for Cockett II and III (12 and 18 cm) perforating veins after an endoscopically monitored incision was made into the deep posterior compartment. The proximal viewing allowed identification of an anteromedial calf Boyd perforating vein. The veins were bluntly mobilized, electrocoagulated, and cut, or, alternatively, perforators were closed with a 5 mm Allport clip (Ethicon Endo-Surgery, Cincinnati, Ohio) before division. A full-limb fasciotomy was performed in patients with thickened fascia, and only subcutaneous and cutaneous closures were employed.

Preoperatively, perforating veins identified by duplex scanning were confirmed at operation. However, additional perforators were identified by the endoscope in nearly every limb. The average number of perforating veins visualized by duplex ultrasound was 1.9. However, the average number of perforating veins obliterated was 3.68. The largest ulcer healed in 90 days, but the mean time to healing was 30.5 days in the remaining limbs. The tendency toward ulcer recurrence manifested by dermatitis or weeping has occurred in limbs with popliteal venous incompetence that persisted following surgery. Preoperative disability scores have decreased in operated limbs. Cellulitis has complicated six procedures, and early subfascial hematoma has occurred in an additional three cases.

Clinical experience suggests that accelerated wound healing is achieved by subfascial perforating vein interruption. Wound complications are significant, but they can be managed on an outpatient basis. This developing experience suggests a broad utility for the procedure in the treatment of patients with severe chronic venous insufficiency.

VENOUS RECONSTRUCTION

Perforator interruption combined with superficial venous ablation has been effective in controlling venous ulceration in 75% to 85% of patients. However, emphasis on failures of this technique has led to a continuing interest in developing techniques of venous reconstruction. A significant breakthrough in direct venous reconstruction was the invention of valvoplasty by Kistner in 1968 and the general recognition of this procedure after 1975.[25] Late evaluation of direct valve reconstruction indicates good to excellent long-term results in more than 80% of the patients.[26]

One cannot overestimate the contributions of Kistner. In addition to valvoplasty, he invented the technique of directing the incompetent venous stream through a competent proximal valve, known as venous segment transfer. After Kistner's developments, surgeons were provided with an armamentarium of procedures that included the venous bypass of Palma,[27] a modification of that procedure using externally supported prosthetic grafts,[28] direct valvoplasty (of Kistner), and venous segment transfer (of Kistner). Further, external valve repair as performed through a number of techniques, including monitoring by endoscopic control, suggests that there will be renewed interest in this form of treatment of venous insufficiency. These procedures preceded by direct, noninvasive visualization of reflux and/or obstruction provide an acceptable therapeutic algorithm for venous stasis disease.

Axillary-to-popliteal autotransplantation of valve-containing venous segments has been of interest since the early observations of Taheri et al.[29] Although excellent results have been reported from some clinics, verification of these results by other groups will require time and effort.

SEPS ANCILLARY PROCEDURES

Sclerotherapy and surgery are no longer considered to be competitive. Detection of axial reflux in the saphenous systems indicates the need for surgical intervention rather than sclerotherapy. Size and location of varicosities and perforating veins also affect this judgment. Small varices, especially those below the knee, where compression therapy is most effective, may suggest treatment by sclerotherapy if saphenous reflux is absent. Large varices, especially those arising in the medial thigh, may dictate treatment by surgery. Perforating veins near the skin lesions of chronic venous insufficiency can be sclerosed, and duplex ultrasound guidance is helpful.

Although reluctance to remove the saphenous vein led to a resurgence of interest in proximal saphenous vein ligation in correction of the gravitational reflux component of venous stasis after 1980, we now know that this is an inferior operation. Repeated comparisons of proximal ligation and stripping of the saphenous vein to the knee continue to show long-term superiority of the latter procedure when used in combination with varicectomy, perforator interruption, or sclerotherapy.[30] Saphenous vein ligation offers the advantage that the patient may return to work or military duty immediately after surgery. In situations in which this factor is requisite, the lesser procedure may be justified.

Thus an exploration of the various options has shown that the one that produces the best long-term results is selective greater saphenous vein stripping to the knee combined with multiple stab avulsions of varices.[31]

Because reflux is the dominant pathologic finding in nearly all cases of venous dysfunction, the first step in surgical treatment is usually directed toward correction of this abnormality. Superficial reflux, rather than deep venous insufficiency, has proven to be an important component of the total problem in more than 50% of legs with the most severe manifestations of chronic venous insufficiency.[32] Therefore removal of the refluxing superficial veins by endoluminal techniques (see next section) is a logical first step in surgical therapy. If this approach is inadequate, surgical venous reconstruction should be considered.

Options in venous reconstruction, which are part of the current armamentarium, include bypass or stenting of physiologically important obstruction, repair or transplantation of venous valves, and redirection of the venous stream through competent proximal valves.[33]

ENDOLUMINAL VENOUS STRIPPING

The technique of saphenous removal (stripping) became endoluminal after Van Der Stricht[34] revived the technique first proposed by Babcock at the turn of the century.[35] In brief, the method includes selection of patients by Doppler or duplex ultrasound to ensure that saphenofemoral reflux is present, introduction of the disposable plastic stripper through an open venotomy in a distal direction after transecting the vein, and ligation of the stump proximally (see Figure 17-2). After the stripper is exposed distally at or just below the knee, a heavy ligature is tied around the vein and the stripper at its proximal end. The vein wall is grasped so that distal traction on the stripper will invert the vein into itself. Further traction allows it to exit through the lower incision. This technique minimizes tissue trauma because the relatively large stripper heads formerly used in saphenous stripping are not used. Thus the procedure accomplishes the objectives and needs of proximal saphenous vein removal and does so, incidentally, in an endovenous fashion.

Although saphenous vein removal has received criticism, it has been tested against the other vein-sparing techniques and remains the best method of preventing persistent distal reflux and recurrent varicosities. Proximal saphenofemoral junction ligation, with or without excision of clusters of varicosities, is the other surgical option. Duplex scanning has determined the natural history of proximal saphenous vein ligation in the treatment of greater saphenous reflux.[36] In 52 of 54 limbs in which actual proximal ligation was achieved, reflux persisted in 24 limbs. Similarly, Rutherford et al.[37] found that 70% of limbs undergoing proximal ligation for venous insufficiency showed persisting reflux, and others[38] have documented a similar experience. Even when the proximal ligation is supplemented by distal sclerotherapy, phlebographically controlled perforator ligation, or even stab avulsion, the results are not as satisfactory as when the same maneuvers are added to removal of the saphenous vein to knee level.[30]

DIRECT VALVE RECONSTRUCTION

Experience with saphenous stripping, varicose vein avulsion, and subfascial perforator vein interruption has uncovered a cohort of patients refractory to these treatments. These are largely patients with true postthrombotic syndrome and severe manifestations of chronic venous insufficiency. Although the vast majority of these patients will have been improved by such manipulations, some will need to be considered for direct valve reconstruction.

Direct valve repair is applicable only to valves with primary reflux, not those of a postthrombotic state. Reconstruction for secondary reflux is virtually impossible because of the serious injury to the valve caused by the previous phlebitis. However, it may be possible to use an adjacent venous segment, such as the deep femoral vein, as an outflow for the diseased superficial femoral vein. This method can be used only when the profunda femoris vein has a competent proximal valve. Another category of possible candidates for venous valvoplasty are limbs that have suffered distal thrombotic disease with destruction of popliteal and distal valves but still have a repairable proximal valve in the superficial femoral vein. Valve repair in this situation yields results that are superior to those obtained by valve transplantation.[26]

Raju,[39] always an innovator, has described a technique for fashioning new valve cusps. He uses a large adjacent tributary vein or perhaps an axillary vein that has been exposed for valve transfer and has been determined unsuitable. Either of these veins yields thin valves that are more supple than those found in a saphenous vein. Raju describes trimming the adventitia and part of the media and injecting the intramural portion of the vein to create semilunar cusps fashioned to fit the recipient vein. He orients the nonintimal surface inward rather than outward. The U-shaped cusps are anchored by three or four strategically placed through-and-through mattress sutures tied outside the vein wall. It is important to emphasize that this technique is experimental.

Although reflux dominates the pathophysiology of chronic venous insufficiency, in fact, obstruction may be present in recalcitrant limbs. The crossover femorofemoral saphenous vein bypasses invented by Palma and used from the 1960s to the present have demonstrated durability and overall patency of approximately 75%.[40] Nevertheless, the procedure yields a long scar on the donor limb and the additional complications of closure of a concomitant arteriovenous fistula. Therefore the advent of catheter-directed thrombolysis and venous stent placement has become a reality. There are sufficient long-term observations of intravenous stents to justify the performance of this procedure when all other approaches have been tried in a patient with chronic venous insufficiency.[41]

REFERENCES

1. Homans J. The late results of femoral thrombophlebitis and their treatment. N Engl J Med 235: 249-253, 1946.
2. Browse NL, Burnand KG. The postphlebitic syndrome: A new look. In Bergan JJ, Yao JST, eds. Venous Problems. Chicago: Year Book Medical Publishers, 1978, pp 395-404.
3. DePalma RG, Bergan JJ. Chronic venous insufficiency. In Dean RH, Yao JST, Brewster DC, eds. Current Diagnosis and Treatment in Vascular Surgery. Norwalk, Conn.: Appleton & Lange, 1995, pp 365-375.
4. Moyses C, Cederholm-Williams SA, Michel C. Haemoconcentration and the accumulation of white cells in the feet during venous stasis. Int J Microcirc Clin Exp 5:311, 1987.
5. Thomas PRS, Nash GP, Dormandy JA. White cell accumulation in the dependent legs of patients with venous hypertension: A possible mechanism for trophic changes in the skin. BMJ 296:1693, 1988.
6. Schmid-Schönbein GW. Granulocyte: Friend or foe? NIPS 3:6, 1988.
7. Scurr JH, Coleridge Smith PD. Pathogenesis of venous ulceration. Phlebology 7(Suppl 1):13-16, 1992.
8. Scott HJ, Coleridge Smith PD, Scurr JH. Histological study of white blood cells and their association with lipodermatosclerosis and venous ulceration. Br J Surg 78:210, 1991.
9. Perthes G. Über die Operation der Unterschenkelvaricen nach Trendelenburg. Dtsch Med Wochenschr 21:253, 1895.
10. Brodie B. Lectures Illustrative of Various Subjects in Pathology and Surgery, vol 12. London: Longmans, Green, 1840.
11. Trendelenburg J. Über die Unterbindung der Vena saphena magna bei Unter-schenkelvaricen. Beitr Klin Chir 91:195, 1891.
12. Hoare MC, Royle JP. Doppler ultrasound detection of saphenofemoral and saphenopopliteal incompetence and operative venography to ensure precise saphenopopliteal ligation. Aust N Z J Surg 54:49-53, 1984.
13. Bergan JJ, Moulton SL, Poppiti R, Beeman S. Patient selection for surgery of varicose veins using venous reflux quantitation. In Veith FJ, ed. Current Critical Problems in Vascular Surgery, vol 4. St. Louis: Quality Medical Publishing, 1992, pp 138-148.
14. van Bemmelen PS, Beach K, Bedford G, Strandness DE Jr. The mechanisms of venous valve closure. Arch Surg 125:617-618, 1990.
15. van Bemmelen PS, Beach K, Bedford G, Strandness DE Jr. Quantitative segmental evaluation of venous valvular reflux with ultrasound scanning. J Vasc Surg 10:425-431, 1989.
16. Bergan JJ. New developments in surgery of the venous system. J Cardiovasc Surg 1:624-631, 1993.
17. Classification of Joint Councils of the American Vascular Societies. J Vasc Surg 21:635-645, 1995.
18. Mayberry JC, Moneta GL, Taylor LM, Porter JM. Nonoperative treatment of venous ulceration. In Bergan JJ, Kistner RL, eds. Atlas of Venous Surgery. Philadelphia: WB Saunders, 1992.
19. Weitgasser H. The use of pentoxifylline (Trental 400) in the treatment of leg ulcers: Results of a double-blind trial. Pharmatherapeutica 3:143, 1983.
20. Barbarino C. Pentoxifylline in the treatment of venous ulcers of the leg. Am Med Res Opin 12: 547, 1992.
21. Lees TH, Lambert D. Patterns of venous reflux in limbs with skin changes associated with chronic venous insufficiency. Br J Surg 80:725, 1993.
22. Hanrahan LM, et al. Distribution of valvular incompetence in patients with venous stasis ulceration. J Vasc Surg 13:805-812, 1991.
23. Shami SK, et al. Venous ulcers and the superficial venous system. J Vasc Surg 17:487-490, 1993.
24. Walsh JC, Bergan JJ, Beeman S, Comer TP. Femoral venous reflux abolished by greater saphenous vein stripping. Ann Vasc Surg 8:566-570, 1994.

25. Kistner RL. Surgical repair of the incompetent femoral vein valve. Arch Surg 110:1336-1342, 1975.

26. Kistner RL. Late results of venous valve repair. In Yao JST, Pearce WL, eds. Long-Term Results of Vascular Surgery. Philadelphia: WB Saunders, 1993, pp 451-466.

27. Palma EC, Esperon R. Vein transplants and grafts in the surgical treatment of the postphlebitic syndrome. J Cardiovasc Surg 1:94-107, 1960.

28. Gruss JD. Zur Modifikation des Femoralisbypass nach May. Vasa 4:59-62, 1975.

29. Taheri SA, Lazar L, Elias S, Marchand P, Heffner R. Surgical treatment of postphlebitic syndrome with vein valve transplant. Am J Surg 144:221-224, 1982.

30. Neglén P, Einarsson E, Eklöf B. The functional long-term value of different types of treatment for saphenous vein incompetence. J Cardiovasc Surg (Torino) 34:295-301, 1993.

31. Sarin S, Scurr JH, Coleridge Smith PD. Assessment of stripping the long saphenous vein in the treatment of primary varicose veins. Br J Surg 79:889-893, 1992.

32. Shami SK, et al. Venous ulcers and the superficial venous system. J Vasc Surg 17:487, 1993.

33. Bergan JJ. Reconstruction of deep veins. In Negus D, ed. Leg Ulcers: A Practical Approach to Management, 2nd ed. London: Butterworth-Heinemann, 1994.

34. Van Der Stricht J. La crossectomie. Quant et pourquoi? Extrait de Phlebologie 39(1):47, 1986.

35. Babcock WW. A new operation for extirpation of varicose veins. N Y Med J 86:1553, 1907.

36. Bergan JJ. Ambulatory surgery of varicose veins. In Goldman MP, Bergan JJ. Ambulatory Treatment of Venous Disease: An Illustrative Guide. St. Louis: Mosby, 1995.

37. Rutherford RB, Sawyer JD, Jones DN. The fate of residual saphenous vein after partial removal or ligation. J Vasc Surg 12:422-428, 1990.

38. McMullin GM, Coleridge Smith PD, Scurr JH. Objective assessment of high ligation without stripping the long saphenous vein. Br J Surg 78:1139-1142, 1991.

39. Raju S, Hardy JD. Technical options in venous valve reconstruction. Am J Surg 173:301-327, 1997.

40. AbuRahma AF, Robinson PA, Boland JP. Clinical, hemodynamic, and anatomic predictors of long-term outcome of lower extremity venovenous bypasses. J Vasc Surg 14:635-644, 1991.

41. Jakob H, Maass D, Schmiedt WAS, Schild H, Oelert H. Treatment of major venous obstruction with an expandable endoluminal spiral prosthesis. J Cardiovasc Surg 30:112-117, 1989.

Chapter 18

Treatment of Varicose Veins Associated With Congenital Vascular Malformations

J. Leonel Villavicencio and Sandra Eifert

Varicose veins in the extremities may be associated with several pathologic entities. The treatment varies considerably, depending on the etiology and severity of the clinical manifestations, the type of varicosities, and the condition of the patient. To treat the problem properly, an accurate diagnosis of the etiology of the varicosities must be made. Varicose veins of the extremities are secondary to one of the following etiologies:

1. Primary, familial, or essential varicose veins appear early in life, sometimes during childhood. Usually, but not always, a strong family history of varicosities is present. Varicose veins may be large and asymptomatic and may involve minimal skin changes. Telangiectasias, venous lakes, and venules are skin blemishes that have a striking familial tendency.

2. Secondary, postthrombotic, or acquired varicose veins appear as sequelae of deep venous thrombosis. The clinical manifestations are usually severe and vary widely, depending on the extent of initial damage to the deep venous system, as well as on the degree of incompetence or obstruction of the main trunks and perforating veins.

3. Congenital malformations of the vascular system, with or without arteriovenous fistulas, often involve other tissues (i.e., muscle, nerves, bone, and skin). Some malformations are predominantly arterial, whereas others are venous, lymphatic, or a combination of the three. Varicosities are either part of the syndrome or may develop as a consequence of arteriovenous shunting.

4. In iatrogenic, or traumatic, arteriovenous fistulas, varicose veins are secondary to venous hypertension. Hemodynamic effects on the vascular system depend on the location, size, and duration of the arteriovenous fistula.

Each type of varicose veins described has a different etiology and requires a specific type of treatment. The etiology must be recognized to establish the appropriate form of therapy.

COMMON CONGENITAL VASCULAR MALFORMATIONS ASSOCIATED WITH VARICOSE VEINS

The presence of varicose veins has been recognized in several congenital malformations of the vascular system. Even though congenital malformations are present in a relatively small percentage of patients attending a vascular clinic, the severity of the clinical manifestations and the magnitude of the problem are challenging. Management of varicose veins associated with congenital malformations of the vascular system requires knowledge of the pathophysiology involved, experience, and common sense.

The most common vascular malformations presenting with varicose veins are the angio-osteo-hypertrophic syndromes such as Klippel-Trenaunay (KTS), Parkes-Weber (PWS), and Maffucci syndromes. Hemangiomas, which are benign tumors of venous predominance, may or may not be present in these syndromes. The presence of hemangiomas usually requires careful assessment of their size, nature, location, and associated symptoms. Management depends on the patient's age, the histologic nature of the lesion, and the severity of the symptoms. Hemangiomas are frequently found in the Maffucci syndrome and less often in PWS or KTS. On occasion, a hemangioma may thrombose spontaneously and as a result produce acute symptoms that require surgical intervention.

The clinical syndrome that was described by Klippel and Trenaunay[1] in 1900 was a congenital vascular malformation with a port-wine stain, varicose veins, and limb hypertrophy occurring in association. Almost 15,000 cases have been reported since 1900, but confusion still exists with regard to nomenclature, cause, and management of this clinical entity.[2] A condition akin to KTS was described by Parkes-Weber[3] in 1907. In 1918 he reported a similar but clinically distinct group of patients with varicose veins, limb hypertrophy, and arteriovenous communications.[4] This report was the first description of the clinical condition subsequently known as Parkes-Weber syndrome.

Although clinically similar, the differences between KTS and PWS are probably a matter of degree. The distinction hinges on the absence of clinically detectable arteriovenous fistulas in KTS, which are present in Parkes-Weber syndrome. The natural history of congenital arteriovenous fistulas and their sequelae highlight their importance in PWS and has made their management the natural focus of treatment. The absence of clinically detectable arteriovenous fistulas in KTS has left the management of this condition without a clear focus. However, recent investigations with radioactive isotopes have allowed the detection of previously subclinical arteriovenous fistulas.[5,6] The finding of arteriovenous fistulas in a small percentage of patients with KTS further blurs the distinction between the two syndromes. As experience with KTS has increased, it has become evident that this condition may be associated with angiomatous involvement of other organ systems, including the eye, gastrointestinal tract, bladder, and external genitalia.[7-10] Dargeon[11] described a child with a bladder hemangioma who also had unilateral lower extremity hypertrophy and a port-wine stain. Kuffer et al.[12] reported the association of visceral angiomas and thrombocytopenia in KTS. Hendry and Vinnicombe[13] reviewed 31 patients with bladder hemangiomas; 10 patients (31%) were younger than 20 years, and two of them had KTS. Of patients with KTS, 3% to 6% suffer from bladder hemangioma.

Involvement of the lymphatic system also is frequently described.[14,15] In addition, KTS has been reported in association with Sturge-Weber syndrome, in which a port-wine stain is present on the upper face and ipsilateral leptomeninges.[16,17] It seems likely that these clinical syndromes may have a common cause and may be regional manifestations of the same genetic disorder.[18]

The cause of KTS is controversial. Servelle[14] stated that the changes seen in this syndrome were the sequelae of obstruction. He based his assumptions on venographic demonstration of venous obstruction. On the other hand, Baskerville et al.[19] reported that most patients had no impairment of venous drainage and suggested that a mesodermal abnormality occurring during fetal development led to the persistence of microscopic arteriovenous fistulas, which resulted in the clinical syndrome. More recently, a theory was advanced suggesting that KTS was the result of either (1) a half chromatid mutation of the zygote before fertilization or (2) an early somatic mutation that allows survival of the cells by mosaicism but produces a lethal gene, preventing its transmission. The sporadic occurrence of KTS, its equal sex incidence, the variations of severity, and the relative rarity of generalized involvement are consistent with this theory. Genetic mutation could account for the spectrum of diseases known as KTS, PWS, and Sturge-Weber syndrome. More recently, investigators have mapped the locus for an autosomal dominant disorder in three generations of a family with manifest venous malformations. The locus was on chromosome 9p. The interferon gene cluster and the putative tumor suppressor genes MTS1 and MTS2 are also included in this region.[20,21]

The surgical management of KTS and PWS has been extensively discussed and is the subject of controversy. In the presence of a severely symptomatic patient with active arteriovenous fistulas, the decision to intervene surgically is less subject to controversy than if the main clinical manifestations are giantism, varicose veins, and sequelae of chronic venous hypertension. Servelle[14] operated on 786 patients with KTS since 1945. He found that elongation of limbs was invariably noted. Varicose veins were present in 36% of the cases, and a cutaneous port-wine stain was present in 32% of these patients. It is interesting that, based on his venographic studies, Servelle demonstrated anomalies of the popliteal vein in 51% of his cases, the superficial femoral vein in 16%, the popliteal and femoral veins in 29%, and the iliac veins in 3%, with inferior vena cava involvement in only 1% of the cases. Servelle considered that deep venous obstruction was the primary cause and that surgery directed to excision of the abnormal superficial varicosities could worsen the condition by increasing the outflow obstruction. Other authors also have cautioned against surgery on this basis.[22,23]

DIAGNOSIS

A thorough diagnosis is necessary for optimal treatment. Diagnosis begins with a careful clinical examination. The clinical diagnosis includes history, inspection, palpation, and auscultation. The length and circumference measurements of the extremities, the extent of the port-wine stain, and the distribution and size of the varicosities must be recorded. Depending on the severity of the malformation, patients may complain of pain, swelling, and symptoms of chronic venous insufficiency including leg ulceration. We have noted considerable variation in the prevalence, extension, and location of the port-wine stain. The stain may occupy the entire length and usually the lateral aspect of one or more limbs, or it may be present only in isolated areas of the extremity (Figure 18-1). A lateral marginal venous collector, which is a remnant of a fetal vein, often can be observed in these patients (Figure 18-2). The affected extremity may be either hypertrophic or hypotrophic. The length discrepancy of the extremities produces scoliosis, which must be recognized and treated in its early stages to prevent severe sequelae.

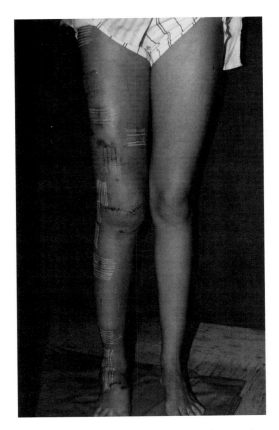

FIGURE 18-1. A 16-year-old girl with Klippel-Trenaunay syndrome shown 1 week after extensive removal of superficial varicose veins, a lateral vein collector, and a large hemangioma over the anterior aspect of the knee. Other hemangiomas present over the dorsum of the foot will require surgery during a second stage. A patent deep venous system was demonstrated through phlebography.

Patients in whom the diagnosis of a venous malformation is suspected must undergo a number of invasive and noninvasive vascular examinations to document the extent and severity of organ involvement in the malformation. Bidirectional Doppler examination is used to assess superficial venous reflux, including reflux into the abnormal marginal vein, as well as perforator incompetence. Strain-gauge plethysmography is used to assess venous outflow and venous capacitance. To evaluate the importance and contribution of the large lateral venous collector in the venous outflow of the extremity, strain-gauge plethysmography readings need to be repeated with compression of the collector shortly before the thigh deflates. A pattern of venous obstruction will be observed after compression if the lateral vein collector plays an important role in the venous outflow. Photoplethysmography measures the venous refilling time and provides information about reflux in the superficial and deep venous systems. Duplex ultrasound scanning and color flow assist in the noninvasive evaluation of the deep venous system and its anomalies. However, the complex nature of the venous circulation, both in the superficial and deep systems of patients with KTS and similar syndromes, often presents a formidable challenge of interpretation.

Both computer tomography (CT) and magnetic resonance imaging (MRI) have been performed selectively to assess the extent and nature of the venous mal-

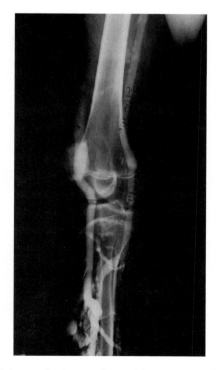

FIGURE 18-2. Ascending phlebography in a patient with a congenital malformation of venous predominance demonstrating a large lateral venous collector with clusters of varicose veins in the lower third of the leg. Excision of all superficial varicosities can be safely performed in one or more stages since there is a patent deep venous system.

formation. Magnetic resonance angiography (MRA) enables the investigator to evaluate the deep and superficial venous channels. MRI and MRA provide us with essential information to determine the prognosis and to select the form of treatment for these malformations. These are useful, noninvasive, easily repeatable diagnostic and screening methods for peripheral and central venous malformations. They have excellent correlation with the conventional invasive angiographic techniques.[24,25]

Often, the noninvasive diagnostic studies provide sufficient information to guide management. However, there are complex malformations in which angiography is essential. Both ascending and descending phlebography, as well as selective varicography, provide essential anatomic and functional information. Varicography aids in localizing the point of drainage of the lateral collector into the deep venous system (Figure 18-3). Due to the large capacity of the superficial venous bed, the deep system may not be well visualized in some malformations such as KTS. In such cases the phlebographic technique requires modification. When poor deep venous filling is observed despite the injection of a large volume of contrast media (>200 ml), the procedure must be repeated after the large

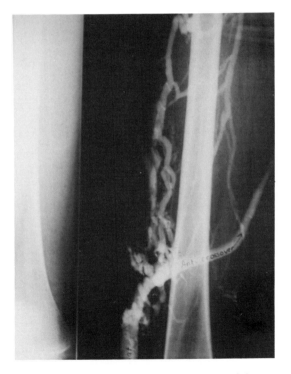

FIGURE 18-3. Varicography is useful in demonstrating the point of drainage of the lateral collector into the deep venous system. A large lateral collector is seen crossing to the medial side to drain into the greater saphenous vein. A thinner plexiform venous channel continues to drain part of the lateral flow into the venous system. A faint femoral vein is seen in the background. A second injection with elastic compression of the superficial system demonstrated a normal superficial femoral vein.

superficial venous bed has been compressed with elastic stockings or elastic bandages.

Contrast or digital arteriography must be done to confirm or rule out the presence of arteriovenous fistulas.

TREATMENT

The most common vascular malformations accompanied by varicose veins and hemangiomas are KTS, PWS, and Maffucci syndromes. The following therapeutic options will be considered in this discussion: conservative treatment, laser therapy, sclerotherapy, embolization, and surgery.[26]

Compression therapy with elastic hosiery, leg elevation, and hygiene of the extremity have been the only forms of management offered to patients with congenital vascular malformations in the past. These methods are valuable and should be used in all patients. However, some patients present with severe symptoms that do not respond to conservative management. Laser therapy should be used in port-wine stains and in some hemangiomas.[27] Small hemangiomas respond well to the flash lamp pump dye laser (wavelength, 585 nm; pulse length, 200-500 microseconds). Larger hemangiomas may be successfully treated with the Nd:YAG laser (wavelength, 1064 nm).[28,29] Sclerotherapy plays an important role in the management of congenital vascular malformations. Small localized venous malformations respond well to repeated injections of 0.75% to 1% polidocanol or sodium tetradecyl sulfate (Sotradecol). Sclerotherapy will not produce good long-term results in the management of the large varicose veins if the points of reflux remain. In such cases ligation and division of the large incompetent perforators followed by sclerotherapy is the treatment of choice and should provide considerable palliation. Sclerotherapy should not be considered for any patient in whom active arteriovenous fistulas are demonstrated. The practice of injecting a sclerosing agent into large arteriovenous shunts carries high risk and may be accompanied by arterial thrombosis, tissue necrosis, and catastrophic consequences. Other sclerosing agents that may be used are sodium tetradecyl sulfate and ethyl alcohol.[30-32] In patients with varicose veins in whom congenital arteriovenous fistulas are demonstrated, catheter embolization of the feeding vessels must be performed before excision of the malformation. Embolization may be carried out using materials such as silicone spheres, polyvinyl alcohol, dura mater, or fascia lata. Steel coils (Gianturco), liquid or semiliquid agents (e.g., pure alcohol, Isobutyl Cyano Acrylate), and amino acids (Ethibloc)[28,33,34] have also been used with different degrees of success.

SURGICAL MANAGEMENT

The large majority of patients may respond to nonoperative treatment or any of the previously described forms of therapy. However, there is a small group of patients with diffuse congenital malformations and severe intractable symptoms for whom surgical treatment must be considered. Surgical excision of the large su-

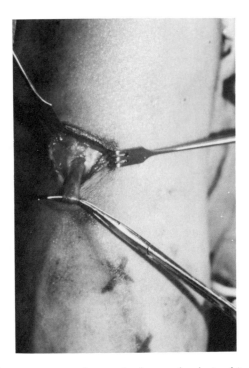

FIGURE 18-4. A 7 mm incompetent perforator is shown clearly in this intraoperative photograph of a patient with Klippel-Trenaunay syndrome. Considerable palliation is achieved after numerous perforators have been divided. Reflux is decreased, ulcers are healed, and varicosities are eliminated.

perficial varices in KTS has been condemned because it is believed that deep venous obstruction frequently results and aggravates venous hypertension. However, surgery must be considered and planned on the basis of both the patient's symptoms and the results of the diagnostic investigations. When duplex scanning or angiographic studies demonstrate a patent deep venous system, we have performed extensive excision of the superficial venous dilatations, including the large marginal vein (lateral venous collector), with ligation and division of the large incompetent perforators routinely present in these patients (Figure 18-4). If hypoplasia and/or obstruction of the deep venous system is diagnosed, the superficial venous system should not be excised. The most common symptoms necessitating intervention are frequent and copious bleeding from skin varicosities, nonhealing venous ulceration, growth deformity, intractable pain, massive edema, recurring thrombophlebitis, and thrombosis of large hemangiomas.

In 614 operated cases, Servelle[14] found the following deep venous anomalies: *compression* of the popliteal vein in 71% of the cases, with a perivenous sheath involving the whole length of the vein in 15% of the patients; *agenesis* or *hypoplasia* of the popliteal vein in approximately 7%; *compression* of the femoral vein in 54%, with a complete perivenous sheath in 2%; and *hypoplasia* and/or *complete agenesis* of the femoral vein in 40% and 3% of the cases, respectively. Ser-

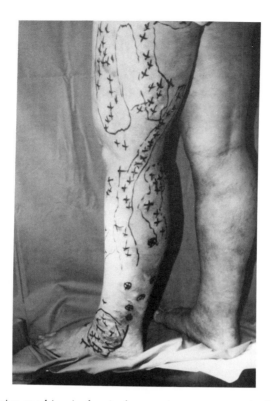

FIGURE 18-5. Preoperative marking is the single most important step in the surgical management of varicose veins. Marking should be done by the operating surgeon. Inadequate preoperative marking increases the chance of recurrence.

velle recommended venolysis and resection of the compressing fibrous sheaths and bands along the entire length of the vein. He reported that the veins were restored to almost normal caliber after this operation. However, we have not had the opportunity to confirm Servelle's observation.

Preoperative Marking

Preoperative marking (Figure 18-5) is the single most important technical step in surgery of the superficial venous system. The examiner must have experience and a thorough knowledge of anatomy, physiology, and pathophysiology. Both careful physical and duplex ultrasound examinations should be performed. Inadequate preoperative marking is not usually listed as a causative factor in recurrent varicose veins; however, an improperly and carelessly marked extremity represents an invitation for recurrence.

Preoperative marking must be performed as follows:
1. The patient must have the extremity washed with an antiseptic soap and water for at least 3 days immediately preceding surgery.

2. The extremity and pubis (if groin exploration is contemplated) should be carefully shaved before marking. This step is especially important in hairy patients.

3. Marking should be done before the administration of any preanesthetic medication. Tracing of the veins requires the patient to stand on a platform under a good source of illumination.

4. Marking should be done with a water-resistant marker so that it will not come off during skin preparation.

5. After the veins have been marked, the patient is advised to wear pajama pants and to avoid direct contact of one extremity with the other, which may lead to ink smearing.

6. Each surgeon develops his or her own technique for marking by using keys, clues, different signs, and tracings to identify perforators and clusters of veins. For this reason surgery must be performed by the surgeon who marks the patient (in teaching centers, the senior surgeon must be present during marking and must assist the resident or fellow with the op-

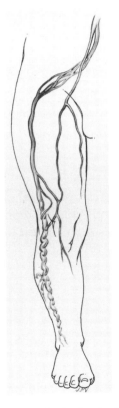

FIGURE 18-6. A lateral collector, a remnant of a fetal vein, is shown draining into the internal iliac venous system. Several degrees of deep venous hypoplasia may or may not be present. When deep venous aplasia is present and the superficial system is the main venous outflow, removal of the abnormal lateral vein may produce acute venous insufficiency, with cases of phlegmasia cerulea dolens and venous gangrene being reported.

eration). An effort should be made to locate the point of entrance of the lateral venous collector into the deep system because this point varies considerably (Figure 18-6).

We have followed the surgical policy of selective segmental excision of the pathologic superficial venous system with division and ligation of incompetent perforating veins. This policy must be followed for all patients in whom evidence of patent deep venous outflow is available. General or regional anesthesia is used in all cases. A pneumatic tourniquet inflated to 250 mm Hg has been employed in all patients with extensive and large varicosities. The operation is usually carried out in 60 to 90 minutes. The procedure involves the *segmental resection* of the lateral collecting vein and its division at the point of communication with the deep venous system. Segmental excision of this trunk is safer than stripping because of the large size of the vein and its tributaries. Indeed, venous aneurysms have been encountered in most patients. These aneurysms require local excision to prevent excessive intraoperative or postoperative bleeding (Figure 18-7). Once the large incompetent perforators have been divided, the clusters of veins can be excised through small incisions. Whenever possible, crochet-hook excision of the superficial clusters of varicose veins should be done to diminish postoperative scarring, even though this aspect of the management is not of particular concern to patients suffering from a congenital vascular malformation. Only one of 19 patients operated on for KTS was found to have incompetence of the long saphenous system. This patient underwent long saphenous vein stripping to a point just below the knee. Superficial venous clusters and venous dilatations can be excised easily in the bloodless field provided by the pneumatic tourniquet. Superficial lymphatic malformations and hemangiomas have been excised in 25% of our patients

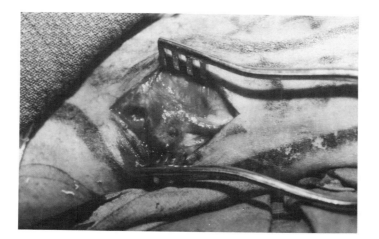

FIGURE 18-7. Large venous aneurysm in communication with an incompetent perforator. This is a common finding in patients with congenital malformations of venous predominance. Since stripping of venous segments connecting with these venous aneurysms may lead to profuse bleeding, segmental excision with direct exposure of the large dilatations is the procedure of choice.

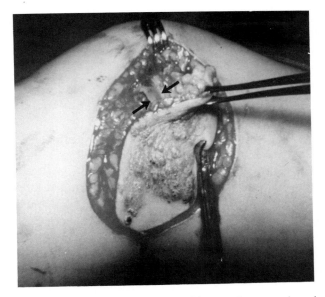

FIGURE 18-8. Localized malformations in the form of hemangiomas or lymphangiomas have been excised in 25% of our patients with congenital malformations of venous predominance. This intraoperative photograph shows en bloc excision of a large lymphangioma that had bled repeatedly. Note the large perforator draining the lesion (between *arrows*).

(Figure 18-8). In those patients with extensive abnormalities, it is wise to have surgery staged over two or three sessions to achieve optimal results. Staging was performed in 16 of our 19 cases. In the postoperative period external compression with elastic hosiery is mandatory.

In the postoperative period sclerotherapy plays an important role in the management of KTS and should begin 2 months after surgery once the postoperative ecchymosis has disappeared.

If the principles of management outlined for patients with diffuse venous malformations are followed, an excellent functional outcome can be expected. Surgery is largely a containment exercise to palliate symptoms. No claims of cure should be made. However, no patient's condition has worsened as a result of excision of the superficial veins. Following the management guidelines described here, no patient has had recurrent varicorrhage, all ulcerations have healed, and the patient's index of satisfaction (ranging from 0 = unsatisfied to 4 = very satisfied) has been 3.5.

Surgery for varicose veins in patients with PWS should not be attempted until the interventional radiologist has completed treatment of the arteriovenous communications by percutaneous catheter embolization. This process may require multiple embolization sessions. Often the elimination of active arteriovenous communications produces sufficient palliation so that the management of the superficial varicosities can be attempted with judicious sclerotherapy.

The clinical manifestations of a diffuse vascular malformation may worsen under certain circumstances, such as pregnancy, puberty, or metabolic disorders.[35,36] Patients with severe, diffuse venous malformations may suffer from pain, anxiety, and psychologic depression, leading to isolation and familial conflicts.[37,38]

MAFFUCCI SYNDROME

Maffucci syndrome is a congenital nonfamilial syndrome that includes both dyschondroplasia (enchondromatosis) and hemangiomatosis. It is a rare disease, with only 200 cases reported in the past 140 years. Recurrent bleeding, pain, and limb disfigurement may lead to vascular consultation. Affected individuals have hemangiomas at birth, and skeletal deformities are noticed later. The diagnosis of Maffucci syndrome is made after clinical, radiologic, and pathologic evidence of hemangiomatosis and enchondromas has been established. Patients with this syndrome frequently have venous dilatations and hemangiomas. Both conditions may be treated by excision. However, larger lesions should be treated only after careful evaluation of the arterial and venous anatomy. Diagnosis of this syndrome must be considered in the evaluation of patients with congenital hemangiomatosis so that the presence of potentially malignant enchondromas will not be missed. We have treated five patients during the last 23 years who presented with signs and symptoms consistent with Maffucci syndrome. All of them complained of pain and heaviness of the involved extremity. All had hemangiomas at birth, skeletal deformities, and enchondromas. In three patients the arterial inflow was evaluated with arteriography; in two others MRI was used. Two patients had excision of hemangiomas, and one had sclerotherapy and compression therapy. All had bone biopsies performed, and none of the enchondromas or the soft tissue lesions demonstrated malignant transformation. Evidence of arteriovenous fistulas was demonstrated in one patient who was submitted to arteriography (Figure 18-9). There was one episode of acute thrombosis of a large chest hemangioma, which was documented by CT scan. CT and MRI scans were useful to evaluate the nature, extent, and vascularity of bone in the lesions. Three of the five patients were children; throughout follow-up ranging from 2 to 20 years, no evidence of malignant degeneration of enchondromas or soft tissue lesions was found. In one patient, however, the extension and complications resulting from the disease process were so severe as to be life-threatening. Malignant degeneration with sarcomatous transformation of the hemangiomas and enchondromas occurs in almost 20% of patients with Maffucci syndrome.[39] The tumors are of mesodermal origin, with the majority being chondrosarcomas. Other malignancies include hemangiosarcomas, lymphangiosarcomas, fibrosarcomas, gliomas, ovarian tumors, and carcinoma of the pancreas.[40]

Benign tumors have also been found in patients with Maffucci syndrome; these include pituitary adenomas, ovarian thecomas, uterine tumors, and multiple fibromas.[41]

Because of the potential for malignant transformation of enchondromas and hemangiomas, biopsies should be performed on suspicious lesions. With soft tissue lesions that are accessible, excisional or incisional biopsy should be rec-

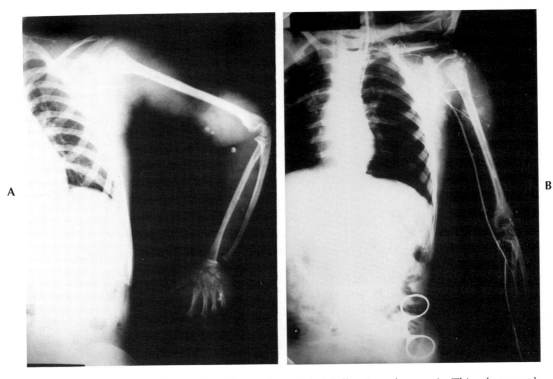

FIGURE 18-9. Radiographic studies of a patient with Maffucci syndrome. **A,** This photograph, taken 5 minutes after arteriography, shows static venous flow where contrast material remained for long periods. True phlebectasia was observed in the phlebographic studies performed. The arm dilatations are hemangiomatous masses. Marked osteoporosis with thinning of bone cortex is clearly observed. The phleboliths shown here are characteristic of this syndrome. **B,** Arteriogram of the same patient. Notice the small arteriectatic zones on the shoulder area. These lesions correspond to small areas of arteriovenous fistulas that responded well to embolization. Resection of hemangiomas under pneumatic tourniquet ischemia resulted in palliation of this patient's symptoms.

ommended because needle biopsies may result in excessive and uncontrollable bleeding.

Management of Maffucci syndrome is palliative. Definitive therapy for vascular lesions is surgical. In an attempt to reduce the size of the hemangiomas, radiation has been used. However, the benefits of this method are questionable. Tumor shrinking with sclerotherapy has been used either alone or followed by surgical excision.

Management of skeletal abnormalities is important during the adolescent period. Procedures for decreasing normal growth in the patient's normal leg may be performed to prevent marked scoliosis and limb asymmetry. Amputation, a course of last resort, may be necessary to relieve the patient of the inconvenient, swollen, and cumbersome extremity. With massive deformities or malignant transformation, disarticulation and wide resection may be indicated.[42] Disarticulation has not been necessary in our series.

SUMMARY

Surgery of the superficial veins in patients with KTS has been controversial because it was believed to result in outflow obstruction. However, our series did not demonstrate these effects. Superficial vein surgery may have been unsuccessful in the past for a number of reasons, the most obvious of which is the initial presence of venous obstruction secondary to aplasia or hypoplasia of the deep system. In such a situation severe venous stasis may result. Adequate demonstration of a hemodynamically sound deep venous system is a crucial prerequisite to superficial venous surgery. In addition, superficial surgery sometimes has been inappropriately directed toward removal of the long and short saphenous vein systems. We found varicosities of the saphenous vein in only 1 of 19 operated cases; therefore we recommend selective saphenous vein surgery only in those patients shown to have overt saphenous vein dilatation, tortuosity, and incompetence. In 18 of our 19 patients, the greater saphenous vein was surprisingly healthy looking in radiographic studies and was found to be competent on Doppler examination. Last, all patients had demonstrable perforator vein competence, often in communication with the large lateral collector vein. Perforator ligation and division should be an integral part of the treatment program. Because of the large diameter of incompetent perforator veins (see Figures 18-4 and 18-7), stripping of any large trunks in patients with KTS should not be done because of the risk of profuse bleeding. Instead, segmental excision through small incisions is the procedure of choice. Patients with intractable symptoms who have a patent deep venous system should be treated with an aggressive surgical policy directed toward the elimination of deep reflux and the excision of the dilated venous clusters. Management of the severe lymphatic anomalies and gross deformities often observed in patients with KTS should be an integral part of the management of this challenging syndrome. Excisional therapy in these cases should be considered to alleviate the heaviness of the affected limbs.

REFERENCES

1. Klippel M, Trenaunay P. Du noevus variqueux et osteo-hypertrophique. Arch Gen Med 185: 641-672, 1900.
2. McKusick KA. Mendelian Inheritance in Man: Catalogues of Autosomal Dominant, Autosomal Recessive and X-Linked Phenotypes, 6th ed. Baltimore: Johns Hopkins University Press, 1983.
3. Parkes-Weber F. Angioma formation in connection with hypertrophy of limbs and hemihypertrophy. Br J Dermatol 19:231-235, 1907.
4. Parkes-Weber F. Hemangiectatic hypertrophy of limbs—Congenital phlebarteriectasis and so-called congenital varicose veins. Br J Child Dis 15:13-17, 1918.
5. Bollinger A, Vogt B, Luthy E, Hegglin R. Flow measurement in patients with multiple arteriovenous fistulae of the extremity. Helv Med Acta 33:76-87, 1976.
6. Haimovici H, Sprayregen S. Congenital microarterio-venous shunts: Angiographic and Doppler ultrasonographic identification. Arch Surg 121:1065-1070, 1986.
7. O'Connor PS, Smith JL. Optic nerve variant in the Klippel-Trenaunay-Weber syndrome. Ann Ophthalmol 10:131-137, 1978.
8. Gloviczki P, Hollier L, Telander RL. Surgical implications of Klippel-Trenaunay-Weber syndrome. Ann Surg 197:353-362, 1983.

9. Hall BD. Bladder hemangiomas in the Klippel-Trenaunay-Weber syndrome. N Engl J Med 285: 1032-1033, 1971.

10. Tjaden BL, Buscema J, Haller JA, Rock JA. Vulvar congenital dysplastic angiopathy. Obstet Gynecol 75:552-554, 1990.

11. Dargeon HW. Tumors of Childhood. New York: Paul B. Hoeber, 1960, p 367.

12. Kuffer FR, et al. Klippel-Trenaunay syndrome, visceral angiomatosis and thrombocytopenia. J Pediatr Surg 3:65-72, 1968.

13. Hendry WF, Vinnicombe M. Hemangioma of the bladder in children and young adults. Br J Urol 43:309, 1971.

14. Servelle M. Klippel-Trenaunay syndrome. Ann Surg 197:365-373, 1985.

15. Baskerville PA, Ackroyd JS, Lea Thomas M, Browse NL. The Klippel-Trenaunay syndrome: Clinical radiological hemodynamic features and management. Br J Surg 72:232-236, 1985.

16. Stewart G, Farmer G. Sturge-Weber and Klippel-Trenaunay syndromes with absence of inferior vena cava. Arch Dis Child 65:546-547, 1990.

17. Furakawa T, Igata A, Toyokura Y, Ikeda S. Sturge-Weber and Klippel-Trenaunay syndrome with nevus of ota and ito. Arch Dermatol 102:640-645, 1970.

18. Happle R. Lethal genes surviving by mosaicism. A possible explanation for sporadic birth defects involving the skin. J Am Acad Dermatol 16:899-906, 1987.

19. Baskerville PA, Ackroyd JS, Browse NL. The etiology of the Klippel-Trenaunay syndrome. Ann Surg 202:624-627, 1985.

20. Boon LM, Mulliken JB, Vikkula M, Watkins H, Seidman J, Olsen BR, Warman ML. Assignment of a locus for dominantly inherited venous malformations to chromosome 9p. Hum Mol Genet 3(9):183-187, 1994.

21. Gallione CJ, et al. A gene for familial venous malformations maps to chromosome 9p in a second large kindred. J Med Genet 32(2):197-199, 1995.

22. Lindenhauer SM. The Klippel-Trenaunay syndrome. Ann Surg 162:303-314, 1965.

23. Vollmar J, Vogt K. Angiodysplasie und Skeletsystem. Chirurg 47:205, 1976.

24. Laor T, Burrows PE, Hoffer FA. Magnetic resonance venography of congenital vascular malformations of the extremities. Pediatr Radiol 26(6):371-380, 1996.

25. Allison JW, Glasier CM, Stark JE, James CA, Angtuaco EJ. Head and neck MR angiography in pediatric patients: A pictorial essay. Radiographics 14(4):795-805, 1994.

26. Mulliken JB, Young AE. Vascular birthmarks. Hemangiomas and malformations. Philadelphia: WB Saunders, 1988, pp 24-37.

27. McClean K, Hanke CW. The medical necessity for treatment of portwine stains. Dermatol Surg 23(8):663-667, 1997.

28. Loose DA, Weber J. Angeborene Gefaessmissbildungen. Periodica Angiologica 21:170-207, 216-313, 1997.

29. Fuchs B, Philipp C, Engel-Murke F, Staltout J, Berlien HP. Techniques for endoscopic intracorporal laser applications. Endosc Surg 1:217-223, 1993.

30. de Lorimier AA. Sclerotherapy for venous malformations. J Pediatr Surg 30(2):188-194, 1995.

31. Van der Stricht J. The sclerosing therapy in congenital vascular defects. Int Angiol 9(3):224-227, 1990.

32. O'Donovan JC, Donaldson JS, Morello FP, Pensler JM, Vogelzang RL, Baner B. Symptomatic hemangiomas and venous malformations in infants, children and young adults: Treatment with percutaneous injection with sodium tetradecyl sulfate. AJR 169(3):725-729, 1997.

33. Jackson JE, Mansfield AO, Allison DJ. Treatment of high-flow vascular malformations by venous embolization aided by flow occlusion techniques. Cardiovasc Intervent Radiol 19(5):323-328, 1996.

34. Yakes WF, Luethke JM, Parker SH, Stavros AT, Kah KM, Hopper KD, Dreisbach JN, Griffith DJ, Seibert CE, Carter DE. Ethanol embolization of vascular malformations. Radiographics 19(5):787-796, 1990.

35. Gotze S, Weitzel H. Praenatale Diagnostik und geburtshilfliches Management bei einem Fall von Klippel-Trenaunay-Weber-Syndrom. Z Geburtshilfe Perinatol 191(1):43, 1987.

36. Rubin SM, Jackson GM, Cohen AW. Management of pregnant patient with a cerebral angioma. A report of two cases. Obstet Gynecol 78(5 Part 2):929-933, 1991.

37. Kohler A, Dirsch O, Brunner U. Venolymphatic angiodysplasias as the cause of recurrent varicose veins. Vasa 26(1):52-54, 1997.

38. Banet GA, Anstine-Bessenecker PL. Arteriovenous malformations of the hand: A case study. J Vasc Nurs 10(4):6-12, 1992.

39. Schwarz HS, et al. The malignant potential of enchondromatosis. J Bone Joint Surg 69A:269-274, 1987.

40. Johnson JL, Webster JR, Sippy HL. Maffucci's syndrome (dyschondroplasia with hemangiomas). Am J Med 228:864-866, 1960.

41. Lewis RJ, Ketchum AS. Maffucci's syndrome: Functional and neoplasm significance. Case report and review of the literature. J Bone Joint Surg 55A:1465-1467, 1973.

42. Sun TS, Swec RG, Shives TC, Unni KK. Chondrosarcoma in Maffucci's syndrome. J Bone Joint Surg 67A:1214-1219, 1985.

SUGGESTED READINGS

Atiyeh BS, Musharrafieh RS. Klippel-Trenaunay-type syndrome: An eponym for various expressions of the same entity. J Med 26:253-260, 1995.

Carr MM, Mahoney JL, Bowen VA. Extremity arteriovenous malformations: Review of a series. Can J Surg 37(4):293-299, 1994.

de Lorimier AA. Sclerotherapy for venous malformations. J Pediatr Surg 30:188-194, 1995.

Jolobe OMP. Klippel-Trenaunay syndrome. Postgrad Med J 72:347-348, 1996.

Paes E, Vollmar J. Diagnosis and surgical aspects of congenital venous angiodysplasia in the extremities. Phlebology 10:160-164, 1995.

Samuel M, Spitz L. Klippel-Trenaunay syndrome: Clinical features, complications, and management in children. Br J Surg 82:757-761, 1995.

Chapter 19

Varicose Veins and Venous Ulceration: Rationale for Conservative Treatment

Gregory L. Moneta and John M. Porter

An examination of the potential relationship between venous ulceration and varicose veins requires consideration of a number of issues, the first of which is the definition of varicose veins. Next, the prevalence of varicose veins in patients with venous ulceration must be determined and accompanied by a careful evaluation of the evidence that varicose veins themselves contribute to the ulcerative process and are not merely another manifestation of abnormal venous hemodynamics that lead to the development of a venous ulcer. In addition, the circumstances under which treatment specifically directed toward varicose veins will lead to prevention, healing, or decreased rate of recurrence of venous ulceration need to be determined. Finally, if a relationship does exist between varicose veins and venous ulcers, various therapies available for treating coexisting varicose veins and venous ulceration must be considered to select optimal treatment for the individual patient.

DEFINITION

Unfortunately, the basic definition of what constitutes a varicose vein is controversial. Most practicing physicians regard any large, tortuous superficial vein as a varicose vein, regardless of the process leading to venous dilation. From this perspective a tortuous superficial vein resulting from an intrinsic defect in the vein wall (a primary varicosity) and one arising as a result of abnormal deep venous hemodynamics (a secondary varicosity) are both considered varicose. It is interesting that the definition of varicose veins given by the World Health Organization is "a sacular dilatation of the veins which are often tortuous." Tortuous dilated veins secondary to previous venous thrombosis or congenital or acquired arteriovenous fistulas are specifically excluded from this definition of varicose veins.[1]

Clearly dilated and tortuous superficial venous channels often are found in patients with previous deep venous thrombosis and either concurrent or prior venous ulceration. Since these dilated superficial veins may contribute to the formation of a venous ulcer, their treatment also will be addressed in this chapter. Therefore, despite the World Health Organization definition, for purposes of the present discussion, we will consider any tortuous dilated superficial vein as a varicose vein, regardless of whether it developed primarily or followed prior deep venous thrombosis. Such a definition is obviously more realistic for the clinician who is evaluating a patient with coexisting dilated, tortuous superficial veins and a venous ulcer. As will be discussed below, however, the use of this definition does not obviate the need to distinguish primary from secondary varicose veins; nor does it diminish the necessity to determine the relative contributions of superficial and communicating vein insufficiency and deep venous insufficiency to the formation of a venous ulcer.

HISTORY

An association between varicose veins and venous ulcers was a recurring theme in the writings of early Greek, Egyptian, and Roman physicians. Celsus (25 BC–AD 50), Galen (AD 130-200), and Aeties (AD 502-574) described bandages for the treatment of venous ulcers.[2-4] In addition, the use of both avulsion and cautery to eliminate varicose veins accompanying venous ulcers was advocated by these early writers. Indeed, it appears that up until the eighteenth century most physicians believed that varicose veins always accompanied venous ulceration. Eighteenth century physicians, however, began to discard the idea that varicose veins were an absolute prerequisite to venous ulceration. Bell[5] and Baynton[6] made no references to varicose veins as a cause of venous ulceration in their discussions of leg ulcers. Spender[7] noted that venous ulcers could occur in the absence of varicose veins provided that the patient's deep veins were damaged by an episode of venous thrombosis. By 1916 Homans[8] clearly recognized the varying etiologies of venous ulceration. He divided venous ulcers into those associated with leg varicose veins (and "cured by the removal of these veins") and the more intractable "postphlebitic" venous ulcer.[9]

Currently, it is clear that venous ulceration may occur with and without associated superficial varicosities. In clinical reports of patients with venous ulcers, the incidence of coexisting varicose veins varies from 30% to 67% (Table 19-1).

ETIOLOGY OF VENOUS ULCERS

A complete discussion of the complex pathophysiology of venous ulceration is presented in Chapter 3. In short, alterations in cutaneous microcirculatory physiology accompany the formation of a venous ulcer. Pericapillary fibrin deposition, alterations in fibrinolysis and/or plasminogen activation, and microcirculatory leukocyte trapping (with associated cutaneous capillary and lymphatic destruction) all appear to interact in a complex and incompletely defined manner to produce local conditions conducive to ulcer formation.[15-18] Although the precise

TABLE 19-1. Associated superficial venous varicosities in patients with venous ulcers

Author	Year	No. of Patients	% With Varicosities
Mayberry et al.[10]	1991	113	32
Gooley and Sumner[11]	1988	15	67
Kitahama et al.[12]	1982	65	33
Cranley[13]	1975	1300	30
Healey et al.[14]	1978	18	67

microcirculatory events leading to venous ulceration have not been determined, there is general agreement that persistent elevation of ambulatory venous pressure is the driving force leading to the microcirculatory changes associated with venous ulceration.

Elevated ambulatory venous pressure (AVP) and shortened venous recovery time (VRT) are clearly associated with an increased incidence of concurrent or past venous ulcer. Nicolaides and Zukowski[19] have demonstrated a virtual absence of venous ulceration in patients with ambulatory venous pressures less than 40 mm Hg. Conversely, patients with an AVP greater than 80 mm Hg are quite likely to have suffered from venous ulceration.

Most patients with venous ulceration have pronounced deep venous valvular insufficiency associated with elevated AVP and shortened VRT. However, severe reflux in the superficial venous system alone may be associated with a markedly elevated AVP and decreased VRT with a normal deep venous system.[20,21] Although it is clear that the large majority of patients with venous ulcers or marked lipodermatosclerosis have both deep and superficial venous reflux, an appreciable minority do not have detectable deep venous insufficiency.[11,20,22,23] The logical conclusion is that isolated abnormalities of superficial and/or perforating veins must be capable of inducing the microcirculatory changes required to produce a venous ulcer without participation of an abnormal deep venous system.

A number of studies suggest that venous ulceration may occur in the absence of detectable deep venous insufficiency. Burnand[24] has demonstrated that incompetent calf perforating veins may be present in patients with normal deep venous hemodynamics. Dodd and Cockett[25] noted an association between leg ulcers and incompetent calf perforating veins and varicose veins in certain patients with phlebographically normal deep veins. Sturrup[26] also has described a subset of patients with venous ulcers who, when standing with a thigh tourniquet, empty their superficial veins with exercise, which implies normally functioning deep veins (Perthes' test). More recently Hoare et al.[20] described 20 patients with venous ulceration and long-standing severe varicose veins who were found to have normal deep venous systems through photoplethysmography, AVP measurements, and Doppler ultrasound. All patients, however, had severe reflux of either the greater or lesser saphenous vein. Moore et al.[21] reported that 10% of their patients with severe venous stasis changes were noted to have isolated superficial venous incompetence on the basis of continuous-wave Doppler examinations.

The problem with these observations is the inability to distinguish in a quantitative fashion perforating and superficial venous incompetence and to determine the relative importance of reflux in the perforating and superficial venous systems with respect to eventual venous ulceration. There is in fact no well accepted method for determining and quantitating reflux in perforating veins. Physical examination, continuous-wave Doppler studies, thermography, and venography all have been found to have either low sensitivities or high false positive rates when compared to the accepted "gold standard" of obvious perforating vein backbleeding at the time of subfascial ligation.[27] Certainly, however, patients with venous ulceration and apparent isolated superficial venous incompetence may have perforating vein incompetence that contributes to their venous ulceration.

The suggestion that varicose veins themselves may cause venous ulceration also is complicated by the observation that 72% of patients with varicose veins and no signs of lipodermatosclerosis and/or ulceration do not have greater or lesser saphenous vein insufficiency.[28] Venous insufficiency, if present at all in such patients, appears to be limited to branches of the greater or the lesser saphenous vein. Conversely, almost all patients with venous ulcers and concurrent varicosities have saphenous or deep venous insufficiency.[10-12,15]

In our view, consideration of the preceding discussion leads to the following conclusions:

1. Varicose veins can be present with or without deep venous insufficiency and with and without greater or lesser saphenous vein insufficiency.
2. Varicose veins are not required for formation of a venous ulcer.
3. Patients with varicose veins and venous ulcers almost always have deep venous insufficiency.
4. The uncommon patient with venous ulceration, varicose veins, and no detectable deep venous insufficiency will virtually always have incompetence of the greater or lesser saphenous veins.
5. Perforating vein insufficiency currently cannot be reliably detected and quantitated.
6. Therefore patients with venous ulcers and apparent isolated greater or lesser saphenous vein insufficiency may have undetected coexisting perforating vein insufficiency.

We therefore believe that there is no evidence that varicose veins themselves, in the absence of deep venous or greater or lesser saphenous vein insufficiency, lead to venous ulceration. The obvious exception is direct pressure necrosis by a varicosity on the overlying skin, which is not a true lipodermatosclerotic ulceration.

TREATMENT OF VENOUS ULCERATION

For a long time compression therapy has been the standard treatment for venous ulceration. Our patients with venous ulceration are treated exclusively with a strict regimen of ambulatory compression through the use of elastic compression stockings. Our policy is to disregard the presence of branch varicosities in the treatment of patients with venous ulcers. Such patients are, however, evaluated through AVPs and VRTs in an effort to identify apparent isolated greater or lesser saphenous vein insufficiency. To date, patients with isolated superficial venous insufficiency and lipodermatosclerosis but not venous ulceration and isolated greater or lesser saphenous vein insufficiency have been identified in our practice. However, patients with isolated superficial venous insufficiency apparently constitute 5% to 20% of the venous ulcer population in the experience of others.[13,20]

With the wide application of ultrasound scanning, a larger population of patients with venous leg ulcer and superficial incompetence has been encountered. At Newcastle Hospital (Newcastle, England), a total of 300 limbs in 153 patients were examined by Doppler ultrasound with color-flow imaging.[29] Of the 98 limbs with hyperpigmentation, lipodermatosclerosis, atrophie blanche, and ulceration, 57% had superficial vein incompetence. Of the 25 limbs with ulceration, 13 had superficial reflux alone and 12 others had deep vein reflux. At the Middlesex Hospital, both limbs of 59 consecutive patients with venous ulceration were assessed by color duplex ultrasound.[30] Isolated deep venous reflux was present in only 12 limbs (15%). A combination of deep and superficial venous reflux was found in 25 limbs (32%), but in 42 limbs (53%) superficial venous reflux was the only abnormality found. In Melbourne, limbs with ulceration more frequently showed superficial reflux, and all limbs with complicated venous problems showed short saphenous reflux.[31] The conclusion of Kenneth Myers, author of the report, was that "most limbs with complications had superficial reflux, either alone or combined with deep reflux. Few had deep reflux alone."

PROTOCOL FOR TREATMENT OF VENOUS ULCERS*

1. Initial bedrest
2. Systemic antibiotics for cellulitis or infection
3. 30 to 40 mm Hg below-knee graduated elastic compression stockings
4. Daily soap-and-water cleansing of ulcer
5. Dry gauze dressing under stocking
6. Treatment of stasis dermatitis with corticosteroid ointment
7. Continued use of graduated elastic compression stockings after healing

*Oregon Health Sciences University, Portland, Ore.

Over the last 15 years we have treated 113 patients with venous ulcers, 32% of whom had associated superficial varicosities, with the method summarized in the box on p. 418.[10] An initial period of bedrest is prescribed until ankle edema resolves as much as possible. In recent years the availability of home health care has greatly diminished the necessity for hospitalization. A brief course of intravenous or oral antibiotics along with local wound care (gentle soap and water scrubs followed by dry gauze dressings changed every 8 hours) also is used during the period of bedrest if periulcer cellulitis or obvious invasive infection, suggested by severe pain in the ulcer, is present.

Edema usually resolves in a few days. The patient then is fitted with an elastic compression stocking and allowed to ambulate. A 30 to 40 mm Hg pressure-gradient below-knee stocking is preferred. The patient is issued two pairs of stockings so that a clean pair is available each day. Wound care is continued with soap-and-water washing of the ulcer daily. A corticosteroid ointment, such as hydrocortisone or triamcinolone in white petrolatum, is applied to areas of stasis dermatitis but not to the ulcer itself. In fact, no additional medications are ever applied to the ulcer. Dry gauze is placed over the ulcer and changed at least twice daily. The gauze is held in place by a nylon stocking to allow the elastic compression stocking to be placed without disturbing the dressing. We also have found stocking application devices, such as the Medi-Butler (medi USA, Elk Grove, Ill.) (Figure 19-1), to be quite helpful in allowing elderly patients to apply their stocking without assistance.

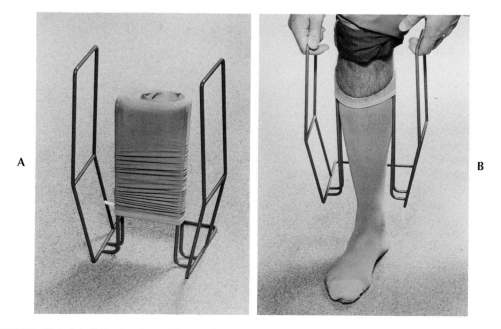

FIGURE 19-1. Medi-Butler device for application of elastic compression stockings. Once the stocking is loaded (**A**), the patient merely steps into stocking and pulls it up to apply it to the leg (**B**).

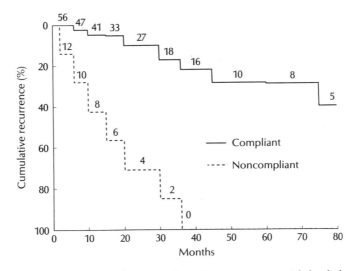

FIGURE 19-2. Life-table recurrence of venous ulceration in patients with healed venous ulcers who were either compliant or noncompliant with the recommendation for continued use of elastic compression stockings. The number of patients at risk in each time interval is printed above the graph. Five-year recurrence rate for compliant patients was 29%. All noncompliant patients had recurrence by 36 months ($p = 0.0001$; chi-square). (From Mayberry JC, et al. Fifteen-year results of ambulatory compression therapy for chronic venous ulcers. Surgery 109:575, 1991.)

TABLE 19-2. Long-term recurrence of venous ulceration after subfascial ligation of communicating veins*

Author	Year	No. of Patients	Total Recurrence (%)	Stockings Worn Postoperatively
Thurston and Williams[36]	1973	89	13	Yes
Bowen[37]	1975	55	32	Yes
Burnand et al.[38]	1976	41	55	?
DePalma[39]	1979	53	6	Yes
Hyde et al.[40]	1981	109	24	Yes
Negus and Friedgood[41]	1983	77	13	Yes
Johnson et al.[42]	1985	37	41 (3 yr)†	?
			51 (5 yr)†	?
Cikrit et al.[43]	1988	27	22	Yes

*Modified from Mayberry JC, et al. Fifteen-year results of ambulatory compression therapy for chronic venous ulcers. Surgery 109:575, 1991.
†Life-table recurrence.

Despite the perception that patients are noncompliant with the use of elastic compression stockings, among our patients we noted 90% compliance. Complete healing of the venous ulcer occurred in 97% of patients who were compliant with the use of stockings. In only 55% of the small number of noncompliant patients did the ulcer heal. Seventy-nine percent of patients having long-term follow-up (n = 73, with mean follow-up of 30 months) remained compliant with the recommendation of lifelong use of stockings. Sixteen percent of these compliant patients developed a recurrence of venous ulcer, a 29% 5-year life-table recurrence rate. All patients who discontinued the use of elastic stockings after initial healing had recurrence of venous ulcers by 36 months (Figure 19-2). Similar results can be obtained by using compression therapy with various paste boots, so-called Unna's boot.[32] However, a cost analysis shows that, at least in our hospital, treatment with elastic compression stockings is considerably less expensive.[33]

Others have attempted to assess the effects of different dressings on venous ulcer healing and have used randomized trials.[34] It has been found that healing was affected significantly by ulcer size and that the paste bandages effected a faster rate of healing than that of limbs treated with a zinc oxide–impregnated stocking or an alginate dressing. The factors of ulceration, sex, and age of the patients had no effect upon ulcer healing in this study. In a review of 24 randomized controlled trials of compression treatment for venous ulcers, it was found that various high-compression regimens are more effective than low-compression regimens but that at this time there is insufficient reliable evidence to indicate which system of high compression is the most effective.[35]

Our results with compression therapy of venous ulceration with elastic compression stockings are at least as good as those obtained with subfascial ligation of communicating veins (Table 19-2). We do not believe that removal of superficial varicosities and/or stripping of an incompetent saphenous system is a mandatory adjunct to effective treatment of venous ulceration. We continue to reserve sclerotherapy or surgical excision of superficial varicosities for indications of cosmesis, hemorrhage, pain in the varicosity itself, and diffuse aching in the extremity that occurs at the end of the day in a leg with hemodynamically normal or nearly normal deep veins.

ADDITIVE SUPERFICIAL AND DEEP VENOUS REFLUX AND VENOUS ULCERS

It has been noted that the results of deep venous reconstructions may be better in patients who also undergo removal of incompetent superficial veins. Ferris and Kistner[44] reported that in patients undergoing valvuloplasty or venous segment transpositions, 58% who also had interruption of the perforating veins had normal postoperative ambulatory venous pressures. AVP was normal in only 11% of patients with deep venous reconstructions who had untreated perforating veins. It has been hypothesized that in a significant number of patients the combination of deep and superficial incompetence may be required to produce a venous ulcer. In an effort to identify these patients and to quantitate venous reflux at varying locations in the superficial and deep veins, investigators have begun using duplex ultrasound to measure reflux volumes or peak velocities.

Quantitative duplex-derived measurements of forward flow in lower extremity veins was reported by Strandness and his group in 1988.[45] These and other investigators subsequently have applied duplex technology to quantify venous reflux in patients with and without the sequela of chronic venous insufficiency.[46,47]

Duplex evaluation of venous reflux is performed with the patient in an upright and non–weight-bearing position with respect to the leg undergoing examination. To allow for application of standard compression, a pneumatic cuff is placed on the thigh and leg and connected to an automatic inflator. The site to be examined is insonated with duplex ultrasound just cephalad to the cuff. The cuff is inflated to a predetermined level for 3 seconds. Then it is rapidly deflated (in <0.5 second). Venous reflux in response to cuff deflation is recorded with the duplex scanner. With this technique, Vasdekis et al.[47] have determined that a total peak reflux volume flow of >10 ml/second correlates well with the presence of venous ulceration and/or lipodermatosclerosis. It is interesting that this correlation appears to hold regardless of whether the reflux is present in the deep or the superficial venous system, or both.[47] Since many patients with venous ulceration have detectable reflux in both the deep and the superficial system, it may be that a critical level (>10 ml/sec) of total reflux exists.

The clinical implication of duplex localization of venous incompetence is that if total reflux were reduced to <10 ml/second, either through removal of incompetent superficial veins and associated varicosities or by various forms of deep venous reconstruction, the patient's propensity to develop venous ulceration would be reduced. Duplex quantification of total venous reflux may provide a method for identifying patients with superficial venous insufficiency, varicose veins, and venous ulceration who are most likely to benefit from obliteration of the greater or the lesser saphenous vein and associated varicosities either by surgery or sclerotherapy. Although this hypothesis has not been formally tested, some clinicians already are incorporating duplex quantification of superficial and deep venous reflux into their vascular laboratory evaluation of patients with varicose veins and venous ulcers.[23] Raju and Fredericks[48] also have noted that total venous reflux appears to be a better predictor of severely symptomatic venous insufficiency than single measurements of AVP or VRT. Whether obliteration of superficial veins selectively identified by duplex scanning as contributing significantly to overall venous reflux will reduce the recurrence rate of a healed venous ulcer awaits the result of a carefully designed clinical trial.

CONCLUSION

Available data suggest that superficial varicosities themselves do not lead to venous ulceration, although associated superficial venous incompetence may serve as the primary source of, or an important contributing component to, the venous reflux necessary for formation of a venous ulcer. If superficial venous insufficiency can be implicated as an important contributing factor to venous ulceration in selected patients, and if such patients can be reliably identified, obliteration of incompetent superficial veins and associated varicosities in patients with venous ulcers may be indicated. However, since we have not identified isolated superficial venous incompetence to be a clinical problem in our patients with venous ulcers, we continue to recommend conservative treatment of venous ulceration with compression stocking therapy. Thus far no other form of therapy has proven superior in the large majority of patients with venous ulcers.

REFERENCES

1. Prerovskly I. Diseases of the Veins. Geneva: World Health Organization, WHO-PA 10964 [internal communication].
2. Celsus AC. Of Medicine in Eight Books. Grieve J, trans. London: Wilson & Durham, 1756.
3. Galen C. Claud: Galeni Opera Omnia. In Kühn CG, ed. Lipsiac: Office Library C Cnobochii, 1821-1833, 22 volumes.
4. Anning ST. Historical aspects. In Dodd H, Cockett FB, eds. The Pathology and Surgery of Veins of the Lower Limb. Edinburgh: Livingstone, 1956.
5. Bell B. Treatise on the Theory and Management of Ulcers. Edinburgh: C Elliot, 1779.
6. Baynton T. A New Method of Treating Old Ulcers of the Legs. Bristol: Emery & Adams, 1799.
7. Spender JK. A Manual of the Pathology and Treatment of Ulcers and Subcutaneous Diseases of the Lower Limbs. London: Churchill, 1866.
8. Homans J. The operative treatment of varicose veins and ulcers, based upon a classification of these lesions. Surg Gynecol Obstet 22:143, 1916.
9. Homans J. The etiology and treatment of varicose ulcers of the leg. Surg Gynecol Obstet 24:300, 1917.
10. Mayberry JC, et al. Fifteen-year results of ambulatory compression therapy for chronic venous ulcer. Surgery 109:575, 1991.
11. Gooley NA, Sumner DS. Relationship of venous reflux to the site of venous valvular incompetence: Implications for venous reconstructive surgery. J Vasc Surg 7:50, 1988.
12. Kitahama A, et al. Leg ulcer: Conservative management or surgical treatment. JAMA 247:197, 1982.
13. Cranley JJ. Venous stasis [letter]. Surgery 77:730, 1975.
14. Healey PJM, et al. Surgical management of the chronic venous ulcer: The Rob procedure. Am J Surg 137:556, 1978.
15. Browse NL, Burnand KG. The cause of venous ulceration. Lancet 2:243, 1982.
16. Leach RD, Browse NL. Effect of venous hypertension on canine hind limb lymph. Br J Surg 72:275, 1985.
17. Thomas PRS, Nash GB, Dormandy JA. White cell accumulation in the dependent legs of patients with venous hypertension: A possible mechanism for trophic changes in the skin. BMJ 296:1693, 1988.
18. Bollinger A, et al. Fluorescence microlymphography in chronic venous incompetence. Int Angiol 8:23, 1989.
19. Nicolaides AN, Zukowski AJ. The value of dynamic venous pressure measurements. World J Surg 10:919, 1986.
20. Hoare MC, et al. The role of primary varicose veins in venous ulceration. Surgery 92:450, 1982.
21. Moore DJ, Himmel PD, Sumner DS. Distribution of venous valvular incompetence in patients with the post-phlebitic syndrome. J Vasc Surg 3:49, 1986.
22. Young J, Moneta GL. Severe primary varicose veins. Postgrad Vasc Surg 1:134, 1990.
23. Schanzer H, Pierce EC II. A rational approach to surgery of the chronic venous stasis syndrome. Ann Surg 195:25, 1982.

24. Burnand KG. The relative importance of incompetent communicating veins in the production of varicose veins and venous ulcers. Surgery 82:9, 1977.

25. Dodd H, Cockett FB. The Pathology and Surgery of the Veins of the Lower Limb, 2nd ed. London: Churchill Livingstone, 1976, p 248.

26. Sturrup H. Ulcus Cruris. Copenhagen: Arne Front-Hansens Forlag, 1950.

27. Nicolaides AN, Sumner DS. Investigation of Patients With Deep Vein Thrombosis and Chronic Venous Insufficiency. Nicosia, Cyprus: Med-Orion Publishing, 1991, pp 50-56.

28. Hanrahan LM, et al. Patterns of venous insufficiency in patients with varicose veins. Arch Surg 126:687, 1991.

29. Lees TA, Lambert D. Patterns of venous reflux in limbs with skin changes associated with chronic venous insufficiency. Br J Surg 80:725, 1993.

30. Shami SK, Sarin S, Cheatle TR, Scurr JH, Coleridge Smith PD. Venous ulcers and the superficial venous system. J Vasc Surg 17:487, 1993.

31. Myers KA, Ziegenbein RW, Zeng GH, Matthews PG. Duplex ultrasonography scanning for chronic venous disease: Patterns of venous reflux. J Vasc Surg 21:605, 1995.

32. Hendricks WM, Swallow RT. Management of stasis leg ulcers with Unna's boots versus elastic support stockings. J Am Acad Dermatol 12:90, 1985.

33. Chitwood RW, Moneta GL, Porter JM. Nonoperative management of chronic venous insufficiency. In Strandness DE Jr, van Breda A, eds. Vascular Diseases: Surgical and Interventional Therapy. New York: Churchill Livingstone, 1998.

34. Stacey MC, Jopp-McKay AG, Rashid P, Hoskin SE, Thompson PJ. The influence of dressings on venous ulcer healing: A randomized trial. Eur J Vasc Endovasc Surg 13:174, 1997.

35. Fletcher A, Cullum N, Sheldon TA. A systematic review of compression treatment for venous leg ulcers. BMJ 315:576, 1997.

36. Thurston OG, Williams HTG. Chronic venous insufficiency of the lower extremity: Pathogenesis and surgical treatment. Arch Surg 106:537, 1973.

37. Bowen FH. Subfascial ligation (Linton operation) of the perforating leg veins to treat postthrombophlebitic syndrome. Am Surg 41:148, 1975.

38. Burnand K, et al. Relation between postphlebitic changes in the deep veins and results of surgical treatment of venous ulcers. Lancet 1:936, 1976.

39. DePalma RG. Surgical therapy for venous stasis: Results of a modified Linton operation. Am J Surg 137:810, 1979.

40. Hyde GL, Litton TC, Hull DA. Long-term results of subfascial vein ligation for venous stasis disease. Surg Gynecol Obstet 153:683, 1981.

41. Negus D, Friedgood A. The effective management of venous ulceration. Br J Surg 70:623, 1983.

42. Johnson WC, et al. Venous stasis ulceration: Effectiveness of subfascial ligation. Arch Surg 120:797, 1985.

43. Cikrit DF, Nichols WK, Silver D. Surgical management of refractory venous stasis ulceration. J Vasc Surg 7:473, 1988.

44. Ferris EB, Kistner RL. Femoral vein reconstruction in the management of chronic venous insufficiency. Arch Surg 117:1571, 1982.

45. Moneta GL, Bedford G, Strandness DE Jr. Duplex assessment of venous diameters, peak velocities and flow patterns. J Vasc Surg 8:286, 1988.

46. van Bemmelen PS, et al. Quantitative segmental evaluation of venous valvular reflux with duplex ultrasound scanning. J Vasc Surg 10:425, 1989.

47. Vasdekis SN, Clarke H, Nicolaides AN. Quantification of venous reflux by means of duplex scanning. J Vasc Surg 10:670, 1989.

48. Raju S, Fredericks R. Hemodynamic basis of stasis ulceration—A hypothesis. J Vasc Surg 13:491, 1991.

Chapter 20

Pelvic and Vulvar Varices: Pelvic Congestion Syndrome

Abraham Lechter

HISTORICAL BACKGROUND

In the past, vulvar and pelvic types of varicose veins were poorly understood; hence their treatment was not rational. With the advent of vascular radiology, ascending and descending phlebography of pelvic and gonadal veins became possible. In 1954, with publication of the classic work by Guilhem and Baux,[1] exploration and invasion of these veins began (see box, p. 426). These vessels were visualized mainly from below in an upward direction; thus the data were inconclusive.

From 1965 through 1968, reports from Ahlberg, Bartley, and Chidekel[2-4] of Scandinavia furnished substantial information about exploration of gonadal veins from above in a downward direction.

In 1975 Craig and Hobbs[5] described the pelvic congestion syndrome. Laparoscopy, popular in the 1970s and 1980s, became instrumental in the diagnosis and clarification of the cause of this syndrome. The laparoscopic approach is the most useful tool for differentiating nonvascular or somatic pathologic conditions from vascular pathologic conditions, specifically varicocele of the gonadal system.

However, as recently as 1991, the medical school of Walter Reed Hospital in Washington, D.C., advocated the internal iliac vein theory of pelvic and vulvar veins.[6,7] At our institution, my colleagues and I studied 450 gonadal vein phlebograms, of which 75% included iliac injection. We have rarely observed a spilling or dumping of dye into the vulva or upper thigh with iliac vein injection. As Hobbs[8] has aptly said, the iliac system is only the "middleman" in the whole picture.

On September 14, 1984, we performed the first operation of bilateral gonadal vein resection with a long median incision and a transperitoneal approach. Since then, 500 operations for varices of pelvic origin and vulvar veins have been performed with a retroperitoneal approach; in addition, 56 operations for pelvic

EVOLUTION OF CONCEPT OF PELVIC VARICES

1. Segmental pelvic varices without direct connection to the saphenous vein were commonly noted.
2. Before elective removal, such varices were studied by varicography, which might show the leakage point at the superficial or deep system through a perforator vein. (The cases described as pelvic varices in this chapter did not show the entrance of contrast material into any vein.)
3. High-pressure escape points from the pelvis into the vulva, labia, and upper thigh, constituting a true pelvic varicocele, were suspected, and positive diagnostic phlebography of gonadal veins confirmed the clinical impression.
4. Excellent surgical results obtained through bilateral resection of gonadal veins and ligation of communications to uterine veins, followed by varicectomy with sparing of the saphenous system, further confirmed the nonsaphenous cause of pelvic varices.

congestion syndrome were performed with this approach. Exceptional cases included three instances of chronic pelvic pain with associated somatic and vascular pathology in which hysterectomy and gonadal resection were simultaneously performed with a transperitoneal approach. Of these 556 operations, 520 included bilateral ligation and excision of both gonadal veins; some of the failures of the early cases could be attributed to unilateral operations of the gonadal system. Both gonadal systems should be operated on, even if the pathologic condition is restricted to one leg or one side of the vulva.[9-12]

The first operations for pelvic congestion syndrome were performed in 1986. Only 56 such procedures have been done by our group in 12 years. Our first male patient underwent surgery in April 1998. Despite excellent results, gynecologists in Colombia and in Europe still consider this treatment a highly controversial issue.[13] More information is needed to approach the problem of pelvic congestion syndrome successfully.

PELVIC VARICES AND GONADAL VEINS

The concept of high back pressure as the cause of varicose veins in the legs was proposed by Trendelenburg in the first decade of the twentieth century and by Dodd and Cockett in the 1940s, relating to their work on the saphenofemoral junction and perforating veins in the leg, respectively. There are, however, varicose veins in the leg that cannot be explained by back pressure. The purpose of this chapter is to present our findings, collected during a 12-year period, from the study and treatment of patients who had high-pressure escape points located in pelvic and abdominal veins.

This group comprised 500 patients included in a prospective study from September 1984 to September 1997. All participants were women aged 31 to 49, with a mean age of 40. All had multiple full-term pregnancies (2 to 14 pregnancies), with an average of 4 deliveries. Their symptoms included pain and often incapacitating heaviness in the thighs and legs. Premenstrual and menstrual pelvic, vulvar, and thigh pain also was present. In addition, pain in the lateral areas of the legs and feet was noted. No trophic changes were observed.

Physical examination of these patients showed the following characteristics:

1. Saphenous veins were "not open," and the saphenofemoral junction was not obviously incompetent, as determined by palpation or Doppler examination.
2. Vulvar varices were frequently present (360 of 500 cases).
3. Varicose veins began at the root of the thigh at the union of the external border of the labia and the inner area of the thigh (Figure 20-1).
4. Two fossae appeared when the patient was recumbent and the thigh and knee were flexed to 45 degrees and slightly abducted (Figure 20-2). The long adductor muscle tendon was prominent and separated the two depressions. The external depression was the saphenous fossa. The inner one was the pelvic fossa, in which varicose extensions of the pelvic veins appeared.
5. The course of the varices did not follow the saphenous system. Typically, it crossed the posterior or anterior area of the thigh to the lateral leg, foot, and popliteal fossa.
6. Small veins often cascaded down the posterior and lateral areas of the thigh and leg. These very superficial veins were usually deep blue or violaceous. They were fragile, prone to ecchymoses and hematomas, and difficult to remove surgically.

Vascular Radiology

Diagnosis is confirmed with invasive phlebography. We rely on direct visualization of pelvic and vulvar veins via the gonadal veins. The ovarian vein has been demonstrated through color-flow imaging.[14]

Fifteen cases were assessed with standard ascending phlebography, and the results were normal. Varicography performed on 25 patients failed to show the site of varicose vein entry into the saphenous or deep venous systems through perforator veins. Of 500 patients, 450 underwent phlebography of the gonadal veins accomplished with the Seldinger technique. With this technique, a catheter inserted under fluoroscopic control reaches the right gonadal vein through the vena cava or the left gonadal vein through the left renal vein; contrast medium is injected intermittently. Both gonadal veins were studied in 320 of the 450 patients. The left gonadal vein was almost always catheterized. Although initially the orifice of the right gonadal vein in the vena cava was difficult to enter, more experience allowed location of this orifice in 80% of the attempts. Catheterization through the arm may help identify the orifices.

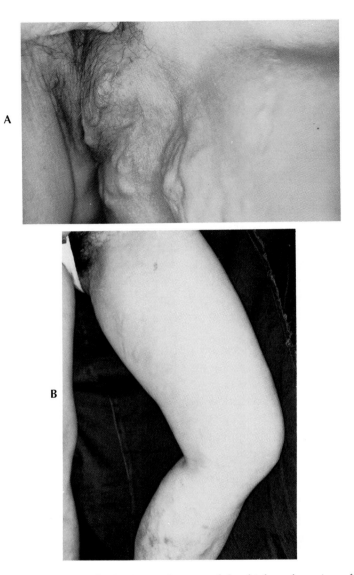

FIGURE 20-1. **A,** Varicose veins beginning at the root of the thigh at the union of the external border of the labia with the inner face of the thigh. **B,** Varicosities cascade down to the leg; they are superficial, deep blue, or violaceous.

One anatomic study revealed variations in the termination of gonadal veins in 22% of cases.[15] Such variations may explain some failures in gonadal phlebography. General findings within our patient group included the following:

1. Dilatation of the utero-ovarian veins with valvular incompetence.
2. Plexiform varicose veins in the pelvis, involving the uterine, vesical, and broad ligament veins (Figure 20-3).

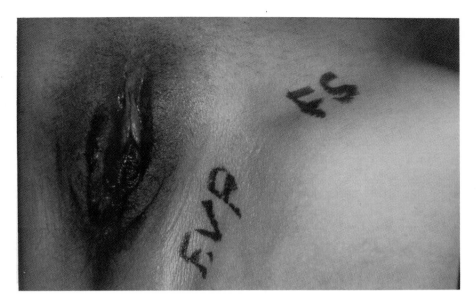

FIGURE 20-2. Two fossae are observed when the patient lies recumbent with the thigh and knee flexed and slightly abducted. Pelvic fossa *(FVP)*; saphenous fossa *(FS)*.

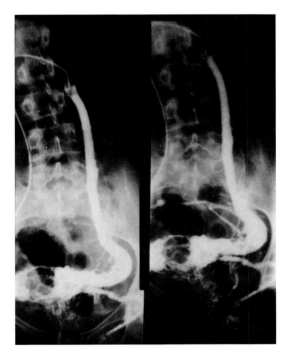

FIGURE 20-3. Dilatation of the left gonadal vein followed by plexiform varices in the pelvis.

3. Varices in the vulva and vagina. "Leaking" of contrast material resulted in filling of varicose veins in the inner and posterior aspects of the thigh (Figure 20-4). This effect has been described as "dumping." We have demonstrated such dumping to knee level by filling varices in this area with injection into the gonadal vein (Figure 20-5). Schobinger[16] has reported examples of dumping from the gonadal veins to varices at the ankle and foot.

4. Drainage of the internal pudendal vein, the obturator veins, and, more rarely, the inferior gluteal vein to the hypogastric vein; drainage of the round ligament vein to the broad ligament veins and of the external pudendal vein to the femoral vein.

5. Filling of the contralateral side in all cases but in varying degrees. Cross-flow explains varices on one side and gonadal insufficiency on the other (Figure 20-6). This situation was present in 11% of our cases.

6. A consistent pattern shows reflux from gonadal veins filling broad ligament veins descending into the vulva and thigh via the obturator, internal pudendal, inferior gluteal, and round ligament veins. Of the last 180 phlebographic studies completed, 140 showed bilateral dilatation and reflux of gonadal veins; 15 studies demonstrated dilatation and reflux only on the left side and 25 only on the right side.

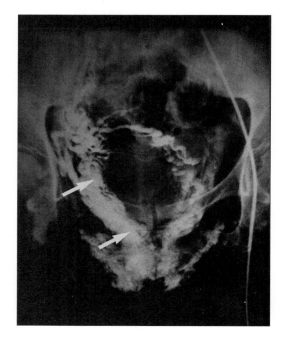

FIGURE 20-4. Vulvar phase of right gonadal phlebography demonstrating filling of vulvar varices via the internal pudendal *(upper arrow)* and the obturator *(lower arrow)* veins. Note filling of both pelvic systems due to pelvic cross-communication and reflux.

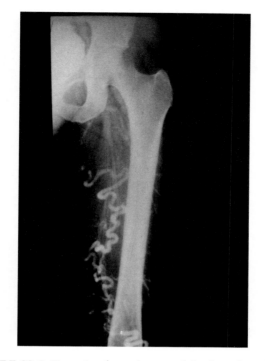

FIGURE 20-5. Dumping from the gonadal vein to knee level.

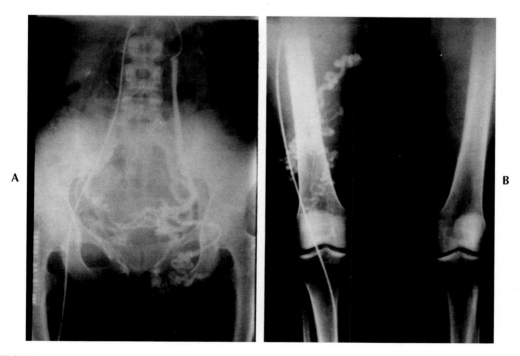

FIGURE 20-6. A, Injection in the left gonadal vein fills veins in the right pelvic and vulvar areas. B, Varices in the right leg are filled from injection in the left gonadal vein.

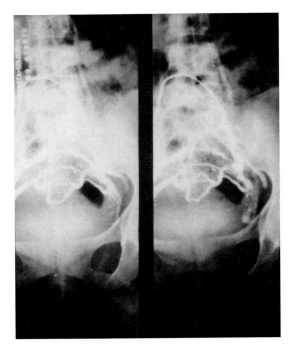

FIGURE 20-7. Pattern of iliac injection. System is competent with no dumping noted.

7. Examination of common, external, and internal iliac veins showed competence. The pattern of iliac injection (Figure 20-7) is different from that of gonadal injection, with 95% of iliac veins being competent.

Surgical Treatment

Gonadal veins are exposed through a curved, almost transverse 6 cm incision located anterior and medial to the anterior iliac spine. Extensive muscle splitting exposes the retroperitoneal space. The gonadal vein is usually attached to peritoneal fat (Figure 20-8). Because the gonadal vein is large and fragile, it is dissected carefully for a few centimeters, ligated, and divided. Hemostats are not used to clamp the vein because they may tear the vessel, producing severe hemorrhage. The ovarian vein is handled with utmost care through the use of atraumatic vascular forceps, and ligatures are passed around and securely tightened above and below the dissected gonadal vein. A careful search for other gonadal veins is performed since at this level the ovarian vein may be double or triple.[15] If a duplication is left unligated, the varicocele may recur. The lower ligature is left long, and dissection of the vein continues into the pelvis (Figure 20-9). As dissection progresses downward, the gonadal vein opens, in an umbrella-like fashion, in front of

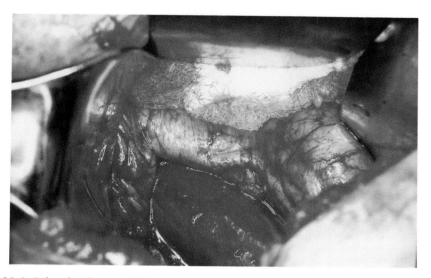

FIGURE 20-8. Dilated right gonadal vein was exposed extraperitoneally. Note the distal bifurcation of the main trunk, psoas muscle, and retroperitoneal fat.

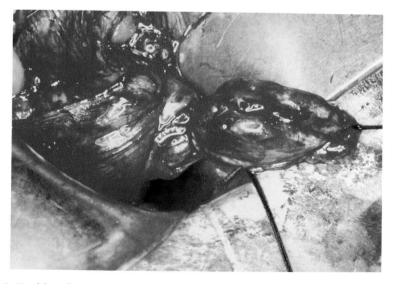

FIGURE 20-9. En bloc dissection and ligature of the gonadal vein into the pelvis anterior to the ovary.

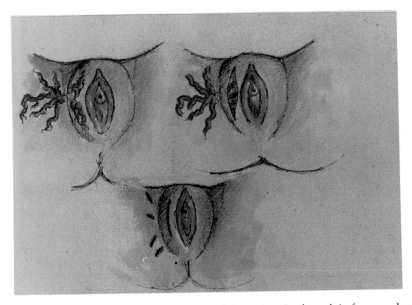

FIGURE 20-10. Varicectomy of vulvar veins. *Upper left:* varices in the pelvic fossa and vulva; *upper right:* vertical incision in the labia to dissect and resect varices; *lower center:* varicectomy completed in the vulva and pelvic fossa with skin sutures shown.

the ovary. Individual ligations are not done because they are difficult, bloody, and time-consuming. Instead, en bloc dissection and ligature are performed at the ovary. At this point, as many as 11 branches usually are found and ligated en masse. A transfixion ligature is applied proximally, near the severed stump.

Muscles and skin are closed in the usual manner. Next, the contralateral gonadal vein is ligated and resected. This step should always be done to avoid failures in the treatment of pelvic and vulvar veins since both gonadal systems communicate freely across the pelvis in the midline. The second part of the operation consists of varicectomy of the vulvar veins (Figure 20-10) and removal of leg veins through small transverse incisions done with the hemostatic technique and varicectomy with crochet-hook needles. Excision of more superficial veins is performed by traction and forcipressure (varicectomy). Alternatively, sclerotherapy can be performed postoperatively. The skin is closed with 5-0 monofilament sutures, and elastic pressure is applied.

Surgical Data and Results

A total of 500 patients presented for treatment. Bilateral gonadal vein ligation was performed in 482 patients (96.4%) (Table 20-1). Unilateral ligations were done in the remaining patients: right gonadal vein resection in 12 patients (2.4%) and left gonadal vein resection in 6 patients (1.2%). During our earliest surgical experience, in 1984 and 1985, my colleagues and I performed ligation

TABLE 20-1. Treatment of pelvic varices in 500 surgical cases, Sept. 1984–Sept. 1997

	No. of Patients	% of Patients
Bilateral resection of gonadal vein	464	92.8
Right gonadal vein resection	24	4.8
Left gonadal vein resection	12	2.4
Vulvar varicectomy	360	72.0
Leg varicectomy (thigh, leg, foot)	500	100.0
Postoperative sclerotherapy	418	90.0

and resection of gonadal veins of the affected side. Currently, we believe that because of cross-communication of pelvic veins and cross-reflux into the vulva and thigh, both gonadal veins should be interrupted. The last 440 patients in our study group had bilateral treatment. Of 80 patients (16%) with saphenous insufficiency, 50 patients (10%) had unilateral insufficiency. The operation was always completed by treating both conditions, pelvic and saphenous. A total of 100 patients (20%) had previous saphenous vein surgery. Among 50 patients (10%), one or more pregnancies followed this surgery and pelvic varices recurred. Recurrent varices after adequate saphenous surgery (24 of our cases) may be treated by gonadal vein resection. Complementary sclerotherapy should be performed on small veins for cosmetic reasons. Most patients (90%) request this additional procedure.

Of the 500 patients, 430 showed excellent results and 50 had good results. A total of 480 patients (96%) had very satisfactory outcomes (Figure 20-11). Sixteen patients had fair outcomes, and four patients showed no improvement, even though the gonadal veins were ligated (both unilateral) and varicose veins were removed (Figure 20-12).

Histopathology*

Microscopic and ultramicroscopic findings. From the inception of the resection of gonadal veins in 1984, we have been gathering gonadal vein tissue for microscopic and ultramicroscopic analysis.

In the process of alteration of the venous wall, the first change is modification of the thickness. Muscular hypertrophy occurs, and the longitudinal fibers of the internal elastic lamella are often disrupted by collagen, which is seen as the

---

*I am grateful to Drs. Fernando Velandia and Esperanza Theuzaba for their help in providing and reading this material on pathology.

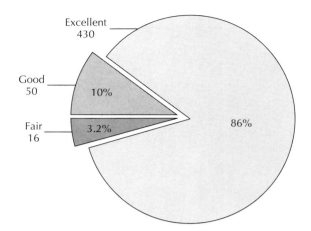

Excellent
430

Good
50

10%

Fair
16

3.2%

86%

FIGURE 20-11. Results of treatment of pelvic varices in 500 surgical cases (Sept. 1984–Sept. 1997).

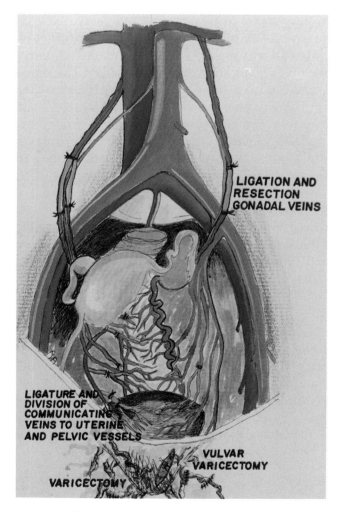

LIGATION AND
RESECTION
GONADAL VEINS

LIGATURE AND
DIVISION OF
COMMUNICATING
VEINS TO UTERINE
AND PELVIC VESSELS

VULVAR
VARICECTOMY

VARICECTOMY

FIGURE 20-12. Artist's view of the complete operation for the treatment of pelvic varices and gonadal veins. Bilateral gonadal resection and ligation with vulvar and leg varicectomy are shown.

orange color dissecting this layer (Figure 20-13). In more advanced cases dilatation of the vein (Figure 20-14) is noted, and herniation of muscular fibers occurs through fibrotic collagen bands, resulting in a pseudoaneurysm and venous dilatation. The trichromic stain shows tortuosity of the wall and sacular dilatation (Figure 20-15). Microscopy of high optical resolution (MOAR) shows replacement, disarray, and disorientation of the muscular fibers, especially in the circular intermediate layer (Figure 20-16). It is very important to stress that inflammation has never been seen in this pathologic material.

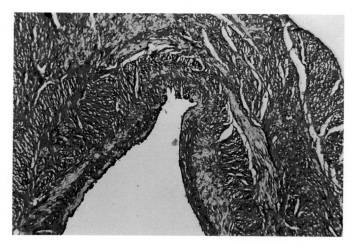

FIGURE 20-13. In muscular hypertrophy collagen fibers disrupt the internal elastic.

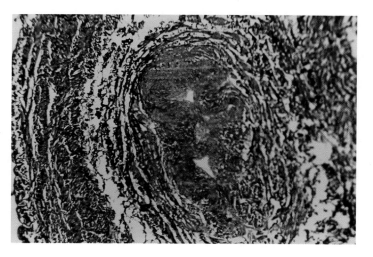

FIGURE 20-14. Dilation of the vein.

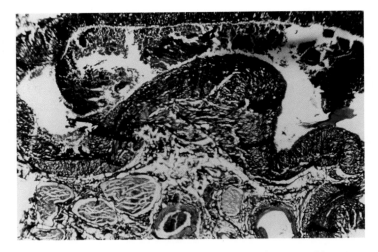

FIGURE 20-15. Tortuosity of the vein wall and venous dilatation.

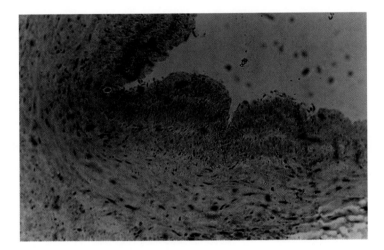

FIGURE 20-16. Replacement, disarray, and disorientation of the muscular fibers.

Electron microscopy shows disorganization of the size of the muscular fiber with increased cellularity and increment of the connective tissue in the media circular layer *(Y)*. Polarity is lost in this layer and is replaced by connective tissue and collagen fibers (Figure 20-17).

The gonadal vein (Figure 20-18) shows circular muscular fibers, cell body, and central nuclei with almost 100% replacement by collagen fibers.

From this study there is ample evidence that the venous wall is abnormal and dilates, giving way secondarily to valve incompetence.

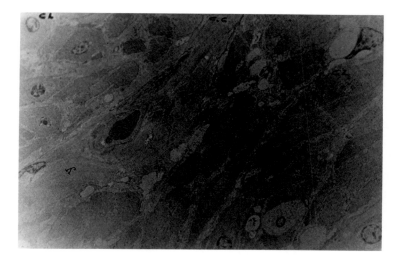

FIGURE 20-17. Magnification (×3000) of increment of connective tissue in media. Circular layer *(Y)* polarity is lost. Replacement is by collagen fibers.

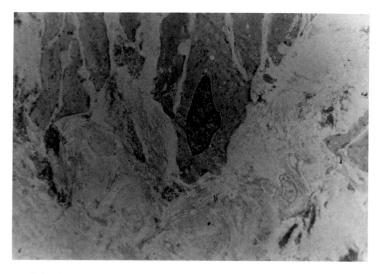

FIGURE 20-18. Cell body, showing central nuclei with almost 100% replacement by collagen fibers.

Discussion

Pelvic veins have been the subject of observation for many years. Lea Thomas et al.[17] described veins that appear during pregnancy in the vulva and labia and on the medial and posterior thigh. The cause was proposed to be from reflux through the internal pudendal and obturator veins from the high-pressure internal iliac vein into the thin-walled vulvar and inner thigh veins, which dilate during pregnancy and occasionally do not disappear. This change was believed to give rise to premenstrual symptoms of vulvar and thigh congestion and pain. Varicectomy was advised as treatment.[18,19]

Craig and Hobbs[5] demonstrated the association of pelvic congestion syndrome and vulvar varices. They advocated vulvar venography to demonstrate drainage into the internal iliac vein via the obturator and internal pudendal veins for visualization of pelvic varicosities in the vesical plexus and broad ligaments. Sumner[20] stated, "Vulvar veins may persist postpartum giving rise to varicosities that extend from the posteromedial thigh down the back of the leg to the posterior and lateral aspect of the thigh and popliteal fossa. They can become congested and painful, especially before the onset of menstruation." Vulvar and leg varicectomy was advised by Craig and Hobbs[5] as treatment.

By performing phlebographic studies in late pregnancy, Kerr et al.[21] showed complete compression of the inferior vena cava and iliac veins against the lumbar spine and psoas muscle, with venous return provided by ascending lumbar and azygous systems and ovarian veins draining the uterus. In 1918 Ivanissevich advanced the theory that varicoceles in males were produced by retrograde flow in the left spermatic vein and described his operation. Interest in the study of pelvic venous circulation increased after the publication of the classic work by Guilhem and Baux[1] in 1954.

Intrauterine phlebography provides considerable information on pelvic pathology and the course of gonadal veins.[22-25] Excellent reviews on pelvic congestion syndrome published by Hobbs,[26] Langeron and Quehen,[27] and many others have aided our understanding of pelvic congestion pain. Retrograde injection techniques, especially selective catheterization of the gonadal vein,[2-4,28] are reliable and successful methods of identifying the anatomy and pathology of these vessels. Ahlberg et al.[4] found that ovarian veins are larger than spermatic veins because of distention of their walls during pregnancy and menses. This dilatation may persist when involution is not complete after pregnancy.

From a review of the literature and confirmation through our experience, we recommend bilateral resection of gonadal veins with ligation of their communications to uterine veins. This procedure interrupts high-pressure reflux into vulvar and thigh veins. The operation represents a radical treatment of varicoceles in females. High ligation should be complemented by complete resection of distal dilated varices, including treatment of insufficiency of the saphenofemoral junction if present. In keeping with this concept, vulvar, thigh, and leg varices should be eliminated at the same time.

PELVIC CONGESTION SYNDROME

The pelvic congestion syndrome is always associated with chronic pelvic pain (pelvagia). It is an elusive and frustrating problem, particularly when no somatic pathologic condition is found. In such a situation the patient is labeled as "psychosomatic" and referred to a specialist in emotional or behavioral problems or to a pain clinic. The emotional impact of pain on the patient may be alleviated by anesthesiologists or psychologists; however, if an organic condition persists, pain resurfaces and a vicious cycle occurs.[29,30]

As a final option, the treating physician frequently resorts to performing a hysterectomy of a normal uterus. This method often fails to relieve the patient's pain. It is believed that approximately 70,000 hysterectomies are performed annually in the United States to alleviate chronic pelvic pain. Although the percentage of normal tissue in this group is unknown, it is believed to be high. Of women referred to the pelvagia clinic at the Naval Hospital in San Diego, 14% had previously undergone hysterectomy and salpingo-oophorectomy with poor results.[31]

Our interest in pelvic congestion syndrome arose from talks with John Hobbs in 1985 about the publication of his article on this syndrome in 1976.[32,33] Our experience covers a 12-year period, from 1986 through 1998. A group of gynecologists was briefed on the coexistence of pelvic varicocele and pelvic pain. They were persuaded not to perform hysterectomies in patients with pelvic varicocele because hysterectomy involves close contact with the uterine body and cervix, resulting in ovarian varicoceles and dilated veins of the broad ligament. Instead, bilateral gonadal vein ligation and resection was suggested for these patients. The steps taken to approach the problem were as follows:

1. Rule out and, if present, treat all organic causes of chronic pelvic pain, such as endometriosis, adhesions, inflammation, tumors, and urinary or rectal pathology.
2. Perform a careful psychologic and/or psychiatric examination.
3. Always perform laparoscopy for positive diagnosis of pelvic varicocele. Gonadal phlebography is rarely required.
4. For optimum results, perform a complete and bilateral gonadal vein ligation and resection.

Fifty-six patients with pelvic congestion syndrome were treated previously for organic problems or had received psychiatric care. Approximately one half of these patients developed relapses from their treatments. Of the 56 patients, 10 had hysterectomies. All patients were women (except our first male patient), ages 24 to 42 years, multiparous (two to four pregnancies), and sexually active. Table 20-2 shows the clinical profile of these patients. This group is distinct from those previously described, who had pelvic varices, varicose leg veins, or vulvar veins. All patients suffered from varying degrees of chronic pelvic pain, which was often incapacitating and at times reflected to the lower back, buttocks, vulva, and upper thighs. To visualize the varicocele, laparoscopy was performed on all patients. Tilting the lower end of the table and having the patient perform a Valsalva maneuver enhanced the varicocele. Only six patients required gonadal vein phlebography to confirm a tentative diagnosis of varicocele through laparoscopy.

Veins at the root of the thigh and the vulval area often became painful, and they dilated before menstruation and after coitus. Vulval symptoms were present in 50% of patients. The most common symptom, except for pelvic pain, was dyspareunia, which was present in 75% of patients. This troublesome condition caused anxiety and depression and was associated with increased marital problems. The frustration associated with dyspareunia is probably the most distressing

TABLE 20-2. Pelvic congestion syndrome: Clinical profile of 56 patients before undergoing bilateral gonadal vein resection

Signs and Symptoms	No. of Patients
Chronic pelvic pain	56
Dyspareunia	40
Vulval symptoms	28
Psychosomatic symptoms	24
Premenstrual syndrome	24
Leg symptoms and varices	20
Vulval varices	18
Dysmenorrhea	16
Urinary symptoms	10
Posthysterectomy	10
Rectal symptoms	6

manifestation of pelvic congestion syndrome and often leads to secondary frigidity. Approximately one half of these patients were incapacitated for several days by premenstrual symptoms and/or dysmenorrhea. One third of this group had vulvar or leg varices with related symptoms. Varicectomy of vulvar or leg veins was performed with gonadal vein surgery in 38 patients. Of particular interest were the 10 patients who had undergone previous hysterectomies for various causes; they all had large varicoceles. Four of these patients had very large dilated veins, all on the right side.

These 56 patients, referred to us by gynecologists, were seen and operated on between May 1986 and April 1998. Six of them underwent laparotomy, hysterectomy, and bilateral gonadal vein ligation. Fifty patients had retroperitoneal dissection of gonadal veins, resection of a segment of 5 to 8 cm of the right and left ovarian veins down to the ovary, and ligation of the upper and lower stumps.

Surgery was followed by an uneventful recovery, with no complications. Both the patients and the physicians were highly pleased with the results. In 40 patients the outcome was excellent; in 16 patients the results were good, with only minor postoperative complaints. To our surprise, patients who had suffered symptoms for 10 years had no further pelvic pain, dyspareunia, or premenstrual symptoms after surgery. Even the emotional characteristics of some patients improved after relief from the pain and other symptoms.

The First Male Patient

This 40-year-old male patient has had repeated episodes of excruciating pain in the right groin irradiating to the right testicle. At presentation, he had bilateral

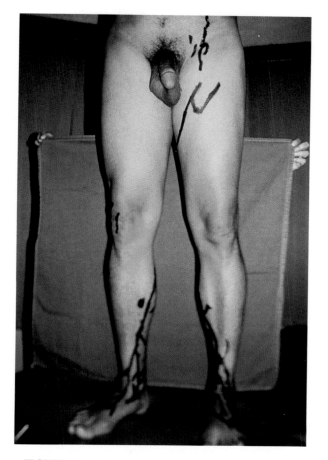

FIGURE 20-19. Varicose veins of the "pelvic" type.

varicose veins of the "pelvic" type and bilateral varicocele (Figures 20-19 and 20-20).

Duplex color echography showed severe reflux and dilatation of the pampiniform plexus bilaterally.

Gonadal phlebography demonstrated insufficiency of both the right and the left gonadal vein and bilateral filling of the varicoceles with dumping into the leg veins (Figures 20-21 and 20-22).

On April 3, 1998, this patient underwent surgery. Bilateral gonadal vein resection and ligation and extensive leg varicectomy were performed with an excellent outcome (Figure 20-23). Pelvic congestion disappeared for 2 months after surgery.

In light of the excellent surgical results we have been able to achieve, we will continue to perform this surgery in well-chosen cases. We recommend that physicians who have patients with chronic pelvic pain associated with varicocele perform bilateral gonadal vein resection and ligation.

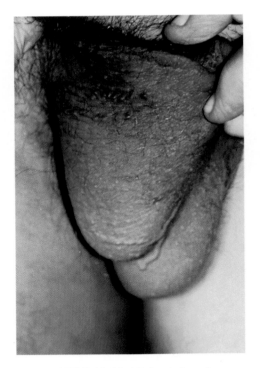

FIGURE 20-20. Right varicocele.

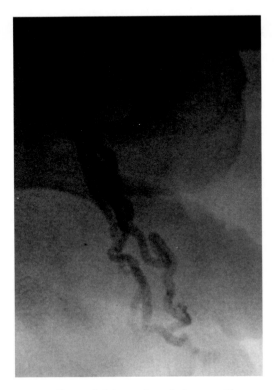

FIGURE 20-21. Filling of right varicocele from orifice at caval wall.

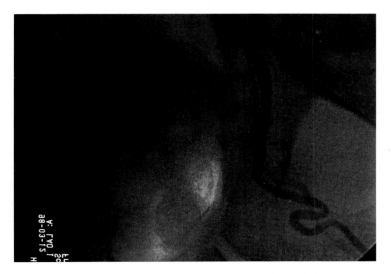

FIGURE 20-22. Filling of left varicocele from orifice at left renal vein.

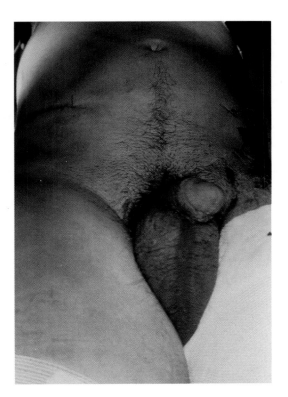

FIGURE 20-23. Postoperative aspect showing incisions and bandages. Varicoceles have disappeared.

REFERENCES

1. Guilhem P, Baux R. La Phlebographie Pelvienne par Voies Veineuse, Osseuse et Utérine. Paris: Masson et Cie, 1954.
2. Ahlberg NE, Bartley O, Chidekel N. Right and left gonadal veins: An anatomical and statistical study. Acta Radiol 4:593-601, 1966.
3. Chidekel N. Female pelvic veins demonstrated by selective renal phlebography with particular reference to pelvic varicosities. Acta Radiol 7:198, 1968.
4. Ahlberg NE, Bartley O, Chidekel N. Retrograde contrast filling of the left gonadal vein. A roentgenologic and anatomical study. Acta Radiol 3:385, 1965.
5. Craig O, Hobbs JT. Vulvar phlebography in the pelvic congestion syndrome. Clin Radiol 25:517, 1975.
6. Gomez ER, Villavicencio JL, Coffey JM, Rich NM. Pathogenesis and surgical management of varicose veins of the vulva and upper thigh: The internal iliac venous insufficiency syndrome. In Veith FJ, ed. Current Critical Problems in Vascular Surgery, vol 2. St. Louis: Quality Medical Publishing, 1990, pp 141-142.
7. Le Page PA, Villavicencio JL, Gomez ER, Sheridan MN, Rich NM. The valvular anatomy of the iliac venous system and its clinical implications. J Vasc Surg 14:678-683, 1991.
8. Hobbs JT. Personal communication. Vienna, 1990.
9. Lechter A. Pelvic varices: Treatment. J Cardiovasc Surg 26:111, 1985.
10. Lechter A, Alvarez A. Pelvic varices and gonadal veins. In Negus D, Jantet G, eds. Phlebology 1985. London: John Libbey, 1986, pp 225-228.
11. Lechter A, Alvarez A, Lopez G. Pelvic varices and gonadal veins. Phlebology 2:181-188, 1987.
12. Lechter A, Lopez G, Franco CA, Martinez C, Camacho J. New concepts in the clinical, radiological and surgical aspects of varices of pelvic origin [abstract]. Vienna: Fifth European American Venous Symposium, 1990.
13. Schraibman IG, Hobbs JT. Pelvic congestion syndrome and ligation of ovarian veins [letter]. Br J Hosp Med 44:14, 1990.
14. Richardson G, Beckwith TC, Sheldon M. Ultrasound assessment in the treatment of pelvic varicose veins. Fort Lauderdale: Third American Venous Forum, 1991.
15. Lechter A, Lopez G, Martinez C, Camacho J. Anatomy of the gonadal veins: A reappraisal. Surgery 109:735-739, 1991.
16. Schobinger RA. Ilio-femoral dumping syndrome [abstract]. Vienna: Fifth European American Venous Symposium, 1990.
17. Lea Thomas M, Fletcher EWL, Andress MR, Cockett FB. The venous connections of vulvar varices. Clin Radiol 18:313, 1967.
18. Dodd H, Payling-Wright H. Vulval varicose veins in pregnancy. BMJ (Clin Res) 1:831-832, 1959.
19. Dixon JA, Mitchell WA. Venographic and surgical observations in vulval varicose veins. Surg Gynecol Obstet 131:458-464, 1970.
20. Sumner DS. Venous dynamics varicosities. Clin Obstet Gynecol 24:743-761, 1981.
21. Kerr MG, Scott DB, Samuel E. Studies of the inferior vena cava in late pregnancy. BMJ 1:532, 1964.
22. Topolanski-Sierra R. Am J Obstet Gynecol 76:44, 1958.
23. Chidekel N, Edlundh KO. Transuterine phlebography with particular reference to pelvic varicosities. Acta Radiol 7:1, 1968.
24. Jaramillo R, Mejia A, Morales H. Flebografía pélvica y varicocele del ligamento ancho. Tribuna Medica 4:1-19, 1965.
25. Mayall RC, Dias Garcia Mayall AC, Moreira Jannuzzi JC. Varices pelviennes de la femme. Phlebologie 36:191-195, 1983.
26. Hobbs JT. Treatment of vulval and pelvic varices. In Bergan JJ, Yao JST, eds. Venous Disorders. Philadelphia: WB Saunders, 1991, pp 250-257.
27. Langeron P, Quehen E. Les algies pelviennes chez la femme. Ann Chir 19-20:1096-1108, 1966.

28. Helander CG, Lindbom A. Varicocele of the broad ligament: A venographic study. Acta Radiol 53:97, 1960.
29. Beard RW, Reginald PW, Pearce S. Pelvic pain in women. BMJ 293:1160-1162, 1986.
30. Beard RW, Highman JH, Pearce S, Reginald PW. Diagnosis of pelvic varicosities in women with chronic pelvic pain. Lancet 2:946, 1984.
31. Reiter RC. Alteraciones somáticas ocultas en mujeres con dolor pélvico crónico. In Pitkin RM, Scott JR, eds. Clínicas Obstétricas y Ginecológicas, vol 1. Apdo: McGraw-Hill Interamericana de México, 1990, pp 155-160.
32. Hobbs JT. The pelvic congestion syndrome. Practitioner 216:529-540, 1976.
33. Hobbs JT. The pelvic congestion syndrome. Br J Hosp Med 43:200-206, 1990.

Editor's Note

Dr. Lechter has elegantly described the classic presentation of pelvic venous congestion. What has been learned since his presentation is that in patients with pelvic pain of venous origin the discomfort is of variable intensity, is worse premenstrually, and is increased by fatigue, standing, and coitus. The condition is well described, and its treatment is nicely illustrated in texts in North America, but it is a well-known fact that physicians, vascular surgeons, and general surgeons have even less knowledge of the condition and its treatment than do gynecologists. For example, the symptom of urinary urgency is actually interpreted as frequency by most surgeons, but in fact it is due to the pressure of pelvic varices on the bladder, giving the feeling that the bladder is full and needs emptying. The postcoital pain is misinterpreted as dyspareunia.

The symptoms lead to sociopsychologic factors that become important in women with chronic pelvic pain.[1] It is thought that in the subgroup of patients with pelvic venous congestion early social experience may play an important role. In particular, the father-daughter relationship may be relevant. Hostility patterns influence the development of the condition.

Because diagnosis is extremely important, imaging methods are of crucial relevance.[2] Although MRI of ovarian reflux is theoretically ideal, in fact the patient is examined in the horizontal rather than the vertical position, which limits the utility of this examination. Ultrasound has been used, and there are defined windows that allow examination of the ovarian veins; however, this requires great expertise.

Ultimately, since radiologic diagnosis that includes contrast media and digital subtraction will define the syndrome exactly, the patient can be counseled on diagnosis and treatment at one stage.[3] The treatment is similar to that of varicocele in men, and transcatheter retrograde venous embolization can be done with a series of coils. What has been learned is that the pelvic pain syndrome disappears in all patients within 4 weeks and that if the treatment is given bilaterally, marked ovarian varices will be obliterated and the chronic pain of pelvic congestion after intercourse and the urinary urgency symptoms can be markedly relieved.

Long-term observation of the initial technical success, which exceeds 95%, declines to 73% at 1 year.[4] Since patients who complain of dyspareunia in particular are not relieved, a clear differentiation between true dyspareunia and postcoital pelvic congestion is necessary. Clearly, pelvic congestion is an important syndrome, and it must be searched for diligently by physicians interested in treating venous disorders.[5]

REFERENCES

1. Fry RP, Beard RW, Crisp AH, McGuigan S. Sociopsychological factors in women with chronic pelvic pain with and without pelvic venous congestion. J Psychosom Res 42:71-85, 1997.
2. Kennedy A, Hemingway A. Radiology of ovarian varices. Br J Hosp Med 44:38-43, 1990.
3. Tarazov PG, Prozorovskij KV, Ryzhkov VK. Pelvic pain syndrome caused by ovarian varices: Treatment by transcatheter embolization. Acta Radiol 38:1023-1025, 1997.
4. Capasso P, Simons C, Trotteur G, Dondelinger RF, Henroteaux D, Gaspard U. Treatment of symptomatic pelvic varices by ovarian vein embolization. Cardiovasc Intervent Radiol 20:107-111, 1997.
5. Sichlau MJ, Yao JST, Vogelzang RL. Transcatheter embolotherapy for the treatment of pelvic congestion syndrome. Obstet Gynecol 83:892-896, 1994.

PART FIVE

Telangiectatic Leg Veins

Chapter 21

Treatment of Telangiectasias

Paul K. Thibault

Lower limb telangiectasias are visible, ectatic dermal veins measuring 0.1 to 1 mm in diameter.[1-4] Initially telangiectasias appear as faint erythematous lines, but with time they become progressively more dilated, tortuous, and elevated above the skin surface and turn blue. The term "venulectasia" is used to describe larger blue telangiectasias measuring 1 to 2 mm in diameter.[5] Invariably telangiectasias are closely associated with either dilated subcutaneous reticular veins or varicose veins[6] (Figure 21-1). Frequently a family history of similar abnormally dilated lower limb veins is noted,[4] but this factor is not invariable. Polygenetic inheritance from maternal or paternal lines is the probable mode of transmission of the susceptibility to form telangiectasias, with hormonal influences (particularly estrogen) being pivotal in the ultimate expression of the disorder. Hence telangiectasias are more common in women; their onset frequently is precipitated by the hormonal surges of menarche and pregnancy.[7] In certain patients telangiectasias may develop or may be aggravated by treatment with oral contraceptives or menopausal hormone replacement therapy.[8] The most common time of presentation for treatment is between the ages of 30 and 50 years, but with the modern trend of emphasizing physical attractiveness, presentation as early as 15 years and as late as 75 years is not unusual. It is uncommon for men to seek treatment for lower limb telangiectasias.

Unattractive or disfiguring visual appearance is the most common presenting symptom of patients with telangiectasias. However, mild to severe pain is also a well-recognized symptom.[5] Isaacs[9] has found that aching/pain, excessive tiredness/fatigue, and throbbing in the legs correlate well with patients presenting with nonbulging reticular veins and telangiectasias compared with a matching control group. Furthermore, these symptoms were independent of the size of the veins. Because the most common reason for requesting treatment is to achieve cosmetic improvement, it is essential that effective treatment be relatively free of adverse sequelae.

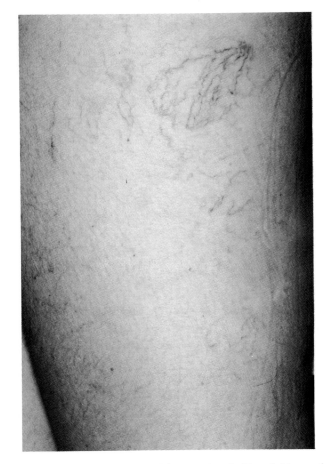

FIGURE 21-1. Lateral thigh telangiectasias with associated dilated blue subcutaneous reticular veins.

HISTORICAL BACKGROUND

In 1934 Biegeleisen[6] described a microinjection technique for treating telangiectasias. He used sodium morrhuate (a mixture of sodium salts of the saturated and unsaturated fatty acids present in cod liver oil), but frequently complications occurred, for example, cutaneous ulceration, pigmentation, and allergic reactions including anaphylaxis. It became clear that there was an obvious need for a mild sclerosing agent free of adverse local and systemic effects.

In 1925 Jausion had recommended chromated glycerin as a sclerosing agent for varicose veins, but because of the mild action of this agent it was eventually discarded for that purpose. However, in France the high safety profile of chromated glycerin for injection of small veins was recognized, and in the 1950s this agent became the most commonly used substance for the treatment of telangiectasias in that country.[10]

Polidocanol was developed in the 1960s as a topical, local, and epidural anesthetic, but its use as an anesthetic was discontinued when it was found to sclerose small-diameter blood vessels through intravascular or intradermal injection. The use of polidocanol as a therapeutic sclerosant for varicose veins was first described by Eichenberger[11] in 1969. Because of its relatively low incidence of adverse effects, polidocanol eventually was popularized as a safe sclerosant for treatment of telangiectasias by Ouvry et al.[12] In the 1970s Foley[13] and Alderman[14] described their experiences with the use of hypertonic saline solution in concentrations of 18% to 20%. Subsequently, the use of hypertonic saline with and without additives soon became popular with North American dermatologists influenced by the absence of antigenicity of unadulterated hypertonic saline solution when compared with other agents.[15]

Sodium tetradecyl sulfate (STS) was first described in 1946,[16] and it was popularized by Fegan[17] for the treatment of varicose veins. However, STS caused an unacceptable incidence of cutaneous ulceration and pigmentation when the commercially produced 1% solution was used for the injection of small veins.[18] Consequently, polidocanol (in Europe) and hypertonic saline solution (in North America) were preferred for the treatment of telangiectasias. Recently, with the correct dilution of STS ranging from 0.1% to 0.2%, this sclerosant has been widely used for treating telangiectasias.

Although steady progress has been made in using sclerotherapy as a therapeutic modality for telangiectasias, other forms of treatment, namely, electrosurgery and laser photocoagulation, have been used. However, they have not achieved acceptance because of their ineffectiveness and adverse sequelae. Electrosurgery of telangiectasias was first used in the early 1900s, but the electrical current required to desiccate cutaneous vessels resulted in dermal necrosis with varying degrees of scarring. Since 1975 various lasers have been used in photocoagulation of lower limb telangiectasias, but enthusiasm for this method has been dampened by the relative ineffectiveness of laser surgery compared with sclerotherapy. Also, laser therapy has been associated with adverse sequelae, including hypopigmentation, hyperpigmentation, cutaneous necrosis, and pain. However, certain lasers have been shown to be safe and effective for fine red telangiectasias <0.1 mm in diameter.[19] Recently a pulsed photothermal device has been shown to give good results in treating leg veins ranging in size from 0.1 to 3 mm in diameter.[20] A complete discussion of laser and intense pulsed-light treatment of leg veins is given in Chapter 22. Hence the remainder of this chapter deals exclusively with sclerotherapy of telangiectasias.

HISTORY AND EXAMINATION

The patient who presents with telangiectasias first should have a directed history taken and a physical examination done. Important information to obtain in the history includes age of onset, possibility of aggravation by past pregnancies, and whether the condition is stable or deteriorating. It is important to note whether the patient's chief complaint is predominantly cosmetic- or pain-related because this factor may significantly influence the patient's expectations regarding treatment outcomes and consequently may affect treatment decisions. History taking should focus on whether the patient has had any bleeding disorders, episodes of superficial thrombophlebitis or deep venous thrombosis, or previous treatment, including surgery and sclerotherapy. Past and present use of hormonal contraceptives and hormonal replacement therapy, cigarette smoking, and allergy to any medications also should be noted. A thorough family history provides valuable information about the potential severity of the telangiectasia.

Examination of the lower limbs is best performed with the patient standing on a platform in front of the physician. Good lighting is essential for a systematic inspection of each aspect of the leg from the groin to the toes. The patterns of telangiectasias and their relationships to underlying reticular and varicose veins must be noted. It is important to remember that patients with cosmetic symptoms associated with lower limb telangiectatic veins may have incompetence of the major superficial veins (long or short saphenous veins). In a study of patients presenting with cosmetic symptoms related to lower limb superficial veins, duplex imaging evaluation of limbs with telangiectasias without clinical evidence of associated bulging varicose veins revealed a significant incidence of incompetence in the long or short saphenous veins (Table 21-1).[21] It is uncommon, however, for telangiectasias to be associated with deep venous incompetence. Therefore after physical examination further diagnostic evaluation with Doppler ultrasound or duplex imaging should be considered if there is clinical suspicion of incompetence of the long or short saphenous systems. For example, telangiectasias occurring on the medial aspect of the leg are frequently associated with incompetence in the long saphenous system.[22] In particular, the appearance of telangiectasias on the proximal medial calf should arouse suspicion of incompetence in the long saphenous vein and necessitate further evaluation with Doppler ultrasound or duplex imaging.[23] In the absence of obvious truncal varices, the incompetence is generally segmental with a competent saphenofemoral junction.

TABLE 21-1. Venous incompetence according to clinical classification*

	Telangiectasias Only (N = 83)	Telangiectasias and Varicose Veins (N = 314)	Varicose Veins Only (N = 84)
Average age (yr)	39.7	41.4	42.5
Superficial incompetence (%)	22.9	49.0	66.7
Deep incompetence (%)	0	1.6	1.2
Perforator incompetence (%)	1.2	10.6	13.1

*Modified from Thibault P, Bray A, Wlodarczyk J. Cosmetic leg veins: Evaluation using duplex venous imaging. J Dermatol Surg Oncol 16:612-618, 1990. Reprinted by permission. Copyright 1990 by Elsevier Science Publishing Co., Inc.

Isolated telangiectasias located on the middle and distal calf should arouse the suspicion of short saphenous vein incompetence. If Doppler examination confirms reflux in the short saphenous system, duplex imaging is required to determine the extent of incompetence and whether the short saphenous vein terminates in the popliteal vein or femoropopliteal vein or as a branch of the thigh segment of the long saphenous vein (Giacomini vein).[23]

Finally, clinical photographs should be taken to document the pretreatment state of all affected areas. This step is essential to assess progress during treatment and to clarify whether adverse sequelae (e.g., telangiectatic matting) have occurred as a result of treatment. A high standard of photography is required, and color transparencies are the preferred medium. Good results normally will be achieved by using a 35 mm single-lens reflex camera with macrolens combined with a macroflash unit. Recently, high-resolution digital cameras have become available. It is likely that in time these will become the preferred means of taking clinical photographs because they allow attachment of clinical photographs to a patient's computerized records, offering significant advantages in storage and retrieval. The background for photographs should be plain and uncluttered. For color photographs a neutral background, such as light blue, is recommended. Progress photographs taken during treatment are necessary only to document unusual or adverse effects.

At the time of initial consultation, the patient should be informed fully about the treatment, the expected outcome, and the nature and likelihood of any adverse effects. This information should be made available to the patient in the form of a comprehensive information leaflet or brochure that the patient can refer to during treatment. Patients with cosmetic symptoms related to telangiectasias often have high expectations for the ultimate outcome, and a realistic goal should be agreed on between patient and physician before treatment is begun.

THE SCLEROTHERAPY ROOM

Since a visit to the sclerotherapist can be a traumatic experience for some patients, a relaxing environment is essential. A warm and neutral decor and soothing background music will assist in relaxing the anxious patient and, in turn, will aid the sclerotherapist in performing his or her work efficiently.

The patient is placed in the supine position on a table positioned in the room so that the sclerotherapist can move around it easily. Such placement minimizes the need to reposition the patient and helps to avoid placing the patient in awkward and uncomfortable postures. Good lighting is essential. Well-placed overhead fluorescent lighting provides shadow-free illumination and obviates the need for additional accessory floor lights, which can become obstacles. Fluorescent lighting also is superior to incandescent lighting for highlighting the blue colors of reticular veins. Overhead "operating" spotlights have been recommended,[24] but such lights are expensive and generate heat in the room, making the temperature uncomfortable for both the patient and the sclerotherapist.

A stool is situated on either side of the treatment table. In general, sclerotherapy of small veins should be performed with the sclerotherapist in the sitting position, which allows the physician to rest his or her arms on the sides of the table for greater steadiness. Either the table or the stool should be readily adjustable in height to optimize the position of the patient relative to the physician. A Mayo stand should be easily accessible to the sclerotherapist, especially if a nurse is not assisting. The stand is equipped with sclerosant solutions, needles, syringes, compression pads, gauze swabs, alcohol solution, and emergency drugs.

TREATMENT PLAN

The presence of telangiectasias should not be considered in isolation from the larger veins into which they drain. If one disregards treatment of reticular veins and proceeds directly to microsclerotherapy of telangiectasias, early recurrence will be noted in most instances because of persisting pressure from proximal sources of superficial venous reflux. There will also be an increased incidence of postsclerotherapy hyperpigmentation and telangiectatic matting. Therefore sclerotherapy of telangiectasias should follow a systematic plan, consisting of the following steps: (1) treatment of associated long or short saphenous vein incompetence (if present), (2) treatment of branch varicosities (if present), (3) sclerotherapy of associated reticular veins, and (4) microsclerotherapy of telangiectasias. Steps 1 and 2 are discussed in Chapters 9, 11, 13, 14, and 15 and therefore are not discussed here.

Treatment of Reticular Veins

The distinction between reticular and varicose veins is arbitrary. In this chapter reticular veins are defined as those abnormally dilated subcutaneous veins that are blue and nonbulging, measure 1 to 3 mm in diameter, and are directly associated with telangiectasias. These reticular veins are seen most commonly over the posterolateral aspect of the thigh and the lateral aspect of the calf. In general, they appear to drain toward the popliteal fossa, with the associated telangiectasias radiating away from the knee (see Chapter 23).

Order of Treatment

As with sclerotherapy of varicose veins, the order of treatment should proceed from proximal to distal, from areas of reflux downstream, and from larger caliber veins to smaller caliber veins.[10,24] A good method is to begin giving injections at the proximal posterior thigh with the patient lying prone and to proceed distally toward the ankle before changing the patient to the lateral position. Again, injections are commenced from proximal to distal points. Next, the anterior and medial aspects of the leg are treated similarly. By using this systematic approach, abnormal veins will not be neglected. Knowing which veins to inject comes with experience, but good lighting will assist in determining the sometimes subtle connections between the cosmetically symptomatic telangiectasias in the dermis and associated abnormally dilated reticular veins in the subcutaneous tissues.

Normally only one limb is treated in a single session, with the number of treatments required determined by the extent and severity of venous dilatation. However, the maximum dose of sclerosing solutions allows complete treatment of reticular veins in one limb to be performed in one or two sessions in approximately 90% of patients.[25] Two different approaches may be used if telangiectasias are extensive and require more than one treatment. The first approach is to treat the reticular veins and associated telangiectasias in one or more adjacent areas in the same session and to leave some untreated until the next session. The second approach is to treat all the reticular veins in the limb in one session and to inject the residual telangiectasias approximately 1 month later.[18] The latter approach often results in fewer injections because many of the telangiectasias fade, either partially or completely, after the source of venous hypertension arising from the reticular veins has been removed. This method has the additional advantage of reducing the incidence of postsclerotherapy hyperpigmentation by allowing a reduction in the strength of sclerosant used when treating the telangiectasias directly.[26]

Injection of Reticular Veins

Two milliliters of sclerosant solution is drawn up in a high-quality, 3 ml plastic disposable syringe fitted with either a 27-gauge or 30-gauge needle, depending on the physician's preference. When injected, the sclerosant should flow easily with a smooth, low-pressure action on the plunger. The advantage of the 27-gauge needle in reducing the plunger pressure is countered by the disadvantage of a slightly more painful skin puncture. Alternatively, a 30-gauge needle is preferred if a slow injection flow rate is required or if the patient is more sensitive to pain or feels anxious. The most common mistake in technique is to transect the vessel on needle insertion. Therefore it is helpful to bend the needle to an angle of 30 to 50 degrees with the bevel up, so that on insertion the bevel will remain pointing upward.

There are two methods of vessel cannulation for reticular veins. The first method is similar to that for injection of telangiectasias, which will be described later. The second method (preferred by many, particularly those who are developing expertise in this field) is to insert the needle slowly but deliberately and to withdraw blood into the hub of the needle (this can be done with both 27-gauge and 30-gauge needles) in order to ensure that the needle bevel is located in the vein lumen before injection. With this method, tissue tension can be achieved by using the dorsal aspect of the nondominant index finger to stretch the patient's skin toward the syringe, which is rested on the pulp of the index finger and distal interphalangeal joint of the middle finger of the nondominant hand (Figure 21-2). If an awkward location (e.g., around the anterior aspect of the knee) prevents adequate tissue tension from being achieved by this method, digital pressure by an assistant may be required. The physician's arms are steadied by either resting

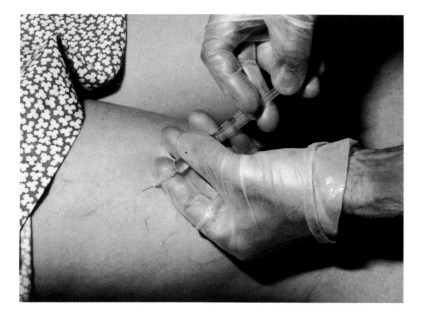

FIGURE 21-2. Blood aspiration technique of injecting reticular veins.

them on the treatment table or, if this is not possible, by gentle pressure of the physician's elbow on the region of the patient's anterior superior iliac spine.

The volume of sclerosant injected depends on ease of flow, concentration of the sclerosant, and diameter of the vein. In general, no more than 0.5 ml should be injected at any one site. Frequently the endpoint is reached when the physician detects a slight increase in resistance to the flow of the solution, denoting vessel spasm. During injection the physician observes the direction of the flow of the sclerosant as the solution replaces blood in the vein and observes for vasospasm. The physician should stop injecting when the desired length of vein has been treated. When a detergent solution is used, the maximum length of a reticular vein that can be treated with one injection is approximately 10 cm. If osmotic solutions are used, more injections may be required because of the more localized effect produced.

During and immediately after injection, the reticular vein undergoes spasm. Within several minutes the vessels and the surrounding skin become erythematous, indicating adequate endothelial damage. This inflammation is more apparent with polidocanol than with STS, hypertonic saline solution, or chromated glycerin. If associated telangiectasias become inflamed during treatment of reticular veins, this effect indicates passage of sclerosant into the telangiectasias, and no further treatment of the telangiectasias is required. However, highly concentrated solutions should not be injected into telangiectasias because this method will result in a higher incidence of postsclerotherapy pigmentation and cutaneous ulceration. Immediately after injection, pressure is applied to the injected veins by using cottonballs with pieces of paper tape stretched firmly over them. Patients usually remark that this method helps to relieve any postinjection pain. Unless the patient has a sensitivity to paper tape, the cottonballs are left in place for 24 to 48 hours.

Microinjection of Telangiectasias

The technique of microinjection of telangiectasias is covered in detail in Chapters 23 and 24. However, a few important points will be described here. As noted earlier, microinjection of telangiectasias can be performed when reticular veins are treated or, alternatively, 4 to 6 weeks later to allow for resolution of venous hypertension from the reticular veins. The order of treatment is identical to that of reticular veins; that is, injection is started proximally and proceeds distally until one particular aspect of the leg has been completed.

Magnifying loupes with powers from 2 to 3.5 magnification are recommended for obtaining good results. However, these may not be necessary for the experienced sclerotherapist. Before injection the skin may be wiped with alcohol. This step changes the refraction coefficient of the skin, making the telangiectasias more visible by indirect lighting. Alcohol also causes some dilatation of the telangiectasias. Disposable 3 ml plastic syringes are used, again filled with 2 ml of sclerosant. All injections are made with a 30-gauge needle, which may need to be changed after three or four injections if it becomes dull. Needles of finer gauge (32- or 33-gauge) can be used for very fine vessels, such as those that occur in telangiectatic matting, but these needles are expensive and dull rapidly.

The physician should be seated in a comfortable position with his or her arms supported as described for injecting reticular veins. Tissue tension can be achieved by using the three-point technique of stretching the patient's skin between the physician's index finger and thumb of the nondominant hand and the fifth digit of the dominant hand, which is holding the syringe (Figure 21-3). Alternatively, two-point tension between the index finger and thumb of the nondominant hand with tension applied diagonally across the line of injection often suffices (Figure 21-4).

The needle should be bent to an angle of 30 to 50 degrees to prevent transection of the vessel. With the physician's dominant hand held steady, the needle tip is rested on the skin surface with the tip initially just piercing the epidermis. A gentle thrust is then made toward the vessel lumen to cannulate the telangiectatic vessel. The feel for this movement develops with experience, and with practice telangiectasias even smaller than the diameter of the needle can be cannulated reliably.[6]

The injection of sclerosant should be slow and limited to a maximum area of approximately 5 cm². Excessive sclerosant concentration or injection pressure is manifested by perivascular blanching followed by acute severe erythema around the telangiectasia. The injection should be stopped at the first indication of extravasation. After one area has been treated, cottonballs fixed with paper tape are applied to the injection sites.

The air-block technique for injecting telangiectasias, in which a small volume of air is injected ahead of the sclerosant, has been recommended by some sclero-

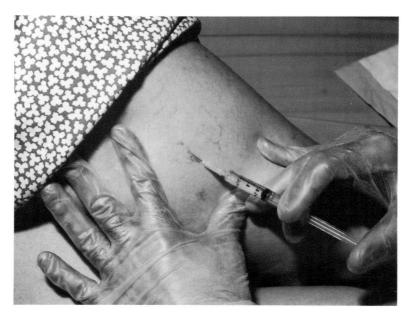

FIGURE 21-3. Three-point tension technique of injecting telangiectasias.

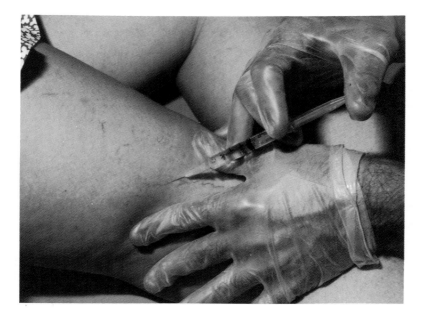

FIGURE 21-4. Two-point tension technique of injecting telangiectasias.

therapists.[2,14] This technique has the advantage of ensuring that the needle tip is located in the vein lumen. In addition, it has been hypothesized that replacement of blood by air results in maximum irritation of the endothelium by the sclerosant. However, this method is usually unnecessary since sclerosant flows in a laminar fashion in vessels <4 mm in diameter,[10] and the experienced physician acquires the "feel" of knowing when the needle tip is located correctly. The air-block technique may be useful for the novice, however, especially when hypertonic saline is being injected because it destroys all cells within its osmotic gradient and therefore is more likely to cause cutaneous necrosis when injected extravascularly.[15] It has been my experience that injecting air with the sclerosant (whether using hypertonic saline or detergent solutions) tends to precipitate visual disturbances or migraines in susceptible individuals.

SCLEROSING AGENTS

The purpose of sclerotherapy is to produce endothelial damage that results in permanent endofibrosis and clinical obliteration of the vessel. The ideal sclerosant would have a highly specific mechanism of action, would be free of adverse effects when used for this purpose, and would not produce allergic reactions. Although many agents have been used in treating telangiectasias, thus far none has completely satisfied the criteria for the ideal sclerosant.

The sclerotherapist should have a sound knowledge of the mechanism of action and the adverse effects of all available solutions in order to select the sclerosant that will optimize results in each patient. The following agents are commonly used in the treatment of telangiectasias.

Osmotic Agents

Osmotic agents exert their effects by dehydrating endothelial cells through osmosis, which results in endothelial destruction. They are hypertonic solutions, and their effect depends on the existence of an osmotic gradient. Because osmotic agents are rapidly diluted in the bloodstream, they lose their potency within a short distance of injection and are less effective in the treatment of veins larger than 3 to 4 mm in diameter.[15]

Hypertonic saline solution. Hypertonic saline is the most commonly used osmotic agent. The advantages of hypertonic saline are its low cost, ready availability, lack of allergenicity of unadulterated solutions, and rapid clinical effect.[13,14,27] It also has been reported to cause less telangiectatic matting compared with polidocanol.[28] The significant adverse effects of hypertonic saline are related to its nonspecific action of destroying cells within its osmotic gradient.[15] Therefore extravascular injection is liable to cause cutaneous ulceration, which can also occur with intravascular injection via diffusion through a damaged endothelium. Diffusion of hypertonic saline through the vein wall also results in irritation of adventitial nerves, causing postinjection pain and transient muscle cramping. Therefore injection technique, concentration, and volume are particularly important when this agent is being used.

Attempts have been made to reduce postinjection pain from hypertonic saline by the addition of local anesthetics such as procaine.[13] However, this practice appears to be counterproductive because the local anesthetics are acidic (and therefore contribute to transient pain on injection) and have known allergenicity, the very properties that proponents of hypertonic saline wish to avoid. The addition of heparin to hypertonic saline in an attempt to prevent thrombosis in larger vessels and to reduce the incidence of thrombophlebitis and postsclerotherapy pigmentation has been found to be of no therapeutic benefit in treating telangiectasias.[29] Concentrations of hypertonic saline used to treat telangiectasias range from 11.7% to 23.4%, the latter being the standard concentration available for use as an abortifacient. The incidence of postinjection pain, muscle cramping, cutaneous ulceration, and postsclerotherapy pigmentation is proportional to the concentration of solution used.[28]

Hypertonic glucose saline solution. Sclerodex (Omega; Montreal, Canada), a mixture of dextrose 250 mg/ml, sodium chloride 100 mg/ml, propylene glycol 100 mg/ml, and phenylethyl alcohol 8 mg/ml, is an osmotic agent used in Canada for the treatment of telangiectasias.[30] The addition of dextrose allows for a reduction of the sodium chloride concentration and osmolarity, which supposedly lessens the pain associated with injection of a more concentrated sodium chloride solution without a reduction in efficacy. The addition of dextrose also may explain its reportedly decreased incidence of postsclerotherapy pigmentation.[15,30] Nevertheless, as with hypertonic saline, particular care needs to be taken with injection technique.

Chromated Glycerin

A chemical irritant, Scleremo (72% chromated glycerin) (Laboratories E Bouteille; Limoges, France) exerts its effect via a direct toxic action on endothelial cells. It has a very mild action and is useful only in sclerosing telangiectasias <0.5 mm in diameter. Use of this agent as a sclerosant has not been approved in the United States or Australia. Postsclerotherapy pigmentation and cutaneous necrosis are rare with this agent, and its use is recommended in those patients who have shown increased sensitivity to other sclerosants. The disadvantages of chromated glycerin are its high viscosity, which results in the solution dripping from the needle tip, and pain on injection. Both of these drawbacks can be overcome partially by dilution with lidocaine.[31] However, this dilution results in a proportional reduction in effectiveness of a solution that already has a very mild action.

Polyiodinated Iodine

Iodine, in the stabilized form of polyiodinated iodine (Sclerodine; Omega, Montreal, Canada) is a chemical irritant with a localized sclerosing effect. Although predominantly used for sclerosing truncal varicose veins using concentrations from 3% to 6%, polyiodinated iodine can be diluted with normal saline or Sclerodex down to concentrations as low as 0.15% to treat telangiectasias. Paravenous injection will cause pain and tissue necrosis, and therefore care should be taken that all injections are totally intravenous. In the treatment of telangiectasias, polyiodinated iodine may be a useful alternative in those patients who are allergic to the detergent solutions.

Detergent Solutions

Detergent solutions include sodium morrhuate, ethanolamine oleate, STS, and polidocanol. These agents act specifically on venous endothelium. They induce sclerosis by damaging the endothelium via interference with cell membrane lipids. They exert their effect along the vessel until either diluted or inactivated by serum surfactants.[15] Only STS and polidocanol are widely used for the treatment of telangiectasias. Table 21-2 gives the approximate equivalent concentrations of STS and polidocanol required for the treatment of lower limb veins. Because of their different mechanisms of action, it is difficult to compare concentrations of detergent solutions with hypertonic saline and Scleremo. However, in the dorsal rabbit ear vein, polidocanol 1% is equivalent in potency to hypertonic saline 23.4%. Scleremo is approximately equivalent in potency to polidocanol 0.25%.[32] Apart from vein diameter, other factors need to be considered in selecting the concentration of solution. Patients younger than 25 years of age generally require weaker solutions to achieve effective sclerosis. Also, care should be taken with elderly patients and cigarette smokers because they may have coexisting diminished cutaneous perfusion, which increases the risk of postsclerotherapy cutaneous necrosis. The area to be treated also influences the choice of concentration. Slightly lower concentrations are required on the medial distal thigh and around the ankle; slightly higher concentrations are needed for treating the lateral and posterior thigh and calf.

TABLE 21-2. Approximate equivalent concentrations of sodium tetradecyl sulfate (STS) and polidocanol required for effective sclerosis of increasing caliber of lower limb vein

Vein Caliber (mm)	STS Concentration (%)	Polidocanol Concentration (%)
0.1-0.5	0.1	0.25
0.5-1	0.2	0.5
1-2	0.3	0.75
2-3	0.5	1
3-5	0.75	2
5-7	1	3

Sodium tetradecyl sulfate. STS is commonly used in concentrations of 0.1% to 0.5% to sclerose lower limb telangiectasias. Concentrations of 0.25% to 0.5% are used to treat reticular veins, and concentrations of 0.1% to 0.2% are used for microinjection of telangiectasias. The appropriate concentrations are achieved by diluting the available strengths of 0.5%, 1%, and 3% with normal saline. Isotonic normal saline is used in preference to hypotonic sterile water to minimize pain on injection.

Injection of STS results in immediate vessel spasm, which aids hemostasis after needle withdrawal. When the correct dilution is used, there is a transient blanching of the vessel followed by mild erythema. Although STS has a predictable and constant effect within the same caliber and type of vein at the same level or area of the leg, there can be variation in sensitivity of effect among patients. Younger patients with veins that have been present for a relatively short time appear to require lower-strength solutions compared with older patients with long-standing venous dilatation. In addition, cigarette smokers may be more sensitive to solution concentration, possibly as a result of chronic endothelial damage and increased endothelial permeability caused by carbon monoxide and nicotine.[33] This increased sensitivity is likely to be directly proportional to the number of cigarettes smoked per day. Systemic reactions to STS, including allergy and anaphylaxis, are extremely rare in the treatment of telangiectasias.

The main disadvantage of STS is the pain it causes for several minutes after injection, especially when the reticular veins are being treated. This pain usually is relieved by applying pressure to the injection sites with cottonballs held firmly in place with paper tape. Alternatively, an ice pack placed over the treated area for several minutes will reduce the pain significantly. The 0.1% to 0.2% solutions used for microinjection cause minor discomfort comparable to that caused by equivalent concentrations of undiluted Scleremo but more than the pain caused by polidocanol. Cutaneous ulceration has been commonly reported when STS is used for the treatment of telangiectasias.[18,30] These high rates of cutaneous ulceration always have occurred when excessive concentrations were used for microinjection. Reiner[16] showed that cutaneous necrosis after intradermal injection of STS in rabbits was concentration-dependent, with 0.313% solution producing no necrosis and 1.25% solution producing necrosis. In the microinjection of telangiectasias, STS rarely causes cutaneous necrosis when diluted to 0.15%.

Polidocanol. Polidocanol is used in concentrations of 0.25% to 2% to sclerose lower limb telangiectasias. Concentrations of 1% to 2% are used to treat reticular veins, and concentrations of 0.25% to 0.75% are used for microinjection of telangiectasias. Polidocanol is available in standard concentrations of 0.5%, 1%, 2%, 3%, and 5%. Other concentrations are achieved by diluting it with normal saline. Experimental evidence in the dorsal rabbit ear vein[31,32] indicates that polidocanol is a weaker agent than STS in producing effective endosclerosis of telangiectasias.

Compared with STS, polidocanol causes less vessel spasm and more erythema, resulting in increased bleeding after needle withdrawal. In part, this effect may be a result of the addition of alcohol 5% to the solution as a preserving agent and for enhancement of its solubility. Like STS, polidocanol has a predictable effect within the same caliber of vein and area of the leg, but a variation in effect occurs among patients. Systemic reactions to polidocanol used in the treatment of telangiectasias have been reported, occurring at a frequency of 0.2% to 0.3%.[34-37]

Because of its inherent local anesthetic properties, polidocanol causes less pain after intravascular injection compared with STS. Cutaneous ulceration is uncommon when concentrations of 0.25% to 1% are used, but it does occur with solutions over 1%. Guex[38] believes that small necroses occurring after injection with polidocanol result from excessive injection pressure and may be avoided by a good technique and using 2.5 ml syringes instead of insulin (1 ml) syringes. Owing to the similar mechanism of action of STS, this advice would also apply to the use of that agent.

ADVANCED TECHNIQUES OF ULTRASOUND-GUIDED SCLEROTHERAPY TO RETICULAR VEINS

Using a high-frequency ultrasound imaging transducer, Somjen et al.[39] have shown that 89% of areas of thigh telangiectasias have associated identifiable incompetent reticular veins. A large proportion of these were found to be associated with deeper subcutaneous vein reflux or perforating vein reflux. Some of the incompetent reticular veins were invisible from the surface, causing treatment failure when standard techniques of sclerotherapy were used. Using high-frequency duplex ultrasound, Forrestal[40] has also observed incompetent reticular veins associated with resistant telangiectasias and telangiectatic matting.

With the use of ultrasound guidance, "invisible" reticular veins can be injected with STS 0.5% to 1% or polidocanol 1%. During the procedure ultrasound can be used to monitor reticular vein spasm to ensure that the entire length of the incompetent vein is being treated. A high-frequency probe of 10 MHz or greater is necessary for this procedure. Following treatment slight erythema of the adjacent telangiectasias will be observed, and venous back pressure in the telangiectasia will be markedly reduced, indicating successful treatment.

In some patients telangiectasias on the medial aspect of the thigh will have associated segmental reflux in the long saphenous vein, usually with a competent saphenofemoral junction.[21-23,39] To achieve best results, ultrasound-guided sclerotherapy to the incompetent segment of the greater saphenous vein proximal to the telangiectasias will be necessary. The technique used is similar to that described for treatment of the incompetent greater saphenous vein in the presence of saphenofemoral junction incompetence.[41]

POSTSCLEROTHERAPY COMPRESSION

Initially described by Orbach[42] and Sigg[43] in the 1950s and popularized by Fegan[17] in the 1960s, a period of continuous compression of varicose veins after injection is now considered essential in producing long-term sclerosis. A number of theories have been suggested to explain why continuous compression improves results in the treatment of telangiectasias.[44] First, adequate compression may result in direct apposition of the treated vein walls to produce a more effective sclerosis. Second, compressing the treated vessels decreases the extent of thrombus formation, helping to prevent recanalization of the treated vessel and decreasing the incidence of superficial thrombophlebitis and postsclerotherapy pigmentation. Third, it has been speculated that thrombus formation contributes to angiogenesis and the development of telangiectatic matting.[45] Therefore it is possible that postsclerosis compression reduces the incidence of this complication.

The optimum cutaneous pressure required to achieve these theoretical benefits in the treatment of telangiectasias has yet to be defined. The benefits of graduated compression hosiery in reducing superficial ambulatory pressures and aiding the optimal unidirectional flow of blood toward the heart have been well documented.[46] However, Allan[47] has shown that a pressure of 80 mm Hg is required to empty blood from cutaneous capillaries in the standing position at a point 5 cm above the medial malleolus. Unfortunately, this degree of pressure results in cutaneous ischemia, especially with recumbency.[44] Therefore a compromise is made by using submaximal graduated compression, which achieves satisfactory patient compliance yet improves the effectiveness of treatment and reduces the incidence of postsclerotherapy pigmentation and telangiectatic matting.

In the treatment of varicose veins, graduated compression stockings that exert a pressure of 35 to 40 mm Hg at the ankle are more effective than bandaging.[48] In the treatment of telangiectasias, Goldman et al.[49] have shown that the incidence of postsclerotherapy pigmentation is greatly decreased when graduated compression stockings that exert a pressure of 30 to 40 mm Hg are used for 3 days after treatment. The same researchers concluded that this degree of compression did not improve the effectiveness of sclerosis in thigh telangiectasias or in vessels with diameters <0.5 mm. Theoretically, the effectiveness of compression by graduated stockings could be improved by the addition of a second stocking for daytime use, resulting in an effective pressure that is equal to or slightly higher than the sum of the individual stocking pressures.[50,51]

The importance of treating the abnormally dilated subcutaneous reticular veins before microsclerotherapy of telangiectasias was emphasized earlier. Continuous compression for 3 weeks is recommended in the treatment of varicose veins.[52,53] Although postsclerosis compression is also recommended in the treatment of reticular veins, empirically it can be assumed that shorter durations of compression will be adequate because of the smaller diameter of these veins. I have found the following protocol to be adequate: 3 to 7 days of continuous graduated compression with a class 2 (30 to 40 mm Hg) compression stocking, followed by a 7-day period of wearing the stocking during the daytime.

MEDICAL RECORD KEEPING

At each treatment session a record of the area and type of vein treated, the sclerosant strength and volume, and the type and duration of postsclerotherapy compression should be made. This information is best documented in the form of

Sclerotherapy progress notes					
	Surname	First name	Sclerosant/strength		
Patient	Smith	Susan		STS	ml
Date	15/9/97		3%	Y / N	0.00
Area treated	Right thigh		0.75%	Y / N	0.00
Description	Reticular veins		0.5%	Y / N	10.00
Compression	Class II graduated		0.3%	Y / N	8.00
Size	4		0.12%	Y / N	0.00
Duration (days)	3 continuous		0.1%	Y / N	0.00
	4 day/night		Polidocanol		ml
	7 daytime		5%	Y / N	0.00
			3%	Y / N	0.00
Notes			2%	Y / N	0.00
Treat left leg in 2 weeks.			1%	Y / N	0.00
			0.5%	Y / N	0.00
			0.25%	Y / N	0.00

FIGURE 21-5. Example of standard progress note.

a standard progress chart to ensure that details are not omitted (Figure 21-5). In this way the progress of the patient's condition can be readily monitored in both short- and long-term follow-up.

FOLLOW-UP CARE

Following the final treatment, patients should be reviewed at monthly intervals until both the patient and the physician are satisfied with the final result. At these visits intravascular coagula should be removed through a small incision made with either a 21-gauge needle or a No. 11 blade. Generally this procedure can be performed without any anesthesia. If this procedure is performed routinely, the treated veins will fade faster and postsclerotherapy hyperpigmentation will be minimized. At the same time areas of telangiectatic matting should be noted; if such areas are present, the physician should look for underlying incompletely treated reticular veins. If the cause of telangiectatic matting or resistant telangiectasias is still not clear, use of duplex examination with a high-frequency probe (10 MHz or higher) should be considered to locate the proximal source of reflux.

REFERENCES

1. de Faria JL, Moraes IN. Histopathology of the telangiectasia associated with varicose veins. Dermatologica 127:321-329, 1963.
2. Bodian EL. Techniques of sclerotherapy for sunburst venous blemishes. J Dermatol Surg Oncol 11:696-704, 1985.

3. Wokalek H, et al. Morphology and localization of sunburst varicosities: An electron microscopic and morphometric study. J Dermatol Surg Oncol 15:149-154, 1989.
4. Goldman MP, Bennett RG. Treatment of telangiectasia: A review. J Am Acad Dermatol 17:167-182, 1987.
5. Weiss RA, Weiss MA. Resolution of pain associated with varicose and telangiectatic leg veins after compression sclerotherapy. J Dermatol Surg Oncol 16:333-336, 1989.
6. Biegeleisen HI. Telangiectasia associated with varicose veins: Treatment by a micro-injection technique. JAMA 102:2092-2094, 1934.
7. Sadick NS. Predisposing factors of varicose veins and telangiectatic leg veins. J Dermatol Surg Oncol 18:883-886, 1992.
8. Vin F, Allaert FA, Levardon M. Influence of estrogens and progesterone on the venous system of the lower limbs in women. J Dermatol Surg Oncol 18:888-892, 1992.
9. Isaacs MN. Symptomatology of vein disease. Dermatol Surg 21:321-323, 1995.
10. Ouvry PA. Telangiectasia and sclerotherapy. J Dermatol Surg Oncol 15:177-181, 1989.
11. Eichenberger H. Resultate der Varizenödung mit Hydroxypolyäthoxy dodecan. Zbl Phlebol 8:181-183, 1969.
12. Ouvry P, Chandet A, Guillerot E. First impressions of Aethoxysklerol. Phlebologie 31:75-77, 1978.
13. Foley WT. The eradication of venous blemishes. Cutis 15:665-668, 1975.
14. Alderman DB. Therapy for essential cutaneous telangiectasia. Postgrad Med 61:91-95, 1977.
15. Goldman MP. A comparison of sclerosing agents: Clinical and histologic effects of intravascular sodium morrhuate, ethanolamine oleate, hypertonic saline (11.7%), and Sclerodex in the dorsal rabbit ear vein. J Dermatol Surg Oncol 17:354-362, 1991.
16. Reiner L. The activity of anionic surface-active compounds in producing vascular obliteration. Proc Soc Exp Biol Med 62:49-54, 1946.
17. Fegan WG. Continuous compression technique of injecting varicose veins. Lancet 2:109-112, 1963.
18. Tretbar LL. Injection sclerotherapy for spider telangiectasias: A 20-year experience with sodium tetradecyl sulphate. J Dermatol Surg Oncol 15:223-225, 1989.
19. Goldman MP, Fitzpatrick RE. Pulsed dye laser treatment of leg telangiectasia: With and without simultaneous sclerotherapy. J Dermatol Surg Oncol 16:338-344, 1990.
20. Goldman MP, Eckhouse S. Photothermal sclerosis of leg veins. Dermatol Surg 22:323-330, 1996.
21. Thibault P, Bray A, Wlodarczyk J. Cosmetic leg veins: Evaluation using duplex venous imaging. J Dermatol Surg Oncol 16:612-618, 1990.
22. Bohler-Sommeregger K, Karnel F, Schuller-Petrovic S, Santler R. Do telangiectases communicate with the deep venous system? J Dermatol Surg Oncol 18:403-406, 1992.
23. Thibault PK. Evaluation of the patient with telangiectasias. In Goldman MP, Bergan JJ, eds. Ambulatory Treatment of Venous Disease. An Illustrated Guide. St. Louis: Quality Medical Publishing, 1993, pp 373-388.
24. Goldman PM. Polidocanol (Aethoxysklerol) for sclerotherapy of superficial venules and telangiectasias. J Dermatol Surg Oncol 15:204-209, 1989.
25. Goldman MP. How many treatments are necessary to sclerose varicose and telangiectatic leg veins? J Dermatol Surg Oncol 17:62, 1991.
26. Thibault P, Wlodarczyk J. Postsclerotherapy pigmentation: The role of serum ferritin levels and effectiveness of treatment with the copper vapor laser. J Dermatol Surg Oncol 18:47-52, 1992.
27. Bodian EL. Sclerotherapy: A personal appraisal. J Dermatol Surg Oncol 15:156-161, 1989.
28. Weiss RA, Weiss MA. Incidence of side effects in the treatment of telangiectasias by compression sclerotherapy: Hypertonic saline vs. polidocanol. J Dermatol Surg Oncol 16:800-804, 1990.
29. Sadick NS. Sclerotherapy of varicose and telangiectatic leg veins: Minimal sclerosant concentration of hypertonic saline and its relationship to vessel diameter. J Dermatol Surg Oncol 17:65-70, 1991.

30. Mantse L. A mild sclerosing agent for telangiectasias. J Dermatol Surg Oncol 11:9, 1985.

31. Martin DE, Goldman MP. A comparison of sclerosing agents: Clinical and histologic effects of intravascular sodium tetradecyl sulphate and chromated glycerin in the dorsal rabbit ear vein. J Dermatol Surg Oncol 16:18-22, 1990.

32. Goldman MP, et al. Sclerosing agents in the treatment of telangiectasias. Arch Dermatol 123: 1196-1201, 1987.

33. Kjeldson K, Astrup P, Wanstrup J. Ultrastructural intimal changes in the rabbit aorta after a moderate carbon monoxide exposure. Atherosclerosis 16:67-82, 1972.

34. Feied CF, et al. Allergic reactions to polidocanol for vein sclerosis. J Dermatol Surg Oncol 20: 466-468, 1994.

35. Conrad P, Malouf GM, Stacey MC. The Australian polidocanol (Aethoxysklerol) study. Results at 1 year. Phlebology 9:17-20, 1994.

36. Conrad P, Malouf GM, Stacey M. The Australian polidocanol (Aethoxysklerol) study. Results at 2 years. Dermatol Surg 21:334-336, 1995.

37. Jaquier JJ, Loretan RM. Clinical trials of a new sclerosing agent, Aethoxysklerol. Soc Franc Phlebol 22:383-385, 1969.

38. Guex JJ. Indications for the sclerosing agent polidocanol. (Aetoxisclerol Dexo, Aethoxysklerol Kreussler). J Dermatol Surg Oncol 19:959-961, 1993.

39. Somjen GM, Ziegenbein R, Johnston AH, Royle JP. Anatomical examination of leg telangiectases with duplex scanning. J Dermatol Surg Oncol 19:940-945, 1993.

40. Forrestal MD. Evaluation and treatment of venulectatic and telangiectatic varicosities of the lower extremities with duplex ultrasound (DUS)–guided injection sclerotherapy. Dermatol Surg 24:996-997, 1997.

41. Kanter A, Thibault P. Saphenofemoral incompetence treated by ultrasound guided sclerotherapy. Dermatol Surg 22:648-652, 1996.

42. Orbach EJ. A new approach to the sclerotherapy of varicose veins. Angiology 1:302-305, 1950.

43. Sigg K. The treatment of varicosities and accompanying complications. Angiology 3:355-379, 1952.

44. Goldman MP. Compression in the treatment of leg telangiectasia: Theoretical considerations. J Dermatol Surg Oncol 15:184-188, 1989.

45. Ouvry PA, Davy A. The sclerotherapy of telangiectasia. Phlebologie 35:349-359, 1982.

46. Christopoulos D, et al. The effect of elastic compression on calf muscle pump function. Phlebology 5:13-19, 1990.

47. Allan JC. The micro-circulation of the skin of the normal leg, in varicose veins and in the post-thrombotic syndrome. S Afr J Surg 10:29-40, 1972.

48. Scurr JH, Coleridge Smith P, Cutting P. Varicose veins: Optimum compression following sclerotherapy. Ann R Coll Surg Engl 67:109-111, 1985.

49. Goldman MP, et al. Compression in the treatment of leg telangiectasia: A preliminary report. J Dermatol Surg Oncol 16:322-325, 1990.

50. Partsch H. Improvement of venous pumping in chronic venous insufficiency by compression on pressure material. Vasa 13:58-64, 1984.

51. Cornu-Thénard A. Réduction à un edeme veineux par bas élastiques. Unique on superposes. Phlebologie 38:159-168, 1985.

52. Batch AJG, et al. Randomised trial of bandaging after sclerotherapy for varicose veins. BMJ 281:423, 1980.

53. Tolins SH. Treatment of varicose veins: An update. Am J Surg 145:248-252, 1983.

Chapter 22

Treatment of Leg Telangiectasias With Laser and High-Intensity Pulsed Light

Mitchel P. Goldman and Robert A. Weiss

The most common reason patients seek treatment for leg veins is cosmetic.[1] Therefore any effective treatment should be relatively free of adverse sequelae. With recent advances, lasers and intense pulsed light (IPL) have become methods for treating telangiectatic vessels with a minimum of adverse effects. However, to be effective and safe, these advanced treatments must be used appropriately.

As detailed in Chapter 16, sclerotherapy has a number of potential adverse effects. Up to 30% of patients treated with sclerotherapy will develop postsclerotic pigmentation[2] and/or telangiectatic matting.[3] These adverse effects can occur even with optimal treatment, but they are more common when an excessive inflammatory reaction occurs. To minimize the risk of an inflammatory response, lasers and IPL act by producing thermal damage, with the ultimate goal being vaporization of the targeted vessel. It is presently believed that thermal effects produce minimal inflammatory response compared with chemical irritation of the vessel wall through sclerotherapy. This chapter addresses the use of light to destroy leg telangiectasias.

An understanding of the appropriate target vessel for each laser and/or IPL is important so that treatment can be tailored to the appropriate target. As detailed in Chapter 21, most telangiectasias arise from reticular veins. Therefore one should treat feeding reticular veins prior to treating telangiectasias. This method will minimize adverse sequelae and enhance therapeutic results. When no apparent connection exists between deep collecting or reticular vessels, telangiectasias may arise from a terminal arteriole or arteriovenous anastomosis.[4] In the latter scenario the telangiectasia may be treated without consideration of underlying forces of hydrostatic pressure.

HISTOLOGY OF LEG TELANGIECTASIA

The choice of proper wavelength(s), degree of energy fluence, and pulse duration of light exposure are all related to the type and size of the target vessel treated. Deeper vessels require a longer wavelength to allow penetration. Large-diameter vessels require a longer pulse duration to effectively thermocoagulate the entire vessel wall, allowing sufficient time for thermal energy to diffuse evenly throughout the vessel lumen. The correct choice of treatment parameters is aided by an understanding of the histology of the target telangiectasia.

Venules in the upper and middle dermis typically maintain a horizontal orientation. The diameter of the postcapillary venule ranges from 12 to 35 μm.[5] Collecting venules range from 40 to 60 μm in the upper and middle dermis and enlarge to 100 to 400 μm in diameter in the deeper tissues. Histologic examination of simple telangiectasias demonstrates dilated blood channels in a normal dermal stroma with a single endothelial cell lining, limited muscularis, and adventitia.[6,7] Most leg telangiectasias measure between 26 and 225 μm in diameter.[6] Electron microscopic examination of "sunburst" varicosities of the leg has demonstrated that these vessels are widened cutaneous veins.[6] They are found 175 to 382 μm below the stratum granulosum. The thickened vessel walls are composed of endothelial cells covered with collagen and muscle fibers. Elastic fibers are also present.

Alternatively, arteriovenous anastomoses may be involved in the pathogenesis of telangiectasias. They have been demonstrated in 1 of 26 biopsy specimens of leg telangiectasias.[4] Red telangiectasias have been found to have an oxygen saturation of 76% compared to blue telangiectasias, which have an oxygen concentration of 69%.[8] Thus each type of telangiectasia may have a slightly different optimal absorption wavelength based on its color in addition to its relative size and depth.

Unlike leg telangiectasias, the ectatic vessels of a port-wine stain are arranged in a loose fashion throughout the superficial and deep dermis. They are more superficial (0.46 mm) and much smaller than leg telangiectasias, usually measuring 10 to 40 μm in diameter. These characteristics may explain the lack of efficacy reported by many physicians who treat leg telangiectasias with the same laser and parameters used for port-wine stain.

LASER TREATMENT OF LEG TELANGIECTASIA

Various lasers have been used in an effort to enhance the clinical efficacy and minimize the adverse sequelae of telangiectasia treatment. Unfortunately, most lasers have also been associated with adverse responses far in excess of those associated with sclerotherapy. This disadvantage is related both to the nonspecificity of the laser used and to the lack of treatment of hydrostatic pressure from the "feeding" venous system.

The optimal light source would have a wavelength that is specific for the vessel treated and be able to penetrate the depth of the vessel through its entire diameter. It has been proposed that this wavelength should be between 600 and 1000 nm. Ideally, a light source should have a pulse duration that would allow the light energy to build up in the target vessel so that its entire diameter is thermocoagulated. Optimal pulse durations have been calculated for blood vessels of various diameters (Table 22-1).

TABLE 22-1. Thermal relaxation times of blood vessels*

Diameter (mm)	Seconds
0.1	0.01
0.2	0.04
0.4	0.16
0.8	0.6
1	1
2	4

*Presented by R.A. Anderson at the Annual Meeting of the North American Society of Phlebology. Washington, D.C., Nov. 1996.

During the process of delivering a sufficient amount of energy to thermocoagulate the target vessel, the overlying epidermis and perivascular tissue should be unharmed. To achieve this effect, some form of epidermal cooling is required. A number of different laser and IPL systems have been developed toward this end.

Carbon Dioxide Laser

The carbon dioxide (CO_2) laser has been used for obliterating venules and telangiectatic vessels.[9-13] The rationale for using the CO_2 laser in the treatment of telangiectasias is to produce "precise" vaporization without significant damage to tissue structures adjacent to the penetrating laser beam. The skin surface, however, as well as the dermis overlying the blood vessel is destroyed. CO_2 laser disruption of vessels has also been reported to cause occasional brisk bleeding from the vessel, requiring pressure bandages for 48 hours.[11] Pain during treatment is moderate to severe, but of short duration. All reported studies demonstrate unsatisfactory cosmetic results. Treated areas show multiple hypopigmented punctate scars with either minimal resolution of the treated vessel or neovascularization adjacent to the treatment site (Figure 22-1). Because of this nonselective action, the CO_2 laser offers no advantage over the electrodesiccation needle and has not been successfully used in treating leg telangiectasias.

Nd:YAG (1064 nm) Laser

The Nd:YAG laser, 1064 nm, has also been used to treat leg telangiectasias.[10] The average depth of penetration in human skin is 0.75 mm, and reduction to 10% of the incident power occurs at a depth of 3.7 mm.[14] Thus this laser should be well suited to treat blood vessels within the middle dermis. However, the 1064 nm wavelength is primarily absorbed by water and to a lesser degree by melanin and hemoglobin. Therefore, as with the CO_2 laser, tissue damage is rela-

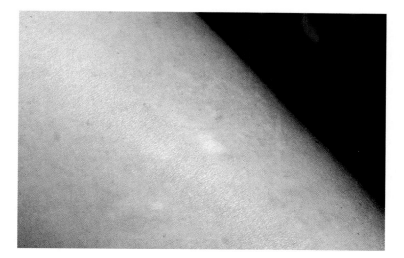

FIGURE 22-1. Appearance after treatment of leg telangiectasia with a CO_2 laser.

tively nonspecific. Apfelberg et al.[10] treated leg telangiectasias with the Nd:YAG laser equipped with a 1.5 mm sapphire contact probe. Treatment complications included linear hypopigmentation and depressions overlying the skin of the treated vessel. Retreatment was needed at 6-week intervals. In addition, the cost is high because the disposable sapphire tips are expensive.

In a recent clinical trial,[14a] 30 patients (50 sites) were enrolled and treated with a new multiple synchronized pulse laser emitting at 1064 nm (Vasculight, ESC Sharplan Medical, Yokneam, Israel). The primary parameter was a single 10- to 16-millisecond pulse or double-synchronized 10-millisecond pulses separated by a 30-millisecond delay. In this study immediate contraction or darkening followed by urtication and visible total vessel closure, as indicated by absence of blanching and visual elimination of the vessel border, occurred in most of the treated sites. Two 3 mm (diameter) vessels were confirmed to be closed without flow by duplex ultrasound visualization with a 10 mHz transducer. Bruising from vessel rupture was seen in approximately 50% of patients. No epidermal injury was noted in any sites, even in Fitzpatrick skin type IV. At 3-month follow-up, 75% improvement was noted at treatment sites.

These promising initial clinical results with a new 1064 nm laser wavelength are in contradistinction to previous studies and provide for immediate closure and subsequent elimination of leg ectatic veins without damage to surrounding tissue. Epidermal injury is unlikely because the near-infrared wavelength has minimal interaction with melanin.

Argon Laser

The argon laser, with output at 488 nm and 511 nm, has wavelengths that are somewhat preferentially absorbed by hemoglobin and to a lesser, although significant, extent by water and melanin. The relatively short wavelength of this laser, combined with a spot size of 1 mm, prevents its penetration much beyond 0.5 mm. When the patient is pigmented or tanned, epidermal melanin will selectively absorb the laser energy, preventing penetration below the epidermis. Thus the argon laser does not have ideal parameters for treating leg veins.

Argon laser treatment of telangiectasias or superficial varicosities of the lower extremities may result in purple or depressed scars. In a report of 38 patients treated by Apfelberg et al.,[10] 49% had either poor or no results from treatment; only 16% had excellent or good results. In addition, almost half of the patients had hemosiderin bruising. In another series Dixon et al.[15] noted significant improvement in only 49% of patients. They speculated that although initially improvement was noted, incomplete thrombosis, recanalization, or new vein formation produced reappearance of the vessels after 6 to 12 months.

In an effort to enhance therapeutic success with leg vein sclerotherapy, the argon laser has been used to interrupt the telangiectasia every 2 to 3 cm prior to injection of a sclerosing agent.[16] Eleven of 16 patients completed treatment. Two patients developed punctate depigmented scars, and three patients developed hyperpigmentation. However, 93.7% of patients were reported to have "satisfactory" results. Cooling the skin simultaneously with argon or tunable dye (577 nm and 585 nm, respectively) laser treatment has been demonstrated to produce improvement in 67% of leg telangiectasias 1 mm in diameter.[17] This effect may be secondary to temperature-related vasomotor changes in blood flow.[18] Overall, argon laser therapy appears to be not only relatively ineffective in treating leg telangiectasias, but also associated with an unacceptably high risk of adverse sequelae.

KTP and Frequency-Doubled Nd:YAG (532 nm) Laser

Modulated krypton triphosphate (KTP) lasers have been reported to be effective at removing leg telangiectasias when pulse durations between 1 and 50 milliseconds are used. The 532 nm wavelength is one of the hemoglobin absorption peaks (Figure 22-2). Although this wavelength does not penetrate deeply into the dermis (approximately 0.75 mm), relatively specific damage (compared to argon laser) can be produced in the vascular target by selecting an optimal pulse duration, enlarging the spot size, and adding epidermal cooling.

Effective results have been achieved by tracing vessels with a 1 mm projected spot. Typically the laser is moved between adjacent 1 mm spots with vessels traced at 5 to 10 mm per second. Immediately following laser exposure, the epidermis is blanched. Lengthening the pulse duration to match the diameter of the vessel is attempted to optimize treatment (see Table 22-1). With this method, West and Alster[19] treated 12 patients with leg telangiectasias. They used a 10-millisecond pulse at 15 J/cm² with a 1 mm handpiece at a repetition rate of 2 pulses per second. The average improvement was 25% to 50% (Figure 22-3).

Quintana et al.[20] treated 19 leg veins <1.5 mm in diameter with the Laserscope KTP Dermastat (Laserscope, San Jose, Calif.). They used a 2 mm diameter handpiece at a fluence of 13 to 15 J/cm² given at a rate of 10 to 15 milliseconds.

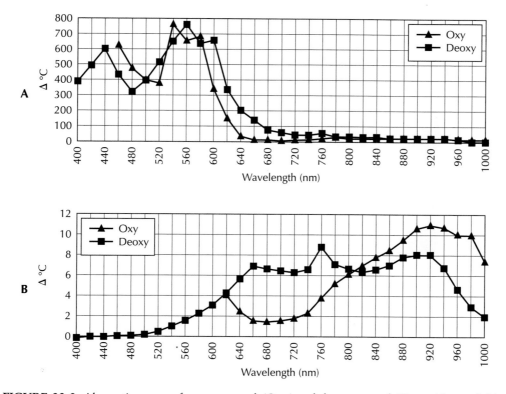

FIGURE 22-2. Absorption curve for oxygenated *(Oxy)* and deoxygenated *(Deoxy)* hemoglobin for blood vessels of different depths and diameters. **A,** Average temperature increase across a 0.2 mm deep, 0.05 mm diameter vessel vs. wavelength. **B,** Average temperature increase across a 2 mm deep, 1 mm diameter vessel vs. wavelength. (From Goldman MP, Fitzpatrick RE. Cutaneous Laser Surgery, 2nd ed. St. Louis: Mosby, 1998. Reproduced with permission. Courtesy of Simon Eckhouse, Ph.D., ESC/Sharplan Medical Systems, Inc., Needham, Mass.)

Patients were treated at 4- to 6-week intervals on four separate visits, with results examined 6 months after the last visit. Only 28% of the patients could be evaluated. Of these patients, 15% achieved 100% clearance, 40% had 75% clearance, 35% had 50% clearance, and 10% had 25% clearance. No scarring was reported, and 25% had transient hyperpigmentation. Therefore this laser is somewhat effective but requires multiple treatments.

A long-pulse 532 nm laser (frequency-doubled Nd:YAG) (Versapulse; Coherent, Inc., Palo Alto, Calif.) has been reported to be effective in treating leg veins <1 mm in diameter that are not directly connected to a feeding reticular vein.[21] When used with a 4° C chilled tip, a fluence of 12 to 15 J/cm² is delivered in a 3 mm diameter spot size as a train of pulses to trace the vessel until spasm or thrombosis occurs. Some overlying epidermal scabbing is noted, with hypopigmentation frequently occurring in dark-skinned patients. There is considerable variation in results reported by individual physicians. Usually, more than one treatment is necessary for maximal vessel improvement, with only rare reports of 100% resolution of the leg vein.[21] We believe that this laser is best used for ves-

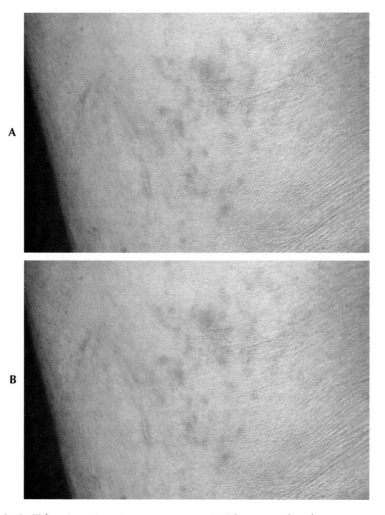

FIGURE 22-3. A, Telangiectasia prior to treatment. **B,** Three months after treatment hyperpigmentation is noted on the telangiectasia treated with the long-pulse FLPDL at 15 J/cm². The side treated with the KTP (532 nm) laser at 15 J/cm² and a 10-millisecond pulse shows no change. (From West TB, Alster TS. Comparison of the long-pulse dye (590-595 nm) and KTP (532 nm) lasers in the treatment of facial and leg telangiectasias. Dermatol Surg 24:221-226, 1998.)

sels that are recalcitrant to other lasers, IPL, and sclerotherapy treatment (Figure 22-4) in Fitzpatrick skin type I and II patients.

McMeekin[22] treated 18 sites of leg veins 0.5 to 1.1 mm in diameter in 10 patients by using the Versapulse laser with a 3 mm diameter spot, 5.5° C cooling at 12 to 16 J/cm² with one to three passes over each vessel. At 1-year follow-up, the patients who had a single treatment showed these results: 6% of patients had complete clearance, 88% had partial clearance, and 6% had no change. Of the partial clearance group, more patients cleared at 16 J than at 12 J. At 16 J/cm²,

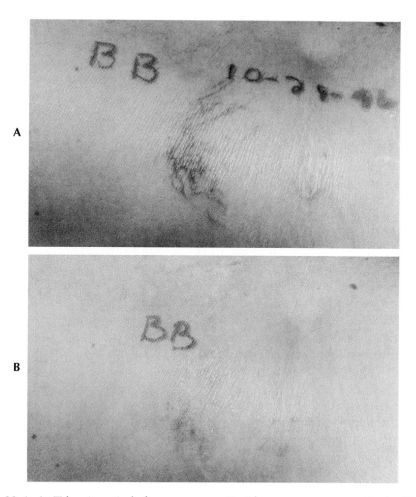

FIGURE 22-4. A, Telangiectasia before treatment. B, After one treatment with the Versapulse at 15 J/cm^2 with a 10-millisecond pulse through a 3 mm diameter spot with the skin chilled through a 4° C quartz tip. (Courtesy of Robert Adrian, M.D.)

37% cleared 25% to 50%; 25% cleared 50% to 75%; and 37% cleared 75% to 100%. Approximately 94% developed hyperpigmentation, which took up to 6 months to resolve. One patient developed blisters and hypopigmented/atrophic scars.

A longer pulse duration of 20 to 50 milliseconds, accompanied by an increase in spot size to 5 mm, with a higher total fluence of 20 J/cm^2, is presently being evaluated. Preliminary results indicate an increase in the efficacy of this laser and reduction in pigmentary changes. Narukar[23] evaluated patients with leg veins <1.5 mm in diameter treated with 2- to 50-millisecond pulses up to 40 J/cm^2 with a 3 to 6 mm diameter spot size and a 4° C chilled tip. He treated patients at 6- to 8-week intervals two to three times. A 45% clearance was found. Interestingly, a

68% clearance was found in patients whose previous sclerotherapy showed a good response. A 32% clearance occurred in patients whose vessels responded poorly to sclerotherapy. At 2-month follow-up, 2% of patients had telangiectatic matting, 4% had hyperpigmentation, and 2% had hypopigmentation.

Flashlamp-Pulsed Dye Laser (FLPDL) (585 nm)

The FLPDL has been demonstrated to be highly efficacious in treating cutaneous vascular lesions consisting of very small vessels, including port-wine stains, hemangiomas, and facial telangiectasias.[24] The depth of vascular damage is estimated to be 1.5 mm at 585 nm. Therefore penetration to the typical depth of a leg telangiectasia may be achieved.[25] However, telangiectasias found over the lower extremities have not responded as well, with less lightening and more post-therapy hyperpigmentation.[26] This result may be due to the larger diameter of leg telangiectasias as compared to dermal vessels in port-wine stains and larger-diameter feeding reticular veins, as described previously. The pulse duration of the first generation of FLPDL was 450 microseconds, optimal for the 50 to 100 μm diameter of port-wine stain vessels. This pulse duration is only effective for treating leg telangiectasias <1 to 2 mm in diameter. Many studies fail to demonstrate satisfactory efficacy. We believe that this situation is due to failure to recognize the importance of high-pressure vascular flow from feeding reticular and varicose veins.

Polla et al.[26] treated 35 superficial leg telangiectasias with the FLPDL. The exact laser parameters were not given, except that vessels were treated an average of 2.1 times with a maximum of four separate treatments. These vessels were described as being either red-purple and raised or blue and flat. No mention was made of the association of reticular or varicose veins with vessel diameter. Fifteen percent of treated vessels had greater than 75% clearing, with 73% of treated areas showing little response to treatment. The only lesions that responded at all were red-pink tiny telangiectasias. Almost 50% of the treated patients developed persistent hypopigmentation or hyperpigmentation.

Vessels that should optimally respond to FLPDL treatment are predicted to be red telangiectasias <0.2 mm in diameter, particularly those vessels arising as a function of telangiectatic matting following sclerotherapy. This prediction is based on knowledge of the type of thermocoagulation produced by this relatively short-pulse laser system. The FLPDL produces vascular injury in a histologic pattern that is different from that produced by sclerotherapy. In the rabbit ear vein approximately 50% of vessels treated with an effective concentration of sclerosant demonstrated extravasated red blood cells (RBCs) (unpublished observations). With FLPDL treatment, extravasated RBCs were apparent in only 30% of vessels treated. Thus the FLPDL may produce less posttherapy pigmentation because of a decreased incidence of extravasated RBCs.

The etiology of telangiectatic matting is unknown, but it has been thought to be related to either angiogenesis[27] or a dilatation of existing subclinical blood vessels by promoting collateral flow through arteriovenous anastomoses.[28] One or both of these mechanisms may occur. Obstruction of outflow from a vessel (which is the end result of successful sclerotherapy) is one of the most important factors contributing to angiogenesis.[29] In addition, endothelial damage leads to the release of histamine and other mast cell factors and vasokines, which promote both the dilatation of existing blood vessels and angiogenesis.[30,31] By its mechanism of endothelial destruction, sclerotherapy provides the means for new blood vessel formation to occur. Indeed, it is remarkable that one does not see a higher incidence of postsclerosis telangiectatic matting with sclerotherapy treatment.

Telangiectatic matting has not been reported to be a side effect of argon, FLPDL, or other laser treatments of any vascular disorders. This situation may be due to the production of intravascular fibrin that occurs during laser treatment.[32-34] This effect is believed to occur through thermal alteration of fibrin complexes or proteolytic cleavage of fibrinogen. Fibrin deposition has been demonstrated to promote angiogenesis.[30] Interestingly, sclerotherapy-induced vascular injury has not been associated with the appearance of fibrin strands (unpublished observations). This finding is explained by the limitation of angiogenesis by factors other than those associated with the absence of fibrin deposition or by intravascular consumption of fibrin-promoting factors in laser treatment of cutaneous vascular disease.

Another possible mechanism for the absence of telangiectatic matting in laser-treated blood vessels is a decrease in perivascular inflammation. Rabbit ear vein treatment with the FLPDL results in a relative decrease in perivascular inflammation as compared to vessels treated with sclerotherapy alone.[34] Multiple factors associated with inflammation have been demonstrated to promote both a dilatation of existing blood vessels and angiogenesis.[31]

Goldman and Fitzpatrick[35] treated 30 female patients with red leg telangiectasias <0.2 mm in diameter. Thirteen of 101 telangiectatic patches were noted to have an associated reticular "feeding" vein between 2 and 3 mm in diameter that was not treated. Seven patients with 25 patches of telangiectatic matting after previous sclerotherapy were also treated. FLPDL 5 mm diameter spots were overlapped slightly, and every effort was made to treat the entire vessel. After treatment, a chemical ice pack (Kwik Kold; American Pharmaseal Co., Valencia, Calif.) was applied to the treated area until the laser-induced sensation of heat resolved (5 to 15 minutes). Thirty-nine telangiectatic patches, chosen randomly, were treated with laser energies between 7 and 8 J/cm² and were compressed with a rubber E compression pad (STD Vascular Products Ltd., Bristol, England); they were fixed in place with Microfoam 100 mm tape (3M Medical-Surgical Division, St. Paul, Minn.). A 30 to 40 mm Hg graduated compression stocking was then continuously worn over this dressing for approximately 72 hours.

As hypothesized, telangiectatic matting and persistent pigmentation did not occur with FLPDL treatment of leg telangiectasias. Post-FLPDL–induced hyperpigmentation completely resolved within 4 months. There were no episodes of cutaneous ulceration, thrombophlebitis, or other complications. However, hypopigmentation occurred in some patients with tanned skin (Figure 22-5). The laser impact sites usually remained hypopigmented for years and in many cases were

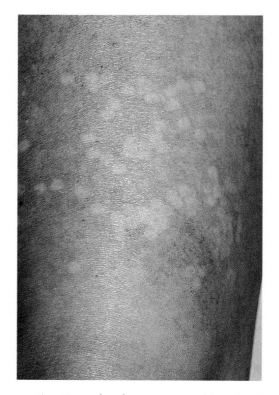

FIGURE 22-5. Hypopigmentation 6 months after treatment of leg telangiectasia with the FLPDL at 7.5 J/cm². (From Goldman MP. Sclerotherapy Treatment of Varicose and Telangiectatic Leg Veins, 2nd ed. St. Louis: Mosby, 1995. Reproduced with permission.)

thought to be permanent. With FLPDL treatment, the most effective fluence appears to be between 7 and 8 J/cm². With these parameters, approximately 67% of telangiectatic patches completely faded within 4 months (Figure 22-6).

There appears to be no difference in the response to FLPDL treatment between linear leg telangiectasias and telangiectatic matting vessels. In these seven patients with 25 sites treated, 72% of the treated sites completely faded at laser fluences between 6.5 and 7.5 J/cm². Telangiectatic matting vessels did not respond to treatment in only one patient with four areas of matting. Less than 100% resolution occurred in 16% of treated areas.

Like telangiectatic matting vessels, progressively ascending telangiectasia represents a network of fine-red telangiectasias usually <0.2 mm in diameter. This condition responds well to the FLPDL at fluences of 7 to 7.25 J/cm².[36] Treatment, however, is tedious, with 2,000 or more 5 mm diameter pulses sometimes necessary to cover the entire affected area.

The reason for greater efficacy of treatment in Goldman and Fitzpatrick's report, as compared to the reports of others,[26,37] may be due to the rigid criteria by which patients were selected for treatment. Patients who responded well to treat-

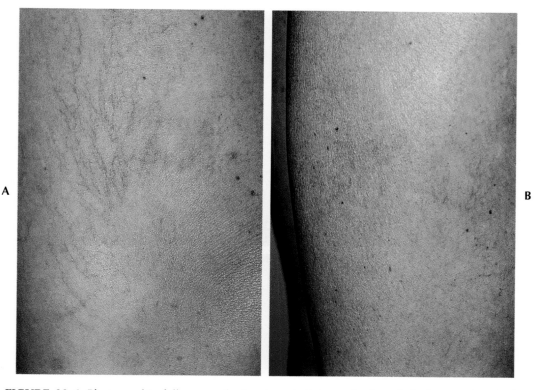

FIGURE 22-6. Photographic follow-up of telangiectatic flair on the lateral thigh treated with the FLPDL at 7 J/cm², 125 pulses. **A,** Before treatment. **B,** Six weeks after treatment. (From Goldman MP. Sclerotherapy Treatment of Varicose and Telangiectatic Leg Veins, 2nd ed. St. Louis: Mosby, 1995. Reproduced with permission.)

ment had red telangiectasias <0.2 mm in diameter without associated "feeding" reticular veins.

Many physicians have found that vessel location may affect treatment outcome, with vessels on the medial thigh being the most difficult to eradicate completely. However, with the FLPDL, vessel location appears to be unrelated to treatment outcome if telangiectatic patches with untreated associated reticular veins are excluded. In addition, there appears to be no obvious difference in efficacy between telangiectatic patches treated with compression and those that are not.

Long-Pulse FLPDL

In an effort to thermocoagulate larger-diameter blood vessels, pulse duration of FLPDL has been lengthened to 1.5 microseconds and the wavelength has been increased to 600 nm. Theoretically, this adjustment permits more thorough heating of a larger vessel. It has been reported that using a 595 nm FLPDL at 1.5 microseconds resulted in >50% clearance of leg veins at a fluence of 15 J/cm² and

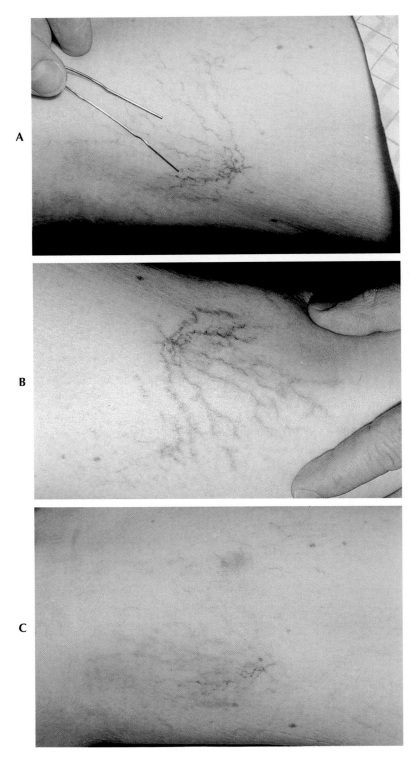

FIGURE 22-7. Treatment of leg telangiectasia with the long-pulse FLPDL. **A,** Before treatment. **B,** Immediately after treatment at 595 nm, 25 J/cm². **C,** Eight weeks after treatment.

approximately 65% clearance at a fluence of 18 J/cm².[38] In this limited study of 18 patients, vessels ranging in diameter from 0.6 to 1 mm were treated with an elliptical spot size of 2 × 7 mm through a transparent hydrogel-based wound dressing. No adverse sequelae were noted at the 5-month follow-up visit (Figure 22-7).

Lee and Lask[39] treated 25 women with leg telangiectasias <1 mm in diameter with the longer-pulse FLPDL (Sclerolaser; Candela Corp., Wayland, Mass.). Each patient had four areas treated: two at a wavelength of 595 nm with fluences of 15 or 20 J/cm² and two additional areas treated with a 600 nm wavelength at 15 or 20 J/cm², respectively. A maximum of three treatments were performed at 6-week intervals. All patients showed improvement. The 595 nm wavelength at 20 J/cm² gave the best results. Treatment response was variable and unpredict-

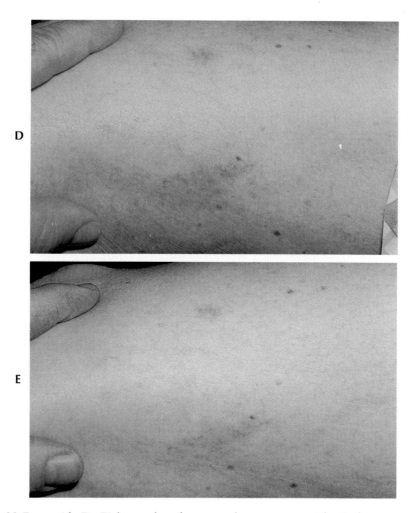

FIGURE 22-7, cont'd. D, Eight weeks after second treatment at identical parameters. **E,** Five months after second treatment. (Courtesy of C.S. Burton III, M.D.)

able, with some patients having complete resolution and some having only slight improvement. Three patients had superficial scabbing that resolved without apparent scarring. Most patients experienced purpura and hyperpigmentation, which resolved after several weeks. Reasons for the variable efficacy were not reported. Thus, at this writing, it is unclear whether increasing the pulse duration to 1.5 milliseconds adds significant efficacy to the treatment of leg telangiectasias >0.2 mm in diameter.

West and Alster[19] used a 590 or 595 nm pulse at 15 J/cm² to treat 12 patients with leg telangiectasias. An average improvement of 75% occurred in these patients. Hyperpigmentation persisted at the 12-week follow-up period in 71% of patients.

Hohenleutner et al.[40] treated 87 patients with the long-pulse FLPDL and either ice cube or gel cooling. They found that cooled Vigilon gel decreases fluence by 35% in addition to decreasing skin temperature 5° C for 1 minute. Ice cube cooling produces a 15° C decrease in skin temperature for 1 minute. With ice cube cooling, clearance >95% occurred in 20% of patients with veins <0.5 mm in diameter but in no veins between 0.5 and 1 mm in diameter treated at 600 nm with 18 J/cm². From 50% to 95% clearance occurred in 82% of veins <0.5 mm in diameter and in 50% of veins between 0.5 and 1 mm in diameter at a fluence of 20 J/cm². Hyperpigmentation and/or hypopigmentation occurred in 48% of patients treated at 20 J/cm² and resolved within 6 months. Thus cooling with ice cubes enhances the clinical efficacy of this laser. Multiple treatments may enhance efficacy even further.

An ultralong-pulse FLPDL has also been developed with a pulse duration of 4 milliseconds and a wavelength of 595 nm (Cynosure; Chelmsford, Mass.). The 4-millisecond pulse duration is created by using two separate laser beams, each emitting a 2.4-millisecond pulse. This laser was used to treat leg veins <1 mm in diameter with a 2 × 7 mm, 5 mm, or 3 × 5 mm spot size. There was no difference in vessel response between a 4-millisecond 16 J pulse, a 4-millisecond 20 J pulse, and a 1.5-millisecond 14.16 J pulse. Approximately 60% improvement was seen. Hyperpigmentation lasting about 12 weeks was seen in 40% to 67% of treated veins. Hypopigmentation lasting about 12 weeks occurred in 20% to 27% of veins.[41]

Long-Pulse Infrared Alexandrite Laser (755 nm) (LPIR)

In order to allow for the deeper penetration required for treatment of larger vessels and the greater thermal diffusion time needed, a new laser system has been developed to allow pulse durations of 20 milliseconds with a spot size of up to 5 mm and a wavelength that theoretically can penetrate 2 to 3 mm. In early clinical trials, Adrian[42] has reported this laser to be effective in clinical and biopsy studies. Unfortunately, comparative studies or statistical evaluation of results have not yet been presented. The success of this method in fulfilling the requirements of selective photothermolysis awaits treatment of a larger number of patients (Figure 22-8).

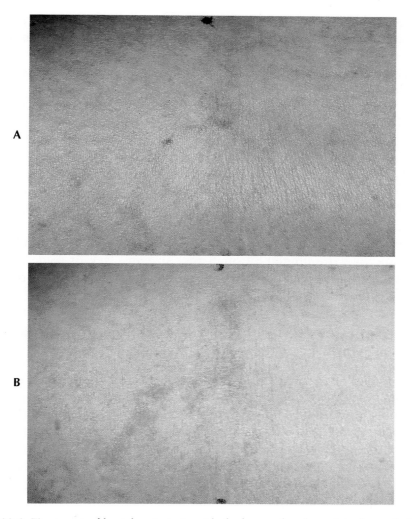

FIGURE 22-8. Treatment of leg telangiectasia with the long-pulse alexandrite laser. A, Before treatment. B, Seven weeks after treatment. (Courtesy of D.H. McDaniel, M.D.)

Diode Lasers

Two new diode pumped lasers have recently entered the U.S. market: a 532 nm laser and 810 nm laser (gallium-arsenide) (LaserLite, Boston, Mass.). Diode lasers generate coherent monochromatic light through excitation of small diodes. These devices are therefore lightweight and portable and have a relatively small desktop footprint. Dierickx et al.[43] evaluated an 800 nm diode laser (Star Medical, Inc., Palo Alto, Calif.) on eight areas of leg veins. The laser was used at 15 to 40 J/cm² given in 5- to 30-millisecond pulses as double or triple pulses separated by a 2-second delay time. Veins were treated every 4 weeks for three sessions and evaluated 2 months after the last treatment. Optimal parameters were

30-millisecond pulses at 40 J/cm². At these parameters vessels 0.4 to 1 mm in diameter showed 100% clearance in 22% of patients, 75% clearance in 42%, and 50% clearance in 32%.

Garden et al.[44] used an 810 nm diode laser with a 750 μm spot size at 40 W and 50-millisecond pulses for a total of 453 J/cm² of fluence delivered. Twelve patients with 58 vessels 0.2 to 0.5 mm in diameter were treated with three to four passes until vessel spasm occurred. Patients were retreated every 2 to 4 weeks. There was a mean clearance of 60% after 2.2 treatments. Eighteen vessels had >70% clearance after three treatments. When a scanner was incorporated into the diode laser so that 15 to 20 mm passes could be given, efficacy increased. In 11 patients treated with the scanner/diode used in two sessions 2 to 4 weeks apart, 18% had 75% to 90% clearance, 21% had 50% to 75% clearance, 18% had 25% to 50% clearance, and 36% had 0% to 25% clearance.

Presently, although these lasers may be less costly to produce and less expensive to operate, they are limited by small spot size and lack of epidermal cooling devices. Therefore judgment on their clinical efficacy for treatment of leg veins awaits larger clinical trials.

EVALUATION OF COMBINED SCLEROTHERAPY/LASER TREATMENT OF LEG TELANGIECTASIA

Goldman and Fitzpatrick[34] also studied the effect of combined sclerotherapy/laser treatment. Twenty-seven patients had either bilaterally symmetrical telangiectatic patches or a large "sunburst" telangiectatic flare, which could be divided into two separate treatment sites. Patients were treated at one site with the FLPDL alone and at the other with FLPDL plus sclerotherapy. Laser fluences were 1 to 2 J/cm² less than those used with FLPDL alone immediately before injection of the telangiectasia with polidocanol (POL), 0.25%, 0.5%, or 0.75%, with a volume of 0.1 to 0.25 ml per injection site.

Forty-four percent of combination-treated areas completely resolved. There appeared to be little difference in efficacy and adverse sequelae with concentrations of POL between 0.25% and 0.75%. There did seem to be an increased efficacy of treatment with laser energies of 7.5 to 7.75 J/cm². As with the FLPDL alone, treatment site did not appear to significantly affect outcome except for an increased incidence of complications in the ankle and knee areas.

The most significant difference between using the FLPDL alone and the combination treatment was the incidence of complications. With combination treatment, posttreatment ulceration and telangiectatic matting occurred in 11% of treated areas compared with no adverse sequelae in the areas treated with FLPDL alone. Six of 23 nonulcerated treatment sites developed persistent pigmentation beyond 1 year. Two of 27 sites developed telangiectatic matting, which lasted more than 1 year. In 4 of 27 treatment sites, superficial ulceration developed. In the patients affected by ulceration, the laser fluences were ≥6.5 J/cm² and the POL concentration was ≥0.5%.

In summary, when pulsed at 450 microseconds, FLPDL is an effective modality for treating red leg telangiectasias ≤ 0.2 mm in diameter. FLPDL treatment is efficacious for both essential telangiectasias and vessels of telangiectatic matting. This form of treatment alone has a low incidence of adverse sequelae. The optimal clinically useful laser fluence is between 7 and 8 J/cm². Treatment is most efficacious if all vessels >0.2 mm in diameter, especially varicose and reticular feeding veins, are treated first with sclerotherapy or another modality. Results are not affected by vessel location. Posttreatment compression of this type of vessel appears unnecessary. Combination treatment seems to offer no advantage to sclerotherapy alone and appears to have a significant degree of complications when treatment is limited to red telangiectasias <0.2 mm in diameter.

In the rabbit ear vein model, preliminary evidence suggests that combination treatment may be more efficacious than either FLPDL or sclerotherapy alone.[34] When used alone, FLPDL was effective only in establishing a histologic and clinical resolution of the vessel when an energy of 10 J/cm² was used. When FLPDL was used in combination with immediate injection of the sclerosant, a significant degree of clinical and histologic resolution of the vessel occurred with all tested laser fluences (8 to 10 J/cm²). Pilot studies using a combination of sclerotherapy with POL 0.25% and laser fluences of 6 and 7 J/cm² demonstrated no endothelial damage in vessels treated with PDL alone at 8 days. Combination-treated vessels at 6 and 7 J/cm² demonstrated endothelial vacuolization. Thus it is possible that FLPDL fluences <5 J/cm² may be successfully combined with sclerotherapy in human leg veins to provide effective therapy. In addition, a relative decrease in the extent of extravasated RBCs and perivascular inflammation was noted in both FLPDL alone and combination treatment.

HIGH-INTENSITY PULSED LIGHT (IPL)

The IPL (PhotoDerm VL; ESC Medical Inc., Newton, Mass.) source was developed as an alternative to lasers to maximize efficacy in treating leg veins. This device permits sequential rapid pulsing and longer-duration pulses and longer-penetrating wavelengths than the laser systems described earlier. Since leg venules are substantially larger and have thicker walls than the ectatic vessels in port-wine stains and hemangiomas, thermal heat diffusion from absorbed RBCs must require longer times to damage the vein wall effectively. This time has been estimated to be 1 to 10 milliseconds or more (see Table 22-1). In addition, leg veins are not mainly composed of oxygenated hemoglobin, as are port-wine stains and hemangiomas. They are filled with predominantly deoxygenated hemoglobin—hence their blue color. Selective wavelengths for deoxygenated as opposed to oxygenated hemoglobin include 545 nm and a broad peak between 650 and 800 nm. Because leg veins are located deeper in the dermis than are telangiectasias, a longer wavelength (and/or greater protection of the epidermis and superficial dermis from thermal damage) is necessary for ideal treatment.

Optical properties of blood are mainly determined by the absorption and scattering coefficients of its various oxyhemoglobin components. Figure 22-2 shows the oxyhemoglobin absorption and scattering coefficient depth of penetration into blood.[45] The main feature to note in the curve is the strong absorption at wavelengths <600 nm, with less absorption at longer wavelengths. However, a vessel that is 1 mm in diameter absorbs more than 67% of light even at wavelengths >600 nm. This absorption is even more significant for blood vessels 2 mm in diameter. Therefore using a light source >600 nm would result in deeper penetration of thermal energy without negating absorption by oxyhemoglobin. This occurs because the absorption coefficient in blood is higher than that of surrounding tissue for wavelengths between 600 and 1000 nm (Figure 22-9).

Theoretically, a phototherapy device that produces a noncoherent light as a continuous spectrum >550 nm should have multiple advantages over a single-wavelength laser system. First, both oxygenated and deoxygenated hemoglobin will absorb at these wavelengths. Second, blood vessels located deeper in the dermis will be affected. Third, thermal absorption by the exposed blood vessels should occur with less overlying epidermal absorption since the longer wavelengths will penetrate deeper and be absorbed less by the epidermis.

With these theoretical considerations, IPL emitting in the 515 to 1000 nm range was used at varying energy fluences (5 to 90 J/cm²) and various pulse durations (2 to 25 milliseconds) to treat venectasias 0.4 to 2 mm in diameter. Clinical trials using various parameters with the IPL, including multiple pulses of variable duration, demonstrated efficacy ranging from over 90% total clearance in vessels <0.2 mm in diameter to 80% in vessels from 0.2 to 0.5 mm and 80% in vessels 0.5 to 1 mm in diameter.[46-48] The incidence of adverse sequelae was minimal, with hypopigmentation occurring in 3% of patients and resolving within 4 to 6 months. Tanned or darkly pigmented (Fitzpatrick type III) patients were likely to

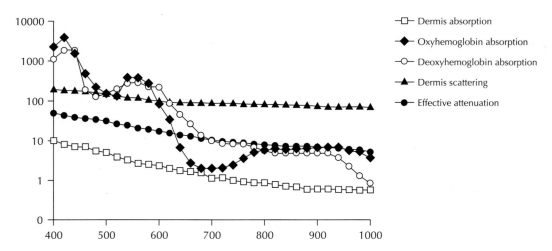

FIGURE 22-9. Coefficient of blood relative to dermis. (Courtesy of ESC/Sharplan Medical Systems, Inc., Needham, Mass.)

develop hypopigmentation and hyperpigmentation in addition to blistering and superficial erosions. These effects all cleared over a few months. Treatment parameters that were found to be most successful ranged from a single pulse of 22 J/cm² in 3 milliseconds for vessels <0.2 mm to a double pulse of 35 to 40 J/cm² given in 2.4 and 4 milliseconds with a 10-millisecond delay. Vessels between 0.2 and 0.5 mm were treated with the same double-pulse parameters or with a 3- to 6-millisecond pulse at 35 to 45 J/cm² with a 20-millisecond delay. Vessels >0.5 mm were treated with triple pulses of 3.5, 3.1, and 2.6 milliseconds with pulse delays of 20 milliseconds at a fluence of 50 J/cm² or with triple pulses of 3, 4, and 6 milliseconds with a pulse delay of 30 milliseconds at a fluence of 55 to 60 J/cm². The choice of a cutoff filter was based on skin color, with a 550 nm filter used for light-skinned patients and a 570 or 590 nm filter used for darker-skinned patients (Figures 22-10 and 22-11).

Weiss and Weiss[49] have reported increased efficacy by lengthening the pulse durations to a maximum of 10 milliseconds in two consecutive pulses separated by a 20-millisecond delay with a 570 nm cutoff filter and fluences of 70 J/cm². They have achieved response rates of 74% in two treatments with an 8% incidence of temporary hypopigmentation or hyperpigmentation. By combining a shorter pulse (2.4 to 3 milliseconds) with a longer pulse (7 to 10 milliseconds) it is theoretically possible to ablate smaller and larger vessels overlying one another in the dermis (Figure 22-12).

Treatment of essential telangiectasia, especially on the legs, is efficiently accomplished with the IPL (Figure 22-13). A variety of parameters have been shown to be effective. We recommend testing a few different parameters during the first treatment session and using the most efficient and least painful ones for subsequent treatments. One study of 14 patients (one of whom had leg telangiectasias) found that a single pulse of 30 J/cm² delivered through a 550 nm cutoff filter in 5 milliseconds was 100% effective.[50] Many other parameters, such as those included in Figure 22-11, are also very effective.

A European multicenter study of 40 women with leg telangiectasias up to 1 mm in diameter involved treatment with various parameters.[51] For vessels up to 0.2 mm in diameter, a 3-millisecond pulse of 22 J/cm² was used. A double pulse of 2.4 milliseconds each separated by a 20-millisecond delay with 35 J/cm² was given for vessels <0.5 mm. A triple pulse of 3.5, 3.1, and 2.6 milliseconds was used with delays of 20 milliseconds and a fluence of 50 J/cm² for vessels <1 mm in diameter. Clearance of 92% occurred in vessels <0.2 mm in diameter. A clearance of 80% was seen in vessels <0.5 mm in diameter. In vessels <1 mm in diameter, 81% clearing was noted. Vessels did not recur in the 1-year follow-up period. Eleven patients had temporary hyperpigmentation. One patient had temporary hypopigmentation, and two patients had a nonscarring blister.

One of the most rewarding conditions to treat is essential telangiectasia. This condition, described previously, responds well to FLPDL, but this therapy can be time-consuming and expensive. With IPL, the large area of involvement can be treated quickly and effectively with many different parameters used.[52]

Text continued on p. 494.

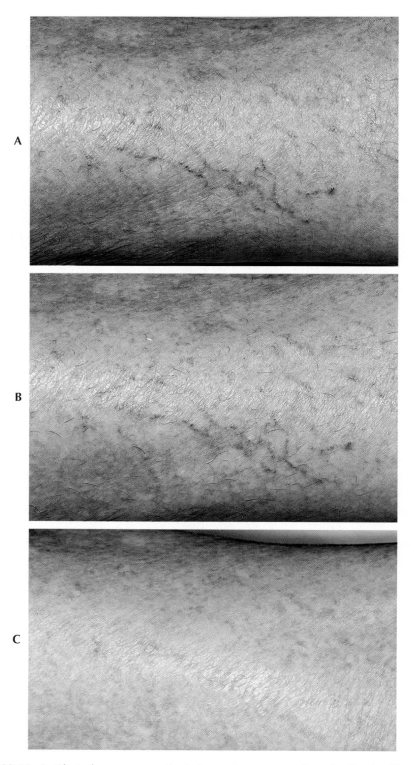

FIGURE 22-10. A, Clinical appearance of a 0.6 mm diameter vessel on the distal calf prior to treatment. **B,** Immediately after treatment with the Photoderm VL with a 590 nm cutoff filter and 41 J/cm² given as a double pulse, 6.5 and 15 milliseconds, with a 10-millisecond delay time. **C,** Ten weeks after treatment resolution is complete. (From Goldman MP. Laser and noncoherent pulsed light treatment of leg telangiectasias and venules. In Goldman MP, Bergan JJ, eds. Ambulatory Treatment of Venous Disease. St. Louis: Mosby, 1996. Reproduced with permission.)

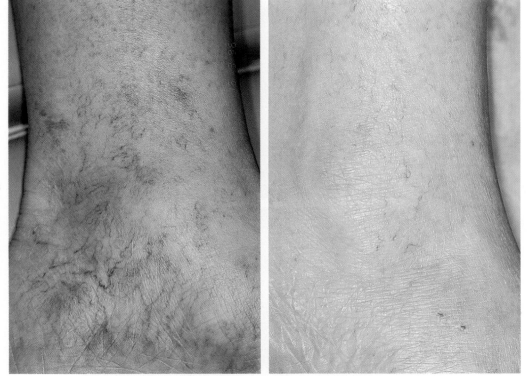

FIGURE 22-11. **A,** Ankle telangiectasia prior to treatment. **B,** Six weeks after a single treatment with the Photoderm VL at 40 J/cm² given as a double-pulse, 2.4 and 4 milliseconds, duration with a 10-millisecond delay. (From Goldman MP, Fitzpatrick RE. Cutaneous Laser Surgery: The Art and Science of Selective Photothermolysis, 2nd ed. St. Louis: Mosby, 1998. Reproduced with permission.)

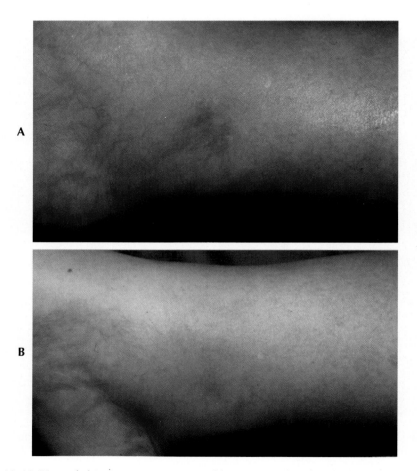

FIGURE 22-12. Tanned skin, type III in 63-year-old woman with isolated telangiectasias without associated varicosities. Previous attempt with sclerotherapy yielded no improvement. **A,** Before treatment. **B,** Ten minutes after treatment with IPL. Parameters were 44 J/cm^2 given at double pulses of 2.4 milliseconds and 7 milliseconds with a 10-millisecond delay through a 570 nm filter.

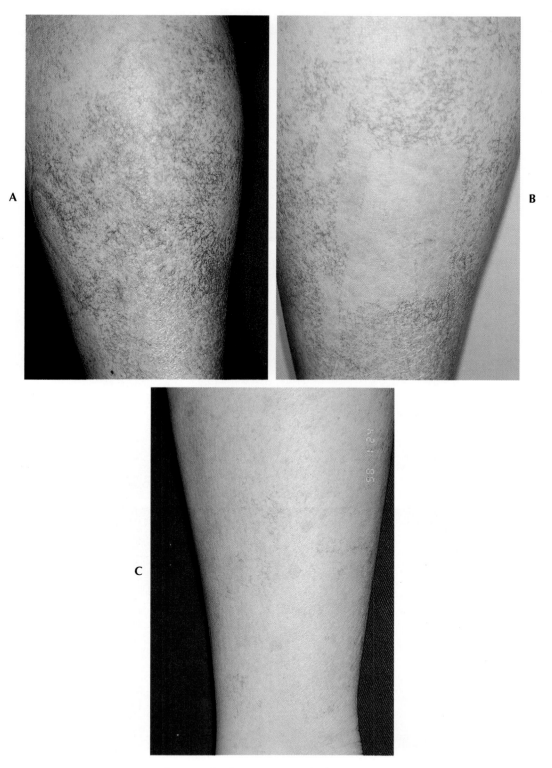

FIGURE 22-13. Treatment of essential telangiectasia with the IPL in a 35-year-old woman. **A,** Before treatment. **B,** After a single treatment at 40 J/cm² delivered in two pulses of 2.4 and 4 milliseconds separated by a delay of 10 milliseconds through a 550 nm filter. **C,** After three treatments at identical parameters, with each treatment covering a different nontreated area, the entire lesion has resolved. A total of 254 pulses was needed to cover the entire area on the leg.

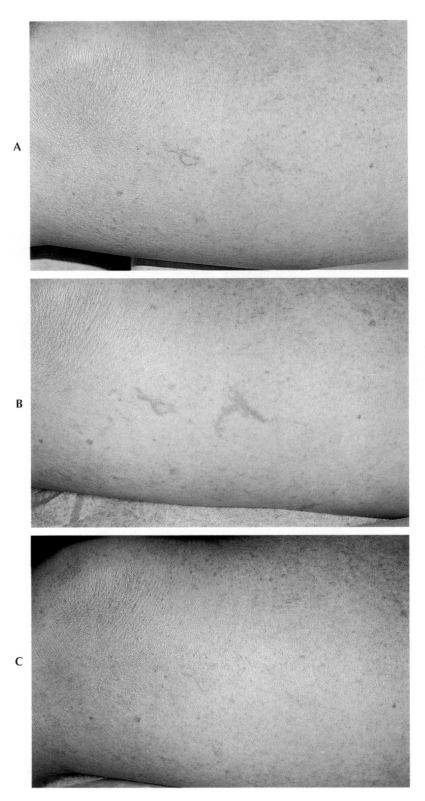

FIGURE 22-14. Ankle of a 55-year-old woman who presented with large varicose veins on the medial aspect of the right leg and telangiectasias at the ankle. The varicose veins, originating from reflux at the hunterian perforator, were eliminated by duplex-guided sclerotherapy. After resolution of the varicose vein, the remaining ankle telangiectasias were treated with IPL. **A,** Before treatment, parameters were 5-millisecond pulse duration, 35 J/cm², single pulse, and 550 nm filter. **B,** Immediately after second treatment. **C,** Resolution 2 months after second treatment.

MERCURY VAPOR FLASHLAMP SYSTEM

Although there are no published studies on this method as of this writing, a mercury vapor flashlamp system is also being promoted for treating leg telangiectasias. This system, OptoDerm (OptoMed, Inc., Austin, Tex.), uses a mercury vapor lamp with wavelength peaks at 436, 546, and 577 nm. The pulse duration is 5 to 50 milliseconds with pulse separation intervals of 2 seconds. An energy fluence of up to 50 J/cm² delivered as a 5 mm, 5 × 20 mm, or 8 × 13 mm spot size can be used.

CONCLUSION

Sclerotherapy treatment is relatively cost-effective as compared to laser or IPL treatment, but when is it appropriate to use this advanced laser therapy? Obviously, patients who are needle phobic will tolerate the use of this technology, even though the pain from both forms of treatment is comparable. Patients who are prone to telangiectatic matting are also appropriate candidates. Vessels below the ankle are particularly appropriate for treatment with light since sclerotherapy has a relatively high incidence of ulceration in this area because of the higher distribution of arteriovenous anastomosis (see Chapter 16). Finally, patients who have vessels that are resistant to sclerotherapy are excellent candidates for laser therapy. Efficacy of 75% clearance with 2 to 3 treatments has been reported in sclerotherapy-resistant vessels.[53] In this study, a novel treatment regimen using a triple pulse of 50 J/cm² in 2, 3, and 4 milliseconds with 50-millisecond pulse delays and a 590 nm cutoff filter was followed 1 minute later by a single 5-millisecond pulse of 35 J/cm² with a 550 nm cutoff filter. This regimen was hypothesized to treat both the deep and the superficial component of the vascular network.

Similarly, Weiss and Weiss[54] have reported enhanced efficacy by combining sclerotherapy with hypertonic saline/dextrose and IPL. This approach compares favorably with the combination sclerotherapy/FLPDL treatment described previously (Figure 22-14).

We believe that optimal efficacy in treating common leg telangiectasias is achieved by using a combination of sclerotherapy followed by laser or IPL with a rationale similar to that described here (sclerotherapy/FLPDL). Sclerotherapy will treat the feeding venous system, and the laser or IPL will effectively seal the superficial vessels to prevent extravasation and consequent pigmentation, recanalization, and telangiectatic matting.

REFERENCES

1. Weiss RA, Weiss MA. Resolution of pain associated with varicose and telangiectatic leg veins after compression sclerotherapy. J Dermatol Surg Oncol 16:333, 1990.
2. Goldman MP, Kaplan RP, Duffy DM. Postsclerotherapy hyperpigmentation: A histologic evaluation. J Dermatol Surg Oncol 13:547, 1987.
3. Duffy DM. Small vessel sclerotherapy: An overview. In Callen J, et al., eds. Advances in Dermatology. Chicago: Year Book Medical Publishers, 1988, p 221.
4. de Faria JL, Moraes IN. Histopathology of the telangiectasias associated with varicose veins. Dermatologica 127:321, 1963.

5. Braverman IM. Ultrastructure and organization of the cutaneous microvasculature in normal and pathologic states. J Invest Dermatol 93:2S, 1989.

6. Wokalek H, et al. Morphology and localization of sunburst varicosities: An electron microscopic and morphometric study. J Dermatol Surg Oncol 15:149, 1989.

7. Bodian EL. Sclerotherapy. Semin Dermatol 6:238, 1987.

8. Sommer A, et al. Red and blue telangiectasia: Differences in oxygenation? Dermatol Surg 23:55, 1997.

9. Bean WB. Vascular Spiders and Related Lesions of the Skin. Springfield, Ill.: Charles C Thomas, 1958.

10. Apfelberg DB, et al. Study of three laser systems for treatment of superficial varicosities of the lower extremity. Lasers Surg Med 7:219, 1987.

11. Frazzetta M, et al. Considerations regarding the use of the CO_2 laser: Personal case study. Laser 2:4, 1989.

12. Landthaler M, et al. Laser therapy of venous lakes (Bean-Walsh) and telangiectasias. Plast Reconstr Surg 73:78, 1984.

13. Apfelberg DB, et al. Use of the argon and carbon dioxide lasers for treatment of superficial venous varicosities of the lower extremity. Lasers Surg Med 4:221, 1984.

14. Glassberg E, et al. The flashlamp-pumped 577 nm pulsed tunable dye laser: Clinical efficacy and in vitro studies. J Dermatol Surg Oncol 14:1200, 1988.

14a. Weiss RA, Weiss MA. Early clinical results with a multiple synchronized pulse 1064 nm laser for leg telangiectasias and reticular veins. Derm Surg [in press].

15. Dixon JA, Rotering RH, Huethner SE. Patient's evaluation of argon laser therapy of port-wine stain, decorative tattoos, and essential telangiectasia. Lasers Surg Med 4:181, 1984.

16. Corcos L, Longo L. Classification and treatment of telangiectases of the lower limbs. Laser 1:22, 1988.

17. Chess C, Chess Q. Cool laser optics treatment of large telangiectasia of the lower extremities. J Dermatol Surg Oncol 19:74, 1993.

18. Tan OT, Kerschmann R, Parrish JA. Effect of skin temperature on selective vascular injury caused by pulsed laser irradiation. J Invest Dermatol 85:441, 1985.

19. West TB, Alster TS. Comparison of the long-pulse dye (590-595 nm) and KTP (532 nm) lasers in the treatment of facial and leg telangiectasias. Dermatol Surg 24:221, 1998.

20. Quintana AT, et al. Removal of leg veins with laserscope potassium titanyl phosphate-532 nm and dermastat 2 mm handpiece. Presented at the 18th Annual Meeting of the American Society of Laser Medicine and Surgery. San Diego, Calif., April 5-7, 1998.

21. Adrian RM. Treatment of leg telangiectasias using a long-pulse frequency-doubled neodymium: YAG laser at 532 nm. Dermatol Surg 24:19, 1998.

22. McMeekin TO. Treatment of spider veins of the leg using a Versapulse Laser at 532 nm. Presented at the 18th Annual Meeting of the American Society of Laser Medicine and Surgery. San Diego, Calif., April 5-7, 1998.

23. Narukar VA. The efficacy of the Coherent Versapulse 532 nm variable pulse laser for the treatment of superficial leg telangiectasia. Presented at the 18th Annual Meeting of the American Society of Laser Medicine and Surgery. San Diego, Calif., April 5-7, 1998.

24. Goldman MP, Fitzpatrick RE. Cutaneous Laser Surgery: The Art and Science of Selective Photothermolysis, 2nd ed. St. Louis: Mosby, 1998.

25. Garden JM, et al. Effect of dye laser pulse duration on selective cutaneous vascular injury. J Invest Dermatol 87:653, 1986.

26. Polla LL, et al. Tunable pulsed dye laser for the treatment of benign cutaneous vascular ectasia. Dermatologica 174:11, 1987.

27. Ashton N. Corneal vascularization. In Duke-Elder S, Perkins ES, eds. The Transparency of the Cornea. Oxford: Blackwell, 1960.

28. Folkman J, Klagsbrun M. Angiogenic factors. Science 235:442, 1987.

29. Ryan TJ. Factors influencing the growth of vascular endothelium in the skin. Br J Dermatol 82(Suppl 5):99, 1970.

30. Dvorak HF. Tumors: Wounds that do not heal: Similarities between tumor stroma generation and wound healing. N Engl J M 315:1650, 1986.

31. Majewski S, et al. Angiogenic capability of peripheral blood mononuclear cells in psoriasis. Arch Dermatol 121:1018, 1985.

32. Nakagawa H, Tan OT, Parrish JA. Ultrastructural changes in human skin after exposure to a pulsed laser. J Invest Dermatol 84:396, 1985.

33. Tan TT, et al. Histologic responses of port-wine stains treated by argon, carbon dioxide, and tunable dye lasers: A preliminary report. Arch Dermatol 122:1016, 1986.

34. Goldman MP, et al. Pulsed dye laser treatment of telangiectasia with and without sub-therapeutic sclerotherapy: Clinical and histologic examination in the rabbit ear vein model. J Am Acad Dermatol 23:23, 1990.

35. Goldman MP, Fitzpatrick RE. Pulsed-dye laser treatment of leg telangiectasia: With and without simultaneous sclerotherapy. J Dermatol Surg Oncol 16:338, 1990.

36. Perez B, et al. Progressive ascending telangiectasia treated with the 585 nm flashlamp-pumped pulsed dye laser. Lasers Surg Med 21:413, 1997.

37. Fajardo LF, et al. Hyperthermia inhibits angiogenesis. Radiat Res 114:297, 1988.

38. Hsia J, Lowery JA, Zelickson B. Treatment of leg telangiectasia using a long-pulse dye laser at 595 nm. Lasers Surg Med 20:1, 1997.

39. Lee PK, Lask GP. Treatment of leg veins by long pulse dye laser (Sclerolaser). Lasers Surg Med (Suppl) 9:40, 1997.

40. Hohenleutner U, et al. Leg telangiectasia treatment with a 1.5 ms pulsed dye laser and ice cube cooling of the skin: 595 vs. 600 nm. Lasers Surg Med [in press].

41. Alora MB, et al. Comparison of the 595 nm long pulse (1.5 ms) and the 595 nm ultra-long pulse (4 ms) laser in the treatment of leg veins. Presented at the 18th Annual Meeting of the American Society of Laser Medicine and Surgery. San Diego, Calif., April 5-7, 1998.

42. Adrian RM. Long pulse normal mode alexandrite laser treatment of leg veins. Presented at the 18th Annual Meeting of the American Society of Laser Medicine and Surgery. San Diego, Calif., April 5-7, 1998.

43. Dierickx CC, Dugue V, Anderson RR. Treatment of leg telangiectasia by a pulsed 800 nm diode laser. Presented at the 18th Annual Meeting of the American Society of Laser Medicine and Surgery. San Diego, Calif., April 5-7, 1998.

44. Garden JM, Bakus AD, Miller ID. Diode laser treatment of leg veins. Presented at the 18th Annual Meeting of the American Society of Laser Medicine and Surgery. San Diego, Calif., April 5-7, 1998.

45. Anderson AR, et al. The optics of human skin. J Invest Dermatol 77:13, 1981.

46. Schroeter CA, et al. Clinical significance of an intense, pulsed light source on leg telangiectasias of up to 1mm diameter. Eur J Dermatol 7:38, 1997.

47. Goldman MP, et al. Photothermal sclerosis of leg veins. Dermatol Surg 22:323, 1996.

48. Behandlung essentieller Telangiektasien durch das Photoderm VL. H + B 71:44, 1996.

49. Weiss RA, Weiss MA. Intense pulsed light revisited: Progressive increase in pulse durations for better results on leg veins. Presented at the 11th Annual Meeting of the North American Society of Phlebology. Palm Desert, Calif., Nov. 1997.

50. Raulin C, Weiss RA, Schonermark MP. Treatment of essential telangiectasias with an intense pulsed light source (PhotoDerm VL). Dermatol Surg 23:941, 1997.

51. Schroeter CA, et al. Clinical significance of an intense light source on leg telangiectasias of up to 1 mm diameter. Eur J Dermatol 7:38, 1997.

52. Raulin C, Weiss RA, Schonermark MP. Treatment of essential telangiectasias with an intense pulsed light source (PhotoDerm VL). Dermatol Surg 23:941, 1997.

53. Weiss RA, Weiss MA. Photothermal sclerosis of resistant telangiectatic leg and facial veins using the PhotoDerm VL. Presented at the Annual Meeting of the Mexican Academy of Dermatology. Monterey, Mexico, April 24, 1996.

54. Weiss RA, Weiss MA. Combination intense pulsed light and sclerotherapy—A synergistic effect. Presented at the 11th Annual Meeting of the North American Society of Phlebology. Palm Desert, Calif., Nov. 1997.

Chapter 23

Painful Telangiectasias: Diagnosis and Treatment

Robert A. Weiss and Margaret A. Weiss

Telangiectatic leg veins may be described as venous spiders, sunburst veins, starburst veins, venous plexuses, dilated venules, venous blemishes, dilated venules and venulectasias, superficial or minor varicosities, essential cutaneous telangiectasias, vanity veins, and cosmetic veins.[1] Despite the cosmetic significance implied by this terminology, all these terms describe the type of telangiectatic networks that may cause physical symptoms of pain and discomfort. Over 50% of patients presenting for treatment of these "spider veins" have aching associated with them.[2] These symptomatic veins are best categorized as arborizing networks (according to the Redisch and Pelzer classification[3]). They are actually combinations or networks of telangiectasias (0.1 to 1 mm) and venulectases (1 to 2 mm). Painful telangiectasias on the leg usually are grouped; they are rarely present as isolated telangiectatic vessels or spider angiomas with a central arteriole. More important, symptomatic telangiectasias and venulectases commonly are associated with slightly larger blue veins, which have been termed "feeder" veins, reticular veins, or minor varicose veins. These small subdermal blue veins may be tributaries of the saphenous system. Reticular veins are most commonly part of a superficial venous system that is separate from either of the saphenous systems, originally described as the "lateral subdermic venous system" by Albanese et al.[4] This chapter discusses common locations and patterns of painful telangiectasias, their intricate association with reticular veins (often comprising the lateral venous system), the type and location of symptoms, and the best approach for eliminating symptoms.

CLASSIFICATION AND ANATOMY

In order to diagnose and treat painful telangiectasias in a logical way, a precise classification is helpful (see box on p. 499). A discussion of painful telangiectasias includes telangiectasias (type I), venulectases (type II), and associated blue

REVISED VESSEL CLASSIFICATION*

Type I

Telangiectasia, "spider veins"
0.1-1 mm diameter
Usually red (rarely may be cyanotic)
> Type IA
>> Telangiectatic matting
>> <0.2 mm diameter network, bright red

Type II

Venulectasia (usually protrudes above skin surface, distinguished from telangiectasia by deeper color and larger diameter)
1-2 mm diameter
Violaceous, cyanotic

Type III

Reticular veins ("minor" varicose veins, "feeder" veins)
2-4 mm diameter
Cyanotic to blue

Type IV

Nonsaphenous varicose veins (primary varicosity of saphenous tributary usually related to incompetent perforator)
3-8 mm diameter
Blue to blue-green

Type V

Saphenous varicose veins (varicosities associated with reflux at saphenofemoral or saphenopopliteal junction or major perforators of saphenous system causing enlargement of long or short saphenous vein)
Usually >8 mm in diameter
Blue to blue-green

---

*Data from Goldman MP. Sclerotherapy treatment for varicose and telangiectatic leg veins. In Coleman WP, Hanke CW, Alt TH, Asken S, eds. Cosmetic Surgery of the Skin. Philadelphia: BC Decker, 1991, pp 197-211; Duffy DM. Small vessel sclerotherapy: An overview. In Callen JP, et al., eds. Advances in Dermatology, vol 3. Chicago: Year Book, 1988, pp 221-242.
Note: This simplified classification eliminates the mixed telangiectasia/varicose category. Since most patients have a combination of multiple varicose vein types, a description of type I in association with type II or type III varicosities is simpler. Classifying varicose veins in this way allows for a more straightforward treatment plan.

reticular veins (type III). In this discussion of painful telangiectasias, it is assumed that reflux from primary varicose veins of type IV and type V has been treated or is absent. It is presently understood that groups of reticular veins, venulectases, and telangiectasias may be subject to forces of stretch and increased venous pressure similar to those that produce major varicosities.[5] A disturbance of normal venous physiology with back pressure and reverse flow or reflux through incompetent valves results in transmission of pressure through reticular veins into venules, causing their expansion into telangiectasias and venulectases.[6]

Arborizing networks of telangiectasias have been shown to be dilated cutaneous venules with intrinsic connections to underlying larger veins of which they are direct tributaries.[7,8] Valves are found throughout the postcapillary venous system regulating flow within the smallest of venules.[9] Thus increased venous pressure is transmitted in a cascade effect; conducted pressure causes increased diameter and incompetence of venous valves from reticular veins to telangiectasias. This effect has been confirmed through Doppler ultrasound demonstration of audible reflux in lateral thigh reticular veins associated with telangiectasias in hundreds of patients who presented for treatment without associated saphenous varicosities.[10] Findings with direct high-resolution duplex ultrasound examination show reflux through knee perforating veins into the lateral thigh reticular veins.[6,11]

Pain associated with telangiectasias may be a consequence of stretching caused by pressure transmitted during reflux through reticular veins and venulectases. In a detailed discussion of symptoms caused by varicose veins, Lofgren[12] states that "the largest varicosities sometimes cause no complaints; other veins of small caliber may give rise to surprising discomfort." One theory that attempts to explain this phenomenon is that compliance of smaller veins may be greater than that of larger ones, with more distensibility and greater stretch resulting in greater stimulation of neural pain receptors. Larger varicose veins develop intramural fibrosis with time, and this change may prevent rapid stretching.[13] In vitro studies of viscoelastic properties of varicose veins demonstrate limited stretch potential of larger varicose veins.[14] Smaller veins such as postcapillary venules may not develop intramural fibrosis. Without this fibrosis, dilatation up to two to four times in diameter may occur. Such dilatation may correlate with the patient's reporting a feeling of "vein breaking." Alternatively, pain in telangiectasias or venulectases may occur with prolonged standing as a direct consequence of slow dilatation through pressure. Potentially increased diameter as a percentage of normal diameter is much greater for venules than for axial veins; hence the increased potential for pain.

LATERAL SUBDERMIC VENOUS SYSTEM

Originally described by Albanese et al.,[4] the lateral subdermic venous system consists of veins that are the size of reticular veins at a depth just below the dermis, longitudinally traversing the lateral thigh and calf and often having complex communications at the lateral knee (Figure 23-1). This system may become varicose even in the absence of saphenous system varicosities. Small perforating veins

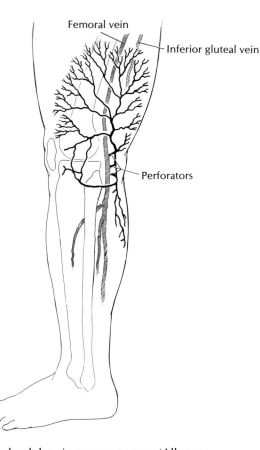

FIGURE 23-1. In the lateral subdermic venous system (Albanese venous system), vein size may range from 3 mm to >1 cm. These veins longitudinally traverse the lateroposterior thigh and lateroposterior calf, often having several direct communications with the deep venous system near the lateral knee. They are often responsible for painful telangiectatic webs seen on the thigh or calf. Reflux is often noted over the sites identified as perforators. An 8 to 10 MHz Doppler probe allows reflux to be heard clearly and loudly through distal compression release or proximal compression. The inferior gluteal vein is shown as a possible tributary to the lateral venous system.

connect the lateral venous system to the deep femoral vein or the popliteal vein, thus serving as the primary source of reflux that propagates the varicosity. Occasionally the lateral system communicates with and is enlarged by reflux through the inferior gluteal vein with a refluxing reticular vein coursing along the posterior thigh. Perhaps a more appropriate term for the Albanese subdermal system would be the "lateral posterior venous system."

Reflux in lateral thigh reticular veins has been traced by Doppler and duplex ultrasound to points near the lateral knee.[6,10] This finding correlates with previously described perforators of the lateral venous system.[4] Reflux may also originate from lateral thigh perforators and the gluteal system. Reflux originating from these and lateral knee perforators are responsible for ultimate dilatation of the telangiectatic bridges seen on the upper lateral and posterior thigh and down the lateral posterior calf. Proposed mechanisms include changes in pressure and shifts in flow with occlusion of veins during sitting. Dramatic shifts in hemodynamics with knee bending have been demonstrated.[15]

Reflux through small perforators at the lateral knee into the lateral venous system combined with lateral thigh perforating veins and posterior sources of reflux from the gluteal system account for the vast majority of painful telangiectatic groups on the lateral and posterior portions of the thigh and the upper calf in patients without reflux at the saphenofemoral junction, saphenopopliteal junction, or "major" perforators associated with the saphenous system. In our experience these lateral minor varicosities are noted initially when the individual is at a younger age (teens through thirties), typically several decades before the onset of major varicosities. This earlier onset may be explained through an examination of venous system embryology of the leg.

Based on anatomic dissections by Hochstetter,[16] the initial venous system of the leg is characterized by a network of superficial veins from which the lateral venous system is derived. The deep venous system then develops in a rudimentary way, accompanied by development of a superficial external saphenous vein that is connected by small perforators to the deep system. When the deep venous system becomes predominant, the external saphenous vein disintegrates at the thigh, but not without leaving a few thigh perforators intact. Albanese et al.[4] speculated that, in areas where the superficial veins do not involute, superficial embryonic veins remain and may become easily and prematurely varicosed. This change occurs for two reasons: (1) because of their superficial location, these veins are poorly supported by surrounding connective tissue; and (2) direct transfascial perforators continue to connect these veins with the deep venous system.

Albanese concluded that when a network of easily varicosed veins occurs on the lateral thigh, it should be considered a developmental defect. With intact lateral knee perforators serving as a direct source for transmission of high pressure from the deep venous system accompanied by a lack of structural support, reticular veins may become stretched and distended easily. The term "minor varicose vein" is fully justified for these lateral thigh reticular veins. A Doppler study of the distribution of varicose veins confirmed the presence of a distinct group of non-saphenous varicosities on the lateral aspect of the thigh and calf that represented the lateral venous system.[17]

Heredity is an important factor in the development of thigh reticular varicose veins,[18] as it is in development of most varicose veins.[19] It is remarkable that reticular varicosities do not increase in frequency with age (as the saphenous types do), which confirms that preexisting factors are of great impact.[18]

DISTRIBUTION

Although painful telangiectasias and venulectases may appear anywhere on the leg, they are most likely to occur near the knee (Figure 23-2). Although a

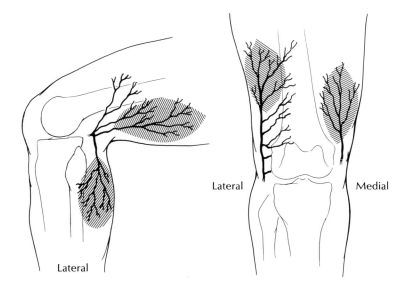

FIGURE 23-2. Regions where painful groups of telangiectasias and venulectases are most likely to occur are shown by the shaded areas. Patients most often complain of focal burning, throbbing, and aching in these regions. The lateral view shows posterior distribution of pain of the lateral venous system associated with telangiectatic webs. Prolonged sitting often produces pain in the posterior thigh, whereas prolonged standing often causes pain in the calf. The anteroposterior view shows less common sites of painful telangiectatic webs on the lateral and medial thigh above the knee. A reticular vein with reflux audible through Doppler ultrasound often is associated with these regions of pain.

bridge of telangiectasias and venulectases on the lateral thigh is the most common pattern, our personal observations in treating 13,000 patients indicate that extension onto the upper calf often is responsible for painful symptoms (Figure 23-3). It is presumed that the latter is caused by the greater effect of gravity during standing. Most of our patients report discomfort along the lateral to posterior calf during standing. The location of pain may be perceived to change during sitting; patients may then relate pain to telangiectatic groups localized on the posterior thigh.

The medial thigh is an especially difficult region because telangiectasias may be observed in association with a reticular vein coursing anterior and inferior to the patella. These telangiectasias may also be a manifestation of reflux originating from larger axial varicosities related to the greater saphenous vein (Figure 23-4). Astute diagnosis of reflux origin is critical when patients report symptoms from telangiectasias in the medial thigh. The physician should not forget that large varicosities connected to the saphenous system may reflux into reticular veins and cause pain in associated telangiectasias.

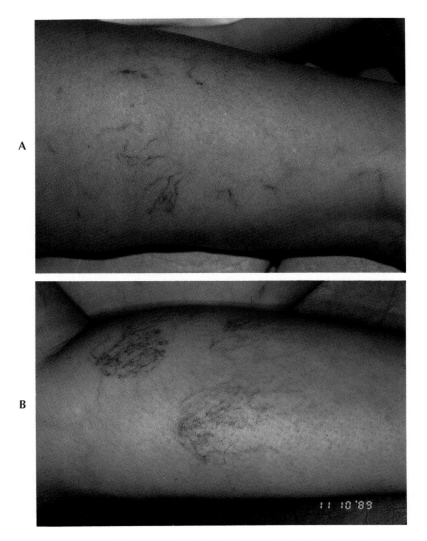

FIGURE 23-3. A, Typical lateral thigh location for a bridge of telangiectasias and venulectases associated with a reticular vein having no symptoms. B, Reticular vein extension onto the upper calf leading to a group or web of telangiectasias and venulectases responsible for symptoms of focal burning.

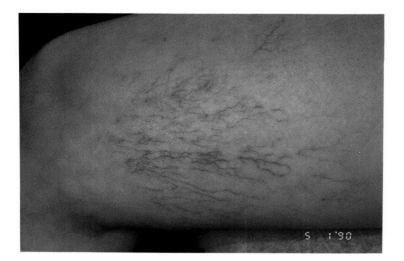

FIGURE 23-4. On the medial thigh, a group of telangiectasias is seen in association with reticular veins that course near the greater saphenous vein. Great caution must be observed in treatment of reticular veins in this region. Telangiectatic matting following treatment often occurs here.

SYMPTOMS

Over the last 5 years, groups of telangiectasias have been accepted as a common cause of leg pain.[20] Table 23-1 lists common symptoms described by patients. Earliest symptoms reported included a sensation of burning discomfort associated with warm weather.[21] Tretbar[22] reported that "although treatment has not been offered to patients for relief of symptoms in the legs, a number of patients have nevertheless reported subjective improvement of aches and pains." Similarly, the association of leg pain with telangiectasias has been made by many of our patients only after telangiectasias, treated initially for cosmetic reasons, completely resolved and the patients subsequently noted far less leg pain and fatigue.

After this initial correlation by patients, we became interested in the details of the therapeutic benefits of sclerotherapy for the relief of pain associated with telangiectasias and venulectases. Many of our patients whose occupations involve long periods of standing have complained of muscle fatigue and aching or localized pain over groups of telangiectasias and/or venulectases. Some relief of symptoms occurs by wearing lightweight support hose.[23]

In order to quantitate the effectiveness of sclerotherapy to relieve leg pain and discomfort, a questionnaire detailing frequency and types of reported symptoms was mailed to 350 patients.[2] The level of pain improvement was recorded and correlated with the extent of cosmetic resolution. Of the patients responding

TABLE 23-1. Symptoms of painful telangiectasias*

Symptom	Overall Incidence (%)	Patients With Posttreatment Improvement (%)
Fatigue, general ache	32	85
Pain in region of telangiectasia or reticular vein	31	86
Focal burning	27	93
Night cramping	21	70
Local edema	19	83
Throbbing sensation (focal or general)	17	86

*Modified from Weiss RA, Weiss MA. Resolution of pain associated with varicose and telangiectatic leg veins after compression sclerotherapy. J Dermatol Surg Oncol 16:333-336, 1990.

to the survey, approximately 53% (114 of 214) had associated symptoms with their telangiectasias and/or venulectases. For all symptoms combined, the overall reported relief of pain following treatment was 85% ($p < 0.001$). The most common symptom was a sensation of fatigue accompanied by a dull, generalized achiness. The second most common symptom was pain at the precise site of a group of venulectases or telangiectasias. A symptom of burning was found frequently in a region of telangiectasias and/or venulectases located at or near the site. Another frequently reported symptom was throbbing or pulsating pain along the leg, usually occurring laterally but not directly associated with a specific group of telangiectasias or venulectases.

Night cramps were reported, and they were improved by sclerotherapy. Edema of a region or engorgement of a telangiectatic group was exacerbated by prolonged standing, but this condition could be reversed by sclerotherapy. Most patients experienced several symptoms. Frequently these symptoms were exacerbated during menses. A small percentage of our patients experienced pain or swelling only during menses.[24] Leg symptoms reported by women have been attributed to the distention of the vein walls induced by hormonal changes of the menstrual cycle.[25]

Many of the symptoms reported for telangiectasias were identical to those reported for larger varicosities. These symptoms include a dull aching of the leg, particularly after prolonged standing, during menses, or as a result of the hormonal changes of pregnancy.[26] According to the Basel study III, approximately 25% of patients with major varicose veins experienced symptoms such as heaviness, swelling, cramps, pain or aching, and restless legs.[27] Estimations of intermittent pain in larger varicosities have been as high as 50%.[28]

Although there are many causes of leg pain, such as arthritis and tendonitis, several clues may be helpful in determining whether leg pain is caused by webs of telangiectasias or venulectases. A dull, throbbing ache or a sensation of heaviness in the legs that occurs at the end of the day but is not noticeable on awakening is very likely to respond to treatment with sclerotherapy. Most commonly, a burning quality to the discomfort that worsens with standing for long hours indicates a venous problem. Focal burning also may occur suddenly, producing a sensation of breakage or rupture. This burning may be the result of decreased breaking strength of already enlarged veins.[29] Tenderness is less likely to be a symptom unless superficial phlebitis is a factor. Other important clues are the relief or improvement of symptoms by the use of support hose or a worsening of symptoms during menses. Pain from telangiectasias, in our experience, is rarely referred to the knee joint or hip. The distribution of pain also may help in diagnosis; for example, pain from a venous source is likely to be located on the lateral to lateroposterior calf or thigh in the distribution of the lateral subdermic venous system varicosities.

Physical examination also is important in determining the source of pain. Obviously, if a patient points to a focal area of pain with an overlying telangiectatic web, the pain is likely to arise from this group (Figure 23-5). Associated reticular veins usually can be identified visually. Transillumination may aid in visualization.[30,31] Doppler ultrasound assists in locating sources of reflux into the telangiectatic group. The method for using the Doppler probe to elicit reflux in varicosities has been described by Schultz-Ehrenburg and Hubner.[32] For reticular veins the method is identical. The patient should be examined while in a sitting or standing position. With a series of manual compressions and decompressions of the calf, the physician moves the Doppler probe over the reticular vein until the loudest flow signal is found. Thus a physiologic site of increased venous pressure into the telangiectasia can be documented and a cause for pain can be identified with greater certainty. The frequency with which reflux into a reticular vein is associated with a group of telangiectasias is quite high.[33] Occasionally, a reflux signal is heard at the point of origin of a telangiectatic group without the visual identification of a reticular vein (Figure 23-6). Presumably the associated reticular vein is just below the surface, preventing its visualization.

Certain occupations that involve long periods of standing carry an increased risk for developing painful telangiectasias. Examples include the work of beauticians, educators, nurses, clerks, assembly line workers, and many others. In our experience such workers complain of symptoms associated with telangiectasias, receive some relief from the use of support hose, and benefit a great deal from sclerotherapy.[2] Even when pain is not a problem with varicosities and telangiectasias, these conditions can be so psychologically disturbing to women that they will not wear shorts or bathing suits at all, thus eliminating major sources of recreation and exercise from their lifestyles.

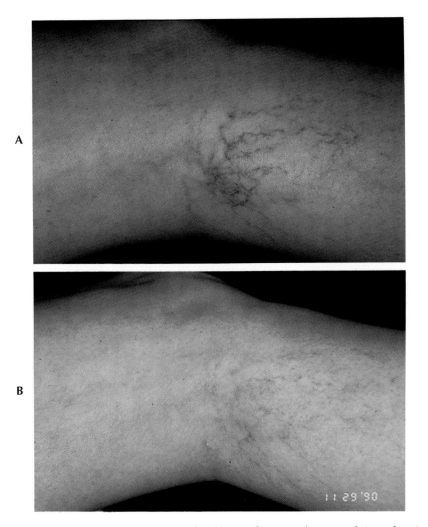

FIGURE 23-5. When a patient points out a focal area of pain with an overlying telangiectatic web, the pain is most likely to arise from this group. **A,** Focal burning pain associated with a telangiectatic web on the proximal lateroposterior calf. Several reticular veins were noted with two sites of reflux identified by Doppler ultrasound. Treatment consisted of 1 ml of 0.2% sodium tetradecyl sulfate (Sotradecol) injected into several points along the reticular veins with an additional injection of 0.5 ml of 0.1% Sotradecol into the telangiectatic web. **B,** Two months later, almost complete cosmetic ablation was noted with complete resolution of pain.

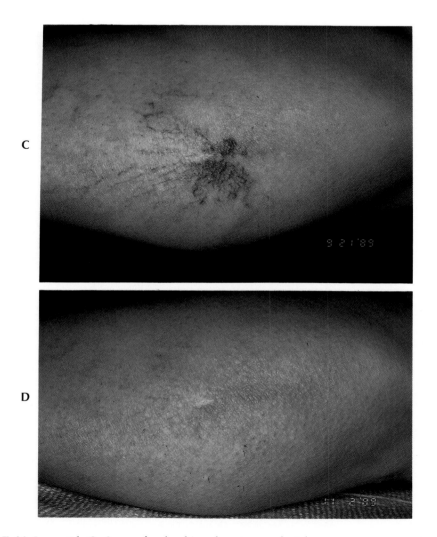

FIGURE 23-5, cont'd. C, Severe focal aching, burning, and night cramps were associated with a telangiectatic web at the site of a previous ligation. A reticular vein (not easily visualized) was traced to the lateroposterior knee. Treatment consisted of 0.75 ml of hypertonic saline (23.4%) injected into the reticular vein, with an additional 0.5 ml of hypertonic saline injected into the web. **D,** Painful symptoms resolved within 1 week. Within 6 weeks, resolution of the dilated venules was seen.   *Continued.*

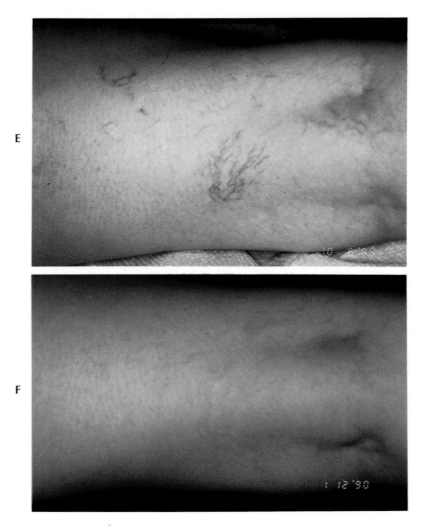

FIGURE 23-5, cont'd. E, Focal aching on the posterior thigh, which worsened with sitting for long periods, was associated with a lateral subdermic venous system reticular vein. The origin of reflux for this telangiectatic web was traced by Doppler ultrasound with distal compression release to a small perforator in the region of the fibular collateral ligament. Treatment consisted of injection of 0.5 ml of 1% polidocanol into the reticular vein and 0.5 ml of 0.5% polidocanol into the telangiectatic web. **F,** A second treatment was necessary to obtain resolution of pain and varicosities at 3 months.

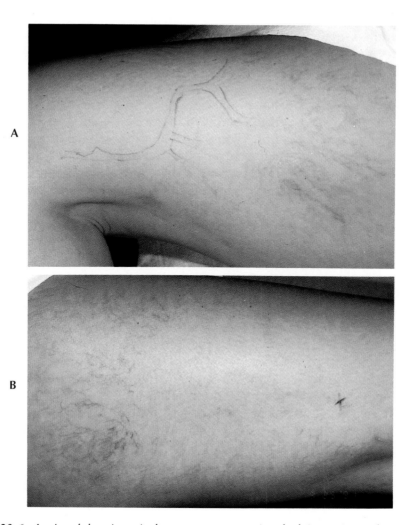

FIGURE 23-6. **A,** A subdermic reticular venous system (marked in pen) can be traced with a 10 MHz Doppler ultrasound probe. **B,** A barely visible lateral venous system reticular vein associated with a bridge of telangiectasias on the thighs is easily identified by Doppler ultrasound. The loudest point of reflux, a good point to initiate injections, is marked with an X.

TREATMENT PROTOCOLS
Painful Telangiectasias

The treatment of painful telangiectasias is identical to that of cosmetic telangiectasias except that particular attention is devoted to associated reticular veins. The basic principle of treatment, proceeding from the largest to the smallest varicosities, holds true. One should first inject the reticular veins, next inject the largest venulectases, and then proceed to the smallest telangiectasias.

The use of Doppler ultrasound helps to identify sources of reflux into telangiectatic groups. Often the Doppler reflux signal may be traced to its loudest point, and the injections can be initiated there. For example, a group of telangiectasias on the lateral thigh may have associated reticular veins that are part of a varicose lateral subdermic venous system; the loudest Doppler flow signal often can be traced to the area distal to the lateral femoral condyle. The injections would be initiated at this site and continued every 3 to 4 cm along the course of the reticular vein. Usually no more than 0.5 ml of sclerosing solution per injection site is necessary, although some longer reticular veins will require 1 ml of solution.

Occasionally, the sclerosing solution is observed to enter the telangiectasia directly from the feeder vein; this occurrence may eliminate the need to inject the telangiectasia directly. Our experience also has shown the reverse situation; that is, when groups of telangiectasias are being injected, occasionally one may visualize sclerosing solution entering the feeder vein from injection through a telangiectasia. This occurrence was demonstrated in 20 patients in whom the flow of sclerosing solution from the telangiectasia into the reticular vein was documented by Doppler ultrasound.[10]

In practical terms the direction of valves in these veins should allow easy flow from smaller to larger veins. However, this method cannot be relied on for treatment of the reticular vein because the development of extravasation at the site of injection in the telangiectatic vein often prevents sufficient sclerosant volume or concentration to enter the larger reticular vein. Therefore the reticular vein would be inadequately treated, and recurrence of the telangiectasia would be more likely. When no clear "feeder" vessel is seen or identified by Doppler ultrasound or transillumination, the point at which the telangiectasias begin to branch out is the site at which injection should be begun. This approach saves time by decreasing the number of injection sites per telangiectatic group.

Based on our experience, simultaneously injecting telangiectasias is more successful than relying solely on sclerosing solution to reach the telangiectasia through reticular vein injection. In the process of flowing from reticular veins into telangiectatic veins, the sclerosing solution may be diluted, inactivated by blood proteins, or lost by leakage through damaged endothelium. The inactivation caused by binding to blood protein is theoretically possible if the elasticity of the venule wall was diminished during the process of becoming enlarged. With this compliance diminished, even elimination of a pressure source would not result in vessel shrinkage.

Reticular Veins

The first treatment session for reticular veins usually is limited to one or two sites in order to (1) observe the patient for any allergic reactions, (2) determine the patient's ability to tolerate the burning or cramping of a hypertonic solution, (3) judge the effectiveness of a particular concentration of sclerosing agent, and (4) observe any reactions to the tape used for compression. The patient returns in

4 to 6 weeks so that the test site can be compared with pretreatment photographs. At each follow-up session the patient is asked if the painful symptoms have decreased. When the symptoms have stopped, the physician can be confident that treatment has been successful, even before visual improvement is recognized. Conversely, if visual improvement is noted but the symptoms have not improved, the source of reflux has not been eliminated and a recurrence in the treated area is highly likely.

Treatment of reticular veins is similar to that of large varicose veins, although the concentration, strength, and volume of the sclerosing solution are decreased. Reticular veins are treated only after all sources of reflux from major varicosities have been treated by sclerotherapy and/or surgery. Doppler ultrasound also may be used as a guide to demonstrate reflux in the reticular veins and to locate those that require treatment.

While the patient is in a recumbent position, a 3 ml syringe with a 27- to 30-gauge needle, bent to an angle of 10 to 20 degrees, is inserted into the reticular vein. Since this vein usually is superficial and visibly blue, it does not require preliminary marking with a pen. When the sensation of piercing the vein is felt, the plunger is pulled back gently with the thumb of the dominant hand until blood is seen beginning to back up into the transparent plastic hub (this is possible even with a 30-gauge needle). If the wall of the reticular vein is very thin, the suction created by pulling back on the syringe may cause the wall to adhere to the needle bevel and prevent aspiration of blood. In this situation the needle can be moved gently forward and backward; if no resistance is felt, the vein probably has been cannulated, and the physician can proceed very cautiously with injection.

We also have observed the reticular vein to shrink spasmodically and virtually disappear from view following an attempt at cannulation. When such shrinkage occurs, another injection site along the reticular vein must be sought. Cannulation of a reticular vein can be more difficult than that of a protuberant venulectasia or telangiectasia.

Usually the volume per injection site is no more than 0.5 ml, but the capacity of long reticular veins may even exceed 1 ml. The progress of the solution can be followed visually, and the injection can be stopped when the entire reticular vein has been cleared of blood and appears to be in contact with the sclerosing solution.

Sclerosing solutions used and their concentrations include the following: (1) 0.5% to 1% polidocanol (Aethoxysklerol; Kreussler & Co., Wiesbaden-Biebrich, Germany) (although not FDA-approved, polidocanol is a forgiving solution in fragile, thin-walled vessels); (2) 0.2% to 0.5% sodium tetradecyl sulfate (Sotradecol; Wyeth-Ayerst Laboratories, Philadelphia, Pa.); (3) 23.4% hypertonic saline, and (4) hypertonic saline with dextrose (Sclerodex; Omega Laboratories, Montreal, Quebec). Until the physician gains experience in cannulating reticular veins, cautious injection cannot be overemphasized. A bruise usually will occur almost immediately, and resistance to injection will be felt when the reticular vein has not been cannulated properly.

Telangiectatic Veins

The injection method for treatment of telangiectasias has been described in detail in other chapters. The concentrations of sclerosing solutions are reduced even further than for reticular veins: 0.25% to 0.5% polidocanol (not FDA-approved) (again, the most forgiving agent, even when a bleb occurs at the injection site); 11.7% to 20% hypertonic saline; hypertonic saline with dextrose; and 0.1% to 0.3% sodium tetradecyl sulfate. The injection technique requires a gentle, precise touch as one learns to appreciate the subtle sensation felt on entering the vessel or to recognize the appearance of needle bevel within the telangiectasia lumen. If these signs are not appreciated immediately, minimal withdrawal of the needle may allow the easy flow of sclerosing solution. A very sharp needle is critical for this fine touch, and the needle is changed often to minimize tearing the vessel. The use of 32- to 33-gauge needles is not advised because such needles dull quickly and are not disposable.

Injection of a tiny bolus of air (<0.05 cc) may be helpful to establish that the needle is within the vein by showing a slight clearing 1 to 3 mm ahead of the bevel. Injection is performed *very slowly.* A small amount of sclerosant (0.1 to 0.5 ml or less) is used, and minimal or no pressure is applied to a 3 ml syringe to maintain filling of the veins for 10 to 15 seconds. Rapid flushing of the vessels with large volumes of sclerosant is not necessary for successful sclerotherapy. Particularly when a hypertonic solution is being used, injection of sclerosant is stopped when blanching in a radius of 2 cm has occurred or when 15 seconds have passed, thus minimizing cramping and burning (e.g., with hypertonic solutions). When painless detergent sclerosants are used (e.g., polidocanol or sodium tetradecyl sulfate), a small volume of the solution with a short interval (10 seconds) of blanching will minimize side effects such as telangiectatic matting.[34]

Occasionally, no blanching occurs at the site of injection, and the sclerosing solution flows easily through the telangiectasia or can be seen flowing through adjacent telangiectasias or reticular veins several centimeters away from the injection site. In this situation the injection is stopped after 0.5 to 1 ml of sclerosant has been injected and gentle massage through immediate manual compression has been applied. Any vessel larger than approximately 0.5 mm or, more important, any vessel that protrudes above the surface of the skin benefits from compression. Cottonballs are secured over the injection sites with paper tape or Transpore tape (3M Medical-Surgical Division, St. Paul, Minn.), and compression is subsequently maintained by graduated compression stockings. Protuberant telangiectasias or telangiectasias associated with reticular veins are treated for 2 weeks with graduated 20 to 30 mm Hg compression support hosiery worn during waking hours. Patients are encouraged to walk, and they are instructed not to restrict their activities (except for heavy weightlifting with the legs). Treatment intervals vary, but allowing 4 to 8 weeks between treatments of identical areas helps to minimize the total number of sessions.

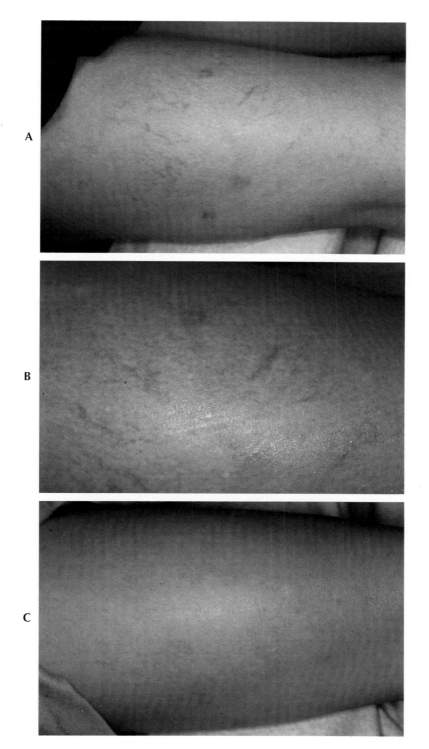

FIGURE 23-7. A, Thigh of a 42-year-old woman who had been treated with sclerotherapy 2 years earlier. Telangiectasias arising from a central reticular vein are noted. **B,** Immediately posttreatment with IPL and sclerotherapy. Edema, erythema, and an urticaria-type reaction is noted over the IPL-treated telangiectasias. The reticular vein was treated with a single injection of hypertonic saline and dextrose (0.5 ml). **C,** Six weeks after a single treatment, complete resolution has occurred.

Combination Sclerotherapy and Intense Pulsed Light

With the addition of intense pulsed light (IPL) for treatment of telangiectasias, a synergistic effect with sclerotherapy has been reported.[35] In this recent study three sites on either leg of a single patient were randomly selected to receive either sclerotherapy alone, IPL alone, or sclerotherapy combined with IPL. Selected sites were as similar as possible based on physical examination, transillumination, and/or Doppler findings. This preliminary study suggested better results with combined therapy (Figure 23-7). The possible synergistic effect may result from the fact that pressure into telangiectatic webs from incompetent reticular varicosities is eliminated by sclerotherapy so that a better response from the IPL treatment of telangiectasias is possible.

REFERENCES

1. Pierce HE. Management of unsightly micro-varicosities. Am J Cosmet Surg 1:45-47, 1984.
2. Weiss RA, Weiss MA. Resolution of pain associated with varicose and telangiectatic leg veins after compression sclerotherapy. J Dermatol Surg Oncol 16:333-336, 1990.
3. Redisch W, Pelzer RH. Localized vascular dilatations of the human skin: Capillary microscopy and related studies. Am Heart J 37:106-111, 1949.
4. Albanese AR, Albanese AM, Albanese EF. Lateral subdermic varicose vein system of the legs. Its surgical treatment by the chiseling tube method. Vasc Surg 3:81-89, 1969.
5. Weiss RA, Weiss MA. Continuous wave venous Doppler examination for pretreatment diagnosis of varicose and telangiectatic veins. Dermatol Surg 21:58-62, 1995.
6. Somjen GM, Ziegenbein R, Johnston AH, Royle JP. Anatomical examination of leg telangiectases with duplex scanning [see comments]. J Dermatol Surg Oncol 19:940-945, 1993.
7. de Faria JL, Moraes IN. Histopathology of telangiectasias associated with varicose veins. Dermatologica 127:321-324, 1963.
8. Wokalek H, Vanscheidt W, Martay K, Leder O. Morphology and localization of sunburst varicosities: An electron microscopic and morphometric study. J Dermatol Surg Oncol 15:149-154, 1989.
9. Braverman IM, Keh-Yen A. Ultrastructure of the human dermal microcirculation. IV. Valve-containing collecting veins at the dermal-subcutaneous junction. J Invest Dermatol 81:438-442, 1983.
10. Weiss RA, Weiss MA. Doppler ultrasound findings in reticular veins of the thigh subdermic lateral venous system and implications for sclerotherapy. J Dermatol Surg Oncol 19:947-951, 1993.
11. Somjen GM, Royle JP, Fell G, Roberts AK, Hoare MC, Tong Y. Venous reflux patterns in the popliteal fossa. J Cardiovasc Surg 33:85-91, 1992.
12. Lofgren KA. Varicose veins: Their symptoms, complications, and management. Postgrad Med 65:131-139, 1979.
13. Maurel E, Azema C, Deloly J, Bouissou H. Collagen of the normal and the varicose human saphenous vein: A biochemical study. Clin Chim Acta 193:27-37, 1990.
14. Psaila JV, Melhuish J. Viscoelastic properties and collagen content of the long saphenous vein in normal and varicose veins. Br J Surg 76:37-40, 1989.
15. Chakfe N, et al. The impact of knee joint flexion on infrainguinal vascular grafts: An angiographic study. Eur J Vasc Endovasc Surg 13:23-30, 1997.
16. Hochstetter F. Morphologisches Jahrbuch 17 Bd. 1891.
17. Goren G, Yellin AE. Primary varicose veins: Topographic and hemodynamic correlations. J Cardiovasc Surg 31:672-677, 1990.

18. Hirai M, Naiki K, Nakayama R. Prevalence and risk factors of varicose veins in Japanese women. Angiology 41:228-232, 1990.
19. Cornu-Thénard A, et al. Importance of the familial factor in varicose disease—Clinical study of 134 families. J Dermatol Surg Oncol 20:318-326, 1994.
20. Weiss RA, Weiss MA. Sclerotherapy of telangiectasia. In Gloviczki P, Yao JST, eds. Handbook of Venous Disorders: Guidelines of the American Venous Forum. London: Chapman & Hall, 1996, pp 355-373.
21. Shields JL, Jansen GT. Therapy for superficial telangiectasias of the lower extremities. J Dermatol Surg Oncol 8:857-860, 1982.
22. Tretbar LL. Spider angiomata: Treatment with sclerosant injections. J Kansas Med Soc 79:198-200, 1978.
23. Ibegbuna V, Delis K, Nicolaides AN. Effect of lightweight compression stockings on venous haemodynamics. Int Angiol 16:185-188, 1997.
24. Weiss MA, Weiss RA, Goldman MP. How minor varicosities cause leg pain. Contemp Obstet Gynecol 36:113-125, 1991.
25. McCausland AM, Holmes F, Trotter AD. Venous distensibility during the menstrual cycle. Am J Obstet Gynecol 86:640-645, 1963.
26. McPheeters HO. The value of estrogen therapy in the treatment of varicose veins complicating pregnancy. Lancet 69:2, 1949.
27. Widmer LK. Peripheral venous disorders: Prevalence and socio-medical importance observations in 4529 apparently healthy persons. Basel study III. Berne, Switzerland: Hans Huber, 1978.
28. Wilder CS. Prevalence of selected chronic circulatory conditions. Vital Health Stat 94:1-2, 1974.
29. Psaila JV, et al. Do varicose veins have abnormal viscoelastic properties? In Davy A, Stemmer R, eds. Phlebologie '89. Blanche, France: John Libbey Eurotext, 1989.
30. Yucha CB, Russ P, Baker S. Detecting I.V. infiltrations using a venoscope. J Intraven Nurs 20:50-55, 1997.
31. Weiss RA, Goldman MP. Transillumination mapping prior to ambulatory phlebectomy. Dermatol Surg 24:447-450, 1998.
32. Schultz-Ehrenburg U, Hubner H-J. Reflux Diagnosis with Doppler Ultrasound [monograph]. Stuttgart: Schattauer, 1989.
33. Weiss RA, Weiss MA. Doppler, veines reticulaires et telangiectasies. Phlebologie 47:333-336, 1995.
34. Goldman MP, Sadick NS, Weiss RA. Cutaneous necrosis, telangiectatic matting, and hyperpigmentation following sclerotherapy. Etiology, prevention, and treatment [review]. Dermatol Surg 21:19-29, 1995.
35. Weiss RA, Weiss MA. Combination intense pulsed light and sclerotherapy: A synergistic effect [abstract]. Dermatol Surg 23:969, 1997.

Chapter 24

Techniques of Small Vessel Sclerotherapy

David M. Duffy

What makes small (0.01 mm to 2 mm in diameter) vessels so interesting is the diversity of their response to treatment. Symmetrically distributed veins of identical size and color can react quite differently to identical treatments. The immediate and long-term results following sclerotherapy are only partially predictable because a large number of host factors play a role. Treatment outcome depends on these factors more than on any combination of treatment strategies. Sclerotherapy is an art, not a science, and many of the controversies regarding "ideal" treatment protocols are rooted in complex, clinically inapparent molecular biomechanisms that are not controllable by changes in technique.

Approximately 98% of our patients are females, and most of them can identify a family member with complaints similar to theirs.[1] This statistical preponderance of females may be related to both male disinterest and the effects of female hormones. These hormones are responsible for a broad variety of vascular phenomena ranging from the response to and release of endogenous vasodilators to cyclical regulation of vessel growth.[2-5] Folkman (personal communication, 1989) notes that "estrogen tends to potentiate certain forms of neovascularization but we have no idea what the biochemical link is."[3,4] An understanding of the mechanisms involved in the development of small lower extremity veins, which worsen with pregnancy, ovulation, and menstruation or appear in large numbers following the trauma of sclerotherapy, may provide clues to unlock the riddle of hormonally mediated vessel growth in wound healing, neoplastic disease, and other pathologic states.[6-8]

Along with juvenile hemangiomas[6] and the vascular component of psoriasis,[9] the occurrence of great numbers of telangiectasias and larger vessels that serve no vital circulatory function suggests that these processes are a benign variant of the broad, but only recently recognized, category of "angiogenic diseases which are caused by disorders of blood vessel regulation."[5,10]

ETIOLOGY
Angiogenesis

Physiologic angiogenesis, which is essential for wound healing, growth, and reproduction, occurs in two forms: cyclical, which takes place during ovulation and menstruation, and sporadic, which occurs normally during wound healing and pathologically in a variety of neoplastic, inflammatory, infectious, and immunologic disorders.[5,9,10] Compared to tissues such as gastrointestinal mucosa, the endothelial cells that line the human vascular tree are relatively quiescent, with turnover times measured in years. Physiologically, males do not require angiogenesis unless pathologic states or wound healing occurs.[8] Despite this deceptive quiescence, the system that controls new vessel growth is as complex as the system that initiates the clotting process in blood. Angiogenesis is poised to initiate rapid proliferation of new vessels, with entire cell populations turning over every 3 to 5 days following exposure to a wide variety of stimuli. These stimuli include hypoxia, venous hypertension, adaptive biomechanical forces,[11,12] tissue trauma, and growth. They operate in many pathologic states, ranging from rheumatoid arthritis to breast cancer.[5,9,10]

Under normal circumstances the "switch" that initiates the stepwise process of new vessel growth is precisely regulated by the dynamic interaction of 50 growth and inhibitory modulators (growth factors) that "turn on" or "turn off" as needed. Patients who need treatment for large numbers of small vessels may have a genetically transmitted, abnormally sensitive response to minimal angiogenic stimuli producing many vessels with minimal provocation (e.g., hypoxia caused by tight clothes or crossed legs, minimal venous reflux, or an exaggerated angiogenic phase of wound healing precipitated by sclerotherapy). This exaggerated response may be abnormally prolonged, intense, and exacerbated by female hormones.[13] It has been postulated that the induction of proliferative vessels, which heal as fast as they are treated, is the major cause of small vessel resistance following sclerotherapy.[14] More recent studies suggest that small vessel resistance following vascular trauma results from both structural changes in the vessel wall (neointimal hyperplasia, migration, and proliferation of smooth muscle cells)[15] and the up-regulation of angiogenic molecular mechanisms to produce proliferative, thick-walled small vessels. Sclerotherapy and other ablative techniques follow an unpredictable angiogenic line balanced between the destruction of targeted vessels and the hyperactivation of the wound healing process in which new, structurally altered, resistant vessels grow.[7,9]

Cellular Memory

Biologic systems have a "memory" for previous events; thus multiple exposures to antigens produce increasingly severe allergic responses to lowered antigenic burdens. Prolonged or repeated painful stimuli produce structural changes in the nervous system, speeding up the transmission of pain impulses.[16] Repeated trauma to the vascular tree in genetically susceptible patients may make it easier to turn on the angiogenic switch. This situation results in a more vigorous and prolonged angiogenic response and diminished benefits for patients who seek treatment for small vessels over the years.

CLINICAL OBSERVATIONS

The notion that small vessels are essentially homogeneous in their response to treatment is false. Vessels between 0.1 mm and 2 mm in diameter are, in fact, an extraordinarily heterogeneous clinical entity. Even small changes in vessel size or location and certain aspects of the patient's history or physical habitus can play an enormous role in treatment outcomes and complications no matter what technique is employed. The following factors can affect treatment outcome.

1. *Vessel size.* There are two classes of small red (0.01 mm to 0.2 mm) telangiectasias: (a) responsive, which often occur in small numbers in previously untreated patients; and (b) resistant, which are often seen in

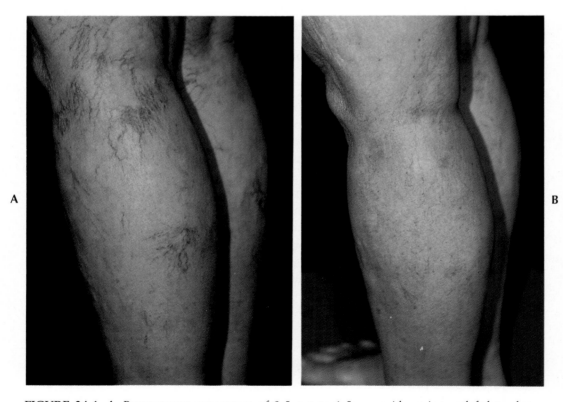

A   B

FIGURE 24-1. **A,** Pretreatment appearance of 0.5 mm to 1.5 mm spider veins on left lateral gastrocnemius muscle and thigh. **B,** Complete disappearance without pigmentation is an unusual occurrence.

large or small numbers following previous sclerotherapy. The mechanisms underlying the difference in response to treatment that occurs in vessels of the same size are outlined later in this chapter. Small (0.1 mm to 0.3 mm) vessels often require multiple treatments and rarely develop pigment no matter what technique is employed. Vessels >0.5 mm are rarely resistant to sclerotherapy and often disappear after one treatment (followed by pigmentation and thrombosis). Articles that discuss the effect of technique changes on the "incidence" of pigmentation or treatment resistance are meaningless unless they specify the size of the treated vessels (Figures 24-1 and 24-2).

2. *Location.* Vessels located in different areas of the body respond quite differently to the same treatment. For example, facial telangiectasias (0.1 mm to 0.3 mm) can be treated with multiple modalities with excellent results; however, vessels of the same size located on the lower extremities often resist these treatment modalities. Ulcerations are most common following treatment of the ankles. Pigmentation rarely occurs above the

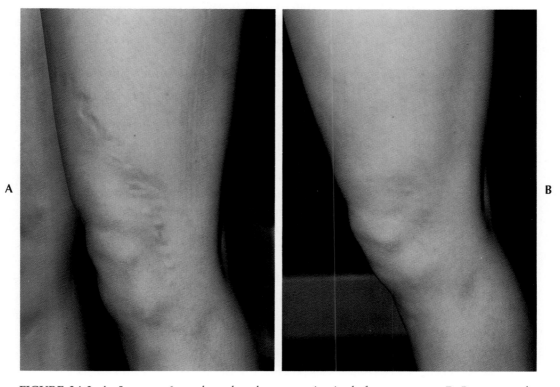

FIGURE 24-2. A, 5 mm to 6 mm lateral saphenous varicosity before treatment. **B,** Prompt resolution without pigmentation is seen 2 months after a single treatment. Although extremely unusual, evolution of healing without pigmentation does occur, demonstrating the inherent variability in treatment of veins.

waist and has never been observed in the treatment of vessels of all sizes involving the hands, breasts, arms, and face.[17-19]

3. *Patient age.* Although patient age is almost never mentioned as an influence on treatment outcome, it has a profound influence. Varicose telangiectasias >0.5 mm in size are more commonly seen in older patients and are often more fragile than vessels of the same size that occur in younger patients. Vessels <0.3 mm are often of more recent origin. Young patients who are *mildly* symptomatic and have a family history of varicose veins invariably have some degree of venous reflux, even though they may present with small numbers of spider veins and no large varicose veins.

4. *Venous reflux/venous hypertension.* Venous reflux and venous hypertension can be contributory or causal factors in the development of small vessels. The effect of venous reflux on the development of spider veins is very slow in the nonpregnant female. Venous hypertension and reflux often result in specific types of vessels (corona phlebectasia) and can contribute to matting and small vessel resistance through several mechanisms. Conversely, telangiectasias that occur in association with large varicose veins can be treated independently with acceptable long-term results,[20] and sclerotherapy or surgical extirpation of larger veins, varicose or reticular, can be followed by resistant telangiectasias.

5. *Obesity and other factors.* Obesity, the use of female hormones, and a history of spider veins occurring during times of hormonal excess are associated with increased telangiectatic matting.[13]

6. *Degree of surface involvement.* Patients with small numbers of telangiectasias routinely achieve more rapid and successful results following sclerotherapy than those who present with large numbers of vessels.

7. *Varicosity.* The word "varicose" means elevated, tortuous, and dilated. Although the term is usually applied to larger vessels, the varicose state routinely occurs in larger (0.6 mm to 0.9 mm), darker telangiectasias and is most commonly seen in older patients. For small vessels varicosity is an excellent marker of fragility. Varicose telangiectasias commonly respond to dilute sclerosants with rapid necrosis, thrombosis, and pigmentation. The presence of varicose telangiectasias should alert the clinician to the possibility of deep venous disease and/or superficial venous reflux.

8. *Vessel wall thickness.* Thin-walled varicose (0.6 mm to 2.5 mm) vessels may respond to treatment (with immediate destruction achieved) with sclerosant concentrations that would be ineffective for the treatment of much smaller vessels.

9. *Symmetrical vessels.* Symmetrical veins are like symmetrical icebergs. Vessels that look alike are not necessarily connected to the deeper venous system in the same way or subjected to identical vascular forces, and therefore they may respond quite differently to identical treatments.

10. *Vessel color.* This characteristic is related to the thickness of the vessel wall, the depth of the vessel beneath the surface of the skin, the color of the overlying skin, the degree of oxygenation of the blood within the vessel, the reflectance of light from constricted or dilated vessels in close proximity, and the reflection of light from the surface of the skin or the transmission of light through vessels where they traverse fascial gaps. Red vessels usually require more treatments than cyanotic or blue-green vessels.

PATTERNS OF RESPONSE TO SCLEROTHERAPY

Some clinical literature suggests that if sclerotherapy temporarily destroys unwanted vessels of all sizes, requires a specific number of treatments, produces "recurrence," or involves certain complications, these results could arise only from bad technique. This misconception oversimplifies the cause of small vessels, their relationship to larger vessels, and the ability to "normalize" the underlying causes of small vessels through specific techniques. I have identified four responses to sclerotherapy: (1) gradual destruction (fading), (2) sudden (immediate) destruction (usually associated with pigment or thrombi), (3) vascular remodeling (second-generation vessels/matting), and (4) recurrence.

Type I—Slow Response

Vessel size is the most important feature in predicting both the outcome of sclerotherapy and the patterns of response observed. Vessels that usually respond to sclerotherapy with gradual fading that is unassociated with pigmentation vary in size from 0.1 mm to 0.3 mm in diameter. Previously untreated ("virgin") veins in this size range usually respond to repeated treatments with progressive diminution in size and lightening in color over several months. Occasionally, telangiectasias treated for the first time may look exactly as they did before treatment. They are, however, partially damaged and can be gradually destroyed by subsequent treatments. I think that the occurrence of hyperpigmentation, thrombosis, and more rapid destruction of vessels up to 0.3 mm in size is unaffected by the use of compression, the injection of reticular veins, or the use of higher concentrations of sclerosants.[21,22] Sclerotherapy for vessels between 0.4 mm and 0.5 mm in size can produce fading or occasionally disappear once without a trace after one treatment (a process commonly seen in 0.4 mm vessels). This type of disappearance, most commonly noted following treatment of patients with a few small patches of telangiectasias, may be a statistical quirk (Figure 24-3). Attempts to accelerate the process of destruction and reduce the number of treatments by using high concentrations of sclerosants occasionally produce more rapid results, but they are often followed by complications associated with increased tissue trauma (e.g., necrosis, pigmentation, thrombosis and matting). Vessels between 0.1 mm and 0.3 mm in diameter are usually treated with 0.75% polidocanol, 23.4% hypertonic saline, or 0.1% to 0.2% sodium tetradecyl sulfate.

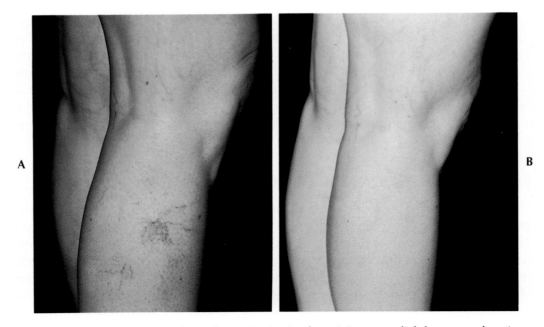

FIGURE 24-3. **A,** A mixture of vessels varying in size from 0.2 mm to slightly greater than 1 mm disappeared immediately after one treatment with 0.75% POL. **B,** Posttreatment appearance 2½ months later.

Type II—Rapid Destruction

Cyanotic vessels between 0.5 mm and 0.9 mm in diameter are rarely resistant to treatment except when associated with incompetent perforators or venous reflux. In this situation, small patches of these vessels are usually located on the anterior or medial thigh and occasionally occur on the gastrocnemius muscle or in the pretibial area (unpublished data). For all vessels >0.5 mm in size, rapid destruction (usually after one treatment) and its sequelae (hemosiderotic hyperpigmentation and thrombosis) are common. My experience is that compression, the injection of reticular veins, and the use of dilute sclerosants do not predictably alter this process. A 2 mm type II vessel in communication with an incompetent saphenofemoral junction may have been responsible for a pulmonary embolism that occurred in an elderly man after treatment[1] (Figure 24-4). Vessels in this size range can be varicose or flat. Varicosity, advanced age, a history of spontaneous bleeding after minimal trauma, and easy bruisability suggest a trial of treatment using low concentrations of sclerosants (e.g., polidocanol 0.25% to 0.5%) for initial treatment. Large numbers of varicose telangiectasias between 0.6 mm and 2 mm in size, either alone or in combination with larger varicose veins, are strong indicators of underlying venous disease and mandate more ex-

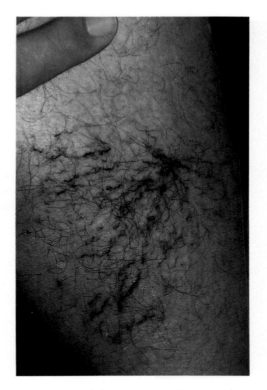

FIGURE 24-4. Sclerotherapy treatment of these 1 mm to 2 mm spider venules may have been partially responsible for a pulmonary embolus in this 73-year-old man, who at a later date was found to have leukemia and a clotting disorder.

tensive laboratory evaluations, particularly when they are associated with venous symptoms.

The concept that as vessels become larger, higher sclerosant concentrations should be used is invalid for treatment of certain types of vessels. Wall thickness and varicosity can be more important than vessel size in determining the degree of response. Varicose thin-walled vessels in the 0.6 mm to 2.5 mm range, particularly when located on the lateral thighs, shins, and ankles, occasionally respond to extraordinarily low concentrations (0.03% polidocanol).[23] Moreover, the presence of fragile vessels in the deep, and therefore invisible, circulation is another reason for using low volumes and concentrations of sclerosants. Although the rate of treatment failure is higher with this approach, fewer complications will occur (Figure 24-5). Sometimes several weeks after treatment, thrombosis can occur in fragile vessels located far from the treated area, particularly in dependent sites such as the ankles and feet, where hydrostatic pressure is highest and sclerosant pooling is likely to take place (Figure 24-6).

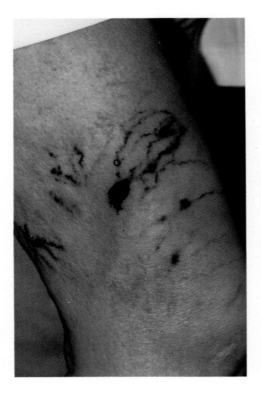

FIGURE 24-5. This elderly patient with veins between 0.5 and 1.5 mm was treated with 1% POL and developed severe tissue necrosis at the injection sites.

FIGURE 24-6. Thrombosis noted on the bottom of the foot following sclerotherapy treatment of the leg. This vessel responded with sudden thrombosis. Several treatments were necessary for complete resolution.

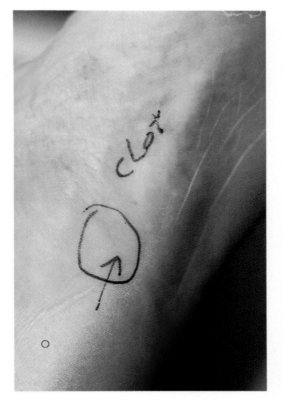

Type III—Vascular Remodeling

Sclerotherapy routinely produces varying numbers of new telangiectasias (0.05 mm to 0.2 mm), which are sometimes larger and darker, as during pregnancy. They may appear identical in size and color to their "virgin" counterparts and are often erroneously described as "recurrences." When vessels of this type occur in large numbers, they are referred to as "telangiectatic matting."[24] When they occur in small numbers, they are designated as "second-generation vessels" included in the spectrum of sclerotherapy-induced neovascularization.[14] Descriptions of this vessel growth and the complicated molecular mechanisms underlying its occurrence have been described.[7,9,25] Vessels are sensory organs that are capable of adapting in a number of ways to vascular trauma and other homeostatic challenges. The influence of previous treatments has been deemed important enough to suggest that vessels <0.2 mm in diameter should be divided into two specific categories: (1) "virgin" veins, which respond to treatment in a predictable way; and (2) resistant small vessels, which usually occur in previously treated patients, in either large numbers (matting) or in smaller numbers (second-generation veins).

Type IV—Recurrence

It is a rare patient who does not develop changes in the clinical appearance, size, and location of small vessels following surgery or sclerotherapy. Excellent clinical and histologic evidence indicates that completely ablated telangiectasias and larger vessels do not recanalize and thus cannot recur in an identical configuration.[26,27] Careful photographic evaluation usually confirms the fact that small red vessels (0.05 mm to 0.2 mm in diameter) will appear in and adjacent to treated sites. These vessels are *new* and can be observed to undergo specific types of "remodeling" when they are observed and photographed over a 20-year period with and without treatment.

Clinically defined by resistance to the same methods of treatment that originally eliminated similar vessels, new telangiectasias can occur in previously treated areas and several centimeters away from them. These vessels may remain fixed in one location (involute with or without treatment) or may appear to migrate and be followed by the intermittent occurrence of similar new vessels at different sites. These vessels have been referred to as "come and go" vessels (Figures 24-7 and 24-8).[22] The occurrence of these small vessels in large or small numbers is seen more frequently on the inner and outer thighs and the inner knees. Exaggerated angiogenesis that occurs in close proximity to the knees may be related to two factors:

1. The postural effects of sleep in which shear receptors located in the vessel walls are activated by prolonged bending of the knees, producing transforming growth factors.[7]
2. The effects of hypoxia, which occurs when the legs are pressed together for long periods of time, resulting in the release of vascular endothelial

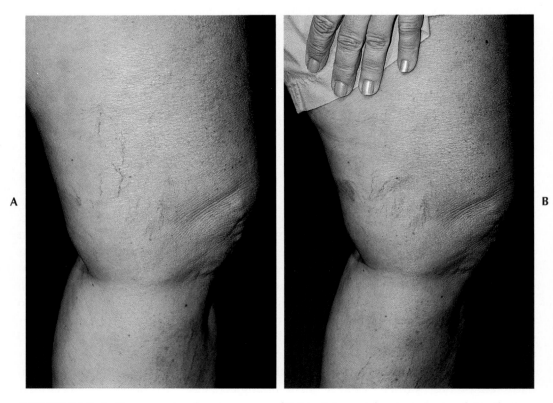

FIGURE 24-7. A, Demonstrates the appearance of 0.3 to 0.4 mm telangiectasias involving the inner knee of this slightly obese 54-year-old woman who had not undergone previous treatment. **B,** This photograph, taken seven months after two treatments, demonstrates the appearance of neovascular vessels (matting) and new vessel growth at an adjacent site (vascular remodeling).

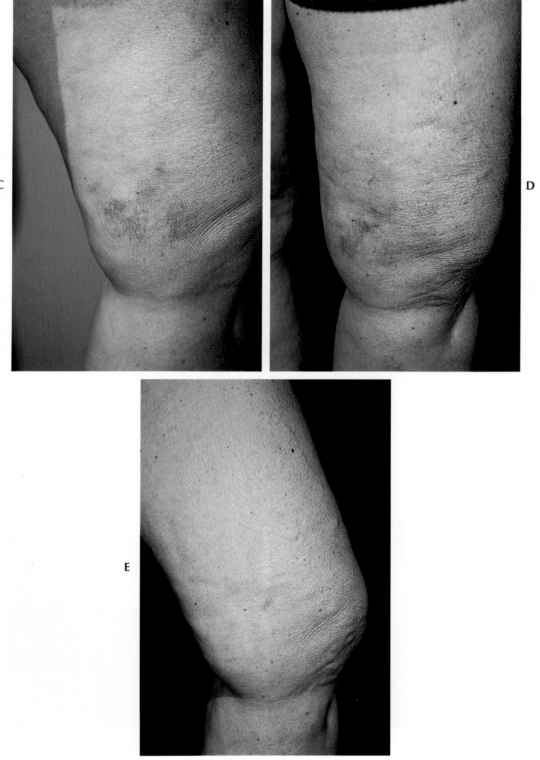

FIGURE 24-7, cont'd. C-D, These photographs demonstrate slow vascular remodeling during a 6-year period in which no treatments were done. A duplex scan revealed saphenofemoral incompetence and incompetence of the proximal portion of the saphenous vein. **E,** This photograph reveals complete resolution of telangiectasia 9 years after the first treatment.

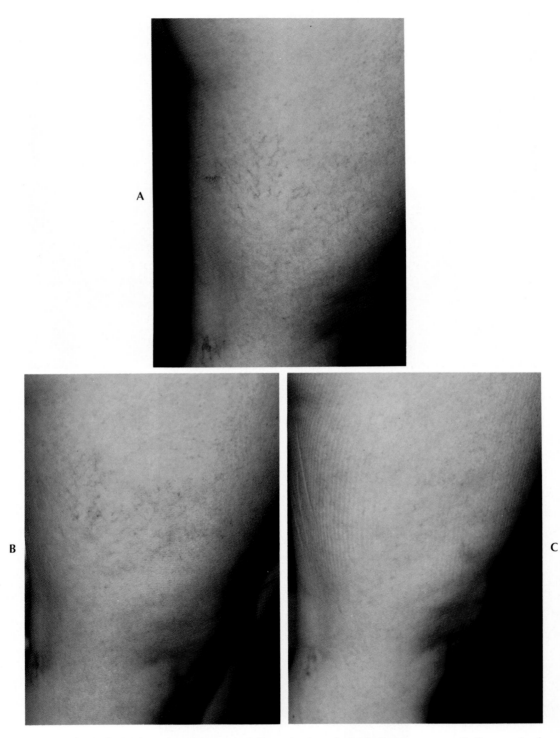

FIGURE 24-8. A, Spider veins, 0.3 mm to 0.5 mm in size, shown before treatment. B, One week after the first treatment, neovascularization (matting) is observed. C, Neovascularization disappeared spontaneously within 2 months after the initial treatment.

growth factor (VEGF), a process similar to the various forms of retinal neovascularization observed in infants and adults.[9] Constant visual changes constitute a dramatic summary of the dynamic vascular processes.

PRETREATMENT GUIDELINES

My colleagues and I ask patients not to shave the affected area for at least 48 hours before treatment because alcohol and dressings can irritate newly shaved skin. Alcohol, when applied to the skin in large quantities, renders the skin more transparent, facilitating the visualization of small vessels.

Moisturizers and the residue of moisturizer-containing soaps leave skin slippery and difficult to grasp. Accordingly, we ask patients to avoid using all forms of moisturizers for approximately 48 hours before treatment. Almost all our patients are women, and they are asked not to wear tight pants and to bring shorts or wear culottes or a full skirt (preferably an older garment because bleeding may result from treatment). We often provide single-use surgical paper shorts to avoid soiling street clothes.

Patients fill out a thorough questionnaire to identify any factors that may place them at greater risk for complications: allergies, medications, symptoms, obesity, female hormone therapy, significant systemic diseases (e.g., collagen vascular disease or diabetes), or a personal or family history of significant venous disease. On the day of treatment, or preferably several weeks in advance by mail, we provide patients with a treatment brochure and a collection of 40 photographs detailing the successes, failures, and complications associated with sclerotherapy and explaining the treatment approaches.

All patients must also sign a written consent form, which informs them of the risks of the procedure and permits their photographs to be used for educational purposes. We inform patients both verbally and in writing of the Federal Drug Administration (FDA) status of the sclerosants employed and our reasons for using them. Our discussions include the advantages and disadvantages of compression and injection of larger vessels; the possibility of discomfort; the need for repeated treatment of small vessels; the sometimes gradual nature of improvement; the effect of location, surface area, hormones, and weight; and the possibility of resistant vessels occurring in previously treated patients or the emergence of new vessels following treatment. Everyone is told to expect minimal discomfort and pruritus, along with redness, bruising, pigmentation, or neovascular vessels, following treatment. In addition, the etiology of telangiectasias and the occasional occurrence of more important complications (i.e., thrombophlebitis, allergies, deep venous thrombosis) are discussed. The impact of the patient's age and general health and the presence or absence of certain symptoms or diseases in regard to treatment outcome are also presented orally and in writing. Patients are routinely warned about the possibility of ulcerations or scars and the areas and circumstances in which they may occur.

There is a public and legal perception that treatment failures, ulcerations, pigmentation, and thrombi associated with sclerotherapy are caused by poor technique. Therefore it is important for patients to know that even with the best technique certain complications can occur.

Patients must be made aware of all possible treatment failures. For example, patients who are genetically predisposed to having spider veins or varicose veins may have a "defective switch" for shutting off vessel growth, which in some cases is triggered by female hormones. These patients must be told that new telangiectasias may occur in conjunction with varicose veins (e.g., with venous hypertension; from trauma, blows, falls, or surgery; after sclerotherapy; with crossing of the legs or wearing of tight hosiery). We also explain that small new vessels may occur after one treatment but that more commonly multiple treatments produce effects similar to those of multiple pregnancies, causing new vessel growth. These new vessels can be resistant to treatment, particularly when they occur on the outer thighs or the inner knees. For patients who sleep on their sides and have numerous vessels on the inner knees, we suggest placing a pillow between the knees during sleep. After careful examination and a review of the patient's records, we discuss patterns of response to sclerotherapy and their relationship to the size of the vessels and other aspects of the patient's history. With the patient paying close attention, we use a clear plastic ruler or a plastic vein calibration card to measure vessels >1 mm in size.

For patients with concerns of "catastrophic" results or those who are terrified of needles, we offer laser treatment or perform sclerotherapy on a small test area at the time of a consultative visit. We often compare both telangiectasia injection and/or injection of reticular veins with or without compression on selected patients on an individual basis.

Finally, all patients are initially photographed, both at close range and at a distance, to demonstrate the nature and extent of vessels present before treatment. This step is done for several reasons. First, patients commonly forget about their pretreatment appearance and often are pleasantly surprised to see how much progress has been made. Second, photographs can help correlate the specific effect of certain regimens on their vessels, which aids the physician in making decisions about the effect of the injection of reticular veins, sclerosant concentration, compression, and treatment frequency. Third, photographs serve to document the long-term (and sometimes unexpected) effects of treatments, often revealing a constantly changing pattern of new small vessel growth.

TREATMENT PROTOCOLS

My careful photographic documentation involving 350,000 images combined with a 20-year experience in the treatment of over 5000 patients suggest that good results can be obtained using a variety of approaches. The complexity of molecular mechanisms controlling blood vessel response to trauma ensures that no simple "recipe" can guarantee reproducible or optimal results in all patients.

Treatment Schedule

Patients with virgin telangiectasias in the 0.1 mm to 0.3 mm range generally require two to four treatments, depending on the surface area of involvement and other host factors, as discussed earlier in the chapter. These treatments are usually carried out at 4- to 6-week intervals. Less frequent (2- to 3-month) treatments may make the gradual fading process more effective and reduce the total number of treatments necessary (Figure 24-9). When patients want faster results, virgin telangiectasias of all sizes can be treated at 1-week intervals; however, we warn these patients that matting and resistant small vessels may be more common under these circumstances. Larger (0.6 to 0.9 mm) telangiectasias usually require only one treatment. Patients are warned that thrombosis and pigmentation may occur, despite the use of compression and the injection of reticular veins. These patients are often seen 1 week after treatment for thrombectomies or for reassurance as necessary. Patients with matting or small numbers of previously treated vessels, up to 0.2 mm in diameter, are treated more slowly, at 3- to 6-month intervals. We prefer to wait at least 6 months following patient treatment at another facility. Matting and second-generation vessels <0.2 mm in size may involute or become responsive if enough time has been allowed to elapse. Treatment for small vessels is not carried out at any time during pregnancy, although it may be safe to do so.[29] For the treatment of resistant telangiectasias, higher sclerosant concentrations are generally no more effective and routinely produce more neovascularization. Recent experience using a high-energy, long-pulsed 532 nm laser[23] with a pulse duration of 50 milliseconds and 20 to 40 J/cm² is sometimes effective for the treatment of resistant telangiectasias in fair-skinned patients (unpublished data, 1998). The 585 nm pulsed-dye laser can also be employed. Often its use is followed by undesirable hyperpigmentation or hypopigmentation.[30] In general, lasers and photooptical devices are not a substitute for sclerotherapy, but occasionally they are useful for resistant telangiectasias.

MATERIALS AND INSTRUMENTATION
Sclerosing Solutions

The choice of sclerosant is influenced by the needs of the patient, the availability and legal status of the agent, and the experience of the sclerotherapist. At the time of this writing, only two drugs are approved in the United States for the treatment of varicose veins of any size involving the lower extremities: sodium morrhuate (approved in 1930) and sodium tetradecyl sulfate (approved in 1946). Sodium morrhuate is more allergenic, more toxic, but no more efficacious for the treatment of small vessels than either hypertonic saline or polidocanol (POL). As experienced sclerotherapists know, sometimes one sclerosant may work better than another on certain veins in certain individuals. All sclerosants can produce pain, unwanted thrombosis (pulmonary emboli or deep venous thrombosis), necrosis, ulceration, and—with the exception of pure hypertonic saline—allergies.

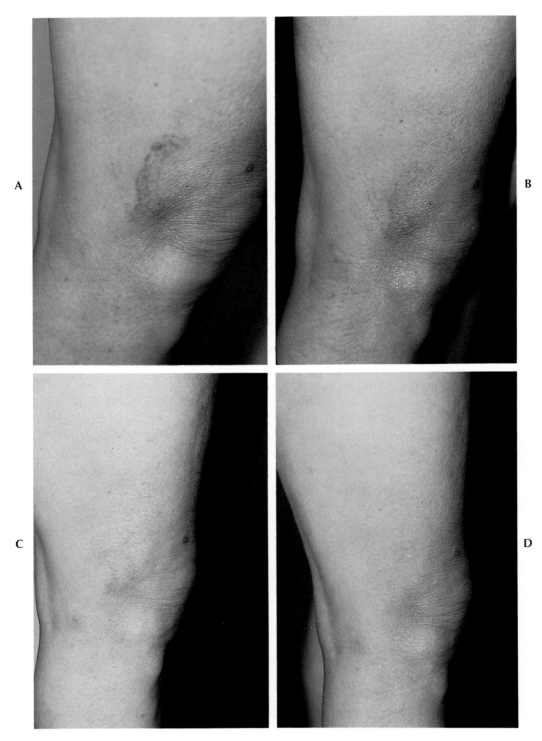

FIGURE 24-9. A, Vessel appearance before treatment. **B,** Thirty days after the first treatment, diminution of the size and number of vessels can be seen. **C,** Three months after the second treatment, further clearing is noted. **D,** Almost complete disappearance of originally treated vessels is seen, but a small area of neovascularization (matting) also appears posterior to the treated area. At this point further treatment should be avoided for at least 3 to 6 months.

For the injection of vessels between 0.1 mm and 0.4 mm in diameter, 0.75% polidocanol or its equivalent (0.25% Sotradecol/23.4% hypertonic saline) are employed. Vessels measuring between 0.5 mm and 0.9 mm in diameter are usually treated with 0.5% or 0.75% polidocanol. All sclerosants, no matter how dilute, can produce immediate destruction or necrosis. The choice of concentrations is based on a clinical assessment of multiple host factors.

The injection of larger vessels as a substitute for, or in association with, the direct injection of telangiectasias has been advocated as a means of reducing complications (e.g., pigmentation, thrombosis, neovascularization, recurrence).[28] For the treatment of flat, thick-walled reticular veins (2 mm to 2.5 mm in diameter), 0.75% to 1.5% polidocanol is usually employed. For varicose, thin-walled reticular veins, 0.5% to 1% polidocanol is used in addition to the direct injection of telangiectasias, followed by compression.

Pure hypertonic saline, which has FDA approval for third-trimester abortions, has the advantage of an absolute lack of allergic responses. It is, however, relatively uncomfortable to use and too weak for treatment of larger vessels. Ulcerations may occur with concentrations of hypertonic saline as low as 10% when the solution is injected intradermally in volumes >0.3 ml.[21] Aching can be minimized by slow injection and massage after treatment. The potential to create devastating ulcers, in the absence of almost perfect technique, makes hypertonic saline less attractive than several other available sclerosants.

Sodium tetradecyl sulfate (Sotradecol) has the advantage of FDA approval, a relatively low incidence of important complications compared to sodium morrhuate, and relative painlessness compared to hypertonic saline. Using a volunteer, my colleagues and I determined that 0.5% Sotradecol, 0.5 cc in volume, injected into the middle dermis did not cause ulcers but that the same volume of 1% solution would cause them (unpublished data, 1990) (Figure 24-10).

POL, or dihydroxypolyethoxydodecane (Aethoxysklerol), is the most "forgiving" of all available sclerosants. An intradermal injection of 0.4 ml of 3% POL leads to mild hyperpigmentation in the region where tiny cutaneous vessels are destroyed (Figure 24-11). It must be remembered that all sclerosants can produce ulcers through mechanisms that are as yet poorly understood. The rate of serious allergies and fatalities reported following the use of POL is lower than that reported for any FDA-approved sclerosant.[22] In low concentrations POL is the most painless of all agents. It should not be used in patients who are being treated with disulfiram (Antabuse) or in patients with certain types of cardiac arrhythmias.

Sotradecol is roughly three to four times as potent as POL on a percentage basis; that is, 0.75% POL is the equivalent of 23.4% hypertonic saline. Individual variability plays a significant role in treatment outcome, and it is difficult to equate one solution strength and type with another absolutely. Certain patients develop pigmentation and thrombosis when extraordinarily dilute solutions (0.03% POL or equivalent) are used, solutions that are roughly 18 times weaker than the same solution that can be used for vessels of approximately the same size (Figure 24-12).

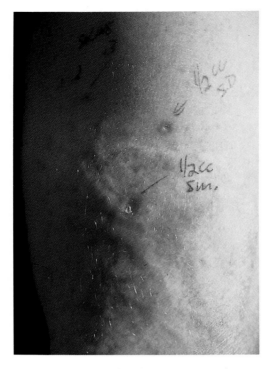

FIGURE 24-10. Ulceration associated with sclerotherapy. Upper ulcer, measuring approximately ¼ inch, resulted from 0.5 ml of 1% Sotradecol administered intradermally. Larger ulcer resulted from administration of 0.5 ml of 5% sodium morrhuate.

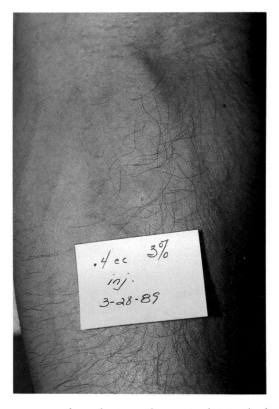

FIGURE 24-11. Skin appearance of a volunteer who received 0.5 ml of 3% POL without tissue necrosis occurring.

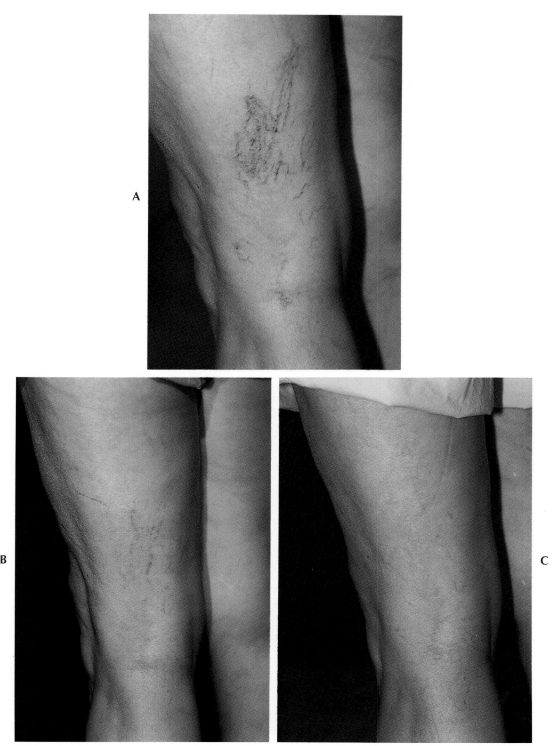

FIGURE 24-12. A, Pretreatment appearance of elevated tortuous and dilated spider varicosities measuring 0.5 mm to 1.5 mm on the left posterolateral thigh. **B,** Pigmentation and a few thrombi were still present after two treatments at 2 months after initiation of treatment. **C,** Almost 2 years after treatment, a good residential result is noted, with no apparent pigmentation. Since vessels of this type routinely undergo sudden destruction with transient pigmentation, patients must be warned of this effect.

Syringes

We fill our syringes in advance with various concentrations of solution and identify the sclerosant concentration by attaching a colored sticker on the piston. Disposable 1 ml to 3 ml syringes (not Luer-Lok) are recommended. The size of the syringe used is a matter of individual preference. Physicians with larger hands sometimes prefer the delicacy and control afforded by the use of a 1 ml syringe, which is a great deal longer than a 3 ml syringe when full. In either size a non–Luer-Lok syringe is a good choice because it facilitates frequent needle changes.

When the needle is put on the syringe, the bevel side is up, positioned exactly 90 degrees to the T-handle. Routinely, the syringe is filled to only 2.5 ml so that the extension of the piston fits the operator's hand exactly. Beginners should experiment to find the exact volume piston extension and syringe that is best for their hand.

Hypodermic Needles

The best and most uniformly finished No. 30 needles seem to be 30-gauge ½-inch hypodermic needles, either a Poly-Kote metal hub needle with a silicone-coated tribeveled point (distributed by Acuderm, Inc., Fort Lauderdale, Fla.) or an Air-Tite 30-gauge ½-inch needle (distributed by Air-Tite of Virginia, Inc., Virginia Beach, Va.). Needles smaller than 30 gauge are often nondisposable and dull and therefore a poor choice. Recently, a high-quality disposable 31-gauge needle has become available (Air-Tite of Virginia, Inc.). However, in experienced hands, a sharp No. 30 needle can be used easily to inject vessels as small as 0.05 mm in diameter.

Following manufacture, needles are not uniformly sharp. Dull needles can produce a scratchy sensation during injection. If this effect is noted on the first injection, the needle should be discarded. If it happens often, another needle brand should be chosen. About 1 in every 500 needles will lack a bevel completely. After multiple injections, the needle tip can become blunt and will require more force to penetrate the skin. When such a needle is observed under the microscope, it is evident that the needle tip is bent. Frequent needle changes, often after every third to fifth injection, are the rule, particularly in areas where the skin is tough and rigid, such as the feet, knees, or ankles.

Ideally, only the tip and the bevel of the needle are placed in the vein. For smaller vessels, only about one half of the bevel is actually inside the vein. The needle lumen can be seen shadowed by the walls of the transparent vessel like a sliver. This visual appearance of the needle, often associated with the sudden reflux of blood and confirmed by the flow of injected sclerosant along the path of the vessels, and the absence of a wheal are the most important factors in determining placement. The amount of force required to initiate sclerosant flow is only slightly less in small vessels than that necessary to inject the skin itself.

Miscellaneous Materials

- Isopropyl alcohol, cottonballs, and a Petri dish. Cottonballs saturated with isopropyl alcohol can be kept in a Petri dish. The alcohol can be applied to treated areas to clarify the skin as an aid in determining the injection point. Alternatively, a drop of sclerosant applied judiciously to a smaller area clarifies the skin, takes less time to apply, and reduces slipperiness.
- Microfoam surgical tape and Micropore 5 mm ½-inch tape (3M Medical-Surgical Division, St. Paul, Minn.) and cottonballs. Microfoam surgical tape is excellent for compression, but in areas where the skin flexes, particularly the popliteal fossa, we use Micropore tape under the Microfoam tape to minimize abrasion and the effects of occlusion.
- Cameras. The N-90 Nikon camera equipped with the SB 24 Nikon Speedlight and the E.D. 105 mm Micro-Nikkor lens, is used with ASA 64 Kodachrome or Ektachrome film. All modern single-lens reflex cameras use through-the-lens flash systems, but autofocus lenses and their dedicated flashes are used to enhance focusing speed and flash precision. Autofocus cameras are routinely used in the manual focus mode, which eliminates the tracking or hunting that occurs when autofocus devices cannot "decide" what small changes in the contrast of cutaneous vessels represent the desirable choice.
- Opticaid magnifiers (2.5 to 5 power magnification) or other similar magnifiers. These magnifiers have the advantage of lightness and ease of use (particularly with eyeglasses) but the disadvantage of the need for a closer working distance. The choice of magnification is an individual matter.
- Gauze pads (4 × 4 inch) and bandages.
- Timer. A timer can be set for the approximate time that injecting is to be continued because it is easy to lose track of time while concentrating on the work.
- Two overhead spotlights that converge on the treated area and are easy to move (even while sitting and injecting the veins). The presence of two lights permits the person injecting the veins to move his or her head in any direction without blocking light.
- Two stools with wheels. Such stools are the right height to permit the person doing the injection to sit comfortably with knees under the table and to move quickly when necessary.
- Power-operated surgical table.
- Vessel measurement. We use a clear plastic ruler to measure all vessels >1 mm in size. For measurement of telangiectasias, only a plastic vessel gauge is used (Coherent Laser, Palo Alto, Calif.) (1-800-367-7899). When this card is used, the patient becomes involved in the measuring process and learns which types of vessels may be expected to fade, to be resistant, or to produce clotting and pigmentation.
- Graduated compression stockings (range: 12 mm Hg to 40 mm Hg). The open-toe type is preferred.
- Disposable paper surgical shorts.

- Solu-Medrol, analeptics, Benadryl, cardiotonics, and normal saline in large (10 ml) syringes attached to 25-gauge ½-inch needles for neutralization when extravasation of sclerosants occurs. A large syringe prevents confusion when neutralization must be achieved.

POSTTREATMENT GUIDELINES

For the treatment of small (<2 mm) type I vessels in young ambulatory patients, few postoperative instructions are necessary. Patients who play vigorous games of tennis are encouraged to avoid that activity for a day or two. Otherwise, their activities are unrestricted. For patients with type II vessels, particularly when they are widespread, postoperative care is a great deal more important. It includes alternating between elevating the legs as much as possible and vigorous walking. For patients with symptomatic vessels who have jobs that require prolonged periods of standing, we routinely advise them to take 2 or 3 days off work. In many cases the use of graduated compression hosiery (20 to 30 mm Hg) is recommended for 1 to 2 weeks.

Patients are instructed to call the office if severe pain develops or if localized tenderness, swelling, scabs, blisters, or anything unusual is noted. The ordinary course of events is described in the treatment brochure given to the patient. Patients also are warned that certain areas are more prone to problems; neovascularization is most common in treatment of the inner knees, ulcerations occur most often on the ankles, and thrombosis is the rule for vessels of a certain size.

COMPLICATIONS

There are three major sources of patient concern, frustration, and dissatisfaction after sclerotherapy for telangiectasia.

1. Thrombi. We characterize the occurrence of slightly tender thrombi following treatment of telangiectasias >0.5 mm in diameter as "good lumps," indicating that the vessel has been destroyed and will not need to be treated again. Patients with vessels ≥0.6 mm are repeatedly told that these vessels often look worse before they look better and that the clots will not break loose and are not dangerous. E.M.L.A. Cream (ASTRA U.S.A., Inc., Westborough, Mass. 01581-4500) or a local anesthetic is used to reduce discomfort when clots are drained, preferably 1 to 3 weeks after treatment. Patients are warned that a delay in draining these liquified thrombi may make them more difficult to eradicate.

2. Pigmentation. Persistent pigmentation can be a major cause of discontent after treatment of larger vessels. During our initial evaluation, we repeatedly point out the type of vessels that are prone to pigmentation while carrying out our measurements of the areas to be treated. Patients are told that pigmentation is rarely permanent and that the occurrence of thrombi and pigmentation is not always controllable by technique and should be viewed as part of the normal healing process. When pigmentation per-

sists past 1 year, Baker's solution or specific lasers may be effective[1,23] (D. Groot, personal communication, 1998).

3. Small vessel problems. Patients who present with previously untreated telangiectasias (up to 0.4 mm in size) are warned that repeated treatment of the same small vessels is usually necessary. The fading process is often slow enough to require careful review of pretreatment photographs to revive patient enthusiasm for treatment. Patients are told that in some individuals the resolution of small vessels is additive, with each treatment producing more noticeable benefits. They are also told that in other cases major benefits will not be seen for the first one or two treatments but that subsequent treatments can produce good results. We call the latter patients "slow responders." Previously untreated patients are told to expect a 95% probability of satisfaction after treatment of small vessels with any technique.

The occurrence of resistant neovascular vessels in large numbers (matting) or in smaller numbers (second-generation vessels) is the number one cause of dissatisfaction with sclerotherapy (Figure 24-13). When they occur in small numbers,

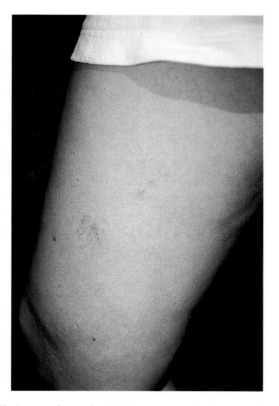

FIGURE 24-13. A small cluster of vessels <0.2 mm occurring in a previously treated patient (second-generation vessels). This vessel resisted all forms of treatment, including injection of reticular vein with high-concentration (3%) polidocanol, compression, and the use of a 532 nm laser.

these vessels often look no different to the patient than the vessels for which they originally sought treatment (with good results).

Typically, patients will travel long distances to our office after having had good results following our treatments and poor results after treatments carried out by physicians at a more convenient location. These patients are convinced that poor technique or the use of a different type of sclerosant was responsible for their disappointment. We tell these patients that the first person to treat very small vessels is the hero and that subsequent treatments are more difficult.

For a favorable patient-physician experience, keep the following important tips in mind:

1. Ask patients to circle the vessels that bother them the most. This approach avoids the phone call several days later claiming that the vein that the patient wanted treated was "missed."
2. Never forget to treat the anterior thighs. Most complaints will come from patients in whom one or two small vessels were missed in an area that they can easily see.
3. Do not treat areas in which ulceration has previously occurred. [AUTHOR'S NOTE: The worst ulcer I ever created occurred on the medial malleolus directly adjacent to a scar caused by a previous ulcer.]
4. Have an open-door policy for the patient's concerns. Tell patients that they will be seen without charge for a brief examination if they are concerned about treatment outcome.
5. Warn patients about increasing resistance with multiple treatments.
6. Do not guarantee results. Talk patients out of compulsively treating every vessel. Explain that more treatments may lead to more vessels.
7. Patients with very large vessels and obvious signs of venous insufficiency are best treated by other means after Doppler and duplex ultrasound examinations reveal axial vein involvement. The younger a symptomatic patient is when she seeks help, the more likely it is that valvular incompetence is to blame.
8. Stress the concept that all patients are different and that each one needs to be treated on an individual basis.
9. Openly discuss the fact that insurance companies should not be asked to compensate patients for cosmetic procedures.

OTHER TREATMENTS
Compression Therapy

Compression therapy is generally recommended for vessels >0.5 mm that communicate with larger varicose veins. Patients who are symptomatic (e.g., edema, fatigue) or present with large varicose veins usually undergo appropriate laboratory evaluation (Doppler or duplex ultrasound) and are treated with compression schedules appropriate for their particular problem. Patients with varicose telangiectasias >0.6 mm in size occasionally note reduced pigmentation or thrombi when Microfoam tape over cottonballs is applied for several days and then compression hosiery (20 to 30 mm Hg) is worn for 1 to 2 weeks. A history of tape allergy and an awareness of the occurrence of folliculitis, or tissue trauma, particularly when tape is applied behind the knees, are discussed with the patient. Micropore tape is routinely applied over cottonballs or sanitary pads before Microfoam tape is applied to the popliteal fossa. Patients with telangiectasias whose work requires long periods of standing (e.g., nurses, flight attendants, grocery store checkers, beauticians, and physicians) tend to become regular users of lightweight (12 to 14 mm Hg) graduated compression hosiery, which substantially reduces fatigue and discomfort. These patients are also encouraged to use this hosiery during menstruation or when forced to sit for many hours during travel. Patients with valvular incompetence who plan to become pregnant in the future often benefit from wearing 20 to 30 mm Hg compression hosiery. Many elect to defer treatment of larger vessels until their families are complete. For patients with small numbers of vessels <0.5 mm in size, vessels are directly injected, with Band-Aids applied as necessary to control bleeding. These patients are sent home with instructions to do a great deal of walking and to avoid high-impact aerobics or exercise, which can traumatize the legs, for at least 24 hours.

For the purpose of comparison, over the years we have routinely used compression therapy (with or without reticular vein injection), using Microfoam tape and cottonballs for several days followed by 1 to 3 weeks of continuous wearing of compression hosiery (20 to 30 mm Hg) on only one leg. We have noted tremendous variability in terms of response to identical treatments and certain paradoxes (i.e., high concentrations of sclerosants sometimes did not work as well as lower concentrations for vessels of the same size) (Figures 24-14 and 24-15).

Currently, we approach compression and/or the treatment of reticular veins as a treatment option for patients with small telangiectasias that are unassociated with larger vessels or a symptom complex. We explain the putative benefits of compression hosiery, providing this treatment as an option to interested patients.

Compression is used for patients:
1. With large varicose veins when only the spider veins are treated
2. Who undergo reticular vein treatment
3. Who are symptomatic
4. In whom venous reflux is detected or suspected

CONCLUSION

While clinicians argue about ideal treatment protocols, molecular biologists are busily identifying and characterizing more than 50 growth modulators that affect vessel growth. Telangiectasias involving the lower extremities of women have been noted to resolve after the use of antineoplastic agents, such as tamoxifen and cyclophosphamide.[13,14] In the future, antiangiogenic drugs such as angiostatin, endostatin, and thalidomide, which are natural inhibitors of angiogenesis, may provide benefits for lower extremity telangiectasias as well as for neoplastic diseases.[31-33]

Research in angiogenesis will revolutionize several fields of medicine. Angio-

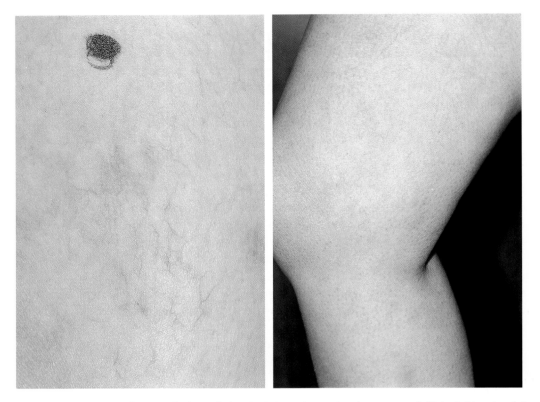

FIGURE 24-14. Complete resolution of tiny (<0.2 mm) previously untreated ("virgin") veins following sclerotherapy. History is as important as appearance in determining treatment outcomes for small telangiectasias.

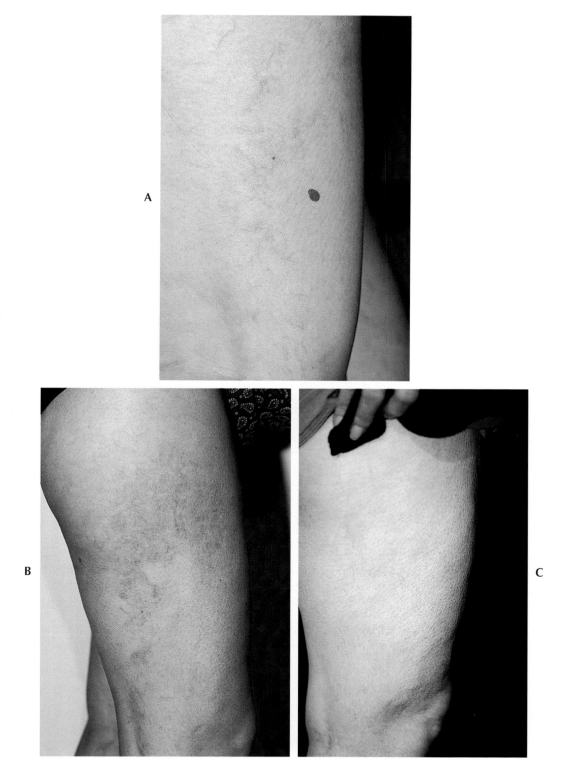

FIGURE 24-15. A, Pretreatment appearance of small telangiectasias on the same patient as in Figure 24-14. On this leg, severe matting occurred following two treatments. The independence of the results obtained from each leg, with identical technique used on identically sized telangiectasias, underscores the inherent variability in treatment outcomes. B-C, The matting observed on the right lateral thigh responded at a later date, as shown in these final photographs taken 13 years after the original treatment, with complete resolution of these spider veins. Note the presence of an untreated reticular vein but its absence with resolution of spider veins.

genic agents have recently been used to induce new vessel growth in cardiac muscles.[34,35] For readers with a scientific bent, literature describing the process of angiogenesis and the molecular biology of the vascular tree provides a wealth of information that can be applied directly to understanding telangiectasia and patient variability in its treatment. Personal experience, gained by using various sclerosants and treatment combinations, is often a better guide than fixed rules. The concept that vessels are sensory organs that can undergo adaptive changes following homeostatic challenges makes it easier to understand both the short- and long-term effects of sclerotherapy.

ACKNOWLEDGMENTS

I would like to thank Cindy Roberts-Smith and Joyce Smith for their careful editing and referencing of this chapter and Robert Weiss, MD, and Mitchel Goldman, MD, for their gracious invitation to contribute to this text.

REFERENCES

1. Duffy D. Small vessel sclerotherapy: An overview. Adv Dermatol 3:221-242, 1988.
2. Skolnick A. Health pros want new rules for girl athletes. JAMA 275:22-24, 1996.
3. Baird A, Hsueh A. Fibroblast growth factor as an intraovarian hormone: Differential regulation of steroidogenesis by an angiogenic factor. Regul Pept 16:243-250, 1986.
4. Torry R, Rongish B. Angiogenesis in the uterus: Potential regulation and relation to tumor angiogenesis. Am J Reprod Immunol 27:171-179, 1992.
5. Folkman J, Klagsbrun M. Angiogenic factors. Science 235:442-447, 1987.
6. Weidner N. Intratumor microvessel density as a prognosis factor in cancer. Am J Pathol 147:9-19, 1995.
7. Duffy D. Sclerotherapy-induced vascular remodeling/neovascularization. Phlebol Dig 1998 [in press].
8. Folkman J, Ingber D. Angiogenic steroids. Ann Surg 206:374-383, 1987.
9. Folkman J. Clinical applications of research on angiogenesis. Seminars in medicine of the Beth Israel Hospital, Boston, Mass. N Engl J Med 33:1757-1763, 1995.
10. Folkman J. The vascularization of tumors. Sci Am 70:58-64, 70-73, 1976.
11. Wickelgran I. Bioengineers view physics as a lever on evolution: The mechanics of natural success. Sci News 135:376-378, 1989.
12. Pennisi E. Thicker than water: Biochemistry blends with fluid dynamics to yield a vascular science. Sci News 140:220-223, 1991.
13. Davis L, Duffy D. Determination of incidence and risk factors for postsclerotherapy telangiectatic matting of the lower extremity: A retrospective analysis. J Dermatol Surg Oncol 16:327-330, 1990.
14. Duffy D. The spectrum of sclerotherapy-induced neovascularization: Clinical features, treatment protocols and commentary. Presented at the Superficial Anatomy and Cutaneous Surgery Conference. University of California–San Diego, Scripp's Clinic, La Jolla, Calif., July 17, 1998.
15. Gibbons GH, Dzau VJ. The emerging concept of vascular remodeling. N Engl J Med 330:1431-1438, 1994.
16. Mantyh PW, DeMaster E, Malhotra A, Ghilardi J, Rogers SD, Mantyh CR, Liu H, Basbaum AI, Vigna SR, Maggio JE, Simone DA. Receptor endocytosis and dendrite reshaping in spinal neutrons after somatosensory stimulation. Science 268:1629-1632, 1995.
17. Duffy D. Sclerotherapy: Broader horizons. J Cutan Aging Cosmet Dermatol 1:263-268, 1991.
18. Duffy D. The role of sclerotherapy in the rejuvenation of aging hands. Cosmet Dermatol 8(10): 1995.

19. Duffy D. Injection of hand veins. Skin Allergy News 1998 [in press].

20. Duffy D. Sclerotherapy-induced remodeling and sclerosants. Presented at the North American Society of Phlebology, Palm Springs, Calif., Nov. 7, 1997.

21. Duffy D. Understanding sclerotherapy. In Lask G, Moy R, eds. The Principles and Techniques of Cutaneous Surgery. New York: McGraw-Hill, 1996, pp 419-436.

22. Duffy D. Sclerotherapy. Clin Dermatol 10:373-380, 1992.

23. Duffy D. Small vessel sclerotherapy: A comparison of protocols. Presented at the American Academy of Dermatology. Orlando, Fla., Feb. 27, 1998.

24. Goldman M. Sclerotherapy: Treatment of Varicose and Telangiectatic Leg Veins, 2nd ed. St. Louis: Mosby, 1995.

25. Duffy D. Misconceptions on spider veins: Sclerotherapy treatment abounds. Dermatol Times 15(9):24, 1994.

26. Bodian E. Technique of sclerotherapy for sunburst venous blemishes. J Dermatol Oncol 11:696, 1985.

27. Holzegel VK. Über Krampfader Verödungen. Dermatol Wochenschr 153:137, 1967.

28. Fronek H. Sclerotherapy of reticular veins. In Goldman M, Bergan J, eds. Ambulatory Treatment of Venous Disease: An Illustrative Guide. St. Louis: Mosby, 1996, pp 49-56.

29. Henry M. Injection sclerotherapy for varicose veins—A view from Ireland. In Goldman M, Bergan J, eds. Ambulatory Treatment of Venous Disease: An Illustrative Guide. St. Louis: Mosby, 1996, pp 99-103.

30. Goldman M. Laser and noncoherent pulsed light treatment of leg telangiectasias and venules. In Goldman M, Bergan J, eds. Ambulatory Treatment of Venous Disease: An Illustrative Guide. St. Louis: Mosby, 1996, pp 89-96.

31. O'Reilly M, et al. Endostatin: An endogenous inhibitor of angiogenesis and tumor growth. Cell 88:277-285, 1997.

32. O'Reilly M, et al. Angiostatin: A novel angiogenesis inhibitor that mediates the suppression of metastases by a Lewis lung carcinoma. Cell 79:315-328, 1994.

33. Barinaga M. Designing therapies that target tumor blood vessels. Science 275:482-484, 1997.

34. Folkman J. Angiogenic therapy of the human heart. Circulation 97:628-629, 1998.

35. Goldman J. Cardiac patient treated by gene therapy. Los Angeles Times, Jan. 6, 1998.

Index

A

Abbas, Haly, 162
Absorption curve for hemoglobin, 475
Adjunctive compression therapy, 131
Adventitia, 30
Age
 small vessel disease and, 522
 telangiectatic matting and, 312
 varicose veins and, 47
Air embolism, 361
Air plethysmography, 96
Albucasis of Cordova, 162
Alexandrite laser for telangiectasis, 484
Allergy to sclerotherapy solution, 333-334
Ambulation after sclerotherapy, 295
Ambulatory venous pressure, 49, 94-95
 ulceration and, 416
Anaphylaxis, sclerotherapy causing, 334
Anastomosis, arteriovenous, 471
Anatomic abnormality, 200, 202
Anatomy, 12-41; *see also* Varicose vein,
 anatomy of
Angina, 324
Angiodysplasia, 134
Angioedema, 333
Angiogenesis
 small vessel disease and, 519
 telangiectatic matting and, 314-315
Angiogenic factor, 61-62
Angio-osteo-hypertrophic syndrome,
 398-409
Anticoagulant, lupus-like, 359
Antihistamine, 324
Argon laser for telangiectasis, 473-474
Arterial injection of sclerotherapy solution,
 346-351
Arteriolar injection of sclerotherapy solution,
 328-329
Arteriovenous anastomosis, 471
Arteriovenous communication, 25-26

Arteriovenous fistula, 397
Asthma, 334-335
Atypical saphenous varices, 115-117
Autotransplantation of vein segment, 392
Avulsion
 instruments for, 205, 206
 technique, 207-210
Axillary-to-popliteal autotransplantation of
 vein segment, 392

B

Back pressure, gravitational, 14-15
Bandage
 compression, 136-141; *see also* Compression
 therapy
 sclerotherapy and, 229, 231
 ulceration and, 421
Beta-glucoronidase, 5
Bleeding, 165-166
Blemish, telangiectatic, 123; *see also*
 Telangiectasis
Blister, tape compression, 318, 320-321
Block, diffusion, 54
Blood flow
 effects of, 47
 turbulent, 36
Boyd perforating vein
 saphenous nerve and, 80
 sclerotherapy of, 290-291
Brodie, Sir Benjamin, 157-158
Bronchospasm, 333

C

Calf
 duplex scanning of, 100
 painful telangiectasis in, 503
Calf muscle pump impairment, 49
Calf perforator vein
 duplex imaging of, 385-387
 role of, 44

Camera, 538
Cannulation of reticular vein, 457
Capillary
    arteriovenous communication and, 26
    hyperpigmentation and, 305
Carbon dioxide laser for telangiectasis,
    472
Cardiovascular disease, 324
Catheter in radiofrequency-mediated
    endovenous shrinkage, 218
CD11b expression, 56, 57
CEAP classification system, 88-92
    disability score and, 91-92
    errors in, 90
    experience with, 88-89
    simplification of, 91
Cell, muscle
    function of, 36
    process of varicosity and, 35
    venous valve and, 20-21
Cellular memory, 519-520
Celsus, Cornelius, 163-164
Chelation for hyperpigmentation, 308
Chemical phlebitis, 279
Chromated glycerin, 230
    allergic reaction to, 341-342
    necrosis and, 328
    telangiectasis and, 462
Chronic venous insufficiency; see Venous
    insufficiency
Chronotherapy for hyperpigmentation,
    310-311
Classification
    of telangiectasis, 498-500
    of varicose veins, 111
        CEAP, 88-91
        disability score and, 91-92
Coagulation
    postsclerotherapy, 306
    sclerotherapy and
        hypercoagulation and, 355
        pigmentation and, 306
Coagulation factors in pregnancy, 357-358
Collagen, endovenous shrinkage and, 217
Collagenous matrix in vein wall, 29
Collagenous tissue in varicose vein, 30
Color of vessel, 499, 523
Color-flow Doppler imaging
    greater saphenous vein incompetence and,
        277
    technique of, 98-103
Common femoral vein, 43
Competence of valve, 38

Complications
    of sclerotherapy, 325-362; see also
        Sclerotherapy, complications of
    of small vessel treatment, 540-542
Compression blister, tape, 318, 320-321
Compression folliculitis, tape, 321-322
Compression sclerotherapy, 247-264; see also
        Sclerotherapy, compression
Compression stockings; see Stockings,
        compression
Compression therapy, 127-145
    adjunctive, 131
    bandage for, 136-141
    contraindications for, 141
    hosiery for, 142-145
    hyperpigmentation and, 309
    indications for, 129-135
        angiodysplasia as, 134
        chronic venous insufficiency as, 130-131
        deep venous thrombosis as, 132-133
        dermatologic disease as, 135
        edema as, 134-135
        lymphedema as, 134
        superficial venous thrombosis as, 132
    Klippel-Trenaunay syndrome and, 403
    postsclerotherapy, 295
        complications of, 355
        excessive, 331
        overview of, 229, 231, 233
        telangiectasis and, 465-466
    small vessel disease and, 542-543
    telangiectasis and, 465-466
    thrombophlebitis and, 345
    ulceration and, 419, 421
Congenital vascular malformation, 397-411;
        see also Vascular malformation
Congestion, pelvic, 425-445, 447; see also
        Pelvic congestion syndrome
Connective tissue
    subendothelial, 30
    of venous wall, 5
Contamination in sclerotherapy, 231
Continuous-wave Doppler–guided
        sclerotherapy, 237-238
Contraceptive, oral, 355-357
Contraction, smooth muscle, 4, 5-6
Contraindications
    for compression therapy, 141
    for sclerotherapy, 227, 278-279
    for surgery, 172, 198-199
Contrast agent, echo-enhanced, 278
Corticosteroid, edema and, 311
Cosmetic issues, 172

Cuff, fibrin, 50-52, 131
Cutaneous disorder, 135
Cutaneous necrosis after sclerotherapy, 325-333
Cutaneous stigmata of venous dysfunction, 383-384
Cyanotic vessel, 524
Cytokine, 60
    venous wall and, 5
Cytoplasm, 35

D

de Chauliac, Guy, 162
Death, sodium tetradecyl sulfate causing, 337
Deep venous reflux, 421-422; *see also* Reflux
Deep venous thrombosis
    after sclerotherapy, 345-346
        amount of injection and, 353-355
        cause of, 353
        compression and, 132-133, 355
        hypercoagulable state and, 355
        inherited factor deficiency and, 358-359
        oral contraceptives and, 355-357
        pregnancy and, 357-358
        prevention of, 359-360
        sclerotherapy and, 345-346
        tamoxifen and, 357
        treatment of, 360
    after surgery, 213
    varicose veins secondary to, 397
Dermatologic disease, 135
Desquamation, 30-31
Detergent sclerosing solution, 332
    telangiectasis and, 462-463
Dextrose/sodium chloride for sclerotherapy, 230
Diagnostic testing, 94-124
    air plethysmography, 96
    ambulatory venous pressure, 94-95
    chronic venous insufficiency and, 117-120
    clinical examination and, 111-112
    color-flow imaging, 98-103
    Doppler ultrasonography, 96-98, 112-117
    duplex scanning, 98-103
    photoplethysmography, 95-96, 112
    saphenous varices and, 120-123
Diffusion block, 54
Dilatation
    gravitational back pressure and, 14-15
    telangiectasis and, 500
Diode laser for telangiectasis, 485-486
Dionis, Pierre, 158-159
Diphenhydramine hydrochloride, 334

Distensibility of vein wall, 36
Dodd perforating vein
    duplex scanning of, 104
    palpation of, 196-197
    patterns of varicosities and, 81
Doppler ultrasound examination; *see* Ultrasound examination, Doppler
Dosage for sclerotherapy agent, 233-234, 283-284
Drainage by perforator vein, 8-9
Dressing
    sclerotherapy-induced ulceration and, 333
    ulceration and, 421
Drug therapy, 64
    hyperpigmentation and, 305-306
    venous insufficiency and, 388
Duplex ultrasound examination; *see* Ultrasound examination, duplex
Dyschondroplasia, Maffucci syndrome and, 409
Dyspareunia, 441-442

E

Echo-enhanced contrast agent, 278
Echo-guided sclerotherapy, 293-295
Edema
    compression therapy for, 131, 134-135
    sclerotherapy causing, 311-312
    ulceration and, 419
Effusion, pleural, 335-336
ELAM-1, 60
Elastase, 56-57, 59
Elastic bandage, 136-141
Elastic stockings, 142-145, 229, 231
Elastic tissue in venous valve, 20-22
Electron microscopy, 32-35
Electrosurgery, of telangiectasis, 453
Embolism, pulmonary, after sclerotherapy
    amount of injection and, 353-355
    cause of, 353
    compression and, 355
    hypercoagulable state and, 355
    inherited factor deficiency and, 358-359
    oral contraceptives and, 355-357
    pregnancy and, 357-358
    prevention of, 359-360
    tamoxifen and, 357
    treatment of, 360
Empty vein technique of compression
    sclerotherapy, 247-264; *see also*
    Sclerotherapy, compression
Enchondroma, 409-410
Endoluminal venous stripping, 393-394

Endoscopic perforator ligation, 102
Endoscopic perforator vein surgery, subfascial, 391-392
Endoscopic sclerotherapy, 239
Endothelial adhesion molecule, 60-62
Endothelial cell
    pregnancy and, 357
    venous ulceration and, 63
Endothelial cell growth factor, 314
Endothelium
    role of, 8
    venous valve and, 20-21
Endovenous shrinkage and occlusion, radiofrequency-mediated, 217-224
    clinical findings in, 219-221
    delivery system for, 218-219
    histology in, 221-223
    indications for, 223-224
    mechanism of action of, 217-218
Energy, radiofrequency, 217-218
Energy metabolism in varicose veins, 45-46
Enzyme, vein wall and, 36
    lysosomal, 5, 45-46
Epinephrine, 334
Equipment
    for avulsion, 205, 206
    for sclerotherapy, 228-231
        compression, 255, 256
        small vessel, 538-540
    for stripping, 166-167
Erythema nodosum, 135
Estrogen
    development of varicose vein and, 16
    telangiectatic matting and, 315
Estrogen replacement therapy, 355-357
Ethamolin, 362
Ethanolamine oleate, 334-335
Ethylenediamine tetraacetate acid, 308
Evaluation of patient; see Diagnostic testing
Exfoliant for hyperpigmentation, 308
External iliac vein, 43
Extravasation of sclerotherapy solution, 325-333
    hyperpigmentation and, 301
    prevention of, 331-332

F

Fat necrosis, membranous, 361-362
Fatality, sodium tetradecyl sulfate causing, 337
Femoral vein, valve incompetence in, 43
Ferritin, 305
Fibrin, 131

Fibrin cuff theory, 50-52, 131
Fibrinolysis, 64, 358
Fibroblast growth factor, 314
Fistula, arteriovenous, 25-26
    congenital malformation and, 397
Flashbulb therapy for hyperpigmentation, 309, 310-311
Flashlamp-pulsed dye laser for telangiectasis, 309, 478-484
Fluorescence capillary videomicroscopy, 53
Flush ligation of saphenous vein, 176-179
Folliculitis, tape compression, 321-322
Foot vein pressure, 49
Frequency-doubled Nd:YAG laser, 474-478
2-Furildioxime, 308-309

G

Galen, 163
Gender, 14, 47
Genetics, 13, 48
Geniculate group of perforating veins, sclerotherapy of, 290
Giacomini vein, 273, 292
Glucose saline solution, hypertonic, 462
Glycerin
    chromated
        allergic reaction to, 341-342
        telangiectasis and, 462
    necrosis and, 328
Gonadal vein, 426-445; see also Pelvic congestion syndrome
Gravitational back pressure, 14-15
Gravitational pressure, postsclerotherapy hyperpigmentation and, 304
Greater saphenous vein; see also Saphenous vein
    duplex scanning of, 101, 102
    photoplethysmography of, 95
    reflux of, classification of, 87
    sclerotherapy of, 265-298; see also Sclerotherapy
Greco-Roman era, 163-164
Groin
    lymph and, 213
    reflux in, 103-104
    surgery on, 202-203
Growth factor, telangiectatic matting and, 314

H

Hair growth, 324
Harvey, William, 159-160
Healing, failure of, 63

Heart rate, anaphylaxis and, 334
Heat, radiofrequency-mediated endovenous
    shrinkage and, 217-218
Height, 48
Hemangioma, 398
    Maffucci syndrome and, 409-410
Hemidesmosome, 35
Hemiparesis, 352-353
Hemoglobin, absorption curve for, 475
Hemosiderin deposition, 301, 302
Heparin
    allergic reaction to, 342-343
    arterial injection of sclerotherapy solution
        and, 350
    deep vein thrombosis and, 359, 360
    low-molecular-weight, compression therapy
        and, 132-133
    telangiectatic matting and, 314
Heredity, 13, 48
Hexosamine, vein wall and, 36
High-intensity pulsed light treatment for
    telangiectasis, 487-493
High-pressure vein, 266
Hirsutism, 324
Histamine-induced endothelial contraction,
    305
Histology, 46, 57-61
    radiofrequency-mediated endovenous
        shrinkage and, 221-223
Histopathology, pelvic congestion and,
    435-439
History of surgery, 150-173
    eighteenth century and, 158-159
    from 1941 to 1953, 151-153
    Greco-Roman era and, 163-164
    Middle Ages and, 162-163
    modern period and, 164-170
    nineteenth century and, 156-158
    seventeenth century and, 159-160
    sixteenth century and, 160-161
    Trendelenburg and, 155-156
    turn-of-the-century and, 153-155
Hormone in development of varicose vein,
    15-16
Hosiery; see Stockings, compression
Hunter, John, 159
Hunter perforating vein
    patterns of varicosities and, 81
    sclerotherapy of, 290
Hyaluronidase injection, 332
Hydrostatic pressure, 15, 26-28
Hypercoagulation, 355-356
Hyperosmotic agent, 327

Hyperpigmentation, postsclerotherapy, 280,
    300-311
    coagula and, 306
    duration of, 306-307
    etiology of, 301-303
    intravascular pressure and, 304
    predisposition to, 304-306
    prevention of, 307-308
    small vessels treatment and, 540-541
    technique of, 304
    treatment of, 308-311
    type of solution and, 303-304
    vessel diameter and, 304
Hypertension, venous
    ambulatory, 49, 94-95
    healing and, 63
    leukocytes and, 55-56, 62
Hypertonic saline, 300
    allergic reaction to, 342
    complications of, 362
    extravasation of, 331
    pain and, 317
    small vessel disease and, 535
    telangiectasis and, 461-462
    ulceration and, 333
Hypertrichosis, 324
Hypertrophy, increased pressure causing, 15
Hypoxia, 54

I
ICAM-1, 60
Iliac vein, 43
Immunohistochemistry, 46
Incision placement, 200, 201
Incompetence
    of perforating vein, 23-25, 167-170
    saphenofemoral, 99, 270-271
        reflux and, 103-104
    of saphenous vein, 102
        sclerotherapy for, 265-298; see also
            Sclerotherapy
    valvular, 17, 38, 43
        examination of, 384-385
Induration, 262-263
Infection
    postsclerotherapy hyperpigmentation and,
        306
    ulcer and, 263
Inflammation
    hyperpigmentation and, 301
    reticular vein and, 458
    sclerotherapy causing, 279
    telangiectatic matting and, 314

Inherited factor deficiency, 358-359
Injection
    arterial, 346-351
    of reticular vein, 457
    sclerotherapy, 232
        arteriolar, 328-329
        of greater saphenous vein, 281-282
        lymphatic, 331
        of saphenofemoral junction, 285-288
        for telangiectatic blemishes, 123
    of small vessel, 533
    of telangiectasis, 459-461
Innervation, venous disease and, 63-64
Instrumentation
    for avulsion, 205, 206
    for sclerotherapy, 228-231
        compression, 255, 256
        small vessel, 538-540
    for stripping, 166-167
Intense pulsed light treatment
    for hyperpigmentation, 310
    for telangiectasis, 310, 316, 487-493
        sclerotherapy with, 516
Interleukins, 60
    white cell trapping theory and, 55
Internal saphenous vein, 170-171
Intrauterine phlebography, 440
Intravascular pressure, 304; see also Pressure
Iodine sodium iodide, 282, 283, 284
    schedule and dosage for, 289
Iron, hyperpigmentation and, 301, 302, 305
Ischemic neurologic defect after sclerotherapy, 352

J

Junction, saphenofemoral
    anatomy of, 266-268
    incompetence of, 270-271, 273, 274

K

Ketotifen, 316
Klippel-Trenaunay syndrome, 398-409
    characteristics of, 398-399
    diagnosis of, 400-403
    treatment of, 403-409
Knee, duplex scanning of, 102
Krypton triphosphate laser for telangiectasis, 474-478

L

Laboratory evaluation, 94-107
Lactoferrin, 56-57, 58
Lamina, 20

Laser therapy
    hyperpigmentation and, 309-310
    Klippel-Trenaunay syndrome and, 403
    for telangiectasis, 316, 453, 471-487
        argon, 473-474
        carbon dioxide, 472
        diode, 485-486
        evaluation of, 486-487
        flashlamp-pulsed dye, 478-484
        krypton triphosphate, 474-478
        long-pulse infrared alexandrite, 484
        mercury vapor flashlamp system for, 495
        Nd:YAG, 472-473
Lateral subdermic venous system, 500-501
Lesser saphenous vein, 105-106
Leukocyte, adhesion of, 62
Leukocyte activation, 55-56
Leukocyte trapping, 383-384
Leukocyte-endothelial interaction, 62
Leukocytoclastic vasculitis, 135
Lidocaine, 343
Ligation
    perforator, endoscopic, 102
    of saphenous vein
        flush, 176-179
        sclerotherapy vs., 186-189
    sclerotherapy and, 235
    technique of, 211
Light
    high-intensity pulsed, for telangiectasis, 310, 316, 487-493
    in sclerotherapy room, 455, 538
Light microscopy of valve, 19-22
Light reflection rheography, 385-387
Lipodermatosclerosis, 55
Liposome, 302
Localized urticaria after sclerotherapy, 318, 319
Long saphenous vein
    flush ligation of, 176-179
    valve incompetence in, 43-44
    vein-saving surgery of, 179-180
Long-pulse flashlamp-pulsed dye laser, 481-482
Long-pulse infrared alexandrite laser for telangiectasis, 484
Low-molecular-weight heparin, 132-133
Low-pressure vein, 266
Lupus-like anticoagulant, 359
Lymphatic injection of sclerotherapy solution, 331
Lymphatics, 213
Lymphedema, 134

Lysosomal enzyme, 5, 45-46
Lytic agent, 360

M

Macrophage, 55
   hyperpigmentation and, 301-302
   perivascular, 63
Maffucci syndrome, 409-410
Magnetic resonance angiography, 402
Magnifier, 538
Main-stem insufficiency, 189-190
Maintenance compression therapy, 127
Malformation, congenital vascular, 397-411;
     see also Vascular malformation
Margination, white cell, 53-54
Marking, preoperative, in Klippel-Trenaunay
     syndrome, 405-406
Mast cell heparin, 314
Materials and instrumentation, 533
Matrix
   collagenous, in vein wall, 29
   muscle cell contact with, 35
Matting, telangiectatic, 312-316, 541-542; *see*
    also Telangiectasis
Mayo Clinic, 165
Meandering syndrome, 27-29
Medial coat of vein, 30
Medical compression hosiery, 142-145
Medical record keeping, 466-467
Melanocyte, 303
Membranous fat necrosis, 361-362
Metabolism of vein wall, 45-46
Methylprednisolone
   allergic reaction and, 335
   edema and, 311
Methylxanthine, 388
Microcirculation
   histology of, 57-61
   injury to, 55
   neuropathy and, 63-64
   venous insufficiency and, 130
Microinjection of telangiectasis, 459-461
Microscopy
   electron, 32-35
   fluorescence capillary, 53
   pelvic congestion and, 437-439
   of valve, 19-22
   valve failure and, 46
Microvarices, 10
Middle Ages, 162-163
Minocycline, 305-306
Monocyte, 63
Morrhuate, 535

Muscle
   in varicose vein, 31-32, 33
   venous valve, 19-20
   venous wall, 4-5, 29
Muscle cell
   function of, 36
   hemidesmosome and, 35
Muscle pump
   compression therapy and, 141
   impairment of, 49
   venous return and, 128

N

N-acetyl-beta-glucaminidase, 5
Nd:YAG laser
   frequency-doubled, 474-478
   Klippel-Trenaunay syndrome and, 403
   for telangiectasis, 473
Necrosis after sclerotherapy, 325-333
   arterial injection of solution and, 349
   membranous fat, 361-362
Needle, sclerotherapy, 229
   compression, 255, 256, 258
   small vessel disease and, 538
Neovascular vessel, resistant, 540-541
Neovascularization, telangiectatic matting
     and, 314
Nerve
   damage, 360-361
   saphenous, 80
Neuropathy, 63-64
Neutrophil
   CD11b expression of, 56, 57
   elastase and, 56, 59
   lactoferrin and, 56, 58
   venous ulceration and, 63
Nonsaphenous vein, sclerotherapy dosage for,
    234
Noradrenaline, 36, 38
Nucleus, cell, 33

O

Occlusion, radiofrequency-mediated
    endovenous, 217-224
Oral contraceptive, 355-357
Osmotic agent, 461-462; *see also* Hypertonic
    saline

P

Pain
   pelvic congestion syndrome and, 440-442
   saphenous vein incompetence and, 269
   sclerotherapy causing, 316-318

Pain—cont'd
  telangiectasis causing, 498-516; see also
    Telangiectasis, painful
  ulcer and, 263
Palpation, 196-197
Paré, Ambroise, 160-161
Parkes-Weber syndrome, 398-399, 408
Patterns of varicose veins, 70-82
  normal anatomy and, 72-75
  perforating veins and, 76-79
  types of, 80-82
Paul of Aegina, 162-163
Pelvagia, 440-442
Pelvic congestion syndrome, 425-445,
    447
  discussion of, 439-440
  histopathology of, 435-439
  history of, 425-426
  in male patient, 442-445
  radiology in, 427-432
  surgery for, 432-435
Pentoxifylline, 64, 388
Perforator vein
  atypical saphenous varices and, 120
  blood flow in, 266
  Boyd, 80
  development of varicose veins and, 8-9
  Dodd
    duplex scanning of, 104
    palpation of, 196-197
  duplex imaging of, 385-387
  endoscopic ligation of, 102
  incompetent, 23-25, 71-72, 272
    surgical history and, 167-170
  patterns of varicosities and, 80-81
  reconstruction of, 392
  role of, 44
  sclerotherapy of, 290-291
  subfascial endoscopy of, 391-392
  superficial reflux and, 389-391
  surgery on, 207
Perineal vein, 288
Perivascular macrophage, 63
Petit, Jean Louis, 158
Phagocytosis, 301-302
Phlebitis
  chemical, 279
  compression sclerotherapy and, 261
  varicose veins after, 39
Phlebography
  intrauterine, 440
  Klippel-Trenaunay syndrome and, 402
  pelvic congestion and, 427

Photoplethysmography, 95-96, 113, 119,
    385-387
Physicochemical factors affecting vein wall,
    36-38
Pigmentation
  postsclerotherapy, 300-311
  small vessel treatment and, 540-541
Plasma elastase, 56-57
Plasma lactoferrin, 56-57
Plasminogen activator, 47
Platelet-derived growth factor, 61
Plethysmography
  air, 96
  photoplethysmography, 95-96, 113, 119,
    385-387
Pleural effusion, 335-336
Polidocanol for sclerotherapy, 230
  allergic reaction to, 339-341
  complications of, 362
  cutaneous necrosis and, 327, 330
  hyperpigmentation with, 300-301
  pain and, 317-318
  small vessel disease and, 535
  telangiectasis and, 315, 462-463,
    465
Polyiodinated iodine
  allergic reaction to, 342
  telangiectasis and, 462-463
Polymorphonuclear leukocyte, 54
Popliteal fossa
  Doppler ultrasound examination of,
    97
  duplex scanning of, 99, 104-106
Popliteal vein
  Doppler ultrasonography and, 115
  Klippel-Trenaunay syndrome and,
    404
Portable Doppler ultrasound, 96-98
Port-wine stain, 471
Postsclerotherapy compression; see
    Compression therapy
Postsclerotherapy hyperpigmentation, 280,
    300-311
Postthrombotic syndrome, 240
Postthrombotic varicose vein, 8, 9
Posture, 14, 48
Postwar trends in surgery, 151-153
Pregnancy, 15-16, 48
  pelvic congestion and, 440
  sclerotherapy during, 239-240
    pulmonary embolism and, 357-358
Preoperative marking in Klippel-Trenaunay
    syndrome, 405-406

Pressure
  ambulatory venous, 416
  compression sclerotherapy and, 251-253,
      258, 259
  compression therapy and, 136, 141
  foot vein, 49
  gonadal veins and, 426
  gravitational back, 14-15
  hydrostatic, 15, 26-28
  postsclerotherapy hyperpigmentation and,
      304
Pretreatment period
  diagnostic testing in, 94-124; see also
      Diagnostic testing
  in Klippel-Trenaunay syndrome, 405-406
  small vessel disease and, 531-532
Procaine, 350
Procoagulant factor in pregnancy, 357-358
Progesterone, 16
Proliferation, vascular, 61-63
Prostaglandin E$_1$, 64
Protein C, 358
Protein S, 358
Pulmonary edema, 335
Pulmonary embolism after sclerotherapy,
      351-360; see also Embolism,
      pulmonary, after sclerotherapy
Pulsation, in varicosity, 26
Pulsed light treatment for telangiectasis, 310,
      316, 487-493
Pulsed photothermal device, 453
Pump
  heart as, 128
  muscle
    compression therapy and, 141
    impairment of, 49
    venous return and, 128
  sponge, 253, 254

Q

Q-switched ruby laser, 310

R

Racial differences in varicosity, 14, 48
Radiofrequency-mediated endovenous
      shrinkage and occlusion, 217-224
Radiographic evaluation of pelvic congestion,
      427-432
Recanalization after sclerotherapy, 123
Reconstruction
  of valve, 394
  venous, 392
Record keeping, 466-467

Recurrence
  causes of, 107
  compression sclerotherapy and, 260
  flush ligation and, 176-179
  sclerotherapy and, 322-323
  in small vessels, 527, 531
Red blood cell, hyperpigmentation and,
      301-303, 306, 307
Refilling time, 95-96, 113
Reflection rheography, 385-387
Reflex, vasovagal, 323
Reflux
  air plethysmography and, 96
  in atypical saphenous varices, 120-122
  classification of, 103-106
  compression sclerotherapy and, 253-255
  dialogue about, 199-200
  Doppler ultrasonography and, 114-115
  in lateral subdermic venous system,
      501-502
  radiofrequency-mediated endovenous
      shrinkage for, 223-224
  in small vessel, 522
  superficial
    testing and, 389
    treatment of, 389-391
  surgical correction of, 393
  ulceration and, 417, 421-422
  venous, 49, 111
Remodeling, vascular, 527
Reticular vein, 456, 499
  injection of, 457-458
  treatment of, 512-513
  varices in, 10
Retinoic acid, 308
Rheography, light reflection, venous
      insufficiency and, 385-387

S

Saline, hypertonic; see Hypertonic saline
Saphenofemoral incompetence, 99
  reflux and, 103-104
Saphenofemoral junction
  anatomy of, 266-268
  incompetence of, 270-271, 273, 274
  sclerotherapy for, 284-288
Saphenous nerve, 80
Saphenous varices
  atypical, 120-122
  typical, 122-123
Saphenous vein
  anatomy of, 266-268
  classification of, 499

Saphenous vein—cont'd
  dialogue about, 193-214
  Doppler ultrasound examination of, 96-97,
      115-117
  duplex scanning of, 99-102
  flush ligation and, 176-179
  internal, 170-171
  lesser, 105-106
  ligation of, sclerotherapy vs., 186-189
  main-stem insufficiency and, 189-190
  patterns of varicosities and, 81-82
  pelvic congestion and, 427
  perforator veins and, 8-9
  photoplethysmography of, 95
  radiofrequency-mediated endovenous
      shrinkage of, 223-224
  sclerotherapy for; see Sclerotherapy
  short
    anatomy of, 266
    incompetence of, 273
    sclerotherapy of, 292
    surgery on, 207-208
  stripping of, 170-171, 393-394
  surgery of, 175-176
    sclerotherapy vs., 180-186
    vein-saving, 179-180
  valve incompetence in, 43-44
  wall weakness in, 27
Scanning, duplex, 98-103; see also Ultrasound
    examination, duplex
Schwartz maneuver, 275
Scintillating scotoma, 361
Scleremo, 362
Sclerotherapy
  above-to-downward approach, 227
  adverse sequelae of, 300-324
    hyperpigmentation as, 300-311
    pain as, 316-318
    recurrence as, 322-323
    stress-related, 323-324
    swelling as, 311-312
    tape compression blister as, 318,
        320-321
    tape compression folliculitis as, 321-322
    telangiectatic matting as, 312-316
    urticaria as, 318, 319
  agents for; see Solution, sclerosing
  approaches for, 227-228
  case history of, 240-244
  complications of, 325-362
    air embolism as, 361
    allergic or toxic reaction as, 333-343
    arterial injection as, 346-351

    cutaneous necrosis as, 325-333
    membranous fat necrosis as, 361-362
    nerve damage as, 360-361
    pulmonary embolism as, 351-360
    scintillating scotoma as, 361
    thrombophlebitis as, 343-346
  compression, 131, 247-264
    complications of, 261-262
    difficult presentations and, 260-261
    follow-up for, 259-260
    for induration and ulceration, 262-263
    initial examination for, 247-251
    patient instructions for, 258-259
    preparation for, 251-253
    thigh reflux and, 253-258
  continuous-wave Doppler–guided,
      237-239
  contraindications for, 227, 278-279
  dialogue about, 199, 212-213
  echo-guided, 293-295
  endoscopic, 239
  equipment for, 228-231
  history of, 153, 154-155, 164-165
  indications for, 226-227
  Klippel-Trenaunay syndrome and, 403
  largest-to-smallest vein approach, 227-228
  mechanism of action of, 225-226
  postthrombotic syndrome and, 240
  in pregnancy, 239-240
  results of, 236-237
  for saphenofemoral junction incompetence,
      284-288
  of saphenous vein, 122-123, 265-298
    anatomy and, 266-268
    classification of incompetence and,
        269-274
    complications of, 296
    discussion of, 297-298
    history of, 265-266
    indications for, 269
    ligation vs., 186-189
    patient selection for, 278-279
    postoperative evaluation of, 296
    postoperative management of, 295
    preoperative evaluation in, 274-278
    technique of, 279-284
  sequential, 288, 290-293
  small vessel, 518-546
    clinical features of, 520-523
    complications of, 540-542
    equipment for, 538-540
    etiology of, 519-520
    patterns of response to, 523-531

posttreatment guidelines for, 540
pretreatment for, 531-532
protocol for, 532-533
solutions for, 535
surgery vs., 180-186
technique of, 231-236
for telangiectasis, 123, 455-467; *see also*
    Telangiectasis
    painful, 505-506, 511-516
ultrasound-guided, 237
Scotoma, scintillating, 361
Secondary varicose veins, 39
Shock, anaphylactic, 336
Short saphenous vein
    anatomy of, 266
    incompetence of, 273
    sclerotherapy of, 292
    surgery of, 207-208
Shrinkage and occlusion, radiofrequency-
    mediated endovenous, 217-224
Skeletal abnormality in Maffucci syndrome,
    410
Skin
    hyperpigmentation of, 280
    microcirculation of, 57-61
    progression of damage to, 63
Small vessel sclerotherapy, 518-546; *see also*
    Sclerotherapy, small vessel
Smooth muscle
    of venous wall, 5-8
    venous wall and, 4-5
Sodium iodide, 290
Sodium morrhuate, 362
    allergic reaction to, 334
Sodium tetradecyl sulfate
    allergic reaction to, 336-339
    angina and, 324
    characteristics of, 282, 283
    compression sclerotherapy with, 255
    dosage of, 284
    hyperpigmentation from, 280
    necrosis and, 327-328
    pain and, 317-318
    schedule and dosage for, 289, 290
    small vessel disease and, 535
    telangiectasis and, 453, 462-463, 465
    use of, for sclerotherapy, 230
Solution, sclerosing, 229, 230, 233-234
    cutaneous necrosis from, 325-333
    hyperpigmentation and, 303-304
    reticular veins and, 514
    schedule and dosage for, 289-290
    small vessel disease and, 533, 535

sodium tetradecyl sulfate for; *see* Sodium
    tetradecyl sulfate
    for telangiectasis, 461-465
Sotradecol; *see* Sodium tetradecyl sulfate
Sponge pump, 253, 254
Stanozolol, 309
Stasis, venous, 387
Stasis ulcer, 263
Stockings, compression
    elastic, 142-145
        pressure of, 199
    nonelastic, 229, 231
    sclerotherapy and, 229, 251-253
    telangiectasis and, 466
    ulceration and, 419, 421
Stress-related sequelae of sclerotherapy,
    323-324
Stretch
    painful telangiectasis and, 500
    venous wall and, 4-5
Stripper, 166-167
Stripping
    dialogue about, 203-205
    history of, 155, 165-166
    of saphenous vein, 393-394
        internal, 170-171
Subdermic venous system, 500-501
Subendothelial connective tissue, 30
Subfascial endoscopy, 391-392
Sunburst varicosity, 471
Superficial reflux
    testing and, 389
    treatment of, 389-391
Superficial thrombophlebitis, 343-346
Superficial vein
    definition of varicose veins and, 414-415
    pressure in, 266
Superficial venous reflux, 421-422
Superficial venous thrombosis, 132
Surgery
    compression therapy after, 131
    contraindications for, 172, 198-199
    dialogue about, 199-213
    general aspects of, 175-176
    history of, 150-173
        1941 to 1953, 151-153
        eighteenth century and, 158-159
        Greco-Roman era and, 163-164
        Middle Ages and, 162-163
        modern period and, 164-170
        nineteenth century and, 156-158
        seventeenth century and, 159-160
        sixteenth century and, 160-161

Surgery—cont'd
  history of—cont'd
    Trendelenburg and, 155-156
    turn-of-the-century and, 153-155
  indications for, 171-172
  Klippel-Trenaunay syndrome and,
    403-409
  modern period and, 164-170
  pelvic congestion and, 432-435
  preparation for, 172-173
  sclerotherapy vs., 180-186
  stripping of internal saphenous vein and,
    170-171
  vein-saving, 179-180
  for venous insufficiency, 387-395; *see also*
    Venous insufficiency
Syringe, sclerotherapy, 255, 258
  compression sclerotherapy and, 229
  small vessel disease and, 538

T

T lymphocyte, 384
Tamoxifen, 357
Tape compression blister, 318, 320-321
Tape compression folliculitis, 321-322
Telangiectasis, 451-467
  examination of, 453-455
  high-intensity pulsed light treatment of,
    487-493
  histology of, 471
  historical background of, 452-453
  laser treatment of, 471-487
    argon, 473-474
    carbon dioxide, 472
    diode, 485-486
    evaluation of, 486-487
    flashlamp-pulsed dye, 478-484
    krypton triphosphate, 474-478
    long-pulse infrared alexandrite, 484
    mercury vapor flashlamp system for, 495
    Nd:YAG, 472-473
  painful, 498-516
    classification of, 498-500
    distribution of, 502-504
    lateral subdermic venous system and,
      500-502
    symptoms of, 505-510
    treatment of, 511-516
  sclerotherapy for, 123, 455-467
    agents for, 461-465
    compression after, 465-466
    facilities for, 455-456
    follow-up care for, 467

    injection of reticular veins and, 457-459
    microinjection and, 459-461
    order of treatment and, 456-457
    record keeping for, 466-467
    of reticular veins, 456
    ultrasound-guided, 465
Telangiectatic matting, 312-316, 541-542
Theophylline, anaphylaxis and, 334
Theory of pathogenesis, 70-72
  fibrin cuff, 50-52
  white cell trapping, 52-55
Thermoregulation, 6
Thigh
  painful telangiectasis in, 503
  reflux in, 253-255
  saphenous trunk sclerotherapy and, 288,
    290
Thrombophlebitis
  compression therapy for, 132
  sclerotherapy causing, 343-346
Thrombosis/thrombus
  after surgery, 213
  postsclerotherapy, 240-244, 322, 345-346
    hyperpigmentation and, 306
    of small vessels, 540
  varicose veins secondary to, 397
Tortuosity of varicose vein, 27-29
Tourniquet
  in ambulatory venous pressure
    measurement, 95
  limitations of, 197
Transcutaneous oxygen tension, 131
Transforming growth factor$_\beta$, 61
Transmission electron microscopy, 32-35
Trendelenburg, Friedrich, 155-156
Tricarboxylic acid, 308
Tumor necrosis factor, 60
  telangiectatic matting and, 316
  white cell trapping theory and, 55
Turbulence, effect of, 36

U

Ulceration, venous, 49-62
  angiogenic factors in, 61-62
  definition of, 414-415
  discussion of, 62-64
  endoscopic surgery and, 391
  etiology of, 415-417
  failure of healing of, 63
  fibrin cuff theory of, 50-52
  histology of, 57-61
  history of, 415
  leukocyte activation and, 55-57

reflux and, 421-422
sclerotherapy and, 332, 536
  compression, 261-263
treatment of, 418-421
white cell trapping theory of, 52-55
Ultrasound examination
  Doppler
    compression sclerotherapy and, 248-249
    perforating veins and, 196-197
    pretreatment, 113-117
    technique of, 96-98
    valve incompetence and, 43-44
    venous insufficiency and, 384
  duplex
    compression sclerotherapy and, 248-249
    dialogue about, 197-198
    of greater saphenous vein, 276-277, 279, 280, 281
    indications for, 119-120
    of perforator vein, 385-387
    technique of, 98-103
    ulceration and, 422
    venous insufficiency and, 385-387
  intravascular, 277-278
Ultrasound-guided sclerotherapy, 237
Urticaria
  sclerotherapy and, 318, 319
  sclerotherapy solution causing, 333

V

Vacuole, 33-34
Vaginal varices, 430
Valsalva maneuver, 275
  Doppler ultrasonography and, 114
Valve, venous
  anatomy of, 17-22
  competence of, 38
  failure of, 46
  incompetent, 70
    in development of varicose veins, 43
  primary incompetence of, 17
  reconstruction of, 394
  ulceration and, 49
  venous insufficiency and, 3-4, 384-385
Varicocele, 444, 445
Varicose vein
  anatomy of, 12-41
    arteriovenous communications and, 25-26
    incompetent perforating veins and, 23-25
    light microscopy and, 30-32
    muscle cell and, 36

physicochemical factors and, 36-38
process of varicosity and, 35
transmission electron microscopy and, 32-35
venous valve and, 17-23
causes of, 13
classification of, 499
congenital malformation and, 397-411; see also Vascular malformation
definition of, 414-415
development of, 8-10, 42-49
discussion of, 62-64
etiology of, 47-49
patterns of, 70-82
  normal anatomy and, 72-75
  perforating veins and, 76-79
  types of, 80-82
process of, 35
recurrent, causes of, 107
sclerotherapy for; see Sclerotherapy
small vessel, 522
theoretical causes of, 70-72
ulceration and, 49-62; see also Ulceration, venous
valves in, 44-46; see also Valve, venous
venous insufficiency and, 3-8, 42-65; see also Venous insufficiency
Variglobin, 362
Vascular endothelial adhesion molecule, 60-61
Vascular endothelial growth factor, 61-62
Vascular malformation
  common, 398-399
  Klippel-Trenaunay syndrome and, 398-409
    characteristics of, 398-399
    diagnosis of, 400-403
    treatment of, 403-409
  Maffucci syndrome, 409-410
Vascular proliferation, 61-63
Vascular remodeling, 527
Vasculitis, compression therapy for, 135
Vasospasm, 329, 331
Vasovagal reflex, 323
Vein
  Giacomini, 273, 292
  gonadal, 426-445; see also Pelvic congestion syndrome
  perforator; see Perforator vein
  saphenous; see Saphenous vein
Vein pressure, foot, 49
Vein wall; see Wall, vein
Venoconstriction, 6
Venodilatation, 6

Venous hypertension, 62
  ambulatory, 49, 94-95
  healing and, 63
  leukocyte, 55-56
Venous insufficiency, 3-8
  classification of, 87-92
  clinical examination of, 111-112
  compression therapy for, 127-145; see also
      Compression therapy
  cutaneous stigmata of, 383-384
  diagnosis of, 384
  Doppler ultrasonography and, 113-117
  duplex imaging in, 385-387
  duplex ultrasonography and, 119-120
  evaluation of, 384-385
  improvable, 118
  microcirculation and, 130
  nonimprovable, 118-119
  plethysmography for, 113, 119
  saphenous varices and, 120-123; see also
      Saphenous vein
  stages of, 112
  surgery for, general aspects of, 175-176
  treatment of, 387-395
    ancillary, 392-393
    endoluminal stripping, 393-394
    options for, 387-388
    reconstructive, 392
    subfascial endoscopic, 391-392
    of superficial reflux, 389-391
    valve reconstruction, 394
  venous valves and, 3-4
  venous wall and, 4-8
Venous pressure, ambulatory, 94-95
  ulceration and, 416
Venous reconstruction, 392
Venous recovery time, 416
Venous reflux; see Reflux
Venous thrombosis
  after sclerotherapy, 345-346
    amount of injection and, 353-355
    cause of, 353

  compression and, 132-133, 355
  hypercoagulable state and, 355
  inherited factor deficiency and,
      358-359
  oral contraceptives and, 355-357
  pregnancy and, 357-358
  prevention of, 359-360
  sclerotherapy and, 345-346
  tamoxifen and, 357
  treatment of, 360
  after surgery, 213
  varicose veins secondary to, 397
Venous ulceration; see Ulceration, venous
Venous valve; see Valve, venous
Venous wall; see Wall, vein
Venule, laser therapy and, 471`
Venulectasia, 499
Viscoelastic property of venous wall, 4
VNUS system, 218
Vulvar varices, 425-445; see also Pelvic
      congestion syndrome

W

Wall, vein
  abnormality of, 29
  anatomy of, 13-17
  blood flow effects on, 47
  chemical changes in, 47
  in development of varicose veins,
      44-46
  endovenous shrinkage and, 217-224
  immunohistochemical study of, 46
  physicochemical factors affecting,
      36-38
  small vessels and, 522
  venous insufficiency and, 4-8
  weakness in, 26-29, 70
Weight, 17, 48
Wheezing, 334-335
White cell trapping theory, 52-55,
      383-384
Wiseman, Richard, 160